Edited by
José M. Vela, Rafael Maldonado, and
Michel Hamon

***In Vivo* Models for Drug Discovery**

Methods and Principles in Medicinal Chemistry

Edited by R. Mannhold, H. Kubinyi, G. Folkers
Editorial Board
H. Buschmann, H. Timmerman, H. van de Waterbeemd, T. Wieland

Previous Volumes of this Series:

Liras, Spiros / Bell, Andrew S. (Eds.)

Phosphodiesterases and Their Inhibitors

2014
ISBN: 978-3-527-33219-9
Vol. 61

Hanessian, Stephen (Ed.)

Natural Products in Medicinal Chemistry

2014
ISBN: 978-3-527-33218-2
Vol. 60

Lackey, Karen / Roth, Bruce (Eds.)

Medicinal Chemistry Approaches to Personalized Medicine

2013
ISBN: 978-3-527-33394-3
Vol. 59

Brown, Nathan (Ed.)

Scaffold Hopping in Medicinal Chemistry

2013
ISBN: 978-3-527-33364-6
Vol. 58

Hoffmann, Rémy / Gohier, Arnaud / Pospisil, Pavel (Eds.)

Data Mining in Drug Discovery

2013
ISBN: 978-3-527-32984-7
Vol. 57

Dömling, Alexander (Ed.)

Protein-Protein Interactions in Drug Discovery

2013
ISBN: 978-3-527-33107-9
Vol. 56

Kalgutkar, Amit S. / Dalvie, Deepak / Obach, R. Scott / Smith, Dennis A.

Reactive Drug Metabolites

2012
ISBN: 978-3-527-33085-0
Vol. 55

Brown, Nathan (Ed.)

Bioisosteres in Medicinal Chemistry

2012
ISBN: 978-3-527-33015-7
Vol. 54

Gohlke, Holger (Ed.)

Protein-Ligand Interactions

2012
ISBN: 978-3-527-32966-3
Vol. 53

Kappe, C. Oliver / Stadler, Alexander / Dallinger, Doris

Microwaves in Organic and Medicinal Chemistry

Second, Completely Revised and Enlarged Edition
2012
ISBN: 978-3-527-33185-7
Vol. 52

Edited by José M. Vela, Rafael Maldonado, and Michel Hamon

In Vivo Models for Drug Discovery

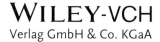

Verlag GmbH & Co. KGaA

Series Editors

Prof. Dr. Raimund Mannhold
Rosenweg 7
40489 Düsseldorf
Germany
mannhold@uni-duesseldorf.de

Prof. Dr. Hugo Kubinyi
Donnersbergstrasse 9
67256 Weisenheim am Sand
Germany
kubinyi@t-online.de

Prof. Dr. Gerd Folkers
Collegium Helveticum
STW/ETH Zurich
8092 Zurich
Switzerland

Volume Editors

Dr. José M. Vela
Laboratorios Dr. Esteve S.A.
Drug Discovery & Development
C/ Baldiri Reixac 4-8
08028 Barcelona
Spain

Dr. Rafael Maldonado
University Pompeu Fabra. PRBB
Neuropharmacology Lab.
c/Dr. Aiguader 88
08003 Barcelona
Spain

Prof. Michel Hamon
University Pierre & Marie Curie
Neuropharmacology, INSERM U894
Site Pitié-Salpetrière 91
75634 Paris, cedex 13
France

All books published by **Wiley-VCH** are carefully produced. Nevertheless, authors, editors, and publisher do not warrant the information contained in these books, including this book, to be free of errors. Readers are advised to keep in mind that statements, data, illustrations, procedural details or other items may inadvertently be inaccurate.

Library of Congress Card No.: applied for

British Library Cataloguing-in-Publication Data
A catalogue record for this book is available from the British Library.

Bibliographic information published by the Deutsche Nationalbibliothek
The Deutsche Nationalbibliothek lists this publication in the Deutsche Nationalbibliografie; detailed bibliographic data are available on the Internet at <http://dnb.d-nb.de>.

© 2014 Wiley-VCH Verlag GmbH & Co. KGaA, Boschstr. 12, 69469 Weinheim, Germany

All rights reserved (including those of translation into other languages). No part of this book may be reproduced in any form – by photoprinting, microfilm, or any other means – nor transmitted or translated into a machine language without written permission from the publishers. Registered names, trademarks, etc. used in this book, even when not specifically marked as such, are not to be considered unprotected by law.

Print ISBN: 978-3-527-33328-8
ePDF ISBN: 978-3-527-67937-9
ePub ISBN: 978-3-527-67936-2
mobi ISBN: 978-3-527-67935-5
oBook ISBN: 978-3-527-67934-8

Cover Design: Grafik Design Schulz, Fußgönheim

Typesetting Thomson Digital, Noida, India

Printing and Binding: Markono Print Media Pte Ltd, Singapore

Printed on acid-free paper

Contents

List of Contributors *XIX*
Preface *XXIX*
A Personal Foreword *XXXI*

Part I Transversal Issues Concerning Animal Models in Drug Discovery *1*

1 The 3Ns of Preclinical Animal Models in Biomedical Research *3*
José Miguel Vela, Rafael Maldonado, and Michel Hamon
1.1 First N: The Need for Use of Animal Models *3*
1.2 Second N: The Need for Better Animal Models *5*
1.2.1 Unbiased Design *8*
1.2.2 Comprehensive Reporting *8*
1.2.3 Selection of the Animal Model Based on Its Validity Attributes *9*
1.2.4 Appropriate Time and Dosing *11*
1.2.5 Use of Biomarkers *12*
1.2.6 Use of Various Animal Models *13*
1.2.7 Quantitative, Multiple, and Cross-Predictive Measurements *14*
1.2.8 Pharmacokinetic–Pharmacodynamic Integration *15*
1.2.9 Predefinition and Adherence to the Desired Product Profile *16*
1.2.10 Comparison with Gold Standard References *18*
1.2.11 Reverse Translation/Backtranslation (Bedside-to-Bench Approach) *18*
1.3 Third N: The Need for 3Rs Guiding Principles *19*
References *22*

2 Alternative Models in Drug Discovery and Development Part I: *In Silico* and *In Vitro* Models *27*
Luz Romero and José Miguel Vela
2.1 Introduction *27*
2.2 *In Silico* Models *34*
2.2.1 Quantitative Structure–Activity Relationship *34*
2.2.2 Biokinetic Modeling *37*

2.2.3	Disease- and Patient-Specific *In Silico* Models *42*	
2.3	*In Vitro* Models *43*	
2.3.1	Primary Cells, Cell Lines, Immortalized Cell Lines, and Stem Cells *44*	
2.3.2	Advanced *In Vitro* Models for the Prediction of Drug Toxicity *46*	
2.3.3	*In Vitro* Tumor Models *47*	
	References *50*	
3	**Alternative Models in Drug Discovery and Development Part II: *In Vivo* Nonmammalian and Exploratory/Experimental Human Models** *59*	
	Luz Romero and José Miguel Vela	
3.1	Introduction *59*	
3.2	*In Vivo* Nonmammalian Models *59*	
3.2.1	Zebrafish *61*	
3.2.2	*D. melanogaster* *66*	
3.2.3	*C. elegans* *71*	
3.3	*In Vivo* Exploratory and Experimental Human Models *74*	
3.3.1	Phase 0 (Exploratory Human Models): Microdosing Studies *76*	
3.3.2	Phase IB/IIA (Proof-of-Concept) Studies: Experimental Human Models *81*	
	References *84*	
4	**Ethical Issues and Regulations and Guidelines Concerning Animal Research** *91*	
	David Sabaté	
4.1	Introduction *91*	
4.2	Current Use of Animals in Biomedical and Pharmaceutical Research *92*	
4.3	Ethical Concerns and Positions on Animal Research *93*	
4.4	General Principles for the Ethical Use of Animals in Research *95*	
4.4.1	The 3Rs Principles (Replacement, Reduction, and Refinement) *95*	
4.4.2	The Principle of Justification *96*	
4.4.3	The Principle of Responsibility *97*	
4.5	Regulatory Framework for Use of Animals in Research *98*	
4.5.1	European Union *98*	
4.5.2	The United States *100*	
4.5.3	Canada *100*	
4.5.4	Japan *100*	
4.5.5	Australia *101*	
4.5.6	India *101*	
4.5.7	China *101*	
4.5.8	Brazil *102*	
4.5.9	Countries without a Specific Legal Framework *102*	
	Acknowledgment *102*	
	References *102*	

5	**Regulatory Issues: Safety and Toxicology Assessment** *107*	
	Antonio Guzmán	
5.1	Introduction *107*	
5.1.1	Animal Testing *107*	
5.1.2	Regulatory Context *109*	
5.1.3	Clinical Context *109*	
5.2	Animal Species in Toxicology Studies *110*	
5.2.1	Rodents *111*	
5.2.2	Nonrodents *112*	
5.2.3	Nonconventional Animal Models *114*	
5.3	Toxicology Studies *114*	
5.3.1	General Principles *114*	
5.3.2	General and Repeated Dose Toxicity Studies *116*	
5.3.3	Safety Pharmacology *118*	
5.3.4	Genotoxicity *119*	
5.3.5	Development and Reproductive Toxicity Studies *122*	
5.3.6	Carcinogenicity Studies *124*	
5.4	Translation to Clinics: Limitations and Difficulties *126*	
	References *127*	
6	**Generation and Use of Transgenic Mice in Drug Discovery** *131*	
	Guillaume Pavlovic, Véronique Brault, Tania Sorg, and Yann Hérault	
6.1	Introduction *131*	
6.2	Improved Mouse Genetic Engineering *133*	
6.2.1	Recent Technical Developments *133*	
6.2.2	The Advent of New Mouse Mutant Resource: One Stop Shop *133*	
6.3	Functional Evaluation and Uses of Mouse Models *136*	
6.3.1	Standardization and Harmonization *136*	
6.3.2	Genetic Background and Environmental Influences *137*	
6.3.3	Challenges Ahead *137*	
6.3.4	Target Identification and Translation to Humans *138*	
6.3.5	Use of GEMMs in Pharmaceutical Industry and Risk Assessment *139*	
6.4	Translation to Clinics: Limitations and Difficulties *140*	
6.5	Perspectives *142*	
	Acknowledgments *143*	
	References *143*	
7	***In Vivo* Brain Imaging in Animal Models: A Focus on PET and MRI** *149*	
	Fabien Chauveau, Mathieu Verdurand, and Luc Zimmer	
7.1	Introduction: Role of Animal in *In Vivo* Imaging *149*	
7.1.1	*In Vivo* Imaging as a Translational Approach for Basic Research *149*	
7.1.2	*In Vivo* Imaging in Animal Models in the Pharmaceutical Industry *150*	
7.1.3	*In Vivo* Imaging in Animal Models and the 3R Principles *150*

7.2	The Choice of the Right Imaging Modality for Brain Imaging	151
7.3	Small Animal Magnetic Resonance Imaging	152
7.3.1	Principles	152
7.3.2	Magnetic Resonance Spectroscopy	152
7.3.3	Magnetic Resonance Imaging	153
7.4	Positron Emission Tomography	155
7.4.1	Basic Principles and Instrumentation	155
7.4.2	PET and Neuronal Metabolism	155
7.4.3	PET and Brain Receptors and Transporters	156
7.4.4	PET and Receptor Occupancy	158
7.4.5	PET and Neurotransmitter Release	159
7.5	Clinical Translation: Limitations and Difficulties	159
7.5.1	Anesthesia	160
7.5.2	Spatial Resolution and Sensitivity	160
7.5.3	The Mass Effect of Injected Tracers	161
7.5.4	Multimodal PET–MRI for Better Clinical Translation	162
	References	163

Part II Animal Models in Specific Disease Areas of Drug Discovery 167

8 Substance Abuse and Dependence 169
Elena Martín-García, Patricia Robledo, Javier Gutiérrez-Cuesta, and Rafael Maldonado

8.1	Introduction	169
8.2	Difficulties to Model Addiction in Animals	170
8.3	Tolerance, Sensitization, and Physical Withdrawal	172
8.3.1	Tolerance	172
8.3.2	Sensitization	173
8.3.3	Physical Manifestations of Withdrawal	174
8.3.4	Affective Manifestations of Withdrawal	175
8.4	Reward and Reinforcement	177
8.4.1	Drug Discrimination	177
8.4.2	Conditioned Place Preference	178
8.4.3	Intracranial Self-Stimulation	180
8.4.4	Self-Administration	182
8.5	Translation to Clinics: Limitations and Difficulties	184
	References	186

9 Mood and Anxiety Disorders 193
Guy Griebel and Sandra Beeské

9.1	Introduction	193
9.2	Animal Models of Anxiety Disorders	194
9.2.1	Preclinical Measures of Anxiety	194
9.2.2	Preclinical Anxiety Models and Endophenotypes	195
9.3	Animal Models of Mood Disorders	197

9.3.1	Major Depressive Disorder *197*	
9.3.1.1	Preclinical Measures of Depression *198*	
9.3.1.2	Endophenotype Models of Depression *199*	
9.3.2	Bipolar Disorder *199*	
9.4	Translation to Clinics: Limitations and Difficulties *200*	
	Acknowledgment *201*	
	References *202*	

10 Schizophrenia *207*
Ronan Depoortère and Paul Moser

10.1	Introduction *207*	
10.2	Models Amenable to Use in Screening *209*	
10.2.1	Models Based on the Use of Pharmacological Agents *209*	
10.2.1.1	Dopaminergic Agonists *209*	
10.2.1.2	NMDA/Glutamate Receptor Antagonists *211*	
10.2.1.3	Other Pharmacological Agents Used to Induce Behavioural Changes *212*	
10.2.1.4	5-HT$_{2A}$ Receptor Agonists *212*	
10.2.1.5	Cannabinoid Receptor Agonists *212*	
10.2.1.6	Muscarinic Receptor Antagonists *213*	
10.2.1.7	Glycine B Receptor Antagonists *213*	
10.2.2	Models Not Based on the Use of Pharmacological Agents *213*	
10.2.2.1	Conditioned Avoidance Response *213*	
10.2.2.2	Potentiation of PPI of the Startle Reflex *214*	
10.2.3	Models More Time Consuming and/or Difficult to Implement *214*	
10.2.3.1	Models Aimed at Reproducing More Complex Symptoms of Schizophrenia *214*	
10.2.3.2	Models Aimed at Reproducing the Chronic Nature of Schizophrenia *216*	
10.2.3.3	Models Based on Genetic Manipulations *218*	
10.2.4	Models for Side Effects *218*	
10.2.4.1	Models for Motor Side Effects *219*	
10.2.4.2	Hyperprolactinemia *220*	
10.2.4.3	Sedation and Motor Incoordination *220*	
10.2.4.4	Models for Cognitive Side Effects *220*	
10.2.4.5	Metabolic Disorders Models *221*	
10.2.4.6	Models for Cardiovascular Effects *221*	
10.3	Translation to the Clinic: Limitations and Difficulties *221*	
10.3.1	Use of "Standard Subjects" *221*	
10.3.2	From Here to . . . ? *222*	
	References *223*	

11 Migraine and Other Headaches *231*
Inger Jansen-Olesen, Sarah Louise T. Christensen, and Jes Olesen

11.1	Introduction *231*	
11.2	Vascular Models *231*	

11.2.1	*In Vitro*	232
11.2.2	*In Vivo*	233
11.3	Neurogenic Inflammation	234
11.4	Nociceptive Activation of the Trigeminovascular System	234
11.4.1	Electrophysiological Recordings on Primary Dural Afferents in Trigeminal Ganglion	237
11.4.2	Electrophysiological Recordings in Trigeminal Nucleus Caudalis	239
11.4.3	Histological Markers after Nociceptive Stimulation of the Trigeminovascular System	239
11.5	Cortical Spreading Depression	240
11.6	Human Experimental Migraine Provoking Models	241
11.7	Animal Experimental Migraine Provoking Models	242
11.8	Transgenic Models	246
11.9	Behavioral Models	246
11.9.1	Allodynia or Hyperalgesia	247
11.9.2	Face Grooming	248
11.9.3	Photophobia	248
11.9.4	Various Behaviors	249
11.10	Translation to Clinics: Limitations and Difficulties	249
	References	250
12	**Nociceptive, Visceral, and Cancer Pain**	**261**
	Christophe Mallet, Denis Ardid, and David Balayssac	
12.1	Introduction	261
12.2	Acute Pain Tests	261
12.2.1	Introduction	261
12.2.2	Electrical Stimulus	263
12.2.3	Thermal Stimulus	264
12.2.4	Mechanical Stimulus	264
12.2.5	Chemical Stimulus	265
12.3	Visceral Pain Models	265
12.3.1	Introduction	265
12.3.2	Pain Achievement Test	266
12.3.3	Animal Models	267
12.3.4	Pathophysiology and Pharmacology	269
12.4	Cancer Pain Models	270
12.4.1	Introduction	270
12.4.2	Pain Assessment in Animal Models of Cancer Pain	270
12.4.3	Animal Models	271
12.4.4	Pathophysiology and Pharmacology	272
12.4.5	Conclusions	272
12.5	Translation to Clinics: Difficulties and Limitations	273
12.5.1	Acute Pain Tests	273
12.5.2	Visceral Pain Models	274

12.5.3	Cancer Pain Models	274
12.5.4	Conclusions	275
	References	275

13 Inflammatory, Musculoskeletal/Joint (OA and RA), and Postoperative Pain 283

Laurent Diop and Yassine Darbaky

13.1	Introduction: Evaluation of Pain in Animal Models	283
13.2	Inflammatory Pain	287
13.2.1	Formalin Test	287
13.2.2	Carrageenan-Induced Hyperalgesia	287
13.2.3	Complete Freund's Adjuvant-Induced Hyperalgesia	288
13.2.4	Capsaicin-Induced Hyperalgesia	288
13.3	Musculoskeletal/Joint Osteoarthritis (OA) and Rheumatoid Arthritis (RA) Pain	289
13.3.1	Osteoarthritis Pain Models	289
13.3.2	Rheumatoid Arthritis Pain Models	293
13.4	Postoperative Pain	297
13.4.1	Incisional Pain	298
13.4.2	Laparotomy	299
13.4.3	Ovariohysterectomy	299
13.4.4	Other Models of Postoperative Pain	299
13.5	Translation to Clinics: Limitations and Difficulties	300
	References	302

14 Neuropathic Pain 305

Said M'Dahoma, Sylvie Bourgoin, and Michel Hamon

14.1	Introduction	305
14.2	Main Types of Neuropathic Pain in Humans	306
14.2.1	Neuropathic Pain Caused by Peripheral Nerve Lesions	306
14.2.1.1	Diabetes-Induced Neuropathic Pain	306
14.2.1.2	Human Immunodeficiency Virus-Related Pain	306
14.2.1.3	Postherpetic Neuralgia	307
14.2.1.4	Neuropathic Pain Caused by Anticancer Drugs	307
14.2.2	Neuropathic Pain Caused by Central Lesions	307
14.2.2.1	Spinal Cord Injury	307
14.2.2.2	The Various Types of Pain in SCI Patients	308
14.3	Modelization of Chronic Pain in Rodents	309
14.3.1	Models of Peripheral Nerve Injury	309
14.3.1.1	Nerve Section	309
14.3.1.2	Nerve Ligation, Compression, and Other Lesion Procedures	310
14.3.1.3	Drug- and Virus-Induced Neuropathic Pain	314
14.3.2	Models of Spinal Cord Injury	318
14.3.2.1	Spinal Cord Contusion	318
14.3.2.2	Clip Compression Injury	319

14.3.2.3	Spinal Cord Transection	*319*
14.3.2.4	Spinal Cord Ischemia	*319*
14.3.3	Neuropathic-Like Pain Evoked by Chemicals Administered at the Spinal Level	*320*
14.3.3.1	Intrathecal Administration of ATP	*320*
14.3.3.2	Intrathecal Administration of BDNF	*320*
14.3.3.3	Excitotoxic Injury to the Spinal Cord	*321*
14.4	Translation to Clinics: Limitations and Difficulties	*321*
	References	*324*

15 Obesity and Metabolic Syndrome *333*
Sunil K. Panchal, Maharshi Bhaswant, and Lindsay Brown

15.1	Introduction	*333*
15.2	Why Metabolic Syndrome?	*333*
15.3	Classical Animal Models of Obesity and Metabolic Syndrome	*335*
15.3.1	Genetic Models of Obesity and Diabetes	*336*
15.3.2	Artificially Induced Metabolic Syndrome in Animals	*337*
15.3.2.1	Monosodium Glutamate-Induced Obesity	*338*
15.3.2.2	Intrauterine Growth-Restricted Rats	*338*
15.4	Human Experimental Models	*344*
15.5	Translation to Clinics: Difficulties and Limitations	*344*
	References	*344*

16 Cognitive Disorders: Impairment, Aging, and Dementia *349*
Nick P. van Goethem, Roy Lardenoije, Konstantinos Kompotis, Bart P.F. Rutten, Jos Prickaerts, and Harry W.M. Steinbusch

16.1	Introduction	*349*
16.2	Pharmacological Models	*349*
16.2.1	Inhibition of Energy/Glucose Metabolism	*350*
16.2.2	Cholinergic Interventions	*350*
16.2.3	Glutamatergic Antagonists	*352*
16.2.4	Serotonergic Intervention	*353*
16.3	Aging and Transgenic Models	*353*
16.3.1	Normal Aging	*354*
16.3.2	Alzheimer's Disease	*355*
16.3.3	Parkinson's Disease	*358*
16.3.4	Huntington's Disease	*358*
16.3.5	Frontotemporal Dementia	*359*
16.3.6	Down Syndrome	*360*
16.4	Translation to Clinics: Limitations and Difficulties	*360*
	References	*362*

17 Stroke and Traumatic Brain Injury *367*
Dominique Lerouet, Valérie C. Besson, and Michel Plotkine

17.1	Introduction	*367*

17.2	Stroke Models	*368*
17.2.1	Global Stroke Models	*368*
17.2.2	Focal Stroke Models	*369*
17.2.2.1	Extravascular Models	*369*
17.2.2.2	Photothrombosis Model	*370*
17.2.2.3	Intraluminal Occlusion Model	*370*
17.2.2.4	Thromboembolic Models	*370*
17.3	Traumatic Brain Injury Models	*371*
17.3.1	TBI Models with Craniotomy	*372*
17.3.1.1	Weight-Drop Model	*372*
17.3.1.2	Lateral Fluid Percussion Model	*372*
17.3.1.3	Controlled Cortical Impact Model	*372*
17.3.2	TBI Models without Craniotomy	*372*
17.3.2.1	Weight-Drop Model	*373*
17.3.2.2	Impact/Acceleration Model	*373*
17.3.2.3	Acceleration/Deceleration Model	*373*
17.3.3	Blast Injury Models	*373*
17.3.4	Repetitive TBI Models	*374*
17.4	Outcome Assessment	*375*
17.5	Translation to Clinics: Limitations and Difficulties	*377*
17.5.1	The Actual Target: From the Neuron to the Neurogliovascular Unit	*377*
17.5.2	From Bench to Bedside to Bench: Recommendations for Improving the Translational Research	*378*
	References	*379*

18 Movement Disorders: Parkinson's Disease *387*
Houman Homayoun and Christopher G. Goetz

18.1	Introduction	*387*
18.1.1	Parkinson's Disease	*387*
18.2	Drug- and Toxin-Based Models of PD	*389*
18.2.1	Reserpine	*389*
18.2.2	Haloperidol	*390*
18.2.3	6-OHDA	*390*
18.2.4	MPTP	*393*
18.2.5	Rotenone	*396*
18.2.6	Paraquat and Other Environmental Toxins	*398*
18.3	Genetic and Functional Models of PD	*398*
18.3.1	Rodent Genetic Models	*399*
18.3.1.1	Adult-Onset Rodent Gene-Based Models	*401*
18.3.2	Rodent Function-Based Models	*403*
18.3.3	Nonrodent Genetic Models of PD	*404*
18.4	Translation to Clinics: Limitations and Difficulties	*405*
	References	*409*

19	**Epilepsy: Animal Models to Reproduce Human Etiopathology** 415
	Isabelle Guillemain, Christophe Heinrich, and Antoine Depaulis
19.1	Introduction 415
19.2	What Animal Species to Use to Model Epilepsy? 416
19.3	Which Type of Models Provide the Most Reliable Information on the Pathophysiology of Epilepsies? 417
19.4	Modeling Four Prototypic Forms of Epilepsy 418
19.4.1	Idiopathic Generalized Epilepsies with Convulsive Seizures 418
19.4.2	Idiopathic Generalized Epilepsies with Absence Seizures 419
19.4.3	Focal Epilepsies Associated with Cortical Dysplasia 420
19.4.4	Modeling Focal Epilepsies Associated with Hippocampal Sclerosis 422
19.5	Translation to Clinics: Limitations and Difficulties 423
	References 425

20	**Lung Diseases** 431
	Laurent Boyer, Armand Mekontso-Dessap, Jorge Boczkowski, and Serge Adnot
20.1	Introduction 431
20.2	Animal Models of Lung Emphysema or Chronic Obstructive Pulmonary Disease 432
20.2.1	Cigarette Smoke-Induced COPD 432
20.2.2	COPD Induced by Tracheal Elastase Instillation 433
20.2.3	Genetically Modified Models of COPD 434
20.2.4	Conclusions 434
20.3	Animal Models of Pulmonary Hypertension 434
20.3.1	Relevance of Experimental Animal Models of PH to Human PH 435
20.3.2	The Monocrotaline Model of Pulmonary Hypertension 436
20.3.3	Fawn-Hooded Rats 437
20.3.4	Hypoxic PH 437
20.3.5	SU5416 Treatment Combined with Hypoxia in Mice 438
20.3.6	PH Related to COPD or Smoke Exposure 439
20.4	Animal Models of Fibrotic Lung Diseases 439
20.4.1	Bleomycin-Induced Pulmonary Fibrosis 439
20.4.2	Other Models 440
20.5	Animal Models of Acute Respiratory Distress Syndrome 440
20.6	Translation to Clinics: Limitations and Difficulties 445
	References 446

21	**Heart Failure** 449
	Jin Bo Su and Alain Berdeaux
21.1	Introduction 449
21.2	Hypertension-Related Heart Failure 450
21.3	Pressure and Volume Overload-Induced Heart Failure 452
21.3.1	Pressure Overload-Induced Heart Failure 452
21.3.2	Volume Overload-Induced Heart Failure 454

21.3.3	Double Pressure and Volume Overload-Induced Heart Failure	454
21.4	Toxic Molecule-Induced Heart Failure	455
21.4.1	Adriamycin-Induced Heart Failure in Rats	455
21.4.2	Monocrotaline-Induced Right Ventricular Heart Failure	455
21.5	Heart Failure Models Related to Myocardial Ischemia and/or Myocardial Infarction	456
21.5.1	Myocardial Ischemia and/or Myocardial Infarction	456
21.5.2	Coronary Microembolization-Induced Heart Failure	457
21.6	Pacing-Induced Heart Failure	458
21.7	Gene Mutation-Induced Cardiomyopathies	460
21.7.1	Cardiomyopathic Hamsters	460
21.7.2	Golden Retriever Muscular Dystrophy Dogs	460
21.7.3	Genetic Modification-Induced Cardiomyopathies in Mice	461
21.8	Translation to Clinics: Limitations and Difficulties	462
	References	462
22	**Endocrine Disorders** 473	
	Thomas Cuny, Anne Barlier, and Alain Enjalbert	
22.1	Introduction	473
22.2	Animal Models in Autoimmune Endocrine Diseases	474
22.2.1	Animal Models of Autoimmune Thyroiditis	474
22.2.2	Animal Models for Addison's Disease	476
22.2.3	Animal Models for Other Endocrine Autoimmune Diseases	476
22.3	Animal Models in Endocrine Tumors	477
22.3.1	Multiple Endocrine Neoplasia Syndromes	477
22.3.2	Adrenal Tumorigenesis	478
22.3.3	Thyroid Tumorigenesis	481
22.3.4	Pituitary Tumorigenesis	482
22.4	Animal Models in Endocrine Physiology: Organogenesis, Reproduction, and Metabolism	485
22.4.1	Pituitary Development Disorders: Lessons from Animal Models	485
22.4.2	Animal Models and Reproductive Function	487
22.4.3	Animal Models Used in Calcium Homeostasis Studies	489
22.5	Translation to Clinics: Limitations and Difficulties	490
	References	491
23	**Gastrointestinal Disorders: A Patho-biotechnology Approach to Probiotic Therapy** 497	
	Roy D. Sleator	
23.1	Introduction	497
23.2	Delivery: Improving Probiotic Resistance to Process-Induced Stresses and Storage Conditions	498
23.3	Survival: Improving Probiotic–Host Colonization	500

23.4	Efficacy: "Designer Probiotics"	*500*
23.5	Translation to Clinics: Limitations and Difficulties	*501*
	Acknowledgment	*502*
	References	*502*

24 Renal Disorders *505*

Dominique Guerrot, Christos Chatziantoniou, and Jean-Claude Dussaule

24.1	Introduction	*505*
24.2	Animal Models	*506*
24.2.1	The RenTg Model of CKD	*507*
24.2.1.1	Benefits of the RenTg Model	*509*
24.2.2	Unilateral Ureteral Obstruction	*510*
24.2.2.1	Technical Aspects	*510*
24.2.2.2	Pathology and Pathophysiology	*511*
24.2.2.3	Clinical Relevance and Limits	*511*
24.2.3	Renal Ischemia–Reperfusion	*511*
24.2.3.1	Technical Aspects	*512*
24.2.3.2	Pathology and Pathophysiology	*512*
24.2.3.3	Clinical Relevance and Limits	*513*
24.2.4	Experimental Alloimmune Glomerulonephritis	*513*
24.2.4.1	Technical Aspects	*513*
24.2.4.2	Pathology and Pathophysiology	*514*
24.2.4.3	Clinical Relevance and Limits	*514*
24.2.5	Angiotensin II-Mediated Hypertensive Nephropathy	*514*
24.2.5.1	Technical Aspects	*515*
24.2.5.2	Pathology and Pathophysiology	*515*
24.2.5.3	Clinical Relevance and Limits	*516*
24.2.6	L-NAME-Mediated Hypertensive Nephropathy	*516*
24.2.6.1	Technical Aspects	*516*
24.2.6.2	Pathology and Pathophysiology	*516*
24.2.6.3	Clinical Relevance and Limits	*517*
24.3	Translation to Clinics: Limitations and Difficulties	*518*
	References	*518*

25 Genitourinary Disorders: Lower Urinary Tract and Sexual Functions *523*

Pierre Clément, Delphine Behr-Roussel, and François Giuliano

25.1	Introduction	*523*
25.2	Lower Urinary Tract Function	*523*
25.2.1	Physiology of Micturition	*524*
25.2.2	Investigation of Lower Urinary Tract Function	*524*
25.2.2.1	Cystometry Evaluation	*524*
25.2.2.2	Evaluation of Urethral Function	*525*
25.2.2.3	Bladder Afferent Recording	*526*
25.2.3	Pathophysiological Models	*527*

25.2.3.1	Bladder Outlet Obstruction	527
25.2.3.2	Overactive Bladder	527
25.2.3.3	Neurogenic Detrusor Overactivity	528
25.2.3.4	Painful Bladder Syndrome/Interstitial Cystitis	528
25.3	Sexual Functions	529
25.3.1	Physiology of Female and Male Sexual Response	529
25.3.2	Models for Sexual Behavior	530
25.3.2.1	Sexual Preference Paradigms	530
25.3.2.2	Copulatory Tests	531
25.3.3	Investigation of the Peripheral Female Sexual Response	532
25.3.4	Investigation of Erection	532
25.3.4.1	Penile Reflex	532
25.3.4.2	Erection in Conscious Animals	533
25.3.4.3	Intracavernosal Pressure Measurement	533
25.3.4.4	Pharmacologically Induced Erection	534
25.3.4.5	Neurally Evoked Erection	534
25.3.5	Investigation of Ejaculation	534
25.3.5.1	Physiological Markers of Emission and Expulsion Phases	534
25.3.5.2	Pharmacologically Induced Ejaculation	535
25.3.5.3	Lumbar Spinothalamic Neurons Electrical Stimulation	535
25.3.5.4	Expulsion Spinal Reflex	535
25.3.6	Pathophysiological Models	536
25.3.6.1	Female Sexual Dysfunctions	536
25.3.6.2	Erectile Dysfunction	536
25.3.6.3	Ejaculatory Disorders	538
25.4	Translation to Clinics: Difficulties and Limitations	538
	References	540

Index *543*

List of Contributors

Serge Adnot
Université Paris-Est Créteil (UPEC)
Faculté de Médecine
Hôpital Henri Mondor
51 Avenue du Maréchal de Lattre de Tassigny
94010 Créteil Cedex
France

Denis Ardid
Clermont Université (Université d'Auvergne)
NEURO-DOL
Faculté de médecine
Place Henri Dunant
63000 Clermont-Ferrand
France

and

INSERM U1107
63001 Clermont-Ferrand
Faculté de médecine
Place Henri Dunant
France

David Balayssac
Clermont Université (Université d'Auvergne)
NEURO-DOL
63000 Clermont-Ferrand
France

and

INSERM U1107
63001 Clermont-Ferrand
Faculté de médecine
Place Henri Dunant
France

and

CHU Clermont-Ferrand
Toxicoloy department
63003 Clermont-Ferrand
France

Anne Barlier
AP-HM, Conception
Laboratory of Molecular Biology
147 Bd Baille
13855 Marseille Cedex
France

and

Aix-Marseille University
Faculté de Médecine Nord
Laboratoire CRN2M, UMR 7286 CNRS
51 Bd Pierre Dramard
13344 Marseille Cedex 15
France

Sandra Beeské
Sanofi
Exploratory Unit
1 avenue Pierre Brossolette
91385 Chilly-Mazarin
France

Delphine Behr-Roussel
Pelvipharm Laboratories
2, avenue de la source de la Bièvre
78390 Montigny le Bretonneux
France

and

University of Versailles-St Quentin
en Yvelines
School of Health Sciences
SIRIUS/EA4501
2, avenue de la source de la Bièvre
78390 Montigny le Bretonneux
France

Alain Berdeaux
Université Paris-Est Créteil (UPEC)
Faculté de Médecine
Laboratoire de Pharmacologie
INSERM U955 (équipe 3 IMRB)
Rue du Général Sarrail, 8
94010 Créteil Cedex
France

Valérie C. Besson
Université Paris Descartes
Faculté de Pharmacie
Laboratoire de Pharmacologie
EA 4475 "Pharmacologie de la
Circulation Cérébrale"
4, avenue de l'Observatoire
75006 Paris Cedex 06
France

Maharshi Bhaswant
Victoria University
College of Health & Biomedicine
St Albans, Melbourne 3021
Australia

Jorge Boczkowski
Université Paris-Est Créteil (UPEC)
Faculté de Médecine
Hôpital Henri Mondor
51 Avenue du Maréchal de Lattre de
Tassigny
94010 Créteil Cedex
France

Sylvie Bourgoin
Université Pierre et Marie Curie
Faculty of Medicine
Neuropsychopharmacology Unit
INSERM U894 – CPN
site Pitié-Salpêtrière
91, boulevard de l'Hôpital
75634 Paris Cedex 13
France

Laurent Boyer
Université Paris-Est Créteil (UPEC)
Faculté de Médecine
Hôpital Henri Mondor
51 Avenue du Maréchal de Lattre
de Tassigny
94010 Créteil Cedex
France

Véronique Brault
Université de Strasbourg
Institut Clinique de la Souris
ICS-MCI, PHENOMIN, GIE CERBM
CNRS, INSERM
1 rue Laurent Fries
67404 Illkirch
France

and

Université de Strasbourg
Institut de Génétique Biologie
Moléculaire et Cellulaire
IGBMC, GIE CERBM
CNRS, INSERM
UMR7104, UMR964
1 rue Laurent Fries
67404 Illkirch
France

Lindsay Brown
University of Southern Queensland
School of Health
Nursing and Midwifery
Toowoomba, Queensland 4350
Australia

Christos Chatziantoniou
Inserm UMR S 1155
Sorbonne Universités
UPMC Univ Paris 06
4 rue de la Chine
75020 Paris
France

and

Université Pierre et Marie Curie
Paris
France

Fabien Chauveau
Université Lyon 1
Lyon Neuroscience Research Center
CNRS, INSERM
59 Bd Pinel
69003 Lyon
France

and

CERMEP-Imagerie du Vivant
Lyon
France

Sarah Louise T. Christensen
University of Copenhagen
Faculty of Health Sciences
Glostrup Hospital
Department of Neurology and
Glostrup Research Institute
Danish Headache Center
Nordre Ringvej 57
2600 Glostrup
Denmark

Pierre Clément
Pelvipharm Laboratories
2, avenue de la source de la Bièvre
78390 Montigny le Bretonneux
France

and

University of Versailles-St Quentin
en Yvelines
School of Health Sciences
SIRIUS/EA4501
2, avenue de la source de la Bièvre
78390 Montigny le Bretonneux
France

Thomas Cuny
University Hospital of Nancy-Brabois
Department of Endocrinology and
Medical Gynaecology
Rue du Morvan
54511 Vandoeuvre-Les-Nancy Cedex
France

and

Aix-Marseille University
Faculté de Médecine Nord
Laboratoire CRN2M, UMR 7286
CNRS
51 Bd Pierre Dramard
13344 Marseille Cedex 15
France

Yassine Darbaky
ANS Biotech
Faculté de Médecine et de Pharmacologie
28, place Henri Dunant
63000 Clermont-Ferrand
France

Antoine Depaulis
INSERM U836
Dynamics of Epileptic Synchronous Networks
38042 Grenoble Cedex 9
France

and

Université Joseph Fourier
Grenoble Institut des Neurosciences
38042 Grenoble Cedex 9
France

Ronan Depoortère
Centre de Recherche Pierre-Fabre
Neuropsychopharmacology Unit
17 avenue Jean Moulin
81106 Castres
France

Laurent Diop
ANS Biotech
Faculté de Médecine et de Pharmacologie
28, place Henri Dunant
63000 Clermont-Ferrand
France

Jean-Claude Dussaule
Inserm UMR S 1155
Sorbonne Universités
UPMC Univ Paris 06
4 rue de la Chine
75020 Paris
France

and

Saint-Antoine Hospital
HUEP, AP-HP
Department of Physiology
184 rue du faubourg Saint-Antoine,
75012 Paris
France

Alain Enjalbert
AP-HM, Conception
Laboratory of Molecular Biology
147 Bd Baille
13855 Marseille Cedex
France

and

Aix-Marseille University
Faculté de Médecine Nord
Laboratoire CRN2M, UMR 7286
CNRS
51 Bd Pierre Dramard
13344 Marseille Cedex 15
France

François Giuliano
Pelvipharm Laboratories
2, avenue de la source de la Bièvre
78390 Montigny le Bretonneux
France

and

University of Versailles-St Quentin
en Yvelines
School of Health Sciences
SIRIUS/EA4501
2, avenue de la source de la Bièvre
78390 Montigny le Bretonneux
France

and

Raymond Poincaré Hospital
Department of Physical Medicine
and Rehabilitation
Neuro-Uro-Andrology
AP-HP
104, boulevard Raymond Poincaré
92380 Garches
France

Christopher G. Goetz
Rush University Medical Center
Department of Neurology
1725 West Harrison Street
Chicago, IL 60612
USA

Guy Griebel
Sanofi
Exploratory Unit
1 avenue Pierre Brossolette
91385 Chilly-Mazarin
France

Dominique Guerrot
INSERM Unit 1096
Rouen University Medical School
22 Boulevard Gambetta
76183 Rouen
France

and

Rouen University Hospital
Department of Nephrology
1 rue de Germont
76031 Rouen
France

Isabelle Guillemain
INSERM U836
Dynamics of Epileptic Synchronous
Networks
38042 Grenoble Cedex 9
France

and

Université Joseph Fourier
Grenoble Institut des Neurosciences
38042 Grenoble Cedex 9
France

Javier Gutiérrez-Cuesta
Universitat Pompeu Fabra
Laboratori de Neurofarmacologia
Parc de Recerca Biomedica de
Barcelona (PRBB)
Dr. Aiguader 88
08003 Barcelona
Spain

Antonio Guzmán
Esteve
Department of Toxicology
Drug Discovery & Preclinical
Development
Parc Cientific Barcelona
Baldiri Reixac 4–8
08028 Barcelona
Spain

Michel Hamon
Université Pierre et Marie Curie
Faculty of Medicine
Neuropsychopharmacology Unit
INSERM U894 – CPN
site Pitié-Salpêtrière
91, boulevard de l'Hôpital
75634 Paris Cedex 13
France

Christophe Heinrich
INSERM U836
Dynamics of Epileptic Synchronous
Networks
38042 Grenoble Cedex 9
France

and

Université Joseph Fourier
Grenoble Institut des Neurosciences
38042 Grenoble Cedex 9
France

Yann Hérault
Université de Strasbourg
Institut Clinique de la Souris
ICS-MCI, PHENOMIN, GIE CERBM
CNRS, INSERM
1 rue Laurent Fries
67404 Illkirch
France

and

Université de Strasbourg
Institut de Génétique Biologie
Moléculaire et Cellulaire
IGBMC, GIE CERBM
CNRS, INSERM
UMR7104, UMR964
1 rue Laurent Fries
67404 Illkirch
France

and

Transgenèse et Archivage d'Animaux
Modèles
TAAM UPS44, CNRS, PHENOMIN
3B rue de la Férollerie
45071 Orléans Cedex 2
France

Houman Homayoun
University of Pittsburgh
Medical Center
Department of Neurology
3471 Fifth Ave, suite 810
Pittsburgh, PA 15213
USA

Inger Jansen-Olesen
University of Copenhagen
Faculty of Health Sciences
Glostrup Hospital
Department of Neurology and
Glostrup Research Institute
Danish Headache Center
Nordre Ringvej 57
2600 Glostrup
Denmark

Konstantinos Kompotis
Maastricht University
School for Mental Health and
Neuroscience
Department of Neuroscience
Universiteitssingel 50
6229 ER Maastricht
The Netherlands

Roy Lardenoije
Maastricht University
School for Mental Health and
Neuroscience
Department of Neuroscience
Universiteitssingel 50
6229 ER Maastricht
The Netherlands

Dominique Lerouet
Université Paris Descartes
Faculté de Pharmacie
Laboratoire de Pharmacologie
EA 4475 "Pharmacologie de la
Circulation Cérébrale"
4, avenue de l'Observatoire
75006 Paris Cedex 06
France

Rafael Maldonado
Universitat Pompeu Fabra
Department of Experimental &
Health Sciences
Laboratory of Neuropharmacology
(NeuroPhar)
Barcelona Biomedical Research Park
(PRBB)
Dr. Aiguader 88
08003 Barcelona
Spain

Christophe Mallet
Clermont Université (Université
d'Auvergne)
NEURO-DOL
Faculté de médecine
Place Henri Dunant
63000 Clermont-Ferrand
France

and

INSERM U1107
Faculté de médecine
Place Henri Dunant
63001 Clermont-Ferrand
France

Elena Martín-García
Universitat Pompeu Fabra
Laboratori de Neurofarmacologia
Parc de Recerca Biomedica de
Barcelona (PRBB)
Dr. Aiguader 88
08003 Barcelona
Spain

Said M'Dahoma
Université Pierre et Marie Curie
Faculty of Medicine
Neuropsychopharmacology Unit
INSERM U894 – CPN
site Pitié-Salpêtrière
91, boulevard de l'Hôpital
75634 Paris Cedex 13
France

Armand Mekontso-Dessap
Université Paris-Est Créteil (UPEC)
Hôpital Henri Mondor
Service de Réanimation Médicale
AP-HP
94010 Créteil Cedex
France

Paul Moser
Centre de Recherche Pierre-Fabre
Neuropsychopharmacology Unit
17 avenue Jean Moulin
81106 Castres
France

Jes Olesen
University of Copenhagen
Faculty of Health Sciences
Glostrup Hospital
Department of Neurology and
Glostrup Research Institute
Danish Headache Center
Nordre Ringvej 57
2600 Glostrup
Denmark

Sunil K. Panchal
University of Southern Queensland
Centre for Systems Biology
Toowoomba, Queensland 4350
Australia

Guillaume Pavlovic
Université de Strasbourg
Institut Clinique de la Souris
ICS-MCI, PHENOMIN, GIE CERBM
CNRS, INSERM
1 rue Laurent Fries
67404 Illkirch
France

Michel Plotkine
Université Paris Descartes
Faculté de Pharmacie
Laboratoire de Pharmacologie
EA 4475 "Pharmacologie de la
Circulation Cérébrale"
4, avenue de l'Observatoire
75006 Paris Cedex 06
France

Jos Prickaerts
Maastricht University
School for Mental Health and
Neuroscience
Department of Neuroscience
Universiteitssingel 50
6229 ER Maastricht
The Netherlands

Patricia Robledo
Universitat Pompeu Fabra
Laboratori de Neurofarmacologia
Parc de Recerca Biomedica de
Barcelona (PRBB)
Dr. Aiguader 88
08003 Barcelona
Spain

and

IMIM-Hospital del Mar Research
Institute
Human Pharmacology and Clinical
Neurosciences Research Group
Neurosciences Research Programme
PRBB
Calle Dr. Aiguader 88
08003 Barcelona
Spain

Luz Romero
Esteve
Drug Discovery & Preclinical
Development
Parc Cientific Barcelona
Baldiri Reixac 4–8
08028 Barcelona
Spain

Bart P.F. Rutten
Maastricht University
School for Mental Health and
Neuroscience
Department of Neuroscience
Universiteitssingel 50
6229 ER Maastricht
The Netherlands

David Sabaté
Esteve
R&D Department Animal Health
Division
Animal Ethics Committee
Avinguda Mare de Déu de
Montserrat, 221
08041 Barcelona
Spain

Roy D. Sleator
Cork Institute of Technology
Department of Biological Sciences
Rossa Avenue
Bishopstown, Cork
Ireland

Tania Sorg
Université de Strasbourg
Institut Clinique de la Souris
ICS-MCI, PHENOMIN, GIE CERBM
CNRS, INSERM
1 rue Laurent Fries
67404 Illkirch
France

Harry W.M. Steinbusch
Maastricht University
School for Mental Health and
Neuroscience
Department of Neuroscience
Universiteitssingel 50
6229 ER Maastricht
The Netherlands

and

Maastricht University
School for Mental Health and
Neuroscience
Department of Neuroscience
Universiteitssingel 50
6229 ER Maastricht
The Netherlands

Jin Bo Su
Université Paris-Est Créteil (UPEC)
Faculté de Médecine
Laboratoire de Pharmacologie
INSERM U955 (équipe 3 IMRB)
Rue du Général Sarrail, 8
94010 Créteil Cedex
France

Nick P. van Goethem
Maastricht University
School for Mental Health and
Neuroscience
Department of Neuroscience
Universiteitssingel 50
6229 ER Maastricht
The Netherlands

José Miguel Vela
Esteve
Drug Discovery & Preclinical
Development
Parc Cientific Barcelona
Baldiri Reixac 4–8
08028 Barcelona
Spain

Mathieu Verdurand
Université Lyon 1
Lyon Neuroscience Research Center
CNRS, INSERM
59 Bd Pinel, 69003 Lyon
France

and

CERMEP-Imagerie du Vivant
Lyon
France

Luc Zimmer
Université Lyon 1
Lyon Neuroscience Research Center
CNRS, INSERM
59 Bd Pinel, 69003 Lyon
France

and

CERMEP-Imagerie du Vivant
59 Bd Pinel, 69003 Lyon
France

and

Hospices Civils de Lyon
Groupement Hospitalier Est
59 Bd Pinel, 69003 Lyon
France

Preface

Once, in a zoo, the chief of a gorilla group had to visit a dentist. He was not easily persuaded and finally, someone advised to mix a "sleeping pill" in his food. This suggestion was fiercely refused by the veterinarians, because they did not want to expose a precarious zoo animal to therapeutics that had been developed for humans.

The anecdote nicely depicts the experts' subliminal discomfort about the comparability of drug action in "humans and mice," which is an ongoing and often an ideological debate in drug development. Many of the arguments in the debate touch fundamental questions as the position of man within the realm of evolution theory [1], or request the full abandonment of any animal test in drug development, since animals that "lead biographical lives" are not different with respect to man's position in evolution [2]. The underlying uncertainty among scientists is raised by the question whether and how animals emotionally judge and reflect on the environments and if so, in which way this activity influences their physiology. Modern brain research has opened Pandora's box by exposing rodents to enriched environment and demonstrating phenotype plasticity [3]. What is then the validity of current animal models of mental disorders?

The work in hand of José M. Vela, Rafael Maldonado, and Michel Hamon paves the ground for addressing these questions in an extended discussion, by rigorously laying out the current approaches in animal testing. The first part is devoted to more general considerations to comprise reflections on the need of animal testing and its replacement, ethical issues, guidelines, and regulation, besides methodological issues as PET and MR imaging of animal brains and the generation and use of transgenic animals. The second part details the methodology of animal models in specific therapeutic areas. According to the fundamental debate, it is of utmost necessity to clarify and differentiate the significance of animal tests in pain research versus obesity therapy and in anxiety disorders versus lung disease. It is the special merit of this book to objectify the discussion on animal tests by elucidating experimental processes and methods in a heterogeneity of pharmacological targets and pointing to the fact that for every animal model a scrutinizing look and critical reflection is inherent in the scientists attitude. Each chapter is concluded by discussion of the translational issues to provide pro and con arguments for the validity and necessity of animal experiments within the specific therapeutic area.

The series editors are indebted to the authors and the editors who made this comprehensive issue possible. We are convinced that the book represents an important contribution to the body of knowledge in a much debated field in drug discovery and that it is of significant value for many researchers who have taken up this promising but difficult field.

In addition, we are very much indebted to Frank Weinreich and Heike Nöthe, both at Wiley-VCH. Their support and ongoing engagement, not only for this book but for the whole series, Methods and Principles in Medicinal Chemistry, adds to the success of this excellent collection of monographs on various topics, all related to drug research.

March 2013
Düsseldorf, Germany
Weisenheim am Sand, Germany
Zürich, Switzerland

Raimund Mannhold
Hugo Kubinyi
Gerd Folkers

References

1 Nagel, N. (2012) *Mind and Cosmos: Why the Materialist Neo-Darwinian Conception of Nature Is Almost Certainly False*, Oxford University Press.
2 Nordgren, A. (2002) Animal experimentation: pro and con arguments using the theory of evolution. *Medicine, Healthcare, and Philosophy* **5** (1), 23–31.
3 Laviola, G., Hannan, A.J., Macrí, S., Solinas, M., and Jaber, M. (2008) Effects of enriched environment on animal models of neurodegenerative diseases and psychiatric disorders. *Neurobiology of Disease* **31**, 159–168.

A Personal Foreword

"Animal research has played a vital role in virtually every major medical advance (. . .) From the discovery of antibiotics, analgesics, antidepressants, and anaesthetics, to the successful development of organ transplants, bypass surgery, heart catheterization, and joint replacement, practically every present-day protocol for the prevention, control, cure of disease and relief of pain is based on knowledge attained—directly or indirectly—through research with animals (. . .) Research leading to almost every Nobel Prize in Medicine awarded since 1901 was dependent on data from animal models"
(National Association for Biomedical Research; http://www.nabr.org/Biomedical_Research/Medical_Progress.aspx).

The first chemical used to treat a specific disease (syphilis) was discovered by Paul Ehrlich through animal experimentation in the early 1900s. Ehrlich and his colleague Sahachiro Hata discovered Salvarsan (also known as arsphenamine or compound 606) by testing compounds in animal models of syphilis. Indeed, the compound was initially called compound 606 as it was the 606th compound screened on infected animals in an attempt to find a treatment for syphilis. Ehrlich and Hata tested the effect of the compound 606 on mice, guinea pigs, and then rabbits with syphilis and they achieved complete cures within 3 weeks, with no dead animals. In 1910, the drug was launched and it made syphilis a curable disease. *In vivo* experimentation was thus credited with starting the pharmaceutical age.

Despite great advances in basic knowledge and the advent of new technologies, drug discovery initiatives often fail to transform this improved understanding and technological progress into truly novel pharmacological approaches to treat disorders. This situation has been partly attributed to the difficulty of predicting efficacy and safety in patients based on results from preclinical studies. Accordingly, the failure of many compounds in clinical trials following demonstration of efficacy and safety in experimental models has called into question the value of the models (and the approach followed in the discovery process in general).

While pointing out the numerous shortcomings of animal research and its limitations when trying to translate the preclinical findings to the clinic, such research remains at the heart of drug discovery and development. Indeed, some important phases of drug discovery and development rely on *in vivo* experiments as a fundamental source of data. The availability of good models reflecting as much as possible the complexity of the human diseases is a key for understanding and exploring disease mechanisms and the achievement of new and better treatments.

Animal models have been especially valuable in coming up with new medicines for a range of conditions and disorders, and it is likely to continue to be and remain an essential part of biomedical research in the foreseeable future. The underlying, unresolved questions are how animal (and alternative) models can contribute most effectively to drug discovery and what are the obstacles and major challenges to overcome in order to increase the probability of achieving clinical benefit based on findings from preclinical research.

This book is dedicated to *in vivo* models used in drug discovery to examine the potential of novel drugs for treating a wide variety of pathological conditions. Almost all the major conditions are reviewed. Current needs regarding the use of animal models (Chapter 1), the available alternatives to animal models (Chapters 2 and 3), ethical aspects and regulations in relation to animal research and 3Rs principles (Chapter 4), requirements of regulatory authorities concerning safety and toxicological testing (Chapter 5), the generation and use of genetically modified mice (Chapter 6), and novel brain imaging tools (Chapter 7) are reviewed in the first part of the book. In the second part, experimental models used to discover new therapeutic strategies in most of the major diseases and conditions have been expertly reviewed (Chapters 8–25). The opportunities offered by *in vivo* models for improving our understanding of the pathophysiology of diseases as well as their particularities and limitations have been depicted. The difficulties when trying to model a human disease are an important issue that has been expertly and critically discussed by the authors of the different chapters (see "Translation to Clinics" section at the end of each chapter), focusing on the limitations in translating to the clinic the discoveries from research using the different models that are currently being used in the search for better treatments for a given human disorder. This is a differentiating piece in this book.

Finally, it is imperative to warmly acknowledge the authors who contributed their excellent chapters and made this book possible. We greatly appreciate their expert opinion and their effort to comprehensively review different aspects of the use of *in vivo* models and their applications in drug discovery in the different research/disease areas.

José Miguel Vela
Rafael Maldonado
Michel Hamon

Part I
Transversal Issues Concerning Animal Models in Drug Discovery

1
The 3Ns of Preclinical Animal Models in Biomedical Research

José Miguel Vela, Rafael Maldonado, and Michel Hamon

In vivo experimentation has played a central role in biomedical research in the past, and it has also been a hot issue of public, scientific, and even philosophical discussion for centuries [1–3]. At present, a paradigm regarding needs, usefulness, and ethical treatment of animals in research has evolved, but discussion is open [3].

It is a matter of fact that the use of animal experimentation is a genuine need for the primary purposes of target validation and estimation of multiple parameters of new therapeutic drugs, including efficacy, margin of safety, and metabolism and pharmacokinetics. It is also obvious that current unmet needs regarding experimentation with animals primarily focus on the development of better animal models, with improved translation to humans, as well as on further advancements of replacement alternatives, minimization of number and suffering of animals used, and continuous improvement of the well-being of laboratory animals [4].

Accordingly, there are three major needs (3Ns) regarding nonhuman animal models in biomedical research: (i) the need for use, (ii) the need for better, and (iii) the need for three Rs (3Rs) – replace, reduce, and refine – guiding principles. Justification of one of these needs does not justify the neglect of or insufficient perseverance with the other two.

1.1
First N: The Need for Use of Animal Models

The use of animal models in biomedical research has been making great contributions to the medical advancements, and it is likely to remain an integral part of research in the foreseeable future.

Animal models (in most cases, rodent models) are well-established tools for both fundamental and applied biomedical research, and thus the main instrument for drug discovery, validation, preclinical, and toxicological studies. They are widely used due to the deep knowledge obtained (e.g., the mouse became the second and the rat the third mammal, after humans, to have its whole genome sequenced), the possibility of genetic (e.g., inbred strains) and environmental standardization, the access to a broad spectrum of strains, genetic modifications (transgenic and gene

---

In Vivo *Models for Drug Discovery*, First Edition. Edited by José M. Vela, Rafael Maldonado, and Michel Hamon.
© 2014 Wiley-VCH Verlag GmbH & Co. KGaA. Published 2014 by Wiley-VCH Verlag GmbH & Co. KGaA.

knockout models available), and pharmacological interventions adapted to address specific scientific problems, and their general – although sometimes controversial – acceptance by the scientific community, patent regulatory bodies, health regulatory authorities, and ultimately a society with unmet medical needs that demands better and safer medicines.

Scientists involved in biomedical research rely on animal models as an important means of generating knowledge and obtaining information on the potential relevance and therapeutic application of their discoveries. Indeed, most biomedical researches, including those grounded in molecular studies, need at some point validation of their findings in a suitable cell, tissue, organ, or preferably whole animal model reproducing or mimicking as much as possible the physiology or behavior under study.

Regulatory authorities require evidence for both efficacy and safety of novel compounds in appropriate animal models. The need for more effective medicines and the emphasis on risk avoidance in our society have resulted in a broad range of regulations intended to guarantee efficacy and safety of new pharmaceutical products. Many of these regulations rely on animal tests. In fact, animal testing is a key element of the product assessment legislative and regulatory procedures: animals used for regulatory requirements for the production and quality control of products and devices for human and veterinary medicine and to satisfy regulatory toxicological and other safety requirements accounted for at least 23% of the total number of animals used for experimental purposes in the European Union in 2008 [1].

From the intellectual property viewpoint, patents are granted for inventions that are novel, involve an inventive step (nonobviousness) with regard to the state of the art, and are useful for or susceptible to application. In order to encourage innovation, the subject matter claimed in a patent application must not be already known or be part of the prior art, and for this reason it is essential to file a priority application before any public disclosure or use of an invention. Waiting too long to file an application threatens the novelty of the invention and inventors may lose forever the chance to obtain a patent if the subject of the invention is revealed prior to the filing date. Accordingly, patent applications for new drugs are usually filed early, during the drug discovery or preclinical development program, before clinical trials would eventually demonstrate safety and efficacy in humans. Experiments in appropriate animal models are thus a main source of data to meet the substantive conditions of patentability and support the claims of the patent application [4].

Finally, the market and ultimately the society demand better medicines based on the differentiation of novel compounds from those already on the market, and potential advantages of new drugs in terms of efficacy and/or safety are usually demonstrated early on during the drug discovery program using appropriate, as much as possible translatable to humans, animal models.

Independent of its acceptance, justification of animal experimentation seems reasonably clear based on the benefits that research relying on animal models has conferred and still confers upon humans. The benefits involved here are understood to include such things as advances in knowledge as well as things more commonly regarded as tangible benefits, such as improvements in disease diagnosis and treatment. There are thousands of evidences showing how valuable data obtained from animal experimentation underlie or have allowed key discoveries and improvements with positive impact on human health. It is important to note that for the purpose of this chapter, it is assumed that either in the short or in the long term (or both), the benefits of research using animal models are substantive, an assumption that is compatible with the possibility that alleged benefits of some research could be considered spurious or that benefit arguments could be debatable [2]. In any case, this is not the place to undertake an analysis of the balance between the costs and benefits of the myriad experimental uses of animals in biomedicine or to philosophically debate over moral quandaries regarding animal experimentation.

Even so, animal models need to be improved as findings arising from current preclinical animal models often poorly translate to human disease and clinical practice. In addition, animal models are not the only source of valuable data supporting new discoveries, and more and better alternative models need to be developed to replace and/or reduce the number of animals used, while increasing their well-being.

1.2
Second N: The Need for Better Animal Models

The translation of novel discoveries from basic research to clinical application is a long and often inefficient and costly course. This goal has resulted over the years in phrases such as "from bench to bedside," "from mouse to man," "from laboratory findings to clinical practice," or "today's science; tomorrow's medicine." The rather recent terms "translational research," "translational pharmacology," and "translational medicine" also highlight this goal, emphasizing the distinctive scientific processes that have to be done to move (or translate) basic research into a finally approved therapeutic agent [5]. Translational research has become a top priority in national and international road maps to human health research.

Translational research is a paradigm for research, an alternative to the dichotomy of basic (or fundamental) and applied research. It is actually a distinct research approach seeking to make findings from basic science useful for practical applications enhancing human health and well-being. It is necessarily a much more multidisciplinary style of research, with low and permeable barriers and much interaction between academic research and industry practice.

Translation almost always involves animal models of disease in order to evaluate the possible therapeutic use of a compound. Appropriate animal models for the evaluation of efficacy and safety of new drugs or therapeutic concepts are thus critical for the success of translational research. Unfortunately, although testing in animal models is a key step, animal models do not always reflect the clinical situation. In fact, translational research frequently fails to replicate in the clinic what has been demonstrated in the laboratory.

Despite great advances in basic knowledge, the improved understanding has not yet led to the proportional introduction of truly novel pharmacological treatment approaches. Transgenic and knockout techniques have revolutionized manipulation of rodents and other species to get greater insights into human disease pathogenesis, but we are far from generating ideal animal models of most human disease states [6]. In addition, rapid advances in modern omic sciences coupled with the high-speed synthetic and high-throughput screening capabilities should provide new targets, new insights into efficacy and risk factors, shortened drug discovery cycle times, and better drug candidates. But this is not (always) the case. Drugs fail at a higher rate in phase II trials, the point at which researchers first test efficacy in humans, and a reason for the high attrition in the clinic has been suggested to be the poor predictive power of animal models for efficacy in humans [7–9]. Indeed, the US Food and Drug Administration (FDA) in its Critical Path Initiative report points to the limited predictive value of currently available animal models as one of the reasons for the recent slowdown, instead of the expected acceleration, in innovative medical therapies reaching patients, and states that better predictive nonclinical screening methods are urgently needed [4]. Altogether, with the increased emphasis on translational medicine, the use of high-quality, predictive, *in vivo* animal models has been recognized as an essential component of modern drug discovery if late-stage failure for lack of clinical efficacy is to be avoided.

Two fundamental reasons for this "lost in translation" problem have been suggested: the "butterfly effect" (intrinsically related to the behavior of many animal models) and the "two cultures" problem (differences between the methodologies for preclinical and clinical research) [10].

It is clear that modeling has intrinsic limitations. An animal model is defined as any experimental preparation developed in an animal for the purpose of studying a human condition, and thus, as implied by the term "modeling," no perfect animal model exists for any disorder [7]. The cross-species predictability is always an issue as the animal response to the pharmacological manipulation may engage different mechanisms/pathways and thus confound the actual human response to pharmacological interventions. The imprecise diagnostic criteria for some illnesses also inevitably lead to problems when trying to model the condition. In addition, the complex nature of human conditions makes it difficult/impossible to reproduce human behaviors and deficits [11]. For example, language deficit plays a major role in autistic spectrum disorders, but rodents do not have language so it is not possible to develop a language-impaired "autistic" mouse. Going further, how predictive specific knockout models are for the effects of acute or chronic pharmacological intervention in patients? How well does locomotor responsiveness to the administration of psychostimulants or altered water maze learning predict the antipsychotic and cognition-enhancing effects of novel compounds in patients? [7].

But not always the failure of apparently promising interventions to translate to the clinic may be caused by inadequate animal data and overoptimistic conclusions about efficacy drawn from methodologically flawed animal studies. The decision to conduct clinical trials is not always supported by reliable evidence of efficacy in animal models [12], and in the clinical setting, improved patient classification, more homogenous patient cohorts in clinical trials, standardized treatment strategies, improved drug delivery systems, and monitoring of target drug levels and drug effects are warranted [13]. Clinical trials should also adopt more practices from basic science and show greater responsiveness to conditions of clinical practice [14]. The disparity between the results of animal models and clinical trials may be explained in some cases by shortcomings of the clinical trials. For instance, these may have insufficient statistical power to detect a true benefit of the treatment under study or allow therapy at later time points, when the window of opportunity has passed [15]. In addition, both positive and negative results contribute to knowledge but, in contrast to many clinical studies, negative studies obtained with animal models are usually not reported. Negative results are often considered by investigators and journal referees and editors as unsuccessful or with low scientific value and attractiveness to be published, although such information is vital [8]. As neutral or negative animal studies are more likely to remain unpublished than negative clinical trials, the impression is that the former are more often positive than the latter, which overstates the disparity between the results of animal models and clinical trials [15].

Unfortunately, the difficulties in developing new compounds, particularly those working through novel mechanisms, are currently leading to a lack of confidence (as many pharmaceutical companies are terminating in-house research, more often in complex conditions such as neurological and psychiatric disorders) and a state of skepticism regarding the usefulness of animal models (will their use only allow discovery of more "me-too" compounds?) [5]. To address this problem, it is not enough to investigate and bring about new models. Changing the way academic researchers, drug developers, and regulatory agencies operate is advised. Instead of moving progressively from simple cultured cell models to imperfect animal models and then into clinical trials [9], future efforts should be focused more on the underlying mechanisms at work in a disease and finding drugs to affect one or the other mechanism. More intensive clinical and preclinical interactions are needed to ensure that basic science knowledge gained from animal models and information from the clinical/human domain converge to develop truly translational measures in both preclinical and clinical testing. Information must flow in both directions from humans to nonhumans and then back again so that it is not lost in translation [16]. In addition, the research should not be stalled at the animal model stage, but instead the clinical trials need to be focused, safe, and ethical, backed up by a robust, translationally relevant preclinical research strategy [17]. This new translational approach combined with the evolving focus on the identification of reliable biomarkers that correlate with clinical and functional endpoints provides a fresh and optimistic framework.

The remaining task of animal model validation is of such magnitude that no single pharmaceutical company or academic center can effectively address the issues relevant even to a specific disease. Consortia from industry and academia (e.g., Innovative Medicines Initiative and Horizon 2020 in Europe) to tackle some of the issues related to preclinical discovery approaches on a precompetitive level (indeed, specific work packages on animal models improvement are included in most disease-focused project IMI consortia) together with the development of mechanisms for data sharing are essential, and both industrial and academic researchers must contribute. This requires a change of mindset of all the stakeholders involved: industry being willing to share more data, resources, and compounds; academia being prepared for some more practically oriented groundwork rather than cutting-edge scientific experimentation leading to high-impact publications; and governments and regulatory authorities promoting such joint initiatives and innovative approaches to improve translation of novel discoveries from basic research to clinical application [7,18].

While recognizing the difficulty of predicting efficacy in patients based on results from preclinical studies, animal models could contribute most effectively to translational medicine and drug discovery. In the following sections, some comments regarding key features and obstacles of animal modeling are depicted, with the aim to encourage preclinical–clinical translation in drug discovery and eventually improve the translational value of animal models and/or enrich the information they provide. This issue has been evaluated expertly and critically previously by other authors [5,7,15,19,20] and key data included herein have been obtained from the information in these excellent review articles.

1.2.1
Unbiased Design

Adequate internal validity of an animal experiment implies that the differences observed between groups of animals allocated to different interventions may, apart from random error, be attributed to the treatment under investigation. The internal validity may be reduced by different types of bias through which differences between treatment groups are introduced. Blinding of the experimenter to the drug administration, randomization of animal subjects, control of variables that may affect outcome and lead to erroneous conclusions, predefined (not determined on a *post hoc* basis) eligibility criteria if animals are excluded (e.g., inadvertent blood loss during surgery or weight loss), control of study conduct, and accurate statistic analysis of the results are always mandatory [5,15].

1.2.2
Comprehensive Reporting

Inadequate or incomplete reporting raises ethical as well as scientific concerns as it reduces the value gained from animal experiments, which can result in unnecessary additional studies, and might hinder the translation of experimental findings to humans by restricting the potential use of systematic reviews and meta-analyses to assess preclinical evidence. In order to maximize the output of research that uses animals, initiatives such as the ARRIVE (Animal Research: Reporting of *In Vivo* Experiments) guidelines have been developed collaboratively by scientists, statisticians, journal editors, and research funders. They consist of a checklist of 20 items with the essential information that should be included in publications reporting animal research to describe a study in a comprehensive and transparent manner, and make recommendations on the reporting of the study design, experimental procedures, animal characteristics, housing and husbandry, and statistical analysis. The ARRIVE guidelines were simultaneously published in a number of bioscience journals in 2010 and, since then, more than 300 journals have adopted them (the full list can be found on the NC3Rs web site at www.nc3rs.org.uk/ARRIVE). Applying guidelines carefully may represent an opportunity to improve standards of reporting and ensure that the data from animal experiments can be fully scrutinized and utilized [12,21].

1.2.3
Selection of the Animal Model Based on Its Validity Attributes

Even if the design and conduct of an animal study are sound and eliminate the possibility of bias, the translation of its results to the clinic may fail because of disparities between the model and the clinical trials testing the treatment strategy. Common causes of such reduced external validity not only are limited to differences between animals and humans in the pathophysiology of disease, which are largely determined by disease-specific factors, but also include differences in comorbidities, the use of comedication, timing of the administration and dosing of the study treatment, and the selection of outcome measures [15].

A primary concern to scientists, working either in academic world or in the industry, is the selection of the most appropriate animal model to achieve the intended research goals. Quite often researchers are confronted with the choice among models that just reproduce the pharmacological effect of treatments on the expression of a specific but sometimes unconnected symptom, models that reproduce cardinal pathological features of the disorders caused by mechanisms that may not necessarily occur in the patients, versus models that are based on known etiological mechanisms but do not reproduce all clinical features.

Traditionally, animal models of human diseases are selected based on three main attributes: (1) the similarity to the specific symptoms of the human phenomena (i.e., face validity); (2) the similarity in response to pharmacological treatment (i.e., predictive validity); and (3) the degree to which a model supports a mechanistic theory between the human disorder and the model itself (i.e., construct validity). Reliability, on the other hand, requires that the outputs of the model are robust and reproducible between laboratories.

Animal models, in addition to being reliable, should ideally exhibit full validity attributes, but in practice this does not happen and every model has its own attributes that determine the purpose it can serve. Accordingly, the criteria each model fulfills to demonstrate its validity are, for practical purposes, largely determined by the objective of the model and its intended use. In this way, animal models commonly used in screening processes during drug discovery tend to be simple and rely on partial face validity (tendency to be biased due to its focus on one or few specific symptoms) and predictive validity (tendency to be biased based on the positive response to known treatments) as principal features, although they should rely not only on the effectiveness of the compounds belonging to the drug class it is being investigated but, more importantly, on the ineffectiveness of drugs known to be devoid of any therapeutic potential in the disease as well [20]. These predictive validity-based experimental models are useful in exploring the effect of pharmacological treatments on the expression of a specific symptom (that although concurrent with the disease may be of poor clinical relevance or unrelated to the underlying pathophysiology) and are valuable to accomplish the generation of "me-too" compounds, but the discovery of new, first-in-class drugs with groundbreaking mechanisms of action requires enhanced understanding that can be better attained via construct validity, by focusing more on the underlying mechanism of the disease to find new drugs neutralizing that mechanism [20]. Hence, construct validity-based models offer better alternatives for target identification and validation as well as for drug candidate profiling (but not for screening of a large number of compounds as these models are normally costly and time consuming). In turn, care should be taken because construct validity-based models may be dependent upon uncertain etiological assumptions and inferences, which could result in taking wrong compounds into clinical trials, particularly when trying to model complex diseases with poor understanding of their etiology.

Animal models need to be optimally selected and data derived from each need to be interpreted and applied most appropriately and effectively to the drug discovery and decision-making processes. A possible strategy could be to establish a sophisticated, construct validity-based model early on for target validation, using already existing compounds that target the novel mechanism of action or other methods (e.g., RNA interfering and knockout technologies) to get information on the sensitivity and specificity of the model. Once the model has been selected and a significant correlation between *in vitro* activity at the target and *in vivo* activity in the model has been demonstrated, advanced lead compounds arising from the discovery program need be tested in the model. If wisely chosen, the preclinical model can aid the design of the clinical trial needed for human studies. Therefore, animal models closely modeling the clinical pathology, although normally sophisticated and time consuming, can be used to increase the confidence in the functional significance of a target (target validation) and determine later on the pathway for further drug development to facilitate the "win or kill" decision-making process. Especially in cases where the predictive validity of a model is relatively unknown because of the absence of clinically active reference drugs, it is critical to avoid using behavioral assays that have limited construct validity simply because they happen to be faster. Such an approach using rapid predictive validity-based models is, when appropriate, complementary and helpful for screening purposes during the intermediate drug discovery process, but not for target validation (at the very beginning) and preclinical candidate selection (at the end of the discovery process) as they would provide for more rapid but wrong decision making. Furthermore, one should exclude models that lead to false positives (effectiveness of drugs known to be clinically inefficacious) and be innovative but cautious when relying on novel but yet untested models in terms of their translational value and potential for a significant clinical outcome.

Current drugs for treating some diseases are mostly variations on a theme that was started several decades ago. Sadly, clinical efficacy has not improved substantially over the years in some areas probably because both clinical and preclinical researchers have focused too much on a specific symptom, which is only one of the hallmarks of the disease [22]. Many strategies employed in the design of animal experiments began with attempts to detect the effect of serendipitously discovered drugs already in clinics. In a simplistic view, this initial backtranslational pharmacological strategy requires the identification of just one symptom (and not necessarily the most relevant) sensitive to the modulation by both the reference drug and the new "me-too" compounds being developed, and thus heavily relies on face and predictive validities. However, the power of these strategies to predict an effective new treatment is unclear. The complexity of the clinical condition inevitably means that even the best animal models are inadequate representations of the condition they seek to mimic. Therefore, to attempt to model complex human disorders where validity is often limited to superficial similarities (referred to as face validity) that often reflect quite different underlying phenomena from the clinical situation is probably overambitious [11]. More information is needed on disrupted mechanisms underlying the pathology. Uncovering these mechanisms is necessary for these models to significantly advance discovery of new prevention or therapeutic strategies. Along this line of thinking, the predictive power of animal models can be increased by improving our ability to (1) systematically and selectively measure disease-relevant processes in rodent models, (2) identify mechanisms underlying these processes, and (3) model putative etiologic or pathogenic mechanisms that lead to these abnormalities [19].

Numerous studies are still focused on better treatment for the symptoms rather than on the causal mechanisms to prevent the development of the disorder [5]. However, when approaching therapeutic indications where there are still great unmet medical needs, we need to shift the focus from overreliance on predictive validity to the reliance on construct/etiological validity. This is certainly a high-risk/high-benefit approach that needs to be viewed as a much-needed long-term investment in the development of the field of translational research that will eventually increase the success rates. In addition, models with good construct/etiological validity could also be used for further target identification and thus provide additional opportunities for drug discovery [7].

1.2.4
Appropriate Time and Dosing

An indication of the timing and progression of the disease is needed so that the treatment may be applied at the appropriate time/age of the animal. In many cases, the progression of the disease is so rapid in the animal model compared with the clinical condition that the narrow time window for intervention decreases the probability of selecting the optimum time for treatment. Similarly, therapeutic changes exerted by drug treatments can be detected very soon following acute administrations in animals, but require much more time and chronic treatments in patients. It is also not easy to estimate whether the time that a biochemical change takes to translate into a measurable behavioral change in the animal model is similar to the time taken to get a clinically relevant change in patients. However, all this information needs to be obtained from the animal model and compared with those in clinics to select the most appropriate time and duration of treatments.

When drugs are administered to the animal before or at the time of the disease model inductor (either drugs or experimental manipulations such as injury or surgery), data obtained best translate into a preventive therapeutic approach, which is relevant in some conditions when the disorder is expected or scheduled (e.g., prevention of nausea before cancer chemotherapy or pain before surgery). However, for regular "curative" approaches, the effect of drugs (usually restoration of normal baseline values) should be assayed in appropriate animal models once the disease has clearly developed, not at the time or soon before or after the inducing insult. Examining the effect of a compound in young (sometimes healthy) animals rather than in old animals with comorbid conditions is also a dangerous simplification when approaching therapeutic effects commonly affecting elderly people.

Finally, numerous drugs have been developed using an acute response measurement, but they are administered to patients requiring long-term treatment. It seems reasonable that if chronic treatments are required in clinical practice (as it is actually the case in most chronic conditions), subchronic/chronic treatments should be assayed in chronic models of the disease. Tachyphylaxis, desensitization, tolerance, and even addiction phenomena need to be anticipated. The system may also need time to react to the drug–receptor interaction to establish a good pharmacological response, and thus the compound needs to be given repeatedly. This is even clearer when therapeutic effects in patients have been reported following repeated but not acute treatments (e.g., antidepressants). In these cases, preclinical data relying heavily on acute behavioral tests (e.g., forced swimming test for serotonin reuptake inhibitor antidepressants) should only be considered of predictive value for "me-too" compounds based on the previous demonstration of the therapeutic effect of the drug class. Otherwise, this approach could hardly provide valuable information leading to the discovery of new first-in-class drugs.

1.2.5
Use of Biomarkers

The translational value (i.e., predictability) attained using animal models of disorders in which the molecular basis of the disease is better understood and disease biomarkers are known is potentially higher. In particular, when suitable quantitative imaging biomarkers or biochemical biomarkers from easily accessible biofluids (e.g., blood and urine) or tissues are available, the same measures used in experimental animals are feasible in patients. This approach is attractive because it potentially relies on the mechanistic action of the drug, and thus allows decisions to be made on the basis of quantitative data in experimental animals that can be later on confirmed in humans. Unfortunately, reliable biomarkers are not available for many complex diseases with unmet therapeutic needs.

Although the ultimate aim of biomarker investigations is to find biomarkers that will most accurately predict disease outcome, the reality is that it is difficult to extrapolate the findings and most proposed candidate biomarkers are not consistent enough to be considered for measurement in routine practice. In fact, changes in the expression of the proposed biomarker in disease states could reflect compensatory or secondary (not causally related) adaptations, far away from the relevant mechanisms underlying the pathology. It is important to note that a biomarker-based approach is not based on "patient outcomes" (i.e., reduction in clinical symptoms or improvement in quality of life), but rather on "improved" hypothesized biomarkers that may be considered more readily amenable to translational work than functional outcome. Here is the risk. For example, if overexpression of protein X in plasma is known to correlate with the severity of a disease, a drug declining plasma protein X levels in a purported animal model of such disease could encourage further development of the molecule. However, this is not black or white as possible outcomes include confirmation of the biochemical hypothesis but no effect of the drug treatment on the behavioral measures, or alternatively, the behavioral measures improve in response to treatment but protein X expression does not change. Some may argue that behavioral measures are less sensitive because they are not measuring the relevant behavioral symptoms or they are measuring responses unrelated to the actual underlying pathology. Alternatively, behavioral measures may be considered more sensitive and more meaningful than the biochemical parameters because the concentration of protein X poorly reflects the molecular and cellular events in the specific pathway that underlies the behavioral deficits. Furthermore, often unknown is to what degree a biomarker should change to allow for reliable predictions of clinical efficacy [7]. Thus, if possible, measurement of reliable clinically recognized biomarkers, more preferably multiple reliable biomarkers identifying different pathophysiological alterations, and most preferably multiple reliable biomarkers together with (behavioral) measurement of clinically meaningful symptoms, is advised.

1.2.6
Use of Various Animal Models

No single animal model can account for the entire disease syndrome it purports to represent and every model has its strengths and weaknesses that should be taken into consideration for determining its applicability. Therefore, given the heterogeneity and etiological complexity of most diseases, the findings emerging from the combined use of different models may ensure replication of findings, provide insight into the various aspects and etiology of the disorder, and lead to better new treatments. Comparison of these findings might also elucidate genuine therapeutic effects rather than effects limited to a specific model that is not necessarily related to the disease. A full suite of animal behavioral tests allows for a comprehensive assessment of the spectrum of symptoms relevant to the disease. The use of multiple experimental manipulations and experimental designs also allows modeling several different inducing conditions and/or engaging several dependent measures. In addition, moving a compound forward to clinical trials represents a considerable investment that many are reluctant to initiate on the basis of the outcome of a single preclinical experiment, however well designed [7].

However, if the predictions from the animal models are mixed (some positive and some negative), what is the global prediction from the aggregate of the preclinical animal data? A priori decisions regarding how many models would be required to show a convincing positive therapeutic response and acceptance of the path to be taken according to the potential outcome of each model would be most appropriate to support moving forward the molecule. This will avoid the feed-forward loop that tends to move ahead lead compounds based on the keenness for some to not give up even when substantial negative outcomes arise from testing in key animal models [7].

1.2.7
Quantitative, Multiple, and Cross-Predictive Measurements

Qualitative assessments of behavior are often subjective. This would lead the investigator to observe what they want to observe, and to render conclusions in line with their expectations. It is thus clear that quantitative assessments based on objective measurements should replace qualitative scores when possible. When not possible, independent assessment by different individuals is required.

It is also clear that multiple readouts are better than single readouts. The use of a multifactorial approach employing several dependent measures, such as imaging, electrophysiological recordings, biochemical and/or neurochemical measurements, and immunohistochemistry, along with different behavioral measures invariably results in an enrichment of the data coming from animal models. A high degree of coherence between multiple dependent variables lends support to the hypothesis, either by indicating the involvement or recruitment of the pathway hypothesized to underlie the disorder or by better defining the active dose range [7].

The predictions from the animal models on the human condition can be only as good as the correspondence between the measures in humans and those in experimental animals. Thus, it is always preferable if the parameter analyzed can be readily measurable in both animals and humans. Identical measures in humans and experimental animals are likely to be analogous or even homologous (in the sense of being mediated by the same substrates) and thus greatly facilitate translation [7]. In particular, if testing approaches applied in human research studies are chosen, measures can have clear conceptual and methodological links to tasks currently in use for nonhuman animal studies and thus have the potential for translation to animal research [23]. Such measures are highly desirable and cross-predictive, but unfortunately not always feasible to design and assess in one or the other population (i.e., experimental animals, healthy human volunteers, and patients). As a caveat, such homologous measures do not necessarily represent clinical trial endpoints as defined in guidelines by health authorities, which adds another level of complexity. In many cases, one may be limited to analogous measures assessing the same/similar process in both experimental animals and humans. Accordingly, current animal models may be very predictive of specific measures and constructs in humans, but unfortunately such measures are not what are currently assessed in the various phases of most clinical trials [7].

An appealing strategy is thus to design tests in animal models as close as possible to those used in humans or, alternatively, to develop human tests more "rodent-like." Not only should the disease or injury itself reflect the condition in humans as much as possible, but age, sex, and comorbidities should also be modeled where possible. The investigators should justify their selection of the model and outcome measures. In turn, human clinical trials should be designed to replicate, as far as possible, the circumstances under which efficacy has been observed in animals [15]. However, it would be unrealistic to expect that animal model tests could be totally aligned to human ones because of dissimilarities between species, differences regarding feasibility and practicability (some measures do not represent clinical endpoints as defined in guidelines by health authorities or are unviable in humans, whereas others rely on elaborated responses that cannot be measured in animals).

1.2.8
Pharmacokinetic–Pharmacodynamic Integration

Pharmacokinetic–pharmacodynamic (PK–PD) integration in pharmacology research is fundamental to improve interpretation of data coming from animal models for different purposes, including target validation or optimizing the development of lead compounds, and has become mandatory for regulatory bodies. The concentration–effect relationship is necessary for translational purposes [24] and it is central to drug discovery in the pharmaceutical industry, but PK–PD integration is still comparatively rare in experimental pharmacology practiced in academic laboratories (in part because drug analysis techniques are not widely available to academic scientists). Its absence diminishes the interpretative value of published experimental data and can allow the presentation of misleading information and inaccurate extrapolation to clinical use [25].

PK–PD integration, also called quantitative pharmacology, focuses on concentration–response and time–response relationships based on drug exposure measurements (drug concentrations in plasma or other compartments such as tissues or organs proposed as the site of action for the drug), plasma protein binding (unbound fraction available for target engagement), exposure–effect relationships (correlation between the time course of the effect and drug exposure), and the measurement of active metabolites. This will provide valuable information to extrapolate to clinical use: plasma levels needed to get a significant therapeutic response (e.g., 80% of effect) and levels that, when exceeded, correlate with the occurrence of adverse effects. If the effect is mediated by an active metabolite, the effect could be delayed with respect to that expected based on the exposure to the parent compound. If this is the case, is the metabolite acting through the same mechanism as the parent compound or through a different, perhaps known, failed mechanism of action? If the pharmacological effect at the same dose is increased in subchronic/chronic versus acute treatment, is the increased effect achieved following repeated administrations due to drug accumulation (pharmacokinetic effect) or does it actually reflect a pharmacodynamic, disease-modifying effect? PK–PD integration can answer these relevant questions. Similarly, toxicokinetic (TK) information can substantially enhance the value of the data generated from toxicity testing. Use of TK information can help to ensure that studies are designed to be of most relevance to assessing potential risk in humans, and avoid the use of excessively high doses that could result in unnecessary suffering in experimental animals [26].

Target engagement is a conglomerate of the compound dose size, systemic exposure to the compound (pharmacokinetics), interaction with the target (affinity and efficacy, pharmacology), and physiological (system) reaction to the target–drug interaction. In fact, a compound may have excellent target binding affinity, but fails to engage its target due to low bioavailability or being cleared rapidly from plasma [25]. It can also be present at outstanding levels, but mostly bound to extracellular matrix proteins or fatty compartments and thus not available to interact with its intended molecular target. To get additional information, receptor occupancy studies (e.g., *ex vivo* binding experiments) can be done to assess the actual engagement of the molecular target onto which the drug supposedly binds and correlate it with the pharmacological effect exerted by the drug [27]. Imagine that 50% of maximum possible efficacy is attained when 100% of receptors are occupied by a drug with full intrinsic functionality. In this case, increasing the dose would not result in higher efficacy (but would probably increase adverse effects), and data could be better interpreted in the sense that engaging solely the selected molecular target by a high-affinity selective drug is not enough to achieve a relevant therapeutic effect.

1.2.9
Predefinition and Adherence to the Desired Product Profile

To ensure that any drug discovery project is addressing the requirements of the patients and health care providers and delivering a benefit over existing therapies, the ideal attributes of a novel drug need to be predefined by a set of criteria called a target product profile [28]. The target product profile is an important strategic planning and decision-making tool that is used to define essential attributes required for a specific drug to be clinically successful and of substantial benefit over existing therapies. The desired profile of a pharmaceutical product is thus a list of key features such as desired mechanism of action (i.e., molecular target and mechanism), efficacy (i.e., acceptable levels of efficacy), therapeutic indications (i.e., target patient population), safety (i.e., acceptable levels of safety), advantages respect to competitors, route of administration and dosing schedule, metabolism, and pharmacokinetics.

The descriptions of the animal models that are to be used in the selection of drug candidates are not necessarily included in the product profile, but efficacy and safety data supporting the attainment of the desired predefined attributes are expected to be obtained in appropriate models of the targeted disease. It is thus important to keep focusing throughout the drug discovery process on the selection of the appropriate models and experimental designs that better translate to the clinic and better inform about the attainment (or not) of the desired predefined attributes, and rely on the data obtained in such key experiments to substantiate strategic go/no-go decisions. In other words, the target (desired profile) must be drawn first and then arrows (compounds) must be fired to try to reach the objective. Alternatively, the arrow is first fired and then the target is drawn around (Figure 1.1). This makes much easier the "attainment of the objective," but the success when moving the compound forward... This is something different (although it can provide interesting opportunities if unintended positive results are obtained by "chance" with a compound).

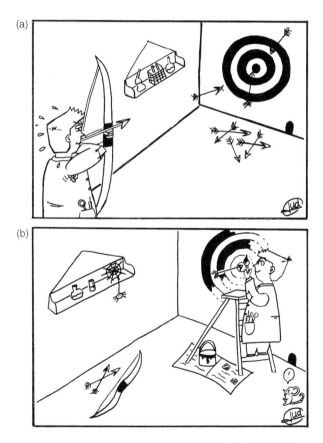

Figure 1.1 Target-driven versus arrow-driven approach for drug discovery. In the target-driven approach (a), the target (desired profile) is drawn first and then arrows (compounds) are fired to try to reach the objective. Alternatively, in the arrow-driven approach (b), the arrow is first fired and then the target is drawn around.

1.2.10
Comparison with Gold Standard References

Competitive advantages of new drugs with respect to existing ones are required (and they should be predefined as key attributes in the target product profile). Animal models allow direct face-to-face comparison of the pharmacological effects of the drug being investigated with a standard best-in-class reference drug, referred to as the "gold standard." The gold standard is often a currently used medication for the targeted disorder that is perceived as being the best, or one of the best, treatment. In the absence of a marketed drug, the gold standard may be a drug acting on the same or different mechanism that has shown efficacy in human studies or is under active preclinical development by competitors for the same therapeutic indication. Differentiation with respect to the reference compound(s) can be attained not only based on improved efficacy and/or better safety profile, but also based on other attributes such as a more convenient route of administration (i.e., oral versus intravenous), dosing (i.e., once a day versus three times a day), faster onset of action, and other differences and innovative features that could be perceived as advantages for patients, physicians, or payers in the context of the particular disease [7].

1.2.11
Reverse Translation/Backtranslation (Bedside-to-Bench Approach)

There is usually a disconnection between the preclinical and clinical teams during drug development, but increasing their interactions and establishing better communication are the best ways to improve translational research. Discussion between preclinical and clinical scientists to improve consistency in preclinical and clinical study designs (e.g., methods, instruments, study groups, study duration, endpoints, and statistical analysis) is highly recommended [10].

In most cases, information flow is unidirectional. The drug discovery workflow is often a progression from *in vitro* to *in vivo* and from preclinical to clinical, with flow of animal data to the clinical domain but not vice versa. Conversely, the product profile is defined primarily clinically and commercially and is provided to guide preclinical research, but no significant preclinical/clinical cross-validation and crosstalk between both disciplines occur. Such a unidirectional flow does not allow maximizing the contribution of animal model data to the process and prevents for any pragmatic and rational modification of animal models to avoid false negatives and positives [7,29].

Emphasis is placed on the need to improve the flow of information from the clinical/human domain to the preclinical domain and the benefits of using truly translational measures in both preclinical and clinical testing. This strategy takes research from bedside to bench, focusing on results from clinical trials to stimulate basic scientific investigation [30]. Traditionally, animal models of human phenomena have been evaluated based on similarity to the human syndrome, response to appropriately corresponding medications, and the degree to which a model supports a common mechanistic theory between the human disorder and the model itself. The "reverse translation" approach relies on patient-based findings to develop suitable animal models, emphasizing their construct validity as a starting point [31]. For example, an individual case report or a small case series in which the clinician notes an unexpected positive response to a drug used for another purpose can be employed to find new therapies. Such bedside-to-bench observations in human disease can help focus the direction of animal research, which in turn will improve the translational process because they are already known to be associated with a clinical endpoint [32]. As focusing on complex clinical phenotypes may be ineffective for the development of novel and effective treatments, new approaches have also been proposed in the form of reverse translation, which include identification and characterization of intermediate phenotypes reflecting defined, although limited, aspects of the human clinical disorder and thereby develop animal models homologous to those discrete human behavioral phenotypes in terms of psychological processes and underlying neurobiological mechanisms [11,33]. All these approaches deserve attention, although the current emphasis on specific dimensions of pathology that can be objectively assessed in both clinical populations and animal models has not yet provided significant successful preclinical–clinical translation in drug discovery [7,34].

1.3
Third N: The Need for 3Rs Guiding Principles

In 1959, the report by Russell and Burch was published as *The Principles of Humane Experimental Techniques*, the basic tenet of their report being that the humanest possible treatment of experimental animals, far from being an obstacle, is actually a prerequisite for a successful animal experiment [35]. The authors proposed the principles of replacement, reduction, and refinement (most often referred to as the 3Rs) as the key strategies to provide a systematic framework to achieve the goal of humane experimental techniques. Today, the principles of the 3Rs are embedded in legislation that governs the use of animals in science across the world.

Replacement as one of the 3Rs is defined as the substitution of conscious living higher animals by "insentient" material. There are a number of alternative methods that can be proposed to replace the use of live animals in either all or part of a project. Replacement can be absolute (techniques that do not involve animals at any point, such as computer modeling, *in vitro* methodologies, or use of human volunteers) or relative (animals are still required to provide cells or tissue, but experiments are conducted *in vitro* using tissue cultures, perfused organs, tissue slices, and cellular or subcellular fractions; alternatively, "phylogenetic reduction" can be applied using other species such as invertebrates or larval forms of amphibians and fish). These methods are well suited and can be cost effective and time saving. They can not only replace but also provide a level of knowledge that complements studies in whole animals.

The goal of reduction, the second of the 3Rs, is to reduce the number of animals used to obtain information of a given amount and precision. It includes methods that minimize animal use and enable researchers to obtain comparable levels of information from fewer animals, or to obtain more information from the same number of animals, thereby reducing future use of animals. Examples could include improved experimental design and statistical analysis, data and resource sharing, and the use of techniques such as imaging. To achieve this, designed studies need to be scientifically and statistically valid with only the minimum number of animals used and not unnecessarily repeated. In fact, improvement of the models to increase their predictive value ultimately results in a reduction of the number of animals and tests needed to reveal the effect. The principle of reduction of number of animals should not be applied at the expense of greater suffering to individual animals and the number of animals used must satisfy statistical requirements (neither too few nor too many). The reductionist approach has been encouraged by the explosion of the genomic and proteomic technologies that opened up new areas of discoveries in biomedical research. The development of early screening *in vitro* techniques, high-content analyses, novel imaging, and analytical techniques has reduced the number of animals that are necessary for an experiment, while simultaneously providing higher quality data. In addition, entirely computerized strategies that use sophisticated algorithms to simulate biology without needing animals at all are being developed.

The third of the 3Rs, refinement, is any decrease in the incidence or severity of "inhumane" procedures applied to those animals that still have to be used. It includes improvements in scientific procedures and husbandry that minimize actual or potential pain, suffering, distress, or lasting harm and/or improve animal welfare in situations where the use of animals is unavoidable. There are two key issues: to assess the impact of any procedure or condition on the well-being of the animal and strategies to decrease invasiveness or eliminate or minimize that impact. Strategies to achieve the goal of refinement often need to be customized to a specific set of circumstances. Examples could include reducing stress by developing new approaches such as training animals, use of noninvasive techniques, or enrichments that improve living conditions. With increasing knowledge and experience, a number of useful guidelines have been developed to assist in minimizing the impact of particular procedures and practices. Refinement is applied to all aspects, including housing, husbandry, and care, techniques used in scientific procedures, periprocedural care, health and welfare monitoring, and experimental design [36]. However, although care is taken to prevent unnecessary suffering in animal experiments, suffering is an inherent aspect of modeling some distressful conditions (e.g., anxiety, depression, posttraumatic stress disorder, and pain), which represent an extra challenge.

This is an area where knowledge is rapidly expanding and collaboration is important to speed up the goals. For example, a European initiative including 18 companies undertook an evidence-based review of acute toxicity studies, where lethality was mentioned as an endpoint in regulatory guidelines, and assessed the value of the data generated. The conclusion of the working group was that acute toxicity studies (the so-called LD$_{50}$ test) are not needed prior to first clinical trials in humans. Instead, information can be obtained from other studies, which are performed at more relevant doses for humans and are already an integral part of drug development. The conclusions were discussed and agreed with representatives of regulatory bodies from the United States, Japan, and Europe, and acceptance of the recommendations effectively led to "replacement" of acute studies in guidelines [37].

These matters are expertly reviewed in different excellent review articles [16,38–48] and a number of web pages (e.g., http://www.ccac.ca/en_/education/niaut/stream/cs-3rs, www.animalethics.org.au/three-rs, http://awic.nal.usda.gov/alternatives/3rs, www.nc3rs.org.uk/page.asp?id=7, www.felasa.eu/recommendations, http://www.forschung3r.ch/en/links/, and http://3rs.ccac.ca/en/about/).

Conducting the 3Rs search is not always easy. Alternative methods are not necessarily covered in the mainstream literature, and methods that may well be relevant to one or more of the 3Rs are not always identified as such. In addition, appropriate keywords may not be used. For these reasons, specialized 3Rs-related databases (visit ecvam-dbalm.jrc.ec.europa.eu/ and www.nc3rs.org.uk/category.asp?catID=3) can be useful to allow a researcher to search in a more focused manner for specific alternative methods (e.g., *in vitro* methods that may replace the use of animals in a given protocol; appropriate anesthesia and/or analgesia to help minimize pain and distress; environmental enrichment techniques; models, simulators, computerized mannequins, and other alternatives to the use of animals for education and training purposes).

The implementation of the 3Rs in biomedical research was analyzed in 14 major biomedical journals between 1970 and 2000. During this period, the total number of articles published annually by the journals more than doubled, but the proportion of studies using animals decreased by 30%. There was also a significant increase in the proportion of animal studies using untreated euthanized animals as donors of biological materials, a gradual decrease in the number of chronic studies, and a 50% decrease in the average number of animals used per published paper. There was an improvement in the reporting of the specification of the animals' husbandry, conditions of care, and environment. Parameters of importance for the evaluation of welfare of the animals were generally poorly reported, but the proportion of papers with adequate information on most of the parameters analyzed increased between 1970 and 2000 [49]. In fact, there are many initiatives that aim to replace, reduce, or refine laboratory animal use. Such efforts are supported by academia, industry, and regulatory authorities, although there is the perception that the implementation of the 3Rs in animal research has not increased as expected [50–52].

It is now more than 25 years since both Council of Europe Convention ETS123 and EU Directive 86/609/EEC (now replaced by Directive 2010/63/EU, with effect from January 1, 2013) on the protection of animals used for scientific purposes were introduced to promote the implementation of the 3Rs in animal experimentation and to provide guidance on animal housing and care. However, full implementation of this legislation depends upon scientists' ability to understand animal welfare issues and to accept the legitimacy of the public's interest in the conduct of science. Education and training of those involved in research and testing is fundamental, and a number of guidelines from different sources including the Federation of European Laboratory Animal Science Associations (FELASA) and the US National Research Council could serve as prototype teaching material. In fact, humane science is good science and this is best achieved by vigorous application of the 3Rs. Animal experiments using the smallest number of animals and causing the least possible pain or distress are consistent with the achievement of a justifiable scientific purpose, and alternative testing methods can have advantages over traditional animal tests, although implementing an alternative from idea to acceptance can take years.

Communication is required between stakeholders, such as regulatory authorities, industry, and academia, about 3R developments and the chances they offer. Sharing test data will help to build up experience with the specific 3R models and facilitate the process of building new experiences, rules, practices, and routines. For example, sharing data and reviewing study designs of pharmaceutical companies and contract research organizations in the United Kingdom have allowed the identification of opportunities to minimize animal use in regulatory toxicology studies [53]. At the end, such a multitude of relatively small steps can lead to a landslide in favor of the 3Rs [50].

References

1 European Commission (2010) Sixth Report on the Statistics on the Number of Animals Used for Experimental and Other Scientific Purposes in the Member States of the European Union. Report from the Commission to the Council and the European Parliament. COM (2010) 511, SEC (2010) 1107 final/2. Brussels, 8.12.2010.

2 Frey, R.G. (2001) Justifying animal experimentation: the starting point, in *Why Animal Experimentation Matters: The Use of Animals in Medical Research* (eds E.F. Paul and J. Paul), Transaction Publishers, New Brunswick, NJ, pp. 197–214.

3 Franco, N.H. (2013) Animal experiments in biomedical research: a historical perspective. *Animals*, 3, 238–273.

4 Food and Drug Administration (2004) Innovation or Stagnation: Challenge and Opportunity on the Critical Path to New Medical Products. US Food and Drug Administration.

5 Green, A.R., Gabrielsson, J., and Fone, K.C. (2011) Translational neuropharmacology and the appropriate and effective use of animal models. *British Journal of Pharmacology*, 164 (4), 1041–1043.

6 Prabhakar, S. (2012) Translational research challenges: finding the right animal models. *Journal of Investigative Medicine*, 60 (8), 1141–1146.

7 Markou, A., Chiamulera, C., Geyer, M.A., Tricklebank, M., and Steckler, T. (2009) Removing obstacles in neuroscience drug discovery: the future path for animal models. *Neuropsychopharmacology*, 34 (1), 74–89.

8 Kola, I. and Landis, J. (2004) Can the pharmaceutical industry reduce attrition rates? *Nature Reviews. Drug Discovery*, 3 (8), 711–715.

9 Horrobin, D.F. (2003) Modern biomedical research: an internally self-consistent universe with little contact with medical reality? *Nature Reviews. Drug Discovery*, 2 (2), 151–154.

10 Ergorul, C. and Levin, L.A. (2013) Solving the lost in translation problem: improving the effectiveness of translational research.

Current Opinion in Pharmacology, **13** (1), 108–114.

11 Stephens, D.N., Crombag, H.S., and Duka, T. (2013) The challenge of studying parallel behaviors in humans and animal models. *Current Topics in Behavioral Neurosciences*, **13**, 611–645.

12 Percie du Sert, N. (2011) Systematic review and meta-analysis of pre-clinical research: the need for reporting guidelines. *European Heart Journal*, **32** (19), 2340.

13 Marklund, N. and Hillered, L. (2011) Animal modelling of traumatic brain injury in preclinical drug development: where do we go from here? *British Journal of Pharmacology*, **164** (4), 1207–1229.

14 Becker, R.E. and Greig, N.H. (2010) Lost in translation: neuropsychiatric drug development. *Science Translational Medicine*, **2** (61), 61rv6.

15 van der Worp, H.B., Howells, D.W., Sena, E.S., Porritt, M.J., Rewell, S., O'Collins, V., and MacLeod, M.R. (2010) Can animal models of disease reliably inform human studies? *PLoS Medicine*, **7** (3), e1000245.

16 Baumans, V. (2004) Use of animals in experimental research: an ethical dilemma? *Gene Therapy*, **11** (Suppl. 1), S64–S66.

17 Fehlings, M.G. and Vawda, R. (2011) Cellular treatments for spinal cord injury: the time is right for clinical trials. *Neurotherapeutics*, **8** (4), 704–720.

18 Germann, P.G., Schuhmacher, A., Harrison, J., Law, R., Haug, K., and Wong, G. (2013) How to create innovation by building the translation bridge from basic research into medicinal drugs: an industrial perspective. *Human Genomics*, **7**, 5.

19 Moore, H. (2010) The role of rodent models in the discovery of new treatments for schizophrenia: updating our strategy. *Schizophrenia Bulletin*, **36** (6), 1066–1072.

20 Fineberg, N.A., Chamberlain, S.R., Hollander, E., Boulougouris, V., and Robbins, T.W. (2011) Translational approaches to obsessive-compulsive disorder: from animal models to clinical treatment. *British Journal of Pharmacology*, **164** (4), 1044–1061.

21 Percie du Sert, N. (2011) Improving the reporting of animal research: when will we ARRIVE? *Disease Models & Mechanisms*, **4** (3), 281–282.

22 Geyer, M.A., Olivier, B., Joëls, M., and Kahn, R.S. (2012) From antipsychotic to anti-schizophrenia drugs: role of animal models. *Trends in Pharmacological Sciences*, **33** (10), 515–521.

23 Alexander, G.E., Ryan, L., Bowers, D., Foster, T.C., Bizon, J.L., Geldmacher, D.S., and Glisky, E.L. (2012) Characterizing cognitive aging in humans with links to animal models. *Frontiers in Aging Neuroscience*, **4**, 21.

24 Taneja, A., Di Iorio, V.L., Danhof, M., and Della Pasqua, O. (2012) Translation of drug effects from experimental models of neuropathic pain and analgesia to humans. *Drug Discovery Today*, **17** (15–16), 837–849.

25 Gabrielsson, J. and Green, A.R. (2009) Quantitative pharmacology or pharmacokinetic pharmacodynamic integration should be a vital component in integrative pharmacology. *The Journal of Pharmacology and Experimental Therapeutics*, **331** (3), 767–774.

26 Creton, S., Saghir, S.A., Bartels, M.J., Billington, R., Bus, J.S., Davies, W., Dent, M.P., Hawksworth, G.M., Parry, S., and Travis, K.Z. (2012) Use of toxicokinetics to support chemical evaluation: informing high dose selection and study interpretation. *Regulatory Toxicology and Pharmacology*, **62** (2), 241–247.

27 Romero, L., Zamanillo, D., Nadal, X., Sánchez-Arroyos, R., Rivera-Arconada, I., Dordal, A., Montero, A., Muro, A., Bura, A., Segalés, C., Laloya, M., Hernández, E., Portillo-Salido, E., Escriche, M., Codony, X., Encina, G., Burgueño, J., Merlos, M., Baeyens, J.M., Giraldo, J., López-García, J.A., Maldonado, R., Plata-Salamán, C.R., and Vela, J.M. (2012) Pharmacological properties of S1RA, a new sigma-1 receptor antagonist that inhibits neuropathic pain and activity-induced spinal sensitization. *British Journal of Pharmacology*, **166** (8), 2289–2306.

28 Wyatt, P.G., Gilbert, I.H., Read, K.D., and Fairlamb, A.H. (2011) Target validation: linking target and chemical properties to desired product profile. *Current Topics in Medicinal Chemistry*, **11** (10), 1275–1283.

29 Mullane, K. (2011) The increasing challenge of discovering asthma drugs. *Biochemical Pharmacology*, **82** (6), 586–599.

30 Ledford, H. (2008) Translational research: the full cycle. *Nature*, **453**, 843–845.

31 Young, J.W., Minassian, A., Paulus, M.P., Geyer, M.A., and Perry, W. (2007) A reverse-translational approach to bipolar disorder: rodent and human studies in the Behavioral Pattern Monitor. *Neuroscience and Biobehavioral Reviews*, **31** (6), 882–896.

32 Levin, L.A. and Bressler, N. (1996) The case report. When small is beautiful. *Archives of Ophthalmology*, **114** (11), 1413.

33 Bradesi, S. and Mayer, E.A. (2009) Experimental models of stress and pain: do they help to develop new therapies? *Digestive Diseases (Basel, Switzerland)*, **27** (Suppl. 1), 55–67.

34 Savonenko, A.V., Melnikova, T., Hiatt, A., Li, T., Worley, P.F., Troncoso, J.C., Wong, P.C., and Price, D.L. (2012) Alzheimer's therapeutics: translation of preclinical science to clinical drug development. *Neuropsychopharmacology*, **37** (1), 261–277.

35 Russell, W.M.S. and Burch, R.L. (eds) (1959) *The Principles of Humane Experimental Technique*, Methuen, London.

36 Buchanan-Smith, H., Rennie, A., Vitale, A., Pollo, S., Prescott, M.J., and Morton, D. (2005) Harmonising the definition of refinement. *Animal Welfare*, **14**, 379–384.

37 Robinson, S., Delongeas, J.L., Donald, E., Dreher, D., Festag, M., Kervyn, S., Lampo, A., Nahas, K., Nogues, V., Ockert, D., Quinn, K., Old, S., Pickersgill, N., Somers, K., Stark, C., Stei, P., Waterson, L., and Chapman, K. (2008) A European pharmaceutical company initiative challenging the regulatory requirement for acute toxicity studies in pharmaceutical drug development. *Regulatory Toxicology and Pharmacology*, **50** (3), 345–352.

38 Zurlo, J., Rudacille, D., and Goldberg, A.M. (1996) The three Rs: the way forward. *Environmental Health Perspectives*, **104** (8), 878–880.

39 Hooijmans, C.R., Leenaars, M., and Ritskes-Hoitinga, M. (2010) A gold standard publication checklist to improve the quality of animal studies, to fully integrate the Three Rs, and to make systematic reviews more feasible. *Alternatives to Laboratory Animals*, **38** (2), 167–182.

40 Balls, M. and Straughan, D.W. (1996) The three Rs of Russell & Burch and the testing of biological products. *Developments in Biological Standardization*, **86**, 11–18.

41 Rowan, A.N. (1980) The concept of the three R's. An introduction. *Developments in Biological Standardization*, **45**, 175–180.

42 Weihe, W.H. (1985) Use and misuse of an imprecise concept: alternative methods in animal experiments. *Laboratory Animals*, **19** (1), 19–26.

43 Orlans, F.B. (1987) Review of experimental protocols: classifying animal harm and applying "refinements". *Laboratory Animal Science*, **37**, 50–56.

44 Bulger, R.E. (1987) Use of animals in experimental research: a scientist's perspective. *The Anatomical Record*, **219** (3), 215–220.

45 Balls, M. and Halder, M. (2002) Progress in applying the three Rs of Russell & Burch to the testing of biological products. *Developments in Biologicals*, **111**, 3–13.

46 Schuppli, C.A., Fraser, D., and McDonald, M. (2004) Expanding the three Rs to meet new challenges in humane animal experimentation. *Alternatives to Laboratory Animals*, **32** (5), 525–532.

47 Baumans, V. (2005) Science-based assessment of animal welfare: laboratory animals. *Revue Scientifique et Technique*, **24** (2), 503–513.

48 Lloyd, M.H., Foden, B.W., and Wolfensohn, S.E. (2008) Refinement: promoting the three Rs in practice. *Laboratory Animals*, **42** (3), 284–293.

49 Carlsson, H.E., Hagelin, J., and Hau, J. (2004) Implementation of the "three Rs" in biomedical research. *The Veterinary Record*, **154** (15), 467–470.

50 Schiffelers, M.J., Blaauboer, B.J., Hendriksen, C.F., and Bakker, W.E. (2012) Regulatory acceptance and use of 3R models: a multilevel perspective. *ALTEX*, **29** (3), 287–300.

51 Obora, S. and Kurosawa, T. (2009) Implementation of the Three Rs in biomedical research: has the turn of the century turned the tide? *Alternatives to Laboratory Animals*, **37** (2), 197–207.

52 Taylor, K. (2010) Reporting the implementation of the Three Rs in European primate and mouse research papers: are we making progress?

Alternatives to Laboratory Animals, **38** (6), 495–517.

53 Sparrow, S.S., Robinson, S., Bolam, S., Bruce, C., Danks, A., Everett, D., Fulcher, S., Hill, R.E., Palmer, H., Scout, E.W., and Chapman, K.L. (2011) Opportunities to minimise animal use in pharmaceutical regulatory general toxicology: a cross-company review. *Regulatory Toxicology and Pharmacology*, **61** (2), 222–229.

2
Alternative Models in Drug Discovery and Development Part I: *In Silico* and *In Vitro* Models

Luz Romero and José Miguel Vela

2.1
Introduction

"The use of animals in medical research and safety testing is a vital part of the quest to improve human health (. . .) Without animal testing, there will be no new drugs for new or hard-to-treat diseases"

[1].

Experiments on animals have been carried out for nearly 2000 years and their use has enabled researchers to make significant advances in many areas of human health and disease (Figure 2.1). Today, animals are used in research and testing for a wide range of purposes. The major uses in the European Union in 2008 were in fundamental biology studies (38.1%) and drug research and development for human and veterinary medicine (22.8%), whereas about 40% of the animals were used for other purposes such as production and quality control of products and devices for human and veterinary medicine, toxicological and other safety evaluation, diagnostics, and education and training (Figure 2.2). Rodents together with rabbits represent more than 80% of the total number of animals used in the European Union. Mice are by far the most commonly used species accounting for 59.3% of the total use, followed by rats with 17.7% [2].

A fundamental of drug discovery and development is the provision of safe and effective medicines. The safety and efficacy of a drug can only be demonstrated through large-scale trials in humans. However, legal and regulatory guidelines involve a plethora of preclinical studies (including experiments in nonhuman animals) to be conducted prior to clinical trials, so that all reasonable steps are taken to mitigate risk to human trial participants. Drug developers also need to provide evidence of the effectiveness of the drug for treating human disease. Scientists have therefore developed nonhuman models that can help in predicting how patients will respond to a drug.

In Vivo Models for Drug Discovery, First Edition. Edited by José M. Vela, Rafael Maldonado, and Michel Hamon.
© 2014 Wiley-VCH Verlag GmbH & Co. KGaA. Published 2014 by Wiley-VCH Verlag GmbH & Co. KGaA.

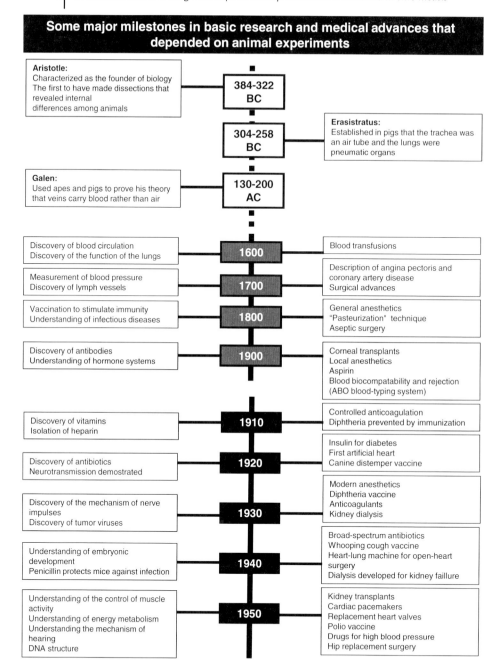

Figure 2.1 Basic research and medical advances: summary timeline.

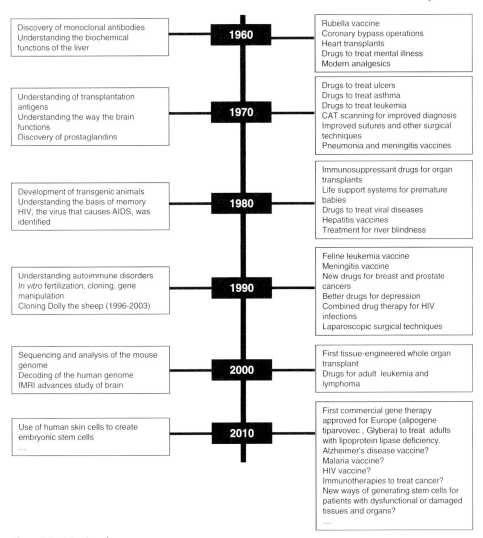

Figure 2.1 (Continued)

The selection of the appropriate animal model is one of the most important steps in the different experimental phases of the drug discovery and preclinical development process. The complex biology of a whole living organism cannot be recreated in a Petri dish, so animals are used to understand how a drug works *in vivo*. Animal models in many cases are excellent models, but they are just models and thus have limitations, particularly when trying to translate to human efficacy and safety data coming from animal studies. These limitations have been acknowledged as a major challenge and a bottleneck in the discovery and development of efficacious and safe therapeutics for some pathologies.

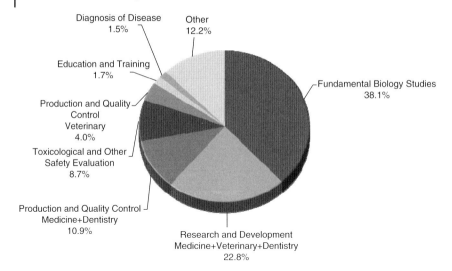

Figure 2.2 Animal usage: purposes of the experiments. Results of the consolidated data of the purposes of the procedures carried out in the 27 member states of the European Union in 2008 [2].

Animals have been used extensively in preclinical testing since laws were passed (e.g., the United States Federal Food, Drug, and Cosmetic Act, 1938) requiring their use in the safety assessment of drugs prior to market approval. Indeed, the use of animals in drug toxicity assessment has played a crucial role in preventing unsafe drugs from entering the market. However, it has been found that many substances that are safe and effective in animal studies are of limited therapeutic benefit or are even toxic in humans. In spite of the rigorous preclinical checks that a drug needs to pass before it can enter in clinical phases, there is a high percentage of attrition during development and withdrawal from the sale, cardiovascular system, hepatotoxicity, and nervous system being the most frequent causes of attrition or withdrawal (Table 2.1). A study in 2002 showed that of the 548 drugs (new chemical entities) approved in the United States between 1975 and 1999, 56 (10.2%) drugs required a black box warning or were withdrawn (45 drugs (8.2%) received one or more black box warnings and 16 (2.9%) were withdrawn from the market) [7]. The United Nations has published a consolidated list of products whose consumption and/or sale have been banned, withdrawn, severely restricted, or not approved by governments. From this list, only about 19% of drugs have been banned worldwide, as there are a number of drugs that have been banned in some countries but are available on the market elsewhere [8]. Examples of drugs that have been withdrawn are troglitazone (Rezulin) and rofecoxib (Vioxx), which were removed from the market in 2000 and 2004, respectively. Both drugs passed through rigorous preclinical checks before their association with elevated risk of liver toxicity and myocardial infarction, respectively, in humans was

Table 2.1 Biological causes of attrition in drug R&D.

Phase	Preclinical	Phases I–III	Postmarketing
Information	Causes of attrition	Causes of attrition	Withdrawal from sale
Source	[3]	[4]	[5]
Sample size	88 CDs stopped	82 CDs stopped	47 drugs
Cardiovascular system	27%	21%	45%
Hepatotoxicity	8%	21%	32%
Hematology	7%	4%	9%
Nervous system	14%	21%	2%
Immunotox; photosensitivity	7%	11%	2%
Gastrointestinal system	3%	5%	2%
Musculoskeletal system	4%	1%	2%
Reprotoxicity	13%	1%	2%
Respiratory system	2%	0%	2%
Renal system	2%	9%	0%
Carcinogenicity	3%	0%	0%
Genetic toxicity	5%	0%	0%
Others	0%	4%	2%

The various toxicity domains have been ranked first by contribution to products withdrawn from sale and then by attrition during clinical development. CDs, compounds. Adapted from Ref. [6].

established [9,10]. The converse of this – substances that are safe and effective in humans but ineffective or toxic in animals – is also true. One clear example is the antibiotic drug penicillin, one of the most important medical discoveries of the twentieth century, that might have never reached the market had it been put through modern preclinical testing because penicillin is ineffective in rabbits and toxic in guinea pigs and hamsters [11].

Limited concordance of the toxicity and efficacy of drugs in humans and animals has contributed to declining productivity in the pharmaceutical industry, and the withdrawal of several approved medications from the market. The questionable scientific value of certain animal experiments, costs associated with animal experimentation, ethical concerns, legislative changes preventing animal tests, education of researchers in the 3Rs (reduction, refinement, and replacement), and the current economic climate have all contributed to a decline in the use of animals in testing and are driving researchers to look for and develop alternative nonanimal research tools. At present, these alternatives cannot replace animals completely as they are unlikely to provide enough information about the complex interactions of living systems. However, technological advances in tissue engineering, "omics" approaches, and *in silico* modeling, for example, are enabling scientists to conduct their research without using animals (or significantly reducing their use) in a broad range of disciplines. The development of alternative empirical (testing) and nonempirical (nontesting) methods to traditional animal testing methods for complex human health effects is a tremendous task. There are possibilities to streamline this process, for example, by sharing cross-company experiences so that the predictive assays that merit further validation as well as those that should be dropped may be identified more readily. Such an experience sharing initiative may also identify gaps for future research investment. Additional information may be gained by learning how failed compounds behaved in *in vitro* or other alternative tests, and through identification of the precise mechanisms that underpinned those failures (so that they can be targeted and avoided in the future). In this way, various initiatives aimed at improving pharmaceutical development, including the US Food and Drug Administration's paper on "Innovation/Stagnation: Challenge and Opportunity on the Critical Path to New Medical Products" [12] and the European Commission and Pharmaceutical Industry partnership, the "Innovative Medicines Initiative" [13], have incorporated the need for alternatives to *in vivo* studies. The International Cooperation on Alternative Test Methods (ICATM) also aims to support more rapid acceptance of new methods and may serve as a resource for validation.

There are multiple drivers for the development of new approaches to replace animal bioassay testing. Position papers in Europe and the United States, legislation for the testing of chemicals and cosmetics, and establishment of validation centers for alternative test methods illustrate the interest in this area of the international community of scientists from academia, pharmaceutical companies and contract research organizations, and regulators and government agencies. New cell and tissue tests, computer models, and other sophisticated methods aiming to replace existing animal tests are continuously being developed. When an alternative method is proposed, it must undergo an internationally recognized validation process before being officially approved as a valid method for safety/toxicology assessment of new chemicals. This procedure is complicated as full regulatory establishment and adoption of a new method typically takes 8–9 years. The alternative methods developed are first put to comparative tests in a number of laboratories (round robin studies) to demonstrate that the results obtained carry as much weight as those of *in vivo* studies, so that these methods provide an equivalent level of safety. The results of these studies are submitted to the responsible scientific committee for evaluation and validation (US Interagency Coordinating Committee on the Validation of Alternative Methods and European Centre for the Validation of Alternative Methods). Once the validity of the method has been recognized by the corresponding scientific committee, the Organisation for Economic Co-operation and Development (OECD) can then officially approve the alternative method and incorporate it into the OECD guideline. It is then up to government authorities to decide whether and to what extent they will accept the use of the alternative to replace, reduce, or refine animal use. Obviously, the opinions of regulators strongly influence the extent to which pharmaceutical companies use available alternatives instead of traditional animal tests, as potential concerns around regulatory acceptance arise when making decisions using novel rather than traditional approaches for safety/toxicology assessment. Indeed, the regulatory validation process of alternative methods to replace an *in vivo* regulatory bioassay may deter scientists from developing them. However, not all scientifically validated methodologies require regulatory acceptance as they can be used as alternative models for basic/discovery biomedical research based on its robustness in providing valuable data on efficacy or safety. This means that focus can be placed on the need for formal validation studies on some occasions, but also on proof of scientific validity on others [14].

Although a number of excellent studies have used mammalian models to discover new compounds, the time and effort involved with screening a large number of candidates are huge. In addition, scientists are unanimous that they would not use animals if alternative models were available for their research. A survey of 1950 individuals (76% scientists and 24% animal care staff; 74% of the scientists worked in academia, 15% in industry, and most of the remaining 11% worked for government bodies) conducted by the UK National Centre for the 3Rs (NC3Rs) (the document can be found on the NC3Rs web site at www.nc3rs.org.uk/page.asp?id=726) in 2007 illustrates interesting trends in the views of scientists on 3Rs. The survey revealed that there is a general good understanding of the definitions of the 3Rs, although there is confusion over the definition of refinement, with 52% of scientists incorrectly defining it as improving experiments to yield better data. When asked to indicate where they had first heard about the 3Rs, most scientists (57%) held that it was during the modular training courses required to attain a project and personal license that they were introduced to the 3Rs. Regarding implementation and the perceived impact on research, the majority of scientists indicated that implementation of the 3Rs would not be detrimental to the quality of their results (82%), but that the complete replacement of animals in research and testing will never be achieved (73%). Approximately one-third of scientists have developed techniques that reduce (34%) or refine (30%) the use of animals. This, however, fell to 12% for replacement techniques. Lack of scientific or technological innovation was seen as the main obstacle to implementing the 3Rs by 33% of scientists. About 77% of scientists involved in designing experiments indicated that they need to look at whole animal system to address their research objectives. The availability of more relevant cell cultures and human tissues, technical advances in tissue engineering, and more predictive computer models were the principal technologies that respondents thought would enable them to address their research objectives without the use of animals. In addition, most scientists identified data sharing or collaboration between research groups (77%) or companies (60%) as one of the factors that would allow fewer animals to be used.

This chapter deals with alternatives to animal models and the concept of 3Rs. Emerging technologies and available alternatives to replace the use of living animals and thus reduce their use in biomedical research (and drug discovery in particular) are depicted. Replacement methods can be absolute or relative (see NC3Rs web site at www.nc3rs.org.uk/page.asp?id=7). This chapter focuses on absolute replacement methods that do not involve animals at any point: computer modeling and *in vitro* methodologies.

2.2
In Silico Models

The high costs of drug development, together with the declining cost of high-performance computing platforms and the availability of improved *in silico* biological models, have been a strong incentive for the development of tests able to detect deficiencies, such as poor absorption, target organ concentration, clearance or efficacy, and toxicity or other adverse effects, early within the drug discovery and development process. The benefits of modeling and simulation during drug design and preclinical assessment can potentially be realized through integration of any available data on physicochemical properties, pharmacokinetics (PK), and pharmacodynamics (PD) [15–18]. Optimal use of PK/PD modeling and simulation will result in fewer failed compounds, fewer study failures, and smaller number of studies needed for registration [17]. In an age of declining productivity, it is hard for drug companies to ignore any technology that could potentially reduce pharmaceutical research and development costs by up to 50%, as was suggested in a 1999 report by PricewaterhouseCoopers [19]. *The Economist*, reporting on the analysis done by PricewaterhouseCoopers, pointed out that the application of modeling and simulation to drug discovery could save US$200 million and 2–3 years in development time for each drug candidate [20]. Computer-aided techniques used in drug design and discovery are summarized in Table 2.2.

For the increased utilization of *in silico* techniques in drug development, further validation studies must be performed. Ideally, this would be achieved via comparison with clinical trial data for a large group of drugs with different mechanisms of action in blinded studies. Such studies should expose any weaknesses in the underlying mathematical models or model parameters, which are only as good as the experimental data on which they are based [21].

2.2.1
Quantitative Structure–Activity Relationship

The relationship between physicochemical structure and biological activity (structure–activity relationship (SAR)) was already recognized in 1894 by Hermann Emil Fischer (Nobel Laureate, 1902) who used the lock-and-key analogy, which may be used to describe the three-dimensional complementarity of drugs with target receptors or enzymes [22]. The discipline of quantitative structure–activity relationship (QSAR) can be considered the very first computer-aided approach in drug discovery and was started in the 1960s by Corwin Hansch and his postdoc Toshio Fujita. QSARs are mathematical descriptions of the relationships between the physicochemical properties of molecules and their biological activities [23], which may be used to predict characteristics at the theoretical, compound design stage [24]. QSAR modeling has been used widely as a key computational tool for predicting physicochemical properties and rationalizing experimental binding data or inhibitory activity of chemical compounds [25]. Typically, QSAR is performed in two

Table 2.2 Computer-aided techniques used in drug design and discovery.

Technique	Roles in drug design and discovery
Docking	Predict binding mode and approximate binding energy of a compound to a target
Structure-based virtual screening	Identify active compounds for a specific target from a chemical library based on docking techniques
Pharmacophore modeling	Perceive and provide description of molecular features necessary for molecular recognition of a ligand by a biological macromolecule
Ligand-based virtual screening	Identify active compounds for a specific target from a chemical library based on pharmacophore modeling techniques
Homology modeling	Build a 3D structure for structure-based drug design for a target for which no crystal structure is available, based on related protein 3D structures
Molecular dynamics	Molecular mechanics-based simulation to understand the dynamic behavior of proteins or other biological macromolecules, to analyze the flexibility of the drug target for structure-based drug design, and/or to calculate the binding affinity of a compound to a target
Two-dimensional quantitative structure–activity relationship	Finding a model that can be used to predict some property from the molecular structure of a compound
Three-dimensional quantitative structure–activity relationship	Technique used to quantitatively predict the interaction between a molecule and the active site of a target; 3D conformation-derived information is utilized in this technique
Quantum mechanics	An electron orbital approach based on first principles to optimize structures of ligands and even protein–ligand complexes, improve the accuracy of docking, and calculate, for example, free binding energy
Absorption, distribution, metabolism, elimination, and toxicity prediction	Prediction of absorption, distribution, metabolism, elimination, and toxicity of chemical substances in the human body to avoid costly later-stage failures in drug development

diverse modes, referred to as two- and three-dimensional QSARs (2D QSAR and 3D QSAR), which are quite different techniques for practical purposes.

Two-dimensional QSAR is conceptually a way of finding a simple equation that can be used to predict some property from the molecular structure of a compound. It is a meaningful correlation (model) between a set of independent variables (chemical descriptors) calculated from chemical graphs and a dependent variable such as binding affinity, log P, or the pK_a value whose value one wishes to predict for the compound of interest [25,26]. Chemical descriptors can be of various kinds such as molecular weight, the number of double bonds, or ionization potential and are classified as constitutional, topological, electrostatic, geometrical, and quantum chemical descriptors [27]. Similar to artificial neural networks (ANNs), a 2D QSAR model is set up by training with a set of compounds having experimentally determined activity to find the descriptors that best explain the activity. Compared with ANNs, QSAR models tend to be much better in extrapolating properties exceeding those of the training set [25].

Two-dimensional QSAR remains a valuable tool for predicting chemical properties of drug-like organic compounds. Hence, it is currently widely employed and an actively pursued methodology in the field of absorption, distribution, metabolism, elimination, and toxicity (ADMET) prediction. Two-dimensional QSAR is best used to compute nonspecific interactions of a compound and its environment such as normal boiling points, passive intestinal absorption, blood–brain barrier permeability, and other pharmacokinetic features. Additionally, 2D QSAR models exist for modeling different types of toxicity such as mutagenicity, carcinogenicity, hepatotoxicity, cardiac toxicity, teratogenicity, bioaccumulation, bioconcentration, acute toxicity, and maximum tolerated dose [25,27].

Many comprehensive drug design packages include their own 2D QSAR modules, with which the users can calculate different molecular descriptors and then build their 2D QSAR models. More stand-alone-type programs in the field include CODESSA (http://www.semichem.com/codessa/default.php), PASS (www.genexplain.com/pass) GUSAR (www.genexplain.com/gusar), DRAGON (www.talete.mi.it), and MOLD^2 (http://www.fda.gov/ScienceResearch/BioinformaticsTools/Mold2/).

Three-dimensional QSAR includes any QSAR approach based on three-dimensional molecular structures. More precisely, 3D QSAR is a technique that uses a three-dimensional grid of points around the molecule, each point having properties associated with it that can vary in a field-like manner from point to point, such as steric interactions or electrostatic potential [25]. Three-dimensional QSAR is mainly used for predicting the binding affinity of a ligand to the active site of a specific target quantitatively even when no information of the active site exists. It often requires three-dimensional structures of the analyzed molecules, plus typically a molecular superposition step [28].

In the early stage of drug design, if the active site of the target is unknown, 3D QSAR is useful to explain activities of existing compounds and to accurately predict the activities of their analogs, whereas pharmacophore searches tend to be more valuable for quickly searching very large chemical databases and thus tend to be better for scaffold hopping to identify novel classes of active compounds. If the geometry of the active site is known, docking tends to replace 3D QSAR and will be the preferred prediction technique in many projects [25,27].

There are several programs developed for 3D QSAR. The most well known among them are comparative molecular similarity indices analysis (CoMSIA) [29], comparative molecular field analysis (CoMFA) [30], and molecular field analysis from Accelrys, which in its approach is similar to CoMFA [31,32]. The models built with the CoMFA or CoMSIA techniques are created to identify a correlation between the molecular fields and biological activity, which can be automatically achieved with a partial least squares (PLS) algorithm. Sheng *et al.* [33] and Salama *et al.* [34] describe the applications of CoMFA and CoMSIA in the drug discovery process.

2.2.2
Biokinetic Modeling

The success of a drug is determined not only by good efficacy but also by an acceptable ADMET profile. Although a large variety of experimental medium- and high-throughput *in vitro* ADMET screens are available, the ability to predict some of these properties *in silico* is valuable. Today, it has been recognized that employing computational ADMET, in combination with *in vivo* and *in vitro* predictions, as early as possible in the drug discovery process helps to reduce the number of safety issues. Moreover, there is a pressure to reduce the number of animal experiments (e.g., the REACH program; http://echa.europa.eu/regulations/reach).

In silico ADMET models are increasingly being utilized. During the past few years, there have been several reviews showing how *in silico* predictions of ADMET processes can be used to help focus medicinal chemistry into more ideal areas of property space, minimizing the number of compounds needed to be synthesized to obtain the required biochemical and/or physicochemical profile [16,18,35–42].

Available tools for modeling and predicting drug ADMET include ADME parameter predictors, metabolic fate predictors, metabolic stability predictors, cytochrome P450 (CYP450) substrate predictors, plasma protein binding interaction predictors, P-glycoprotein (P-gp) inhibition predictors, hERG blockade predictors, physiology-based pharmacokinetic (PBPK) or physiology-based biokinetic (PBBK) modeling software, and so on. Repeat-dose toxicities (chronic toxicity, reproductive toxicity, and cancer) represent the largest challenge. Here, no *in silico* approaches are evident yet [37]. Available ADMET prediction programs are summarized in Table 2.3.

Traditionally, data modeling methods, such as expert systems and QSAR or quantitative structure–property relationship (QSPR) [38,43], have been used to investigate ADMET properties. These methods use statistical and learning approaches, molecular descriptors, and experimental data to model complex biological processes (e.g., oral bioavailability, intestinal absorption, permeability, and mutagenicity) [35,43]. The rules for drug-likeness, lead-likeness, or metabolite-likeness [44,45], relying on simple physicochemical properties, are also well known and implemented in commercially and freely available packages [35,46,47]. Limitations of all these approaches come from the fact that high-quality experimental data are seldom available, and that the approaches tend to neglect direct structural information about the proteins involved in ADMET processes [42,48]. *In silico* approaches based on the three-dimensional structures of these proteins could therefore be an attractive alternative or could complement ADMET data modeling techniques [42,49,50]. The increasing availability of three-dimensional structures provides the means to explore the value of molecular understanding gained by taking into account the ligand and/or protein interactions. The report by Moroy *et al.* [42] focuses on recent *in silico* studies across a breadth of

Table 2.3 ADME/toxicity prediction software packages.

Software	Provided by	Prediction spectrum
Discovery Studio ADMET Software	Accelrys	The ADMET Collection provides components that calculate predicted absorption, distribution, metabolism, excretion, and toxicity properties for collections of molecules: human intestinal absorption aqueous solubility, blood–brain barrier penetration, plasma protein binding, CYP2D6 binding, hepatotoxicity, filter sets of small molecules for undesirable function groups based on published SMARTS rules
Discovery Studio TOPKAT Software	Accelrys	Cross-validated models for the assessments of chemical toxicity from chemical's molecular structure: rodent carcinogenicity, Ames mutagenicity, rat oral LD_5, rat chronic LOAE, developmental toxicity potential, skin sensitization, fathead minnow LC_{50}, daphnia magna EC_{50}, weight of evidence rodent carcinogenicity, rat maximum tolerated dose, aerobic biodegradability, eye irritancy, log P, rabbit skin irritancy, rat inhalation toxicity LC_{50}, rat maximum tolerated dose
ACD/ADME Suite	ACD/Labs	Predicts ADME properties from chemical structure, such as P-gp specificity, oral bioavailability, passive absorption, blood–brain barrier permeation, distribution, P450 inhibitors, substrates and inhibitors, maximum recommended daily dose, Abraham-type (Absolv) solvation parameters, and so on
ACD/DMSO Solubility	ACD/Labs	Predicts solubility in DMSO solution
ACD/PhysChem Suite	ACD/Labs	Predicts basic physicochemical properties, such as pK_a, log P, log D, aqueous solubility, and other molecular properties
ACD/Tox Suite	ACD/Labs	Collection of software modules that predict probabilities for basic toxicity endpoints. Several modules including hERG inhibition, CYP3A4 inhibition, genotoxicity, acute toxicity, aquatic toxicity, eye/skin irritation, endocrine system disruption, and health effects
PK-Sim	Bayer Technology Services	Software tool for whole-body physiologically based pharmacokinetic modeling
KnowItAll ADME/Tox Edition	Bio-Rad	Prediction of ADMET properties using consensus modeling
PreADME	BMDRC	Calculates molecular descriptors. Predicts druglikeness. ADME predictions
PredictFX	Certera	Program to identify and address safety issues. Predicts the profile of affinities against a panel of biological targets, the profile of side effects, and the link between side effects and target profile

Metabolizer Preview	ChemAxon	Enumerates all the possible metabolites of a given substrate, predicts the major metabolites, and estimates metabolic stability. It can be used for the identification of metabolites by MS mass values, discovery of metabolically sensitive functionalities and toxicity prediction, and providing information related to the environmental effects of chemicals by bacterial degradation
HazardExpert Pro	CompuDrug	Predicts the toxicity of organic compounds based on toxic fragments: oncogenicity, mutagenicity, teratogenicity, membrane irritation, sensitivity, immunotoxicity, and neurotoxicity
MetabolExpert	CompuDrug	Predicts the most common metabolic pathways in animals, plants, or through photodegradation
MEXAlert	CompuDrug	Identifies compounds that have a high probability of being eliminated from the body in a first pass through the liver and kidney
pKalc	CompuDrug	Indicates acidic and basic pK_a
PrologP/PrologD	CompuDrug	Predicts the log P/log D values using a combination of linear and neural network methods
ToxAlert	CompuDrug	Predicts the toxicity of organic compounds based on toxic fragments
Cloe PK	Cyprotex	Human, rat, and mouse PK prediction using physiologically based pharmacokinetic modeling
Cloe PREDICTION	Cyprotex	Human intestinal absorption prediction using solubility, pK_a, and Caco-2 permeability data
ADMEWORKS ModelBuilder	Fujitsu Limited	Builds QSAR/QSPR models that can later be used for predicting various chemical and biological properties of compounds. Models are based on values of physicochemical, topological, geometrical, and electronic properties derived from the molecular structure, and can be imported into ADMEWORKS Predictor
ADMEWORKS Predictor	Fujitsu Limited	QSAR-based virtual screening system intended for simultaneous evaluation of the properties of compounds
MetaDrug	GeneGo	Predicts toxicity and metabolism of compounds using >70 QSAR models for ADMET properties
ToxTree	IdeaConsult Ltd	Full-featured and flexible user-friendly open source application to estimate toxic hazard by applying a decision tree approach
Leadscope	Leadscope	Estimates toxicity using QSAR
Derek Nexus	Lhasa Limited	Predicts toxicity properties using QSAR and other expert knowledge rules
Meteor	Lhasa Limited	Predicts metabolic fate of chemicals using expert knowledge rules in metabolism
Molcode Toolbox	MolCode, Ltd CompuDrug	Allows prediction of medicinal and toxicological endpoints for a large variety of chemical structures, using proprietary QSAR models. Molcode

(*continued*)

Table 2.3 (Continued)

Software	Provided by	Prediction spectrum
		is taking part in the European Chemicals Registration (REACH) program
MetaSite	Molecular Discovery	Computational procedure that predicts metabolic transformations related to cytochrome-mediated reactions in phase I metabolism
ADRIANACode	Molecular Networks	Program to calculate physicochemical properties of small molecules: number of H-bonds donor and acceptors, log P, log S, TPSA, dipole moment, polarizability, and so on
isoCYP	Molecular Networks	Predicts the predominant human cytochrome P450 isoform by which a given chemical compound is metabolized in phase I
CASE Ultra	MultiCASE Inc.	Predicts bioactivity/toxicity
META	MultiCASE Inc.	Predicts metabolic paths of molecules
StarDrop	Optibrium	Allows the identification of the regions of a molecule that are the most vulnerable to metabolism by the major drug metabolizing isoforms of cytochrome P450
PASS Online	PharmaExpert	Predicts over 4000 kinds of biological activity, including pharmacological effects, mechanisms of action, toxic and adverse effects, interaction with metabolic enzymes and transporters, influence on gene expression, and so on
IMPACT-F	PharmaInformatic	Expert system to estimate oral bioavailability of drug candidates in humans. IMPACT-F is composed of several QSAR models to predict oral bioavailability in humans
MolScore-Drugs	PharmaInformatic	Expert system to identify and prioritize drug candidates
q-ADME	Quantum Pharmaceuticals	Predicts the following properties: drug half-life ($t_{1/2}$), fraction of oral dose absorbed (FA), Caco-2 permeability, volume of distribution (VD), and octanol/water distribution coefficient (log P)
q-TOX	Quantum Pharmaceuticals	Computes toxic effects of chemicals solely from their molecular structure (LD_{50}, MRDD, side effects)
QikProp	Schrödinger	Provides rapid ADME predictions of drug candidates
Filter-it	Silicos-it	Command-line program for filtering molecules with unwanted properties out of a set of molecules. The program comes with a number of preprogrammed molecular properties that can be used for filtering
SimCYP	SimCYP	Platform for the prediction of drug–drug interactions and pharmacokinetic outcomes in clinical populations. Also available for iPhone (SimCYP for iPhone)

GastroPlus	Simulation Plus, Inc.	Simulates intravenous, oral, oral cavity, ocular, intranasal, and pulmonary absorption, pharmacokinetics, and pharmacodynamics in humans and animals. The underlying model is the advanced compartmental absorption and transit (ACAT) model
MedChem Studio	Simulation Plus, Inc.	Cheminformatics platform supporting lead identification and prioritization, *de novo* design, scaffold hopping, and lead optimization. Fully integrated with MedChem Designer and ADMET Predictor
ADMET Predictor	Simulations Plus, Inc.	Software for advanced predictive modeling of ADMET properties. ADMET Predictor estimates a number of ADMET properties from molecular structures, and is also capable of building predictive models of new properties from user's data via its integrated ADMET Modeler module
MedChem Designer	Simulations Plus, Inc.	Tool that combines molecule drawing features with a few free ADMET property predictions from ADMET Predictor
ADMET Modeler	Simulations Plus, Inc.	Integrated module of ADMET Predictor that automates the process of making high-quality predictive structure–property models from sets of experimental data. It works seamlessly with ADMET Predictor structural descriptors as its inputs, and appends the selected final model back to ADMET Predictor as an additional predicted property
VolSurf	Tripos	Calculates ADME properties and creates predictive ADME models
SMARTCyp	University of Copenhagen	Predicts the sites in molecules that are most liable to cytochrome P450-mediated metabolism
Virtual LogP	University of Milano	Bernard Testa's Virtual log P calculator. The virtual log P is obtained by the molecular lipophilicity potential (MLP) that is calculated projecting the Broto–Moreau lipophilicity atomic constants on the molecular surface
FAF-Drugs2	University of Paris Diderot	Package for *in silico* ADMET filtering
COMPACT	University of Surrey, Guildford, UK	Computer-optimized molecular parametric analysis of chemical toxicity (COMPACT) identifies potential carcinogenicity or toxicities mediated by CYP450s
KOWWIN – EPI Suite	US Environmental Protection Agency (EPA)	Estimates the log P of chemicals using an atom/fragment contribution method
OncoLogic	US EPA	Evaluates the likelihood that a chemical may cause cancer, using SAR analysis, experts' decision mimicking, and knowledge of how chemicals cause cancer in animals and humans

ADMET proteins and through a case study explores the value of this approach. The report also acknowledges the challenge caused by the promiscuous nature of some of the proteins involved in ADMET. Chen *et al.* [50] provide a detailed examination of these challenges in the case of P-glycoprotein, which interacts with a large number of structurally diverse compounds and has multiple binding sites.

The goal of the *in silico* tools is not to produce a series of models to be used in place of laboratory tests, but rather to improve both the design and the strategic use of test methods [51] and further integrate different methodologies to improve overall mechanistic understanding and predictivity [37,41,42,52]. There are several examples to show how some *in silico* approaches can be used to derive new drugs or even new uses for approved drugs [52–54]. Recent advances in physiologically based pharmacokinetic and/or pharmacodynamic modeling [55] that integrate these *in silico* tools to predict needed parameters to describe and give better understanding of the pharmacokinetics and pharmacodynamics of complex mixtures are steps in the right direction. Other recent works have demonstrated that *in silico* methods will have a crucial role in bringing together new types of data for novel nonanimal approaches to risk assessment [56,57].

2.2.3
Disease- and Patient-Specific *In Silico* Models

Several large collaborative programs are underway to develop disease- and patient-specific *in silico* models, which should ultimately assist in the development of novel medical devices and drugs. For example, researchers involved in the euHeart project (www.euheart.eu) [58,59] are developing computational cardiac physiology models to facilitate the understanding of cardiovascular disease (CVD) progression and to improve the diagnosis and treatment of CVD, the leading cause of morbidity in the western world. Another initiative is HepatoSys Competence Network – Systems Biology of Hepatocytes (www.hepatosys.de) [60], which focuses on a quantitative understanding of complex and dynamic cellular processes in detoxification, endocytosis, iron regulation, and regeneration in mammalian hepatocytes. The aim is both to arrive at a holistic understanding of these life processes and to be able to present and make these processes accessible *in silico*.

Drug metabolism in the liver can convert some drugs into highly reactive intermediates that, in turn, can adversely affect the structure and functions of the liver. Drug-induced liver injury (DILI) is therefore one of the most important reasons for drug development failure at both preapproval and postapproval stages. A list of approximately 300 drugs and chemicals with a classification scheme based on clinical data for hepatotoxicity has been assembled previously by Pfizer in order to evaluate an *in vitro* human hepatocyte imaging assay technology (HIAT), which had a concordance of 75% with clinical hepatotoxicity [61]. This example represents the first large-scale testing of a machine learning model for DILI that uses a similarly sized training and test set. The overall concordance of the model is lower (∼60–64% depending on test set size) than that observed previously for *in vitro* HIAT (75%) [61]. However, the test set statistics are similar to those reported elsewhere using structural alerts [62]. This work suggests that currently available data can be used to predict, with reasonable accuracy, future compounds and their potential for DILI (for review, see Refs [63,64]).

An *in silico–in vitro* approach was used to predict compounds likely to cause time-dependent inhibition (TDI) of P450 3A4 in human liver microsomes. The Bayesian classification approach [65], along with simple interpretable molecular descriptors as well as FCFP_6 descriptors [66], was used to classify P450 3A4 TDI. The models used 1853–2071 molecules and were tested with molecules excluded from the models [67]. All of the receiver operator characteristic curves show better than random ability to identify the TDI positive molecules, and these models were integrated into the Pfizer testing paradigm [67].

Scientific research creates and consumes tremendous volumes of data; however, the data available on human toxicities make up only a small fraction. Many industries have realized that they cannot do everything in-house and have developed complex networks of collaborators or partners throughout R&D. Current areas of major interest are Open Innovation, Collaborative Innovation, Open Source, and Open Data. Of relevance to toxicity prediction are the e-Tox (www.etoxproject.eu/), OpenTox (www.opentox.org/), OECD toolbox (www.oecd.org/document/54/0,3746, en_2649_34379_42923638_1_1_1_1,00.html), OCHEM (ochem.eu/), and Open PHACTS (www.openphacts.org/) initiatives that promote a collaborative research and data sharing agenda. As research costs increase, all scientists will be driven to collaborate more and this will require novel databases and tools to selectively share data [68,69] and perhaps create a new business model [70]. The continued utilization of computational models for human toxicity will be critical to any researcher developing new molecules and to regulators and decision makers on all sides [64].

There is no doubt that *in silico* approaches are increasingly being utilized. Their overall accuracy and the underlying understanding have increased over time [36,38,40,42,55]. In comparison with *in vitro* and cell culture methods, which began more than 100 years ago and have been usefully deployed since the 1960s in the discovery of new chemicals, it should be acknowledged that *in silico* tools have been in existence for a relatively short time and have only taken up a pace in the past 20 years. Given the enormous speed of these *in silico* technologies, a much quicker development can be expected as these tools become increasingly user-friendly and transparent. As more examples of successful applications are shown and they are integrated with *in vitro* screening, it seems highly probable that *in silico* approaches will evolve rapidly. There is a need for these computational chemistry tools to align with other information sources (e.g., from systems biology, hazard, metabolites, and exposure) to develop real or virtual models of tissues, organs, and physiological processes that could be used for the risk assessments [60].

2.3
In Vitro Models

In vitro test systems offer many advantages in comparison to whole animal (*in vivo* test systems). They have the potential to be more rigorously standardized than *in vivo* testing. These test systems are more reliable since quality data can be

Table 2.4 Alternative *in vitro* models.

Models available	Advantages	Disadvantages
Subcellular preparations	Molecular level studies Toxic metabolite formation and covalent binding to macromolecules can be assessed	Only quantitative information available
Isolated cells (e.g., primary cultures, cocultures)	Retain original capabilities and properties Mimic *in vivo* response	Loss of influences such as hormones, immunity
Multicellular tissue (slices, cubes, aggregates, and explants)	Retention of 3D structure Cell–cell interaction	Poor retention of viability Oxygen and chemicals cannot penetrate
Isolated organs	High reproducibility	Short period of viability
Stem cells	Pluripotent	Can form tumors
Cell lines	Can be maintained for a prolonged period	Prolongation results in decreased metabolic capacity and altered cellular function
Immortalized cell lines	Capable of extended and indefinite growth *in vitro*	Immortalization alters their characteristics and functions

generated. Also, these are less expensive. There is an additional advantage of human cells being directly used in *in vitro* test systems. They also offer good experimental control of the cellular doses of chemicals [71,72]. The advantages and disadvantages of *in vitro* models (systems) and techniques available for *in vitro* testing are summarized in Table 2.4.

2.3.1
Primary Cells, Cell Lines, Immortalized Cell Lines, and Stem Cells

Cell culture can be an alternative for replacing animals in biomedical research. *In vitro* assays using human immortalized cell lines (HICLs) and primary cells are an important tool in preclinical drug screening.

Primary cell cultures are isolated directly from animal tissues, often using proteolytic enzymes. Their major advantages include tissue-specific functions and retention of capacity for biotransformation. However, cellular isolation can result in damage to cell membrane integrity, with loss of, or damage to, membrane receptors and cellular products. Fortunately, during the interval necessary to establish monolayer cultures from cell suspensions, such cell damage is often repaired [18,73]. Due to the adverse changes that occur within primary cultures maintained for prolonged periods, it may be necessary to isolate new cells for each experiment. Primary cells are desirable because they can most closely recapitulate *in vivo* characteristics. However, their high cost, limited supply, short-term viability *ex vivo*, and donor-specific issues make these cells unsuitable for routine use.

Cell lines are cells that have undergone mutations to allow a cell type that would not normally be able to divide to proliferate *in vitro*. Cell lines provide an unlimited and relatively homogenous supply of cells and have proved valuable for research in several fields. However, cell lines have their own limitations. Many commonly used cell lines are derived from cancerous tumors and have undergone significant mutations so that they divide indefinitely. As a consequence, these cell lines cannot fully recapitulate characteristics of the healthy adult cell types from which they were derived. For example, hepatocarcinoma cell lines do not typically express the full range of metabolizing enzymes in adult hepatocytes, and so these cells must be used with caution when studying metabolism-mediated drug toxicity. Moreover, extended periods of culture over many years can result in decreased metabolic capacity and altered cellular function. Widely used animal-derived cell lines, such as Chinese hamster ovary cells and mouse lymphoma L5178Y cells, suffer from variation in phenotype and behavior between laboratories, even with respect to chromosome numbers [18,73].

Immortalized cell lines are capable of extended, and often indefinite, growth *in vitro*. They are generated by introducing viral oncogenes such as SV40 large T, polyoma virus large T, and adenovirus EIA into primary cells, using calcium phosphate or electroporation treatment. Many immortalized cell lines from various tissues are shown to exhibit the unique characteristics of tissue functions, and they should be useful as an *in vitro* model of various tissues for physiological and pharmacological investigations [18,73–75]. Examples of cells that have been immortalized include rabbit kidney cells, mouse macrophages, rat hepatocytes, and human lymphocytes and osteoblasts. Immortalization, however, may significantly alter their characteristics and function [74–76].

Stem cells are characterized by their ability for self-renewal (i.e., maintaining their undifferentiated state during several rounds of cell division) and their potency (i.e., the ability to differentiate into specialized cell types). The two main stem cell types are embryonic stem cells (ESCs) and adult stem cells (i.e., somatic stem cells). Other types, such as induced pluripotent stem cells (iPSCs), are produced in the laboratory by reprogramming adult cells to express ESC characteristics [77–79]. Stem cells, including human embryonic stem cells (hESCs) and human induced pluripotent stem cells (hiPSCs), potentially offer an alternative to primary cells and cell lines as they are immortal, thereby avoiding the supply issues associated with primary cells, and pluripotent stem cells have the capacity to give rise to any cell type in the body, which could have important implications for research on cell types that are in limited supply (e.g., pancreatic beta cells for diabetes research). hESCs raise considerable ethical and sociological concerns because they are derived from human embryos. However, hiPSCs are less controversial because they can be created from adult cell types via a genetic reprogramming step that returns them to an embryonic state. Stem cells can provide a closer phenotypic match to human cells than to animal material. Much of the considerable interest in stem cell research centers on their potential to replace lost tissue or functional cells, for example, in degenerative diseases [76]. In a related application, stem cell research has helped to elucidate some of the proliferation and differentiation mechanisms involved in hematopoiesis (blood cell production) and, particularly, several hematopoietic cytokines, which are now used in the treatment of cancer patients undergoing chemotherapy and radiation therapy [76]. The ability of hiPSCs to recapitulate pathological tissue formation *in vitro* could open new avenues of research into diseases where suitable animal models do not exist. hiPSCs might also be used to generate patient-specific *in vitro* disease models for personalized medicine approaches, such as the models of inherited metabolic disorders of the liver that were reported by Rashid *et al.* in 2010 [80]. Pluripotent stem cell-derived hepatocyte-like cells offer a means of creating physiologically relevant drug screening assays that could serve as an additional method of detecting toxicity in the lead optimization phase of the drug development process [81]. A recent report by Siller *et al.* [82] discusses the utility of pluripotent cell technology for the modeling of human diseases, such as cancer and infectious disease, and they also spell out the technical and scientific challenges to be addressed if the field is to deliver on its potential and produce improved patient outcomes in the clinic.

Undoubtedly, iPSC technology will provide unprecedented opportunities in drug discovery, biomedical research, and regenerative medicine. However, several challenges remain before stem cells achieve widespread use in the laboratory. Methods for the expansion and reliable differentiation of hESC into desired adult cell types need further development to provide appropriately scaled and reproducible production systems. Further research must also be done to establish whether stem cell-derived adult cells reliably mimic *in vivo* cellular characteristics and responses.

2.3.2
Advanced *In Vitro* Models for the Prediction of Drug Toxicity

Drug-induced liver injury is one of the most common causes of market withdrawal of pharmaceuticals and a leading cause of drug attrition in the pharmaceutical industry [83,84]. According to the US Acute Liver Failure Study Group, DILI accounts for more than 50% of acute liver failure. More than 900 marketed drugs have been associated with DILI [85,86], with clinical manifestations ranging from mild asymptomatic changes in biochemistry to liver failure. DILI is responsible for 5% of hospital admissions [87], and there is a 60–80% mortality rate in patients with drug-induced liver failure if they do not receive a liver transplant [88]. Drugs withdrawn for DILI include iproniazid (1959), bromfenac (1998), and troglitazone (2000). Many other drugs have label warnings and precautions regarding DILI. Thus, with DILI being such a serious and common problem in drug development, there is considerable need to develop a better understanding of models for DILI and to devise strategies to address DILI, early in the drug discovery/development process.

Drugs that cause dose-dependent, reproducible DILI (e.g., acetaminophen) can typically be identified using current preclinical models [89]. The challenge lies in identifying drugs that do not produce dose-dependent effects and only give rise to DILI in susceptible patients. Occurrence of idiosyncratic DILI ranges from 1 in 10 000 to 1 in 100 000; due to this low occurrence, many hepatotoxic drugs fail to be detected during clinical trials (maximum patient tests are ∼5000). It is postulated that to detect a single case of DILI (with 95% confidence), the study would require 30 000 patients, which would make drug development economically unfeasible. If clinical studies cannot be used to identify patient susceptibility, more effective preclinical screens must be sought.

The development of advanced *in vitro* assays, including three-dimensional cell cultures and cocultures of human cell lines and primary cells, might offer one solution. Three-dimensional liver models, such as those developed by Zyoxel (TissueFlex) and RegeneMed (RegeneTOX), and micropatterned coculture systems developed by Hepregen (HepatoPac) enable hepatocytes to be cultured in a more *in vivo*-like environment [90,91]. This enables cells to be cultured for much longer periods (weeks) while remaining highly metabolically competent. Three-dimensional and coculture systems can be used in long-term (chronic) drug toxicity studies and in the evaluation of drug effects at concentrations more comparable to therapeutic *in vivo* levels. In the near future, the combination of these advanced cell culture models with hiPSC techniques could potentially be used to study and understand patient DILI susceptibility and the influence of environmental factors such as diet, smoking, alcohol, and chemical exposure on DILI susceptibility and in the design of safer drugs.

2.3.3
In Vitro Tumor Models

The past decade has seen an explosion in the understanding of cancer biology and with it many new potential disease targets. Yet the ability to translate these advances into therapies is poor, with a high failure rate [92,93]. Only 5% of cancer drugs that have an Investigational New Drug (IND) application eventually go to the market [94]. Lack of safety or efficacy accounts for about 90% of drug failures during clinical trials [95–97]. Both safety and efficacy determinations rely on animal models. The poor performance of most investigational cancer drugs implies that the standard preclinical disease models are faulty or, at least, improperly used. Many cancer drugs have progressed into human trials only to reveal that they offer no clinical benefit. This high failure rate and the huge cost of drugs failing in the clinic mean that fewer drugs are available to patients and less money is available to develop new drugs. Some proposed approaches to improve anticancer drug development are summarized in Table 2.5.

The standard models for testing cancer drugs include cultured human tumor cell lines and rodent xenografts that comprise many of the same lines grown subcutaneously in immune-compromised animals (Table 2.6).

Two-dimensional cell cultures are used in anticancer drug screening. However, these simple systems neglect the cell–cell and cell–matrix interactions that have been shown to play a critical role in tumor drug response. Three-dimensional primary tumor models have been demonstrated to provide more clinically relevant results than the typical monolayer cell line models [118]. Tumor xenograft models are the gold standard method for testing the efficacy and toxicity of anticancer drugs. However, these models are time consuming, expensive, and technically

Table 2.5 Some proposed approaches to improve anticancer drug development.

Traditional approach	Proposed approach	References
Employ preclinical cell culture models at pH 7.4 and ambient oxygen (21%)	Employ preclinical cell culture models at physiological tumor pH (6.5–7.0) and oxygen (0–5%)	[98]
Rank compounds by effective concentration (IC_{50}, ED_{50})	Rank compounds by effective exposure ($C^n \times T$)	[99]
Screen for antitumor activity against bulk tumor	Screen for antitumor activity against tumor stem cells	[100]
Screen for antitumor activity against primary tumors in murine subcutaneous xenografts	Screen for antitumor activity against metastatic disease in orthotopic models or genetically engineered mice with cancer-specific mutations	[101]
Optimize drug candidates by standard ADMET parameters	Optimize drug candidates according to charge dynamics that exploit the tumor pH gradient	[102]
Rely on rodent models to predict clinical activity	Utilize three-dimensional culture of primary human tumors and biomarker-driven phase 0 trials to predict pharmacokinetics and activity	[103]
Focus on oncogenic molecular pathways as biomarkers for drug response	Incorporate tumor drug uptake and retention as a primary marker for drug response	[104]
Design drug carriers to improve formulation	Design drug carriers for tumor-specific delivery and for imaging drug delivery: theranostics	[105,106]
Use plasma pharmacokinetics to model drug delivery to solid tumors	Measure tumor pharmacokinetics directly for drug or drug carrier; apply miniaturized, implantable imaging technology	[104]
Treat all patients with the same dose and schedule	Treat patients based on their unique tumor physiology (e.g., level of hypoxia) and pharmacogenomics; utilize therapeutic drug monitoring for pharmacokinetically guided dose adjustment	[107]
Create drug combinations based on discreet MOA and nonoverlapping toxicities; use standard maximum tolerated dose (MTD)	Create drug combinations based on synergy in preclinical models; use ratiometric dosing with optimal sequence of administration	[108,109]
Traditional phase I/II trial designs to establish the MTD according to Response Evaluation Criteria in Solid Tumors (RECIST)	Biomarker-driven adaptive or continual reassessment designs; randomized phase II/III trials	[110]

Table 2.6 Commonly used cancer models.

Type	Subtype	Example	Reference
Human tumor cell line	Native	HCT116 colon	[111]
	Engineered	FLT3-dependent BaF/3 cells	[112]
Human xenograft	Subcutaneous	PC-3 prostate	[113]
	Orthotopic	PC-3 prostate implanted in prostate	[114]
Mouse tumor	Syngeneic implant	B16 melanoma	[115]
	Induced	Radiation-induced skin tumors	[116]
	Genetically engineered	RIP-Tag mouse pancreatic islet	[117]

challenging to develop, making them unsuitable for routine testing. Because these models are necessarily low-throughput, they have been overshadowed by high-throughput screening (HTS) technologies that can rapidly generate large databases of information for biostatistical analyses that yield the now familiar pathway or heat maps of drug response [93].

Advanced *in vitro* models aim to replicate the structural, functional, and mass transport properties of tumors by culturing (and coculturing) cells in three dimensions. Three-dimensional models, including multicellular tumor spheroid (MCTS) models [119–121], can reproduce many characteristics of the *in vivo* tumor microenvironment and better replicate the barrier to drug penetration, which is presented by dense tumors. Companies including Precos Ltd (Preclinical Oncology Services Limited) have developed coculture three-dimensional microtumor models and these have been shown to more closely replicate characteristics of tumors *in vivo*. The use of cancer stem cell versus traditional bulk tumor models in drug development might improve our ability to hit the root cause of disease. For example, several agents targeting the hedgehog pathway, which regulates cancer stem cell survival and the tumor microenvironment, are now in clinical trials with promising early results [122]. Likewise, a novel monoclonal antibody that targets the Wnt signaling pathway (vantictumab or OMP-18R5) has advanced to phase I testing by OncoMed Pharmaceuticals Inc. in 2011 (clinical trial information: NCT01345201). The presentation at the Annual Meeting of the American Society for Clinical Oncology (ASCO, June 2013), entitled "First-in-human evaluation of the human monoclonal antibody vantictumab (OMP-18R5; anti-Frizzled) targeting the Wnt pathway in a phase I study for patients with advanced solid tumors" (Abstract 2540) [123], was the first clinical presentation of this novel agent. In the ongoing trial of 24 patients, vantictumab was generally well tolerated up to the current dose of 10 mg/kg every 3 weeks. A bone protection strategy has been successful in ensuring bone health. Pharmacodynamic effects of vantictumab on the Wnt pathway in patient samples have been noted. Three patients with neuroendocrine tumors (NETs) experienced prolonged stable disease for 110, 316+, and 385+ days. Based on these data, OncoMed has advanced vantictumab into three phase 1b trials in specific tumor indications to study its safety in combination with standard-of-care chemotherapy. These trials will initiate in 2013 (http://www.oncomed.com/releases/press_release_2013_06_03.pdf).

Models or screening based on cancer stem cells is not facile due to their small population and the difficulty of maintaining and expanding these cells in culture without losing their pluripotent nature. However, the quality of information they yield may be more valuable than the quantity. The same may be said for *in vivo* models, in which the ability of murine xenografts to predict clinical toxicity or activity remains controversial even with the advent of genetic engineering [93,124–126]. A new approach is the "co-clinical trial" concept of Pandolfi and coworkers in which preclinical trials in genetically engineered mice are conducted in parallel with human phase I/II clinical trials [127]. This approach has proved successful in acute promyelocytic leukemia (APL), where APL mouse models recapitulated not only the biological and pathological features of human disease but also the drug response profile.

In summary, preclinical models of cancer should focus on primary or low-passage human tumors preferably maintained in three-dimensional culture. Alternatively, studies should be conducted in the appropriate cancer stem cell model if one is available. Gupta *et al.* recently reported a HTS that revealed selective inhibitors of breast cancer stem cells [128]. A notable hit was salinomycin, an agricultural antibiotic in use for over 30 years. Salinomycin has now been shown to inhibit Wnt signaling and induce apoptosis in stem cells from leukemia, osteosarcoma, and colon, lung, gastric, prostate, and pancreatic carcinomas [129].

References

1 Editorial (2004) Animal research is a source of human compassion, not shame. *Lancet*, **364** (9437), 815–816.

2 European Commission (2010) Report from the Commission to the Council and the European Parliament. Sixth Report on the Statistics on the Number of Animals Used for Experimental and Other Scientific Purposes in the Member States of the European Union. COM(2010) 511. SEC (2010) 1107 final/2. Brussels, December 8, 2010. Available at http://ec.europa.eu/environment/chemicals/lab_animals/pdf/sec_2010_1107.pdf (accessed September 9, 2013).

3 Car, B.D. (2006) Enabling technologies in reducing drug attrition due to safety failures. *American Drug Discovery*, **1**, 53–56.

4 Olson, H., Betton, G., Robinson, D., Thomas, K., Monro, A., Kolaja, G., Lilly, P., Sanders, J., Sipes, G., Bracken, W., Dorato, M., Van Deun, K., Smith, P., Berger, B., and Heller, A. (2000) Concordance of the toxicity of pharmaceuticals in humans and in animals. *Regulatory Toxicology and Pharmacology*, **32** (1), 56–67.

5 Stevens, J.L. and Baker, T.K. (2009) The future of drug safety testing: expanding the view and narrowing the focus. *Drug Discovery Today*, **14** (3–4), 162–167.

6 Redfern, W.S., Bialecki, R., Ewart, L., Hammond, T.G., Kinter, L., Lindgren, S., Pollard, C.E., Rolf, M., and Valentin, J. (2010) Impact and prevalence of safety pharmacology related toxicities throughout the pharmaceutical life cycle. *Journal of Pharmacological and Toxicological Methods*, **62**, e29.

7 Lasser, K.E., Allen, P.D., Woolhandler, S.J., Himmelstein, D.U., Wolfe, S.M., and Bor, D.H. (2002) Timing of new black box warnings and withdrawals for prescription medications. *The Journal of the American Medical Association*, **287** (17), 2215–2220.

8 Ninan, B. and Wertheimer, A.I. (2012) Withdrawing drugs in the U.S. versus other countries. *Innovations in Pharmacy*, **3** (3), Article 87, 1–12.

9. Langton, P.E., Hankey, G.J., and Eikelboom, J.W. (2004) Cardiovascular safety of rofecoxib (Vioxx): lessons learned and unanswered questions: we need processes in place to follow up suspicions about serious adverse events. *The Medical Journal of Australia*, **181** (10), 524–525.
10. Gale, E.A. (2006) Troglitazone: the lesson that nobody learned? *Diabetologia*, **49** (1), 1–6.
11. Morris, T.H. (1995) Antibiotic therapeutics in laboratory animals. *Laboratory Animals*, **29** (1), 16–36.
12. US Food and Drug Administration (2004) Innovation/Stagnation: Challenge and Opportunity on the Critical Path to New Medical Products. Available at http://www.fda.gov/downloads/ScienceResearch/SpecialTopics/CriticalPathInitiative/CriticalPathOpportunitiesReports/ucm113411.pdf (accessed September 4, 2013).
13. Magda, G., Vaudano, E., and Goldman, M. (2012) The rational use of animals in drug development: contribution of the innovative medicines initiative. *Alternatives to Laboratory Animals*, **40** (6), 307–312.
14. Chapman, K.L., Holzgrefe, H., Black, L.E., Brown, M., Chellman, G., Copeman, C., Couch, J., Creton, S., Gehen, S., Hoberman, A., Kinter, L.B., Madden, S., Mattis, C., Stemple, H.A., and Wilson, S. (2013) Pharmaceutical toxicology: designing studies to reduce animal use, while maximizing human translation. *Regulatory Toxicology and Pharmacology*, **66** (1), 88–103.
15. Lave, T., Parrott, N., Grimm, H.P., Fleury, A., and Reddy, M. (2007) Challenges and opportunities with modelling and simulation in drug discovery and drug development. *Xenobiotica*, **37** (10–11), 1295–1310.
16. Wishart, D.S. (2007) Improving early drug discovery through ADME modelling: an overview. *Drugs in R&D*, **8** (6), 349–362.
17. Rajman, I. (2008) PK/PD modelling and simulations: utility in drug development. *Drug Discovery Today*, **13** (7–8), 341–346.
18. Knight, A. (2008) Non-animal methodologies within biomedical research and toxicity testing. *ALTEX*, **25** (3), 213–231.
19. Pharma (2005) Silicon Rally: The Race to e-R&D. PricewaterhouseCoopers. Available at http://www.pwc.com/en_GX/gx/pharma-life-sciences/pdf/silicon_rally.pdf (accessed September 5, 2013).
20. Anonymous (2005) Models that take drugs. *The Economist*, June 11, 2005. Available at http://www.economist.com/node/4031248 (accessed September 5, 2013).
21. Sceat, E. (2011) Improving the human relevance of preclinical trials: technologies to replace animal testing. *International Pharmaceutical Industry*, **3** (2), 36–40.
22. Vedani, A., Lill, M.A., and Dobler, M. (2007) Predicting the toxic potential of drugs and chemicals *in silico*. *ALTEX*, **24**, 63–66.
23. Comber, M.H., Walker, J.D., Watts, C., and Hermens, J. (2003) Quantitative structure–activity relationships for predicting potential ecological hazard of organic chemicals for use in regulatory risk assessments. *Environmental Toxicology and Chemistry/SETAC*, **22** (8), 1822–1828.
24. Vedani, A., Dobler, M., Spreafico, M., Peristera, O., and Smiesko, M. (2007) VirtualToxLab: *in silico* prediction of the toxic potential of drugs and environmental chemicals: evaluation status and Internet access protocol. *ALTEX*, **24** (3), 153–161.
25. Liao, C., Sitzmann, M., Pugliese, A., and Nicklaus, M.C. (2011) Software and resources for computational medicinal chemistry. *Future Medicinal Chemistry*, **3** (8), 1057–1085.
26. Sprous, D.G., Palmer, R.K., Swanson, J.T., and Lawless, M. (2010) QSAR in the pharmaceutical research setting: QSAR models for broad, large problems. *Current Topics in Medicinal Chemistry*, **10** (6), 619–637.
27. Young, D.C. (2009) *Computational Drug Design: A Guide for Computational and Medicinal Chemists*, John Wiley & Sons, Inc., Hoboken, NJ.
28. Clark, R.D. (2009) Prospective ligand- and target-based 3D QSAR: state of the art 2008. *Current Topics in Medicinal Chemistry*, **9** (9), 791–810.
29. Klebe, G., Abraham, U., and Mietzner, T. (1994) Molecular similarity indices in a comparative analysis (CoMSIA) of drug molecules to correlate and predict their

biological activity. *Journal of Medicinal Chemistry*, **37** (24), 4130–4146.

30 Cramer, R.D., Patterson, D.E., and Bunce, J.D. (1988) Comparative molecular field analysis (CoMFA). 1. Effect of shape on binding of steroids to carrier proteins. *Journal of the American Chemical Society*, **110** (18), 5959–5967.

31 Liu, J., Zhao, M., Cui, G., Zhang, X., Wang, J., and Peng, S. (2008) Methyl (11a*S*)-1,2,3,5,11,11a-hexahydro-3,3-dimethyl-1-oxo-6*H*-imidazo-[3′,4′:1,2] pyridin[3,4-*b*]indol-2-substituted acetates: synthesis and three-dimensional quantitative structure–activity relationship investigation as a class of novel vasodilators. *Journal of Medicinal Chemistry*, **51** (15), 4715–4723.

32 Patil, R., Das, S., Stanley, A., Yadav, L., Sudhakar, A., and Varma, A.K. (2010) Optimized hydrophobic interactions and hydrogen bonding at the target–ligand interface leads the pathways of drug-designing. *PLoS One*, **5** (8), e12029.

33 Sheng, C., Zhang, W., Ji, H., Zhang, M., Song, Y., Xu, H., Zhu, J., Miao, Z., Jiang, Q., Yao, J., Zhou, Y., Zhu, J., and Lu, J. (2006) Structure-based optimization of azole antifungal agents by CoMFA, CoMSIA, and molecular docking. *Journal of Medicinal Chemistry*, **49** (8), 2512–2525.

34 Salama, I., Hocke, C., Utz, W., Prante, O., Boeckler, F., Hubner, H., Kuwert, T., and Gmeiner, P. (2007) Structure–selectivity investigations of D2-like receptor ligands by CoMFA and CoMSIA guiding the discovery of D3 selective PET radioligands. *Journal of Medicinal Chemistry*, **50** (3), 489–500.

35 van de Waterbeemd, W.H. and Gifford, E. (2003) ADMET *in silico* modelling: towards prediction paradise? *Nature Reviews. Drug Discovery*, **2** (3), 192–204.

36 Dearden, J.C. (2007) *In silico* prediction of ADMET properties: how far have we come? *Expert Opinion on Drug Metabolism & Toxicology*, **3** (5), 635–639.

37 Hartung, T. and Hoffmann, S. (2009) Food for thought . . . on *in silico* methods in toxicology. *ALTEX*, **26** (3), 155–166.

38 Gleeson, M.P., Hersey, A., and Hannongbua, S. (2011) *In-silico* ADME models: a general assessment of their utility in drug discovery applications. *Current Topics in Medicinal Chemistry*, **11** (4), 358–381.

39 Gleeson, M.P., Modi, S., Bender, A., Robinson, R.L., Kirchmair, J., Promkatkaew, M., Hannongbua, S., and Glen, R.C. (2012) The challenges involved in modeling toxicity data *in silico*: a review. *Current Pharmaceutical Design*, **18** (9), 1266–1291.

40 Raunio, H. (2011) *In silico* toxicology: non-testing methods. *Frontiers in Pharmacology*, **2**, 33.

41 Modi, S., Hughes, M., Garrow, A., and White, A. (2012) The value of *in silico* chemistry in the safety assessment of chemicals in the consumer goods and pharmaceutical industries. *Drug Discovery Today*, **17** (3–4), 135–142.

42 Moroy, G., Martiny, V.Y., Vayer, P., Villoutreix, B.O., and Miteva, M.A. (2012) Toward *in silico* structure-based ADMET prediction in drug discovery. *Drug Discovery Today*, **17** (1–2), 44–55.

43 Michielan, L. and Moro, S. (2010) Pharmaceutical perspectives of nonlinear QSAR strategies. *Journal of Chemical Information and Modeling*, **50** (6), 961–978.

44 Lipinski, C.A., Lombardo, F., Dominy, B.W., and Feeney, P.J. (2001) Experimental and computational approaches to estimate solubility and permeability in drug discovery and development settings. *Advanced Drug Delivery Reviews*, **46** (1–3), 3–26.

45 Dobson, P.D., Patel, Y., and Kell, D.B. (2009) 'Metabolite-likeness' as a criterion in the design and selection of pharmaceutical drug libraries. *Drug Discovery Today*, **14** (1–2), 31–40.

46 Lagorce, D., Sperandio, O., Galons, H., Miteva, M.A., and Villoutreix, B.O. (2008) FAF-Drugs2: free ADME/tox filtering tool to assist drug discovery and chemical biology projects. *BMC Bioinformatics*, **9**, 396.

47 Lagorce, D., Villoutreix, B.O., and Miteva, M.A. (2011) Three-dimensional structure generators of drug-like compounds: DG-AMMOS, an open-source package. *Expert Opinion on Drug Discovery*, **6** (3), 339–351.

48 Bhogal, N., Grindon, C., Combes, R., and Balls, M. (2005) Toxicity testing: creating a

revolution based on new technologies. *Trends in Biotechnology*, **23** (6), 299–307.

49 Vedani, A. and Smiesko, M. (2009) *In silico* toxicology in drug discovery: concepts based on three-dimensional models. *Alternatives to Laboratory Animals*, **37** (5), 477–496.

50 Chen, L., Li, Y., Yu, H., Zhang, L., and Hou, T. (2012) Computational models for predicting substrates or inhibitors of P-glycoprotein. *Drug Discovery Today*, **17** (7–8), 343–351.

51 Veith, G.D. (2004) On the nature, evolution and future of quantitative structure–activity relationships (QSAR) in toxicology. *SAR and QSAR in Environmental Research*, **15** (5–6), 323–330.

52 Ekins, S., Williams, A.J., Krasowski, M.D., and Freundlich, J.S. (2011) *In silico* repositioning of approved drugs for rare and neglected diseases. *Drug Discovery Today*, **16** (7–8), 298–310.

53 Bisson, W.H., Cheltsov, A.V., Bruey-Sedano, N., Lin, B., Chen, J., Goldberger, N., May, L.T., Christopoulos, A., Dalton, J.T., Sexton, P.M., Zhang, X.K., and Abagyan, R. (2007) Discovery of antiandrogen activity of nonsteroidal scaffolds of marketed drugs. *Proceedings of the National Academy of Sciences of the United States of America*, **104** (29), 11927–11932.

54 Bisson, W.H. (2012) Drug repurposing in chemical genomics: can we learn from the past to improve the future? *Current Topics in Medicinal Chemistry*, **12** (17), 1883–1888.

55 Zhao, P., Zhang, L., Grillo, J.A., Liu, Q., Bullock, J.M., Moon, Y.J., Song, P., Brar, S.S., Madabushi, R., Wu, T.C., Booth, B.P., Rahman, N.A., Reynolds, K.S., Gil, B.E., Lesko, L.J., and Huang, S.M. (2011) Applications of physiologically based pharmacokinetic (PBPK) modeling and simulation during regulatory review. *Clinical Pharmacology and Therapeutics*, **89** (2), 259–267.

56 Maxwell, G. and Mackay, C. (2008) Application of a systems biology approach to skin allergy risk assessment. *Alternatives to Laboratory Animals*, **36** (5), 521–556.

57 Davies, M., Pendlington, R.U., Page, L., Roper, C.S., Sanders, D.J., Bourner, C., Pease, C.K., and Mackay, C. (2011) Determining epidermal disposition kinetics for use in an integrated nonanimal approach to skin sensitization risk assessment. *Toxicological Sciences*, **119** (2), 308–318.

58 Smith, N., de Vecchi, A., McCormick, M., Nordsletten, D., Camara, O., Frangi, A.F., Delingette, H., Sermesant, M., Relan, J., Ayache, N., Krueger, M.W., Schulze, W.H., Hose, R., Valverde, I., Beerbaum, P., Staicu, C., Siebes, M., Spaan, J., Hunter, P., Weese, J., Lehmann, H., Chapelle, D., and Rezavi, R. (2011) euHeart: personalized and integrated cardiac care using patient-specific cardiovascular modelling. *Interface Focus*, **1** (3), 349–364.

59 Weese, J., Ayache, N., and Smith, N.P. (2013) Personalized cardiac modeling and simulations in euHeart. *Medical & Biological Engineering & Computing*, **51** (11), 1179–1180.

60 Abbott, A. (2010) Germans cook up liver project. *Nature*, **468** (7326), 879.

61 Xu, J.J., Henstock, P.V., Dunn, M.C., Smith, A.R., Chabot, J.R., and de Graaf, D. (2008) Cellular imaging predictions of clinical drug-induced liver injury. *Toxicological Sciences*, **105** (1), 97–105.

62 Greene, N., Fisk, L., Naven, R.T., Note, R.R., Patel, M.L., and Pelletier, D.J. (2010) Developing structure–activity relationships for the prediction of hepatotoxicity. *Chemical Research in Toxicology*, **23** (7), 1215–1222.

63 Valerio, L.G., Jr. (2011) *In silico* toxicology models and databases as FDA Critical Path Initiative toolkits. *Human Genomics*, **5** (3), 200–207.

64 Ekins, S. and Williams, A. (2012) The future of computational models for predicting human toxicities. Altex Proceedings, 1/12, Proceedings of WC8, pp. 559–554.

65 Xia, X., Maliski, E.G., Gallant, P., and Rogers, D. (2004) Classification of kinase inhibitors using a Bayesian model. *Journal of Medicinal Chemistry*, **47** (18), 4463–4470.

66 Jones, D.R., Ekins, S., Li, L., and Hall, S.D. (2007) Computational approaches that predict metabolic intermediate complex formation with CYP3A4 (+b5). *Drug Metabolism and Disposition*, **35** (9), 1466–1475.

67 Zientek, M., Stoner, C., Ayscue, R., Klug-McLeod, J., Jiang, Y., West, M., Collins, C., and Ekins, S. (2010) Integrated *in silico–in vitro* strategy for addressing cytochrome P450 3A4 time-dependent inhibition. *Chemical Research in Toxicology*, **23** (3), 664–676.

68 Hohman, M., Gregory, K., Chibale, K., Smith, P.J., Ekins, S., and Bunin, B. (2009) Novel web-based tools combining chemistry informatics, biology and social networks for drug discovery. *Drug Discovery Today*, **14** (5–6), 261–270.

69 Ekins, S., Hohman, M., and Bunin, B.A. (2011) Pioneering use of the cloud for development of the Collaborative Drug Discovery (CDD) database, in *Collaborative Computational Technologies for Biomedical Research* (eds S. Ekins, M.A.Z. Hupcey, and A.J. Williams), John Wiley & Sons, Inc., Hoboken, NJ.

70 Bunin, B.A. and Ekins, S. (2011) Alternative business models for drug discovery. *Drug Discovery Today*, **16** (15–16), 643–645.

71 Watanabe, M. (1995) Required effort to evolve toxicity testing using *in vitro* methods. *AATEX*, **3**, 81–84.

72 Bhanushali, M., Bagale, V., Shirode, A., Joshi, Y., and Kadam, V. (2010) An *in-vitro* toxicity testing: a reliable alternative to toxicity testing by reduction, replacement and refinement of animals. *International Journal of Advances in Pharmaceutical Sciences*, **1**, 15–31.

73 Broadhead, C.L. and Bottrill, K. (1997) Strategies for replacing animals in biomedical research. *Molecular Medicine Today*, **3** (11), 483–487.

74 Obinata, M. (2007) The immortalized cell lines with differentiation potentials: their establishment and possible application. *Cancer Science*, **98** (3), 275–283.

75 Eglen, R.M., Gilchrist, A., and Reisine, T. (2008) The use of immortalized cell lines in GPCR screening: the good, bad and ugly. *Combinatorial Chemistry & High Throughput Screening*, **11** (7), 560–565.

76 Luttun, A. and Verfaillie, C.M. (2006) A perspective on stem cells as a tool for *in vitro* testing. *ALTEX*, **23** (special issue), 388–392.

77 Stadtfeld, M. and Hochedlinger, K. (2010) Induced pluripotency: history, mechanisms, and applications. *Genes and Development*, **24** (20), 2239–2263.

78 Zhou, H. and Ding, S. (2010) Evolution of induced pluripotent stem cell technology. *Current Opinion in Hematology*, **17** (4), 276–280.

79 Zhang, W., Ding, Z., and Liu, G.H. (2012) Evolution of iPSC disease models. *Protein Cell*, **3** (1), 1–4.

80 Rashid, S.T., Corbineau, S., Hannan, N., Marciniak, S.J., Miranda, E., Alexander, G., Huang-Doran, I., Griffin, J., Ahrlund-Richter, L., Skepper, J., Semple, R., Weber, A., Lomas, D.A., and Vallier, L. (2010) Modeling inherited metabolic disorders of the liver using human induced pluripotent stem cells. *The Journal of Clinical Investigation*, **120** (9), 3127–3136.

81 Greenhough, S. and Hay, D. (2012) Stem cell-based toxicity screening. *Pharmaceutical Medicine*, **26** (2), 85–89.

82 Siller, R., Greenhough, S., Park, I.H., and Sullivan, G.J. (2013) Modelling human disease with pluripotent stem cells. *Current Gene Therapy*, **13** (2), 99–110.

83 Ballet, F. (1997) Hepatotoxicity in drug development: detection, significance and solutions. *Journal of Hepatology*, **26** (Suppl. 2), 26–36.

84 Stepan, A.F., Walker, D.P., Bauman, J., Price, D.A., Baillie, T.A., Kalgutkar, A.S., and Aleo, M.D. (2011) Structural alert/reactive metabolite concept as applied in medicinal chemistry to mitigate the risk of idiosyncratic drug toxicity: a perspective based on the critical examination of trends in the top 200 drugs marketed in the United States. *Chemical Research in Toxicology*, **24** (9), 1345–1410.

85 Friedman, S.E., Grendell, J.H., and McQuaid, K.R. (2003) *Current Diagnosis and Treatment in Gastroenterology*, Lang Medical Books, New York, pp. 664–679.

86 Pandit, A., Sachdeva, T., and Bafna, P. (2012) Drug-induced hepatotoxicity: a review. *Journal of Applied Pharmaceutical Science*, **2** (5), 233–243.

87 McNally, P.F. (2006) *GI Liver Secrets*, C.V. Mosby, Saint Louis, MO.

88 Antoine, D.J., Williams, D.P., and Park, B.K. (2008) Understanding the role of

reactive metabolites in drug-induced hepatotoxicity: state of the science. *Expert Opinion on Drug Metabolism & Toxicology*, **4** (11), 1415–1427.

89 Bessems, J.G. and Vermeulen, N.P. (2001) Paracetamol (acetaminophen)-induced toxicity: molecular and biochemical mechanisms, analogues and protective approaches. *Critical Reviews in Toxicology*, **31** (1), 55–138.

90 Cui, Z.F., Xu, X., Trainor, N., Triffitt, J.T., Urban, J.P., and Tirlapur, U.K. (2007) Application of multiple parallel perfused microbioreactors and three-dimensional stem cell culture for toxicity testing. *Toxicology In Vitro*, **21** (7), 1318–1324.

91 Chan, T., Yu, H., Moore, A., Khetani, S., and Tweedie, D.J. (2013) Meeting the challenge of predicting hepatic clearance of compounds slowly metabolized by cytochrome P450 using a novel hepatocyte model, HepatoPac^{TM}. *Drug Metabolism and Disposition*, **41** (12), 2024–2032.

92 Kamb, A. (2005) What's wrong with our cancer models? *Nature Reviews. Drug Discovery*, **4** (2), 161–165.

93 Adams, D.J. (2012) The Valley of Death in anticancer drug development: a reassessment. *Trends in Pharmacological Sciences*, **33** (4), 173–180.

94 Kummar, S., Kinders, R., Rubinstein, L., Parchment, R.E., Murgo, A.J., Collins, J., Pickeral, O., Low, J., Steinberg, S.M., Gutierrez, M., Yang, S., Helman, L., Wiltrout, R., Tomaszewski, J.E., and Doroshow, J.H. (2007) Compressing drug development timelines in oncology using phase '0' trials. *Nature Reviews. Cancer*, **7** (2), 131–139.

95 Kola, I. and Landis, J. (2004) Can the pharmaceutical industry reduce attrition rates? *Nature Reviews. Drug Discovery*, **3** (8), 711–715.

96 Arrowsmith, J. (2011) Trial watch: phase III and submission failures: 2007–2010. *Nature Reviews. Drug Discovery*, **10** (2), 87.

97 Arrowsmith, J. (2011) Trial watch: phase II failures: 2008–2010. *Nature Reviews. Drug Discovery*, **10** (5), 328–329.

98 Pencreach, E., Guerin, E., Nicolet, C., Lelong-Rebel, I., Voegeli, A.C., Oudet, P., Larsen, A.K., Gaub, M.P., and Guenot, D. (2009) Marked activity of irinotecan and rapamycin combination toward colon cancer cells *in vivo* and *in vitro* is mediated through cooperative modulation of the mammalian target of rapamycin/hypoxia-inducible factor-1alpha axis. *Clinical Cancer Research*, **15** (4), 1297–1307.

99 Millenbaugh, N.J., Wientjes, M.G., and Au, J.L. (2000) A pharmacodynamic analysis method to determine the relative importance of drug concentration and treatment time on effect. *Cancer Chemotherapy and Pharmacology*, **45** (4), 265–272.

100 Gupta, P.B., Onder, T.T., Jiang, G., Tao, K., Kuperwasser, C., Weinberg, R.A., and Lander, E.S. (2009) Identification of selective inhibitors of cancer stem cells by high-throughput screening. *Cell*, **138** (4), 645–659.

101 Nardella, C., Lunardi, A., Patnaik, A., Cantley, L.C., and Pandolfi, P.P. (2011) The APL paradigm and the "co-clinical trial" project. *Cancer Discovery*, **1** (2), 108–116.

102 Gleeson, M.P., Hersey, A., Montanari, D., and Overington, J. (2011) Probing the links between *in vitro* potency, ADMET and physicochemical parameters. *Nature Reviews. Drug Discovery*, **10** (3), 197–208.

103 LoRusso, P.M. (2009) Phase 0 clinical trials: an answer to drug development stagnation? *Journal of Clinical Oncology*, **27** (16), 2586–2588.

104 Wolf, W., Presant, C.A., and Waluch, V. (2000) ^{19}F-MRS studies of fluorinated drugs in humans. *Advanced Drug Delivery Reviews*, **41** (1), 55–74.

105 Kelkar, S.S. and Reineke, T.M. (2011) Theranostics: combining imaging and therapy. *Bioconjugate Chemistry*, **22** (10), 1879–1903.

106 Yoo, J.W., Irvine, D.J., Discher, D.E., and Mitragotri, S. (2011) Bio-inspired, bioengineered and biomimetic drug delivery carriers. *Nature Reviews. Drug Discovery*, **10** (7), 521–535.

107 van den Bongard, H.J., Mathot, R.A., Beijnen, J.H., and Schellens, J.H. (2000) Pharmacokinetically guided administration of chemotherapeutic agents. *Clinical Pharmacokinetics*, **39** (5), 345–367.

108 Mayer, L.D., Harasym, T.O., Tardi, P.G., Harasym, N.L., Shew, C.R., Johnstone, S.

A., Ramsay, E.C., Bally, M.B., and Janoff, A.S. (2006) Ratiometric dosing of anticancer drug combinations: controlling drug ratios after systemic administration regulates therapeutic activity in tumor-bearing mice. *Molecular Cancer Therapeutics*, **5** (7), 1854–1863.

109 Mayer, L.D. and Janoff, A.S. (2007) Optimizing combination chemotherapy by controlling drug ratios. *Molecular Interventions*, **7** (4), 216–223.

110 Yap, T.A., Sandhu, S.K., Workman, P., and de Bono, J.S. (2010) Envisioning the future of early anticancer drug development. *Nature Reviews. Cancer*, **10** (7), 514–523.

111 Bressan, A., Bigioni, M., Bellarosa, D., Nardelli, F., Irrissuto, C., Maggi, C.A., and Binaschi, M. (2010) Induction of a less aggressive phenotype in human colon carcinoma HCT116 cells by chronic exposure to HDAC inhibitor SAHA. *Oncology Reports*, **24** (5), 1249–1255.

112 Kazi, J.U., Sun, J., and Ronnstrand, L. (2013) The presence or absence of IL-3 during long-term culture of Flt3-ITD and c-Kit-D816V expressing Ba/F3 cells influences signaling outcome. *Experimental Hematology*, **41** (7), 585–587.

113 Kaighn, M.E., Narayan, K.S., Ohnuki, Y., Lechner, J.F., and Jones, L.W. (1979) Establishment and characterization of a human prostatic carcinoma cell line (PC-3). *Investigative Urology*, **17** (1), 16–23.

114 Sankpal, U.T., Abdelrahim, M., Connelly, S.F., Lee, C.M., Madero-Visbal, R., Colon, J., Smith, J., Safe, S., Maliakal, P., and Basha, R. (2012) Small molecule tolfenamic acid inhibits PC-3 cell proliferation and invasion *in vitro*, and tumor growth in orthotopic mouse model for prostate cancer. *Prostate*, **72** (15), 1648–1658.

115 Freedman, V.H., Calvelli, T.A., Silagi, S., and Silverstein, S.C. (1980) Macrophages elicited with heat-killed bacillus Calmette-Guerin protect C57BL/6J mice against a syngeneic melanoma. *The Journal of Experimental Medicine*, **152** (3), 657–673.

116 Phillips, J., Moore-Medlin, T., Sonavane, K., Ekshyyan, O., McLarty, J., and Nathan, C.A. (2013) Curcumin inhibits UV radiation-induced skin cancer in SKH-1 mice. *Otolaryngology: Head and Neck Surgery*, **148** (5), 797–803.

117 Hager, J.H., Hodgson, J.G., Fridlyand, J., Hariono, S., Gray, J.W., and Hanahan, D. (2004) Oncogene expression and genetic background influence the frequency of DNA copy number abnormalities in mouse pancreatic islet cell carcinomas. *Cancer Research*, **64** (7), 2406–2410.

118 Furukawa, T., Kubota, T., and Hoffman, R.M. (1995) Clinical applications of the histoculture drug response assay. *Clinical Cancer Research*, **1** (3), 305–311.

119 Yuhas, J.M., Tarleton, A.E., and Harman, J.G. (1978) *In vitro* analysis of the response of multicellular tumor spheroids exposed to chemotherapeutic agents *in vitro* or *in vivo*. *Cancer Research*, **38** (11 Part 1), 3595–3598.

120 Ma, H.L., Jiang, Q., Han, S., Wu, Y., Cui, T.J., Wang, D., Gan, Y., Zou, G., and Liang, X.J. (2012) Multicellular tumor spheroids as an *in vivo*-like tumor model for three-dimensional imaging of chemotherapeutic and nano material cellular penetration. *Molecular Imaging*, **11** (6), 487–498.

121 Nagelkerke, A., Bussink, J., Sweep, F.C., and Span, P.N. (2013) Generation of multicellular tumor spheroids of breast cancer cells: how to go three-dimensional. *Analytical Biochemistry*, **437** (1), 17–19.

122 Harris, L.G., Samant, R.S., and Shevde, L.A. (2011) Hedgehog signaling: networking to nurture a promalignant tumor microenvironment. *Molecular Cancer Research*, **9** (9), 1165–1174.

123 Smith, D.C., Rosen, L.S., Chugh, R., Goldman, J.W., Xu, L., Kapoun, A., Brachmann, R.K., Dupont, J., Stagg, R.J., Tolcher, A.W., and Papadopoulos, K.P. (2013) First-in-human evaluation of the human monoclonal antibody vantictumab (OMP-18R5; anti-Frizzled) targeting the WNT pathway in a phase I study for patients with advanced solid tumors. *Journal of Clinical Oncology*, **31**, Abstract 2540.

124 Olson, H., Betton, G., Robinson, D., Thomas, K., Monro, A., Kolaja, G., Lilly, P., Sanders, J., Sipes, G., Bracken, W., Dorato, M., Van Deun, K., Smith, P., Berger, B., and Heller, A. (2000) Concordance of the toxicity of pharmaceuticals in humans and in animals. *Regulatory Toxicology and Pharmacology*, **32** (1), 56–67.

125 Rangarajan, A. and Weinberg, R.A. (2003) Opinion: comparative biology of mouse versus human cells: modelling human cancer in mice. *Nature Reviews. Cancer*, **3** (12), 952–959.

126 Bracken, M.B. (2009) Why animal studies are often poor predictors of human reactions to exposure. *Journal of the Royal Society of Medicine*, **102** (3), 120–122.

127 Nardella, C., Lunardi, A., Patnaik, A., Cantley, L.C., and Pandolfi, P.P. (2011) The APL paradigm and the "co-clinical trial" project. *Cancer Discovery*, **1** (2), 108–116.

128 Gupta, P.B., Onder, T.T., Jiang, G., Tao, K., Kuperwasser, C., Weinberg, R.A., and Lander, E.S. (2009) Identification of selective inhibitors of cancer stem cells by high-throughput screening. *Cell*, **138** (4), 645–659.

129 Naujokat, C. and Steinhart, R. (2012) Salinomycin as a drug for targeting human cancer stem cells. *Journal of Biomedicine & Biotechnology*, **2012**, 950658.

3
Alternative Models in Drug Discovery and Development Part II: *In Vivo* Nonmammalian and Exploratory/Experimental Human Models

Luz Romero and José Miguel Vela

3.1
Introduction

Animal model systems are an intricate part of the discovery and development of new medicines. Mammalians such as rats, mice, dogs, and rabbits are classically used to test the effects of compounds before they are tried in humans, but other animal species have also contributed to the generation of biomedical knowledge and have application in different phases of the drug discovery and development process.

Methods to replace the use of animals can be absolute (i.e., *in silico* and *in vitro* methods) or relative (i.e., phylogenetic and/or ontogenetic reduction) (see NC3Rs web site at www.nc3rs.org.uk/page.asp?id=7). This chapter deals with relative replacement methods that avoid or replace the use of "protected" animals (all living vertebrates and cephalopods) by using invertebrates (e.g., *Drosophila* or nematode worms) or immature forms of vertebrates (e.g., embryos or larval forms of zebrafish). It is important to note that the use of a "lower" species (phylogenetic reduction) is often considered to be a refinement, but such a judgment can only be made if assessment of the available scientific evidence suggests that the lower species is less sentient/likely to suffer less (one can never know with certainty what any nonhuman animal species experiences). In addition to relative replacement by model organisms other than mammals (i.e., invertebrates and fish embryos and larvae), absolute replacement by "nonanimal" alternatives using human volunteers or patients (e.g., noninvasive studies in experimental human models) is considered in this chapter.

3.2
In Vivo Nonmammalian Models

The advancement of genetics and the recognition that many biological mechanisms and protein functions are highly conserved have led to the relatively recent integration of model organisms other than mammals into the drug discovery process. These include bacteria and yeast, which are classically utilized in drug discovery mainly to produce complex organic molecules in large quantities for testing. They are also valuable for genetic studies as well as many other studies at the molecular and cellular levels. However, unlike unicellular organisms such as bacteria or yeast, multicellular eukaryotic organisms also allow studies at the tissue, organ, and whole complex organism levels.

Whereas the history regarding the use of rodents and other mammals in drug discovery and development is long, the history for other small animals such as the fish (*Danio rerio*), the fruit fly (*Drosophila melanogaster*), and the nematode (*Caenorhabditis elegans*) is short, although they have been studied for decades by basic scientists to understand some biological mechanisms of eukaryotes. The use of these small animal models to study human disease is based on the molecular conservation during evolution and validated by the sequencing of their entire genomes. Indeed, many cellular biochemical pathways regulating metabolism, proliferation, cell death, and cell survival are highly conserved among eukaryotic organisms.

They are increasingly used and, in the next future, these small animal models may become cornerstones of modern drug discovery programs and be used to discover new drugs and dissect human diseases. Nonmammalian model organisms can be used at all stages of drug discovery, including early identification and validation of targets, *in vivo* efficacy, safety and toxicological evaluation, pharmacodynamics (PD), and identification of the mechanism of action of drugs. The nematode *C. elegans*, the fruit fly *D. melanogaster*, and the fish *D. rerio* are gaining momentum as screening tools. These organisms combine genetic amenability, low cost, and growth conditions that are compatible with large-scale screens. The main advantage with respect to cell-based screens is to allow high-throughput screening (HTS) in a whole-animal context as most biologically active molecules cause complex responses in animals that cannot be predicted by cell culture models. Accordingly, drug screening in these model organisms offers to fill the gap between *in vitro* and *in vivo* mammalian model testing by eliminating compounds that are toxic or have reduced bioavailability and by identifying others that may boost unknown but effective mechanisms of action in a whole-organism setting. Classical animal studies remain too slow and their analyses are often limited to only a few readouts. In contrast, a library of small molecules can easily be assayed *in vivo* in multiwell plates containing the whole small organism and thus changes in the phenotype upon treatment can be analyzed. Screens can be performed that are based simply on the morphology, but others score complex phenotypes using whole-mount *in situ* hybridization, fluorescent transgenic reporters, and even tracking of movement and other behaviors. The availability of many mutants also enables the discovery of chemical suppressors of genetic phenotypes. Moreover, their use is not dependent on the prior identification of a target and permits the selection of compounds with an improved safety profile. Cooperation among academic and industry laboratories is needed to develop standard operating procedures and widely accept these alternative models using nonmammalian vertebrates (i.e., zebrafish; in most cases, embryos) and invertebrates (i.e., nematode worms and flies) to predict the response of mammalian vertebrates (normally adult humans). However, these organisms are poised to make an enormous impact on the future of drug discovery.

In the following sections, we will briefly review some of the most common uses of these model organisms in drug discovery and development.

3.2.1
Zebrafish

The zebrafish, a small, tropical freshwater species native to Pakistan and India, has been a popular pet for decades and has become a model organism due to its many advantages as an experimental vertebrate. Some have labeled the zebrafish the "vertebrate *Drosophila*," due to its genetic tractability, small size, low cost, and rapid development. Zebrafish embryos and larvae are small, transparent, and undergo rapid development *ex utero*, allowing *in vivo* analysis of embryogenesis and organogenesis. These characteristics can also be exploited by researchers interested in disease processes to model human diseases and can be used in different phases of the drug discovery and development process. There are, therefore, potential advantages of using this species to replace or reduce the use of mammals.

Its use for research increased substantially by the end of 1990s, following the demonstration that it is amenable to large-scale forward genetic screens (previously limited to invertebrates such as flies, worms, and yeast). The zebrafish genome has been sequenced by the Sanger Center, and there has been substantial annotation of the genome through the Trans-National Institutes of Health Zebrafish Genome Initiative. Collections of full-length zebrafish cDNAs are available, as are multiple DNA microarrays for expression profiling experiments. Gene expression can be rapidly analyzed using whole-embryo *in situ* hybridization, and gene function can be rapidly and robustly studied using antisense morpholino oligonucleotides. Furthermore, techniques for generating transgenic lines, targeted mutations (reverse genetics), and cloning by nuclear transfer have been developed. Genetic mutants affecting a wide range of biological processes, including development, behavior, metabolism, vision, immunity, and cancer, have been identified [1–3].

Genetic disease-related screens have been carried out in zebrafish to identify mutations that cause a number of diseases [2]. Similarly, the developmental roles of individual genes have been determined by injection of morpholino oligonucleotides into zebrafish embryos to cause a robust knockdown of gene function. On this basis, therapeutic targets can be identified by forward genetic (phenotype to genotype) or morpholino oligonucleotide screens, although the relevance of most of the identified genes to disease pathology remains poorly established. Alternatively, small-molecule screens to identify suppressors of zebrafish disease phenotypes can be done even before the identification of a validated target (i.e., phenotypic screening). Indeed, for diseases for which the optimal therapeutic targets have not yet been identified, zebrafish offer a rapid phenotype-based approach to discover compounds that modify the disease phenotype, regardless of the specific molecular target. Zebrafish can also be a useful model for HTS phenotype-based lead discovery once a therapeutic target has been identified and validated. That is, small-molecule screening in zebrafish represents an *in vivo* approach to identify not only molecular targets, but also new chemical tools and drug leads. In the forward approach, "phenotype-based small-molecule discovery," a library of compounds can be screened for a specific phenotype in the animal, and from this the target(s) can be identified. Conversely, the reverse approach entails testing chemical compounds with known molecular targets for specific phenotypes in the zebrafish [1,4,5]. Structure–activity relationships (SARs) in zebrafish are also possible. In contrast to traditional *in vitro* SAR in cells or membranes where structural changes that improve potency are pursued (but changes might have detrimental effects on absorption or toxicity), SAR studies in zebrafish couple the analysis of binding affinity and ADME/toxicity.

The strength of the zebrafish resides in the analysis of phenotype. Perhaps no other organism (and certainly no vertebrate) is better suited to high-throughput phenotyping, and the scale that can be achieved in zebrafish experiments is impressive by vertebrate standards. Zebrafish have several inherent advantages for drug screening: they are small, inexpensive to maintain, and easily breed in large numbers. Breeding pairs can produce over 200 embryos each week that are fertilized outside of the mother and can be easily collected from the breeding tank. Embryonic development from a single cell, and the rapid formation of discrete tissues and organs with physiological similarity to their human counterparts, can be viewed in real time under a light microscope. Organ progenitors can be observed by 36 h postfertilization, and hatching occurs at 48–72 h postfertilization. By 120 h postfertilization, zebrafish develop discrete organs and tissues, including brain, heart, liver, pancreas, kidneys, intestines, bone, muscles, nerve systems, and sensory organs. Independent feeding occurs by 5 days postfertilization. Adult zebrafish are 3 cm long. Larvae, which are only 1–4 mm long, can live for 7 days in a single well of a standard 96- or 386-well microplate supported by nutrients stored in the yolk sac. Administration of drugs is simple: zebrafish larvae absorb small molecules diluted in the surrounding water through their skin and gills. The transparency of zebrafish for several days postfertilization enables *in vivo* observation of live or whole-mount fixed specimens, including the visualization of vital dyes, fluorescent tracers, antibodies, and riboprobes. In contrast to conventional *in vitro* assays using cultured cells, results obtained in zebrafish can be more predictive of results *in vivo* as they involve ADME properties. In this way, many of the *in vitro*/cell-based screens may fail to detect metabolic conversion into inactive and/or secretable compounds or, alternatively, conversion from inactive to active compounds (prodrugs). In contrast, compounds undergoing metabolic conversion are potentially identified in zebrafish screens.

Drug screening assays using zebrafish are becoming increasingly popular [6] and used as a platform for *in vivo* HTS drug discovery [7]. Zebrafish have been more and more used for toxicological assessment, particularly cardiotoxicity, hepatotoxicity, neurotoxicity, and developmental toxicity [8–11].

Unforeseen cardiotoxicity is a major problem that can result in drug withdrawal (e.g., cisapride, rofecoxib, and terfenadine). New compounds are usually screened in assays that measure cardiac electrophysiological activity in cells or in whole-animal mammalian models. Zebrafish offers an interesting alternative. The heart is the first organ to develop and function in zebrafish and a beating heart forms by 22 h postfertilization. By 48 h postfertilization, the cardiovascular system is fully functional and exhibits a complex repertoire of ion channels. Zebrafish ERG (ether-a-go-go-related gene) is expressed in the early stages of zebrafish development, and the amino acid sequences of the pore-forming domain of zebrafish ERG and human ERG are 99% conserved. The zebrafish have been shown to be an excellent model for assessing drug-induced cardiotoxicity, although zebrafish and mammalian hearts differ in structure and zebrafish lack a pulmonary system. However, they exhibit similar functional characteristics, including blood flow, valves, a rhythm regulated by electrical system, and heart beat associated with pacemaker activity. Cardiac functions such as heart rate, contractility, rhythmicity, and gross morphology can be visually assessed and some biomarkers can be evaluated using live animals at 48 h postfertilization using a dissecting microscope because they are transparent. Importantly, pharmacological responses to a number of well-characterized cardiotoxins are strikingly similar to responses in humans. hERG inhibitors and other drugs that produce prolongation of the QT interval in humans, which is associated with an increased risk for torsade de pointes (a serious heart arrhythmia that may lead to death), consistently cause bradycardia and 2:1 atrioventricular block in zebrafish embryos. Accordingly, these assays are simple and well suited for predicting adverse cardiotoxic drug effects in humans. Additionally, electrocardiograms in adult zebrafish have been done demonstrating that heart functions in adult zebrafish are similar to heart functions in humans [10,12].

Hepatotoxicity is also a major toxicological problem. Drug-induced hepatotoxicity is usually assayed *in vitro* using cytochromes, liver microsomes, or hepatocytes and *in vivo* in laboratory animals, by serum enzyme tests, hepatic excretory tests, assessment of alterations in the chemical constituents of the liver, and histological analysis. Again, zebrafish offer an interesting alternative as they exhibit mechanisms equivalent to mechanisms in mammals, including enzyme induction and oxidative stress as a general defense against xenobiotic chemicals [10,13]. Many zebrafish homologs of mammalian lipid metabolizing enzymes are present in the zebrafish liver. Since zebrafish complete primary liver morphogenesis by 48 h postfertilization and liver is fully formed and functioning by 72 h postfertilization, zebrafish can be used as a convenient model for assessing hepatotoxicity. Drug effects on zebrafish liver tissue, including liver necrosis, can be assessed visually as an initial screen for drug-induced hepatotoxicity. Histopathology can also be performed on zebrafish samples after drug treatment in adult animals. Liver function enzymes can be assessed in serum and enzyme reporter assays and cytochrome P450 assays (orthologs of CYP3A have been characterized in zebrafish) are also possible.

Neurotoxicity is another leading cause of drug withdrawal that can be assayed in zebrafish. Current approaches for assessing neurotoxicity use mammals and rely mainly on labor-intensive behavioral and morphological (neurohistopathology) assays. Zebrafish are transparent for several days postfertilization and specific neurons and axon tracts can be visualized *in vivo* using differential interference contrast microscopy or by injecting live dyes. In fact, the ability to examine the entire nervous system visually, including the brain, in live animals makes zebrafish a convenient model for assessing neurotoxicity. Specific types of neurons and glial cells as well as apoptotic and neurotoxicity markers can also be visualized in fixed intact zebrafish by immunohistochemistry or *in situ* hybridization. The small size of early-stage zebrafish permits performance of whole-animal assays in a 96-well microplate format for neurotoxicity screening. Finally, locomotor activity can be analyzed visually or by continuous image acquisition to assess the number of movements, duration, and distance traveled in a given time period. At the larval stage, locomotion occurs in short episodes punctuated by periods of rest and drug effects on locomotion can be evaluated, either by manual analysis or by using a program (ZebraZoom) to automatically track larvae, detect episodic movement, and extract large-scale statistics on motor patterns to produce a quantification of the locomotor repertoire in a high-throughput format, as required for large screens. Seizures in zebrafish have also been shown when treated with a convulsion-inducing agent [10,14,15].

Developmental toxicity can also be assessed in zebrafish. Established protocols used for assessing drug effects on reproduction and development involve some *in vitro* assays using cell cultures or rodent whole-embryo culture test, the *in vivo* frog embryo teratogenesis assay, and the gold standard assays exposing pregnant animals, usually rats or rabbits, to compounds and subsequently assessing toxic effects on fetuses. Zebrafish has been shown to be sensitive to compounds that exhibit teratogenicity *in vivo* in mammals and, in contrast to rodent embryo culture that is limited to early organogenesis, zebrafish embryos can be cultured up until advanced organogenesis to assess morphological and functional endpoints that are similar to those used in conventional mammalian reproductive toxicity studies. In addition, the zebrafish genome is well characterized, and dysmorphology phenotypes linked to genomic targets can potentially enable rapid identification of mechanisms of action for compound-induced teratogenicity [10,16]. In addition, approaches for assessing drug effects on apoptosis have been developed in transparent zebrafish using microscopy and morphometric image analysis, particularly in the context of developmentally regulated apoptosis. The effects of neuroprotectants in a chemical-induced disease model and the effects of radio-protectants in irradiated whole animals using a conventional 96-well microplate format have also been investigated [17].

Zebrafish have also emerged in the last decade as a valuable system for modeling human disease. New tools and methods for phenotypic screening, including zebrafish models, for different therapeutic indications have been developed. For example, the rewarding effect of drugs of abuse has been assessed in a conditioned place preference zebrafish model [18]. Psychotropic compounds, including hallucinogens, have been screened in both adult and larval zebrafish models [19]. Zebrafish embryos, in particular zebrafish dystrophin mutants, have been used to screen a chemical library of small molecules to identify compounds that modulate the muscle phenotype and ultimately discover novel human muscular dystrophy therapeutics [20]. Zebrafish models have also been proposed to study drug effects on cancer [21–23], serotonin syndrome [24], EAST (epilepsy, ataxia, sensorineural deafness, and tubulopathy) syndrome [25], cognitive function [26], bipolar disorder [27], epilepsy [28], modulation of appetite [29], and inflammation [30], among other diseases. Finally, robotic platforms for zebrafish handling/sorting at HTS scale [31] and methods for automatic capture and high-throughput phenotype analysis have been described [32].

Altogether, zebrafish is a unique vertebrate system that has become a widely used model organism because of its fecundity, its morphological and physiological similarity to mammals, the existence of many genomic tools, and the ease with which they can be manipulated by a range of forward and reverse genetics techniques to facilitate gene discovery and functional studies. The transparency of the embryo, external development, and the many hundreds of mutant and transgenic lines available add to the allure. In addition, zebrafish can be used for screening of compound libraries in the discovery process of promising new therapeutics: zebrafish and their embryos and larvae are small, easily accessible, and relatively low cost, making them pertinent for *in vivo*, whole-organism phenotype-based, high-content and high-throughput small-molecule screening in partially or fully automated drug screening platforms. Moreover, their physiological and developmental complexity provides accurate models of human disease to underpin mechanism of action and *in vivo* validation studies. Because of these attributes, the zebrafish might also provide opportunities to accelerate the process of drug discovery. Target identification and validation, assay development, disease modeling, chemical screens, SAR studies, lead compound discovery, and toxicology have been identified as main steps of the drug discovery and development process of pharmaceutical research where zebrafish can more likely contribute [1–3, 5–11,33–36]. Zebrafish embryo screens can be used in the preregulatory phases as an intermediate step between cell-based evaluation and conventional animal testing and can be very valuable to streamline the drug development timeline, discard compounds with potential toxicological problems, and prioritize drug candidates for animal testing, thus reducing the need for mammalian studies (i.e., reducing the number of compounds reaching conventional toxicological assessment in rodents and other mammals). While recognizing the growing importance of zebrafish, there are, however, several limitations and drawbacks in the zebrafish model. The main one is inherent to its ability as a model: the potential of zebrafish models as efficient preclinical models of disease and drug-induced states in humans needs/remains to be proven. Another is its very rapid development, which means that screening with zebrafish is analogous to "screening on a runaway train." Therefore, zebrafish embryos need to be precisely staged when used in acute assays, so as to ensure a consistent window of developmental exposure. As an additional limitation, it is important to note that highly hydrophobic compounds, large molecules, and proteins are not absorbed, and they need to be injected into the yolk sac, the sinus venosus, or the circulation. Drugs can also be delivered by oral intubation in adult zebrafish. It is also unclear how ADME after drug delivery in fish water compares with ADME after delivery by other routes of administration.

In addition, reported results show that there are some inter- and intralaboratory variations, confounding interpretation of drug-induced toxicity and limiting wider acceptance of this model organism. Further efforts are necessary to fully validate the model and for effective replacement of classical animal models.

3.2.2
D. melanogaster

For more than 100 years, Drosophila genetics has been a central contributor to research on inheritance and genome organization. In 1910, Morgan made the fortunate and historical decision to work on Drosophila based on their short life cycle and ease and low cost of maintenance. Within 10 years, Morgan and students formulated the central concepts of heredity and the first genetic maps. Fruit flies, in hindsight to Morgan, had fortuitous experimental properties of a very few (four) chromosomes and "polytene" chromosomes in the salivary gland. Polytene chromosomes have a reproducible banding pattern that reveals an unparalleled chromosomal cytology, allowing a physical map to be linked to a genetic map. In 1927, Muller introduced the use of ionizing radiation to cause genetic damage and to induce mutations, allowing chromosomal deletions, inversions, and duplications to be physically mapped on polytene chromosomes. By 1970, an ordered set of deletions and duplications covering 70% of the Drosophila chromosomes was already available, which laid the foundation of genetic screens that identified mutations with developmental phenotypes. By 2000, targeted gene disruption methods using gene replacement by homologous recombination and post-transcriptional RNAi techniques were developed to generate gene knockout phenotypes. To generate transgenic Drosophila, ectopic expression systems utilizing a promoter that drives either constitutive or regulated expression of the gene of interest (i.e., mutations generated by gene overexpression) have also been developed. In summary, since the work of Morgan, the fly community has continued a strong tradition of developing innovative research tools to dissect biological and genetic networks. Numerous mutant phenotypes have been discovered that disrupt developmental, physiological, and behavioral processes, and genes have been identified as responsible for the mutant phenotypes [37].

Drosophila offers many versatile advantages for target discovery and validation, including genome-wide genetic mutations and genome-wide expression studies. The convergence traditional tools with new advances are increasing the ease, speed, and value of Drosophila research. The complete sequence of the Drosophila genome is available from 2000. This information, combined with the ability to map genes and to study function by mutation or transgenesis, allows scientists to study the relationship of genotype with phenotype. A simple BLAST scan shows a sequence similarity of 50% between fly and mammalian proteins. Interestingly, 77% of human disease-associated genes are clearly related to genes in Drosophila, which indicates that genes important to human diseases, such as cancer, diabetes, and inflammation, are highly conserved from Drosophila to humans in both structure and function. The conservation of biological processes suggests that Drosophila research will be an important tool for human health. Nevertheless, comparative analysis of the genome of this model invertebrate organism reveals that about 30% of fly genes do not appear in sequences of yeast, worms, or mammals and are suspected to be insect specific. In addition, there are exceptions related to the distinct physiology that are not preserved across species. For example, flies have no erythrocytes and, therefore, hemoglobin homologs are absent [37].

Drosophila research has developed the versatile tools needed to understand the biological function of virtually every gene. The ability to screen thousands of mutations is an important approach toward identifying new genes important for a biological function. Initially, conventional genetic screens (genomes are mutagenized using chemicals or ionizing radiation to create random mutations) were performed to identify mutations that effect processes such as viability, morphogenesis, or determinate behaviors. Later, most genetic screens used targeted gene approaches and were developed to look for changes in specific cellular markers and molecular pathways. Today, the more common approaches to genetics screens are transposon-based genetic modifier screens, clonal screens, or a combination of any of these techniques [37].

Emerging genomic technologies are being applied in *Drosophila*. RNAi technologies are used as a "knockout" tool not only to study gene function but also to perform cell-based "genetic" screens as *Drosophila* cell-based systems are extremely amenable to RNAi (dsRNA added to *Drosophila* cell lines, even without transfection, is 95% effective in ablation of protein expression). The use of RNAi in S2 cells has allowed rapid and deep characterization of complex functions of proteins involved in a variety of signaling pathways. The combination of high-throughout RNAi and small-molecule screens also represents an interesting approach for drug target identification in *Drosophila* cells [38]. Transcriptional profiling using microarrays has also been developed in *Drosophila* and it represents an invaluable tool for comparing the RNA expression profiles of different samples. The advantage of using *Drosophila* is that a genome-wide expression analysis in most animal species tends to result in the detection of a vast number of genes that are differentially regulated, whereas, in *Drosophila*, experiments can be designed to compare samples that are carefully matched in terms of developmental stage and genetic background, which allows identification of true biologically relevant changes in gene expression [37].

D. melanogaster is a model system for drug discovery. The relevance of this small fruit fly is not limited to genetics-based target identification and validation. Chemical genetics as defined by using small molecules as probes of biological function is an emerging discipline that can be applied to *Drosophila* by designing drug screens based on the concept that, if a mutation in one gene makes animals resistant to a chemically induced phenotype, the chemical is likely to target the same biological network as the mutant gene product. Many examples of mutations in *Drosophila* orthologs of mammalian genes that are responsive to pharmacological agents have been found. The conservation of pharmacology combined with the genetic tools available in *Drosophila* can be used to identify the pathway of drug action.

Drosophila has been used as a model organism of a variety of human diseases, either to investigate the biological basis of the disease or to identify therapeutic drugs for the disease. Phenotypic screenings are feasible and a number of simple and robust behavioral assays for determining larval locomotion, adult climbing ability, or courtship behaviors of Drosophila have been developed [39].

In the cancer field, Drosophila has made seminal contributions to many of the pathways and mechanisms that are fundamental to the cancer process. In addition, some tumor suppressors were identified in flies and Drosophila is expected to make a major impact on drug discovery of anticancer drugs in the future [40,41]. Drosophila allows large-scale screening for rapid and economical identification of novel, bioavailable antitumor chemicals using in vivo tumor models. It has been demonstrated by using a Drosophila Ras-driven tumor model that tumor overgrowth can be curtailed by feeding larvae with chemicals that have the in vivo pharmacokinetics essential for drug development and known efficacy against human tumor cells. In a screen of 2000 compounds, a glutamine analog acivicin with known activity against human tumor cells was identified as a potent inhibitor of Drosophila tumor formation. Through RNAi-mediated knockdown of candidate acivicin target genes, an enzyme involved in pyrimidine biosynthesis was identified as a possible crucial target of acivicin-mediated inhibition. On this basis, Drosophila has been considered a powerful and economical tool for in vivo screening of large libraries for anticancer drug discovery [42].

D. melanogaster has been proposed to be a model organism to study obesity and insulin resistance [43]. Diet composition, alone and in combination with overall caloric intake, modulates fat deposition and also life span in flies [44]. Larvae reared on a high-sugar diet were hyperglycemic, insulin resistant, and accumulated fat (hallmarks of type 2 diabetes) compared with those reared on control diets. Excess dietary sugars, but not fats or proteins, elicited insulin-resistant phenotypes. Expression of genes involved in lipogenesis, gluconeogenesis, and β-oxidation was upregulated in high-sugar-fed larvae [45]. Regarding food intake, different studies highlight the conservation of molecular mechanisms controlling appetite in Drosophila and provide a method for unbiased whole-organism drug screens to identify novel drugs and molecular pathways modulating food intake. For example, a high-throughput whole-organism screen has been done in D. melanogaster larvae to identify drugs that modulate food intake. Metitepine, a nonselective serotonin (5-HT) receptor antagonist, was identified as a potent anorectic drug. By screening fly mutants for each of the 5-HT receptors, the serotonin receptor 5-HT2A was identified as the sole molecular target for feeding inhibition by metitepine [46].

Nociception, allowing animals to detect and avoid potentially harmful stimuli (i.e., warning of injury that should be avoided), serves an important protective function in animals that is under stringent evolutionary pressure and is evolutionarily conserved across species. Accordingly, D. melanogaster avoids noxious stimulus and can be used in nociception research. It is now considered as an emerging model organism for studying the conserved genetics of nociception, particularly with respect to recently developed high-throughput Drosophila "pain" paradigms using thermal and mechanical stimulation [47]. Genetic screening for mutants defective in noxious heat response has identified a gene, painless, that encodes a molecule distantly related to the human pain processing vanilloid receptor TRPV1 that is required for thermal and mechanical nociception, but not for sensing light touch, in *Drosophila* larvae [48]. Other genes, including TRPA1 and the Ca^{2+} channel straightjacket (stj; α2δ3 ortholog), have been identified using genome-wide neuron-specific RNAi knockdown based on avoidance of noxious heat in a behavioral paradigm in *Drosophila* [49,50]. Local and global methods of assessing thermal nociception and qualifying and quantifying nociceptive responses in *Drosophila* larvae have been described [51]. The thermal nocifensive response is also known to differ depending on the larval developmental stage [52]. Thermal allodynia and hyperalgesia following ultraviolet irradiation-induced tissue damage have also been shown in a *Drosophila* model following thermal nociceptive sensitization [53]. Moreover, pharmacological techniques and noxious heat were used to assay antinociceptive behavior in intact adult *Drosophila* [54]. *Drosophila* is thus an interesting, ethically acceptable animal model for combined genetic and pharmacological analgesia research.

In neurodegenerative diseases and psychiatric disorders, *Drosophila* has been instrumental in understanding disease mechanisms and pathways as well as being an efficient tool in drug discovery studies. Different strategies using *Drosophila* to study complex psychiatric disorders such as schizophrenia, autism, and attention-deficit hyperactivity disorder (ADHD) are available [55]. A *Drosophila* model of fragile X syndrome has been developed and used to assess the effects of treatments on multiple neural circuit morphological defects and to investigate mechanistic hypotheses [56]. Regarding memory, a circuitry of chemosensory processing, odor–tastant memory trace formation, and the "decision" process to behaviorally express these memory traces has been suggested from a series of behavioral experiments. Interaction between olfactory and gustatory pathways during the establishment and behavioral expression of odor–tastant memory traces was found to operate as a part of the chemobehavioral system in larval *Drosophila* [57]. Olfactory, visual, and place memory paradigms that restrict behavioral choice as well as genes involved in memory formation in the fly have been investigated [58]. *Drosophila* has also recently emerged as a model of Alzheimer's disease with neural features and assessable learning and memory. Transgenic flies that express human amyloid-β in the nervous system develop age-dependent short-term memory impairment and neurodegeneration [59]. In this way, two independent approaches, including synaptic plasticity-based analysis and behavioral screening of synthetic compounds, have been used for identifying compounds that are capable of rescuing the amyloid-β-induced memory loss in transgenic fruit fly [60]. Finally, a Parkinson's disease model *Drosophila* showing locomotor dysfunction as the age progresses has been developed by expressing normal human α-synuclein in the neurons. Measurement of the climbing ability of parkinsonian flies was used to evaluate the efficacy of the treatment added to the diet [61]. The "curative" effect of some treatments on the behavioral symptoms of the flies and on the α-syn aggregation in their brain has been investigated [62]. A transgenic *D. melanogaster* model of

Huntington's disease is also available and has been used to assess the therapeutic potential of treatments [63].

The fruit fly *D. melanogaster* has also become a valuable system to model the rewarding properties of drugs [64]. Cocaine induces motor behaviors in flies that are remarkably similar to those observed in mammals. Repeated cocaine administration also induces behavioral plasticity, and a key role for dopaminergic systems in mediating cocaine's effects has been demonstrated through both pharmacological and genetic methods. Interestingly, unbiased genetic screens have identified several novel genes and pathways in cocaine behaviors [65]. Regarding alcohol addiction, flies show hyperactivation upon exposure to a low to medium dose of alcohol, whereas high doses can lead to sedation. In addition, when given a choice, flies will actually prefer alcohol-containing food over regular food. Recent studies have demonstrated that the larvae of *Drosophila* show conserved alcohol tolerance and withdrawal phenotypes indicating that *Drosophila* genetics can be used in studying alcohol addiction. The genes and biochemical pathways implicated in controlling these behavioral responses in flies also participate in determining alcohol responses and drinking behavior in mammals [66,67].

Drosophila has also been used to discover new anti-infective drugs. Traditionally, chemical libraries are screened using *in vitro* culture systems to identify small molecules with antimicrobial properties. Nevertheless, almost all compounds passing through *in vitro* screening fail to pass preclinical trials. Drug screening in *Drosophila* offers the possibility to eliminate compounds that are toxic or have reduced bioavailability and identify others that may boost innate host defense or selectively reduce microbial virulence in a whole-organism setting [68–71]. Interestingly, several genetic screens for microbial pathogenicity in *Drosophila* identified virulence traits shown to be important for infection in mammals that may serve as targets for future drug development. In addition, conventional antimicrobial agents retain full activity in *Drosophila* infection models, which may pave the way for use of this minihost for high-throughput antimicrobial drug screening. Finally, the availability of genetic tools that allow for conditional inactivation of almost every gene in *D. melanogaster* is anticipated to result in the discovery of novel immunomodulatory mechanisms of action of newly identified antimicrobial compounds. Overall, the powerful genetics of and capacity for large-scale screening in this fly make this minihost a promising complementary model that may result in a new paradigm in antimicrobial drug discovery [72].

In conclusion, the common fruit fly *D. melanogaster* is a well-studied and highly tractable genetic model organism for understanding molecular mechanisms of human diseases. Many basic biological, physiological, and neurological properties are conserved between mammals and *Drosophila*, and nearly 75% of human disease-causing genes are believed to have a functional homolog in the fly. *Drosophila* research offers a mammalian relevant system where orthologous proteins can be studied by mutations and other genetic tricks to modify functional pathways to reveal their function. Once hooked into a pathway, many new genomic tools can be brought to bear on a problem. Advances in *Drosophila* research allow the combination of genome sequence information, genome-wide cDNA, mapping protein interactions, gene expression profile, and genome-wide mutations in an unprecedented dissection of a complex organism. The use of sophisticated genetic approaches combined with emerging genomic technologies suggests that the fly has much to offer as a tool for understanding basic cellular processes and provides an attractive and complex model system for exploring the molecular basis of human diseases and discovering new therapeutics. The incorporation of *Drosophila* into the therapeutic discovery process holds tremendous promise. *Drosophila* (as wild type or manipulated genetically or pharmacologically) has been proposed as a model organism to identify disease-causing genes/proteins (target identification) as well as drug therapeutics in a variety of diseases. *Drosophila* has emerged as an interesting whole-animal model of human diseases. This small fly provides several unique features such as powerful genetics, highly conserved disease pathways, and very low comparative costs. The fly can effectively be used in low- to high-throughput drug screens as well as in target discovery. However, drug discovery in such heterologous, phylogenetically disparate invertebrate as the fruit flies would still require further validation in mammalian models. Additional limitations include a lack of reliable tests to study complex disease phenotypes in flies and difficulties in translating disease symptoms into the animal model [37,73–75].

3.2.3
C. elegans

The small roundworm *C. elegans* has become a research tool, but with much less of a history and tradition in drug discovery than other model systems such as *Drosophila* or zebrafish (and of course rodents and other mammals). *C. elegans* was the first multicellular organism to have its genome completely sequenced [76] and along with the bacterial genome efforts served as a proving ground for the methods that were successfully utilized in the sequencing of the human genome. Preliminary analysis indicated that 74% of the human genome sequence had *C. elegans* matches [76] and this number does not take into account that DNA or amino acid alignments sometimes fail to detect conserved function and three-dimensional protein structure.

While containing a mere total of 959 somatic cells, this nematode contains complex structures, such as a digestive tract, a nervous system, muscles, and complex behaviors. The worm is optically clear, enabling the entire process of development to be visualized under the microscope, and is hermaphroditic, enabling genetically identical individuals to be cloned. *C. elegans* also has a rapid life span, with a 3- to 5-day life cycle depending on the temperature, with an individual worm being capable of producing more than 500 progeny over that period of time. They are inexpensive to grow. With their daily diet consisting of bacteria, they can be grown both on solid substrates such as agar and in liquid culture, the latter making them amenable to higher throughput handling appropriate for an industrial setting. The larval stages of *C. elegans* may also be frozen down, allowing the archiving of individual strains [37].

The availability of the genomic information has enabled the broader application of "reverse genetics" approaches to biological questions. Reverse genetics is a process that starts with a gene sequence and then investigates the function of that gene by removing it from an organism. In "forward genetics," one starts from a mutation and then progresses to revealing the gene responsible. The ability to know the function of every gene will be enormously useful in understanding human diseases and in identifying novel targets for drug discovery. However, finding the molecular target that is responsible for a disease or that mediates drug's effects is not an easy task. For instance, additional activities of the antidepressant fluoxetine (Prozac) were identified in *C. elegans* [77]. Fluoxetine is a known inhibitor of presynaptic reuptake of the neurotransmitter serotonin, but its complete mechanism of action involves other activities. Fluoxetine exerted a neuromuscular effect on *C. elegans* distinct from inhibition of serotonin reuptake. By screening for mutants resistant to this effect, a novel gene family that encodes over a dozen multipass transmembrane proteins was identified. Such type of information may have clinical implications for the mechanism of action of drugs and, interestingly, for the discovery of new molecular targets to develop novel treatments. The ability to find all of the potential targets of a given drug is a key advantage as many drugs that fail in clinical trials have strong efficacy but have intolerable side effects and, in many of these cases, the side effects are due to the interaction of the compound with multiple targets, some of which are responsible for the efficacy and some for the toxicity. The use of genetic systems to tease out all of the possible targets of a compound allows the design of specific secondary screens. Secondary screens enable the identification of more specific compounds that interact with and modify the beneficial targets only. The end result is less toxic, more efficacious drugs. *C. elegans* tools have become more sophisticated and faster over the last 5 years, and their application to gene function and drug discovery is just beginning to bear fruit. Novel tools for analyzing the result of loss of gene function and the ability to look at global protein–protein interactions and transcript levels on a whole-genome scale will be drivers of future discoveries in *C. elegans* [37].

In addition to genetic studies, this nematode has been used as a model for human disease and pathway identification in some therapeutic areas, including cancer (e.g., oncogenes discovered in *C. elegans* have been involved in the control of cell growth and transgenic worms have been generated that harbor wild-type or mutant forms of genes involved in human cancer to rapidly assess the role of cancer-specific gene mutations in the context of a whole organism) [78] and aging and age-related disorders (e.g., environmental factors and genetic manipulations that control the longevity in *C. elegans* have been identified) [79]. Its use has also been described in toxicology (neurotoxicology, reproductive and developmental toxicology, and environmental toxicology), for both mechanistic studies and HTS approaches, including genome-wide screening for molecular targets of toxicity and rapid toxicity assessment for new chemicals. This could hopefully lead to an increased use of *C. elegans* in complementing other model systems in toxicological research [80]. *C. elegans* is also a suitable host model for the evaluation and characterization of antimicrobial drug effects and a number of innovative antimicrobial drug screens have been carried out successfully in *C. elegans* [81]. Classical identification of new drugs with antimicrobial activities is done by screening large libraries of molecules directly for their capacity to block the growth of bacterial or fungal monocultures. However, both the efficacy and its potential cytotoxicity are assessed by using *C. elegans* as an *in vivo* infection system. In addition, infection of *C. elegans* induces a number of defense mechanisms, some of which are similar to those seen in mammalian innate immunity. Furthermore, it has been demonstrated that several microbial virulence mechanisms required for full pathogenicity in mammals are also necessary for infection in nematodes. Other utility is the study of the nervous system as *C. elegans* has a nervous system that mediates a large number of complex behaviors, including responses to mechanical and environmental stimuli. The nervous system of *C. elegans* utilizes many of the same neurotransmitters, such as acetylcholine, dopamine, and GABA, and *C. elegans* does respond to many of the drugs that affect the chemistry of the human brain [37]. In the case of Alzheimer's disease, *C. elegans* homologs of human presenilin genes allowed the biological function of the mutant human presenilin genes to be investigated. In addition, *in vivo* screening in *C. elegans* has been described as a drug discovery approach in Alzheimer's disease. In brief, accumulation of amyloid-β within the brain is a hallmark in Alzheimer's disease and, although various *in vitro* and cell-based models have been proposed for high-throughput drug screening, *C. elegans* offers a convenient *in vivo* system for rapid and cheap examination of amyloid-β accumulation and toxicity in a complex multicellular organism. For this purpose, a new transgenic strain of *C. elegans* that expresses full-length amyloid-β was generated. The amyloid-β accumulates *in vivo* and stains positive for amyloid dyes, consistent with *in vivo* fibril formation. Interestingly, PBT2, an investigational therapeutic shown to be neuroprotective in mouse models of Alzheimer's disease and significantly improve cognition in patients, provided rapid and significant protection against the amyloid-β-induced toxicity in *C. elegans* [82]. Currently, *C. elegans* has numerous models of both amyloid-β- and tau-induced toxicity, the two prime components observed to correlate with Alzheimer's disease pathology, and these models have been applied to the discovery of numerous Alzheimer's disease-modulating candidates [83].

In summary, nematode worm *C. elegans* is a simple model organism that provides attractive platforms for devising and streamlining efficient drug target identification and drug discovery. Its biology has been investigated to an exceptional level. This, coupled with effortless handling, a notable low cost of cultivation and maintenance, and the ease of performing *in vivo* whole live animal HTS as well as genetic manipulations and biochemical studies to identify proteins targeted by specific drugs and molecular pathways involved in the mechanism of drug action, makes *C. elegans* well positioned to aid in the discovery of new therapies [84–87]. On the downside, protein divergence between invertebrates and humans and the difficulty to model complex diseases and translate findings to humans are main limitations. In any case, invertebrate model organisms such as *C. elegans* are an imperfect yet much needed tool to bridge the gap between traditional *in vitro* and preclinical animal assays.

3.3
In Vivo Exploratory and Experimental Human Models

> "Today's drug discovery and development paradigm is not working, and something needs to be done about it (. . .) Such failure was due, at least in part, to the failure of experiments on animals to predict out-comes in human patients (. . .) It may well be that the drug mechanisms for which animals can provide some useful prediction of potential efficacy and safety in man have already been exploited, so the proportion for which they are less useful, or even frankly misleading, is increasing (. . .) So, if animals can no longer be relied upon, what alternatives are there? I suggest that the answer, at least in principle, is startlingly simple: We should focus on the target species, i.e. humans" [88].

On this basis, Coleman [88] has proposed to move away from reliance on animal surrogates and focus on biological *in vitro* tests using human biomaterials (human cells, tissues, and even organs). This approach benefits from the availability of advanced technologies to assay such biomaterials *in vitro*, analyze data, and construct *in silico* models based on the ever-increasing amount of human data available. However, this approach has several limitations. There are disease conditions that are too complex and/or intractable to lend themselves to a relatively simple *in vitro* approach, and where *in vivo* studies in nonhuman species seem the only way forward. Such approaches are also expensive and low throughput (although there is nothing more expensive and delaying in drug discovery and development than getting a wrong answer). At the logistic level, there is an additional difficulty as such an approach requires biomaterial obtained from clinical volunteers or patient donors of cells, tissue, and organs following surgery or postmortem [88,89]. In any case, *in vitro* methods using human biomaterial actually represent a very interesting alternative to replace and ultimately reduce the use of animals in drug discovery and development (see *in vivo* alternatives in Chapter 2).

There are many ways in which human biology can be accessed and exploited for the purpose of the discovery and development of more efficacious and safer medicines. Information coming from observations in the human domain and clinical practice, mainly based on the unexpected effect of natural products or drugs developed for other diseases, has played a major role in the discovery of new medicines and repositioning of known ones to new indications. In fact, human models, in particular pharmacologically induced human models, although unintended most of the time, have hugely contributed to the understanding of disease pharmacology. For instance, the major neuropharmacological theories of schizophrenia have their origins in studies of the effects of drugs of abuse in humans. Research into the effects of LSD initiated the serotonergic model, amphetamines the dopamine hypothesis, and PCP and ketamine the glutamatergic hypothesis of schizophrenia [90].

This chapter and this section in particular deal with the intended use of *in vivo* human models. These are collectively recognized as exploratory and experimental human trials. They are not a part of the classical pathway involving phase I–IV clinical studies on human volunteers and patients, but they may provide valuable answers to some relevant questions regarding the suitability of the pharmacological properties of drug leads or candidates in humans or the drug's mechanism of action. They are also convenient to identify disease biomarkers for diagnostic purposes or to monitor disease progression and therapeutics.

Exploratory investigational studies with new drugs, the so-called phase 0 studies, can be done before traditional phase I trials. In many cases, for the purpose of phase 0 exploratory, first-in-human trials, subtherapeutic doses of the new drug are given to a small group of patients (typically fewer than 15 human volunteers) for roughly a week at a maximum to determine basic pharmacokinetic (PK) properties. No therapeutic benefit can be conferred by the small doses given in such phase 0 studies, and while taking part patients are not allowed to enroll in a trial with therapeutic intent.

The recognition by drug regulatory agencies of exploratory pre-phase I studies (now the term phase 0 studies has been coined) is a stepping stone in the direction of obtaining human data in the preclinical stage. Because exploratory studies present fewer potential risks than do traditional phase I studies that look for dose-limiting toxicities, exploratory investigations can be initiated with less or different preclinical support than is required for traditional studies with new drugs. Exploratory human studies can have multiple goals: understanding mechanism of action, PK, or lead compound selection. The main aim is to help identify, early in the process, promising candidates for continued development and eliminate those lacking promise. Different examples of exploratory investigational new drug application studies are considered by the FDA:

- Microdosing studies, which involve single exposure to microgram quantities of test compounds, designed to evaluate drug PK or imaging of specific targets, but not to induce pharmacological effects.
- Trials to study pharmacological effects of candidate compounds. Since such studies would involve pharmacologically relevant doses, they would require more extensive preclinical support than would microdose studies.
- Clinical studies to evaluate mechanism of action.

It is important to note that conducting such exploratory studies is an option and not a requirement by regulatory authorities, that the scope is limited to a few purposes under singular scenarios, and that ethical issues have also arisen. However, the benefits are clear: earlier (before formal phase I studies) identification of drugs with the good or wrong (e.g., unsuitable PK in human) profile would increase the efficiency of drug development, making drugs available to patients sooner and at reduced costs.

Pre-phase I trials were not unheard before the term phase 0 was coined, but they were rare. Nowadays, in spite of limitations, exploratory/experimental studies in humans are increasingly done for multiple purposes. These include exploratory phase 0 studies, but also investigational studies after phase I (or after a more extensive, phase I-like safety/tox preclinical support has been obtained) that aim to get data predictive of drug effects (before phase II clinical trials) or explore the drug's mechanism of action, or even drug-free studies to explore disease mechanisms or to identify disease biomarkers. This is in a way gradually shifting the focus of early drug development away from animal studies toward safe and ethical studies in human, which could also yield more relevant and reliable data (at least in terms of translation and species differences-related issues). This enables go/no-go decisions to be based also on human models and not only on animal data. In the context of replacement, this approach represents an attractive alternative, and regarding reduction of studies with animals, exploratory and experimental studies in humans would reduce the number of animals ultimately needed to select an appropriate clinical candidate. The number of human subjects ultimately needed would also be reduced. In the following sections, we will briefly review two of the most common uses of *in vivo* human models in drug development.

3.3.1
Phase 0 (Exploratory Human Models): Microdosing Studies

The concept of microdosing first appeared in the late 1990s as a method of assessing human pharmacokinetics prior to full phase I clinical trials [91] and the first data appeared in the literature in 2003 [92].

A 2001 workshop, organized by Volunteers in Research and Testing in the United Kingdom, addressed the possibility of conducting early human studies using microdosing techniques (exploratory IND, phase 0 or pre-phase I studies) to replace laboratory animals [93]. It was considered that conducting pre-phase I studies, very low dose human studies could enable drug candidates to be assessed earlier for *in vivo* human pharmacokinetics and metabolism, on the basis of a reduced preclinical animal toxicity package. Moreover, accelerator mass spectrometry (AMS), nuclear magnetic resonance (NMR) spectroscopy, and positron emission tomography (PET) were presented as potentially useful spectrometric and imaging methods enabling microdosing studies. These studies would permit less promising compounds to be eliminated and promising candidates to be selected before extensive animal tests begin and before exposing humans to escalating dose studies in classical phase I trials. Phase 0 studies would also enable early rational selection of the appropriate species for subsequent animal tests, on the basis of human pharmacokinetic and metabolic data.

The workshop proposed that very early studies in volunteers would be conducted using microdoses, calculated to be subtoxic and also below the dose threshold for measurable pharmacological or clinical activity. A microdose was defined as "the lowest dose in human subjects that yields useful data by whatever analytical method is used (e.g., depending on detection limits). This would not exceed 1% of the minimum pharmacologically active dose obtained from the most sensitive pharmacological model. In the absence of these data, the microdose would not exceed 1 μg per person." The workshop considered that microdosing studies in healthy volunteers, providing *in vivo* human ADME data, should be introduced into the drug development process where they add value to a compound's selection or subsequent development, or where they lead to a reduction in animal use, without compromising the scientific quality of the data obtained [93].

The regulatory authorities in Europe, the United States, and Japan have introduced new guidelines describing the steps necessary to conduct human microdosing studies with limited safety studies in animals: a position paper from the European Medicines Agency in 2004 [94], guidelines from the FDA in 2006 [95], and guidance from Japanese Ministry of Health, Labor and Welfare in 2008 [96]. These efforts were then standardized through a multidisciplinary scientific guideline following agreement on a harmonized approach between Europe, the United States, and Japan by the International Conference on Harmonisation of Technical Requirements for Registration of Pharmaceuticals for Human Use [97].

Currently, microdosing methodology is referred to as a new viable "tool" in the drug development "toolbox." Phase 0 studies represent the first administration of the novel agent to humans, at limited doses (less than 1/100 of the test substance calculated to yield a pharmacological effect, with a maximum dose of 100 μg), on a small number of patients (often $n < 10$) and over a short period (<7 days). In microdosing studies, with drug levels in the picogram to femtogram range, pharmacokinetic analysis requires positron emission tomography or accelerator mass spectrometry – techniques that rely on the assessment and analysis of radioisotopes incorporated into the test drug (e.g., carbon-14) [92].

The main objective of microdosing studies is to validate preclinical development in order to better justify the scientific rationale [98,99]. The original concept of microdosing was to provide PK data as early as possible in humans, which could be used to assess the PK at higher therapeutic doses. Microdosing trials are thus designed to evaluate PK, bioavailability, metabolism, and/or distribution of a drug or its metabolite. The properties of two or more structurally similar analogs aimed at the same molecular target can be determined. Based on a recent review, there are currently a total 35 compounds where microdose and therapeutic dose data have been compared (oral and intravenous, human and animal). Of the 35 compounds (human and animal), 27 tested orally (79%) and 100% of those tested intravenously showed scalable PK between a microdose and a therapeutic dose [99].

Besides purely PK prediction, microdosing is now being extended into other areas of drug development. In fact, the application of microdosing as a tool in drug development is expanding into different and hitherto unexpected fields [100]. The technique has been extended to assess the magnitude of potential drug–drug interactions and early indications of the metabolic profile of the drug as well as in the study of polymorphisms and transporters. Microdosing can also be used to assess if the drug is reaching its intended target tissues in human subjects [99]. In addition, microdosing emerges as an attractive approach for the study of new and existing drugs in vulnerable populations (children, pregnant women, elderly, and hepatically and renally impaired), who are routinely excluded from clinical trials due to safety concerns [99]. Exploration of the utility of microdosing in vulnerable populations will likely become attractive with regulatory and societal pressures increasing in favor of equity of science and therapeutic development.

In addition to microdosing studies, originally described as clinical trials to determine drug PK, phase 0 studies also include (1) clinical trials to establish pharmacologically relevant doses and (2) clinical trials to study the mechanisms of action. In the first case, phase 0 trials are used to determine a dose regimen for molecular targeted compounds or biomodulators meant for use along with other drugs such as conventional chemotherapeutic agents. They do not determine the maximum tolerated dose, but they can be designed to determine a sequence of administration and a dose range for subsequent combination trials [101,102]. In the last type of phase 0 trials, the mechanisms of action of drugs are related to drug efficacy (the PD effect of a drug is thereby evaluated). It especially holds significance in the field of oncology for the evaluation of molecular targeted chemotherapeutic drugs [101–103].

Phase 0 microdosing trials have potential for improving the efficiency of drug development, although they do not replace traditional phase 1 trials [103] and do not provide any evidence for clinical efficacy and safety. However, industry is increasingly accepting the phase 0 concept to identify promising agents, with many pharmaceutical giants becoming pioneers in this field [104]. Phase 0 studies also open an opportunity for research-based small biotech companies by early demonstration of proof of principle for speedy development of own molecules or to attract investors for further clinical development [102]. However, both benefits and limitations need to be considered (Table 3.1). Maximum benefit of phase 0 trials could be realized by identifying the most promising candidate or relatively promising candidates, establishing PK–PD correlation for the candidate, use of phase 0 results in go/no-go decision making, logical selection of combination regimens, and design of further clinical trials. As phase 0 trials enable assessing human PK and PD very early in the development process, it is hoped that these can be an effective addition to drug development armamentarium [105].

Microdosing studies enable testing times and costs to be reduced. The cost involved in typical toxicology and phase I studies for a new drug is estimated to be 4–6 million dollars [106]; therefore, the cost saved, even after considering the phase 0 cost, would be significant by eliminating the poor molecules in addition to even larger time and opportunity cost. In a human microdose study, a subpharmacologically active dose of drug is administered and samples (typically plasma) are collected and analyzed for parent drug or metabolites. Since the very small doses administered are of low toxicological risk (the potential for adverse side effect to a human subject in the clinical study is considered to be minimal), regulatory agencies allow a microdose to be administered to human subjects based upon a reduced safety package compared with that required for a full phase I clinical trial

Table 3.1 Benefits and limitations of phase 0 clinical trials.

Benefits
- Explore clinical characteristics of a candidate agent with very low number of patients in a short duration of time
- Could improve success rate of overall new drug development
- Guide go/no-go decisions for subsequent clinical development
- Provide better approximation of active and safe starting dose for phase 1 trials
- Could expedite clinical development bypassing single-drug phase 1 studies, better informed designs of later clinical studies, and use of biomarkers
- Serve as a candidate selection tool by distinguishing most promising candidate from a set of analogs
- By early elimination of non-promising molecules could save valuable patient resources; cost, time, and resources
- Shift resource utilization toward promising candidates
- Require lesser preclinical testing data than what is mandated for traditional phase 1 studies
- Closely related agents can be evaluated under single exploratory IND
- Provide opportunity to develop potential biomarkers
- Decrease human toxicity due to minute dose of the test substance and shorter duration of administration/exposure to the drug (since they mostly involve a single-dose administration compared with a dose escalation study in the traditional phase 1 trials)
- Less number of humans/animals are used
- Small quantity of the test drug is required
- Test drug may be prepared as per the principles of the good laboratory practices unlike good manufacturing practices compliance as required for the traditional phase 1 studies
- Any route of administration is possible
- Drug can be assessed in vulnerable patients such as patients with renal impairment, women in their reproductive age, cancer patients, and so on
- Assessment of the test drug for its modulator effects on the targets in a tumor
- Select the best animal species for the long-term toxicological studies based on the inference drawn from the MD metabolite profiling data
- Reduce overall cost of conducting a microdosing study compared with that of a conventional phase 1 study

Limitations
- Nonlinear PK, if exists, can pose problems for dose extrapolations
- False-negative results can lead to discontinuation of promising candidates
- Every drug may not be a suitable candidate for phase 0 trials
- Absence of any therapeutic and/or diagnostic intent
- Motivating volunteers to become a part of the trial is difficult as there is no therapeutic intent
- Very few validated biomarkers are available for predicting the anticancer activity
- Ultrasensitive and high-tech equipment such as AMS and PET are required, which are scarcely available
- Predicting the absorption characteristics at the microdose levels is challenging since certain drugs dissolve easily at low doses; however, they display limited solubility at higher doses
- Unnecessarily extend the process and increase the expenditure as phase I study still needs to be carried out

(i.e., normally with no genotoxicity investigations and a single-dose rodent toxicology study) [107]. As a result, only an abridged nonclinical package is required to support a microdosing clinical study. This makes the microdosing concept attractive when a speedy decision on drug candidate selection around PK and drug metabolism is critical, particularly when clear decisions cannot be made based on *in vivo* animal and *in vitro* preclinical PK data.

The microdosing approach offers the opportunity of early human screening of many more drug candidates offering greater predictability versus animal and/or *in vitro* models. Hence, human microdosing studies offer the promise of (1) improved candidate selection, (2) reduced attrition rates, (3) safer clinical studies, and (4) a potential reduction in the use of animals in early clinical development. The microdosing approach could by this means potentially reduce the time of preclinical testing from 12–18 to 6–8 months and cut down the associated expenses by 10 times [99,108,109]. The comparison between microdosing and conventional studies in drug development is given in Table 3.2.

Table 3.2 Comparison of microdosing strategy with conventional studies.

Features	Microdosing strategy	Conventional approach
Time from selection of preclinical candidate to finalized first-time-in-man study	5–8 months	12–18 months
Cost from selection of preclinical candidate to finalized first-time-in-man study	$0.3–0.5 million	$1.5–3.0 million
Minimum amount of compound required and qualification	<100 mg in GLP quality only	~100 g (GMP qualified for phase I)
Predictive power for pharmacokinetic parameters at pharmacologically effective doses	Generally good if mass effects and/or protein binding make no significant contributions	Definite
Need for ^{14}C-labeled compound for first-time-in-man study	Yes (if AMS is used), no (if LC–MS/MS is used)	No
Available options for outsourcing	Use of AMS requires certification of clinical CRO for ^{14}C work; analytics restricted to a handful of highly specialized providers	Huge number of certified preclinical and clinical CROs and analytical laboratories in all major pharmaceutical markets
Standardization and degree of establishment of regulatory path	Very new – authorities and developers are on a learning curve; US and European regulations not identical in some points	Firmly established and internationally harmonized through ICH guidelines; few if any variations possible

Microdosing not only allows selection of drug candidates more likely to be developed successfully but also helps in determination of the first dose for the subsequent phase I clinical studies. Microdosing is thus a promising front-runner in the search for alternatives to animals in drug discovery and development and, if scientifically validated, it has potential advantages for animals, patients, and the pharmaceutical companies developing life-saving drugs for the future [109]. Stakeholders (regulatory, industry, and academia) should collaborate to systematically validate microdosing as a drug development approach. In a recent study, Yamane et al. [110] assessed the cost effectiveness of three microdose-integrated strategies (categorized by analytical methods: microdose-LC–MS/MS, microdose-AMS, and microdose-PET) compared with a conventional drug development strategy without microdose clinical trials. They showed that in a hypothetical scenario where 100 drug candidates were selected under either one of the three microdose-integrated strategies or a conventional one, the incremental cost effectiveness ratio per one additional drug approval was JPY 12.6–12.9 billion, which was lower than the threshold (JPY 24.4 billion), suggesting that implementing microdosing clinical trials would be cost effective.

In summary, microdosing has reached its first decade and at present it does have a place in drug development. It may provide human data to a phase of development where the majority of decision making is currently based on nonhuman data. The concept has been extended from a purely PK predictive method toward addressing other questions, such as drug–drug interactions, polymorphism, and looking at whether a drug is likely to reach its site of action. Moreover, microdosing is an attractive approach for the study of new and existing drugs in vulnerable populations (children, pregnant women, elderly, and hepatically and renally impaired), who are routinely excluded from clinical trials due to safety concerns. Microdosing may yet have more to offer in unanticipated directions and provide benefits that have not been fully realized to date.

3.3.2
Phase IB/IIA (Proof-of-Concept) Studies: Experimental Human Models

Formal traditional phase I clinical trials are designed to assess the safety, tolerability, PK, and some basic PD of a drug. For this purpose, the drug is tested for dose ranging on healthy volunteers (usually 20–100) at ascending doses until precalculated PK levels are reached or intolerable side effects start showing up (at which point the drug is said to have reached the maximum tolerated dose). Phase I typically includes single and multiple ascending dose studies as well as investigation of the food effect on the absorption of the drug. In contrast, phase II studies are designed to assess if and how well the drug works, as well as to continue phase I safety assessments. Phase II studies are thus powered to detect a clinically significant improvement in patients (usually 100–300), often utilizing multiple dose arms (including placebo) and multiple clinical sites. Phase II studies are sometimes divided into phase IIA and phase IIB. Phase IIA is specifically designed to assess dosing requirements (how much drug should be given). Phase IIB is specifically designed to study efficacy (how well the drug works at the prescribed dose).

In 1997, Sheiner [111] identified two distinct activities in clinical development: learning and confirming, each with different goals, study designs, and analysis modes. Whereas the traditional, confirmatory approach to clinical drug development is useful to categorize activities, learning trials aim to understand a new drug candidate to maximize its medical value and determine whether it justifies continued investment. Recommendations including adjustments in dose level or refinements in formulation or patient subgroups could also be done based on learning. Because key hypotheses are tested during the learning trials, these trials are smaller, more flexible, and able to adapt to the evolving clinical safety and efficacy data than are the traditional confirmatory phase I and phase II trials. On this basis, confirmatory trials represent a cost-effective verification of the knowledge derived in the learning trials about the drug's safety, efficacy, and, ultimately, ability to serve an unmet clinical need.

Learning trials are done frequently at the "interphase" between formal, traditional, confirmatory phase I and II clinical trials, with wide variation in practice as to what is done, with both healthy volunteers and patient populations, before going on to full phase II studies [112]. Model-based methods are commonly used for learning (i.e., establishing proof of concept) in phases IB–IIA biopharmaceutical developments. It is important to have a clear understanding that clinical trials performed for learning are not pivotal, confirmatory (regulatory) trials and that the data, ultimately, are for gaining incremental knowledge to advance (or not) compounds (i.e., internal decision-making purposes). For instance, in the case of a compound acting on a novel target, this period before full phase II trials is argued to be the phase during which exploratory work for learning should be done [111]. The improved performance of healthy subjects, exposed or not to a mechanistic, disease-related manipulation (i.e., experimental human model), would be a surrogate for improvement in disease at the appropriate dose. In the more usual case of a variation on an existing mechanism, this is the period to verify which dose produces the desired effect so as to move as quickly as possible into phase II trials with doses that one is confident will work. In the latter instance, a direct accessible biochemical measure or the occurrence of a drug class-related behavior becomes a surrogate for an effect that is hypothesized to produce the clinical benefit. Biomarkers and surrogate markers providing a prognostic indication of a clinically relevant endpoint are very valuable and are increasingly used in proof-of-concept phase IB/IIA studies [113]. Unfortunately, good surrogates and biomarkers for drug development are not always available (in fact, they are essentially missing for many important clinical indications).

A wide variety of experimental human models have been developed in healthy volunteers. These include experimental gingivitis model, experimental models of inflammation and allergic responses, experimental endotoxemia model, experimental bacterial and viral infection/challenge models, experimental headache, experimental dyspnea, experimental upper airway obstruction, experimental acute stress model, experimental increase of intraocular pressure, experimental model of insomnia, and experimental models of hyperalgesia and pain (see, for example, clinicaltrials.gov; advanced search query: "experimental" and "model" in title section). Numerous clinical trials have been done in these experimental human disease models mainly to assess and anticipate the effect of pharmacological interventions but also for other purposes, including understanding disease-underlying biological mechanisms or biomarker investigation. Experimental interventions to induce the clinical model are very variable: no oral hygiene (e.g., gingivitis model), administration or injection of chemicals or biologics (e.g., endotoxemia model), or application of external stimuli (e.g., pain models).

As a case example, human experimental pain models represent one of the most extended uses of experimental models in humans. Human experimental pain models are widely used both to understand pain mechanisms and to test analgesic compounds. They are particularly relevant for both the clinician and the scientist as they allow exploring the effect of specific treatments on different pain-generating mechanisms and hence reach a pain treatment tailored to each individual patient and pain characteristics. Experimental pain models offer the possibility to explore the pain system under controlled settings. Experimental models to evoke pain and hyperalgesia are available for most tissues. Standardized stimuli of different modalities (i.e., mechanical, thermal, electrical, or chemical) can be applied to sensitized or nonsensitized skin, muscles, and viscera for a differentiated and comprehensive assessment of various pain pathways and mechanisms. In healthy volunteers, the effect of acetaminophen is difficult to detect unless neurophysiological methods are used, whereas the effect of nonsteroidal anti-inflammatory drugs could be detected in most models. Anticonvulsants and antidepressants are sensitive in several models, particularly in models inducing hyperalgesia. For opioids, tonic pain with high intensity is attenuated more than short-lasting pain and nonpainful sensations. In general, the sensitivity to analgesics is better in patients than in healthy volunteers, but the lower number of studies may bias the results. However, what about their value to translate basic science to clinical pain research? Are models actually predictive of analgesic efficacy of a drug for a particular condition? Experimental models have variable reliability, and validity should be interpreted with caution. The validity of the prediction increases with the increase in the number of analgesic drug classes tested. Models including deep, tonic pain and hyperalgesia are better to predict the effects of analgesics. From available evidence, only five clinical pain conditions were correctly predicted by seven different pain models for at least three different drugs. Assessment with neurophysiological methods and imaging is valuable as a supplement to psychophysical methods and can increase sensitivity. Altogether, human experimental pain models have value to link animal and clinical pain studies, providing new possibilities for designing successful clinical trials. However, current human pain models cannot replace patient studies for studying efficacy of analgesic compounds, although being helpful for proof-of-concept studies and dose finding [114–119].

References

1 Zon, L.I. and Peterson, R.T. (2005) *In vivo* drug discovery in the zebrafish. *Nature Reviews. Drug Discovery*, **4** (1), 35–44.

2 Lieschke, G.J. and Currie, P.D. (2007) Animal models of human disease: zebrafish swim into view. *Nature Reviews. Genetics*, **8** (5), 353–367.

3 Gibert, Y., Trengove, M.C., and Ward, A.C. (2013) Zebrafish as a genetic model in preclinical drug testing and screening. *Current Medicinal Chemistry*, **20** (19), 2458–2466.

4 Taylor, K.L., Grant, N.J., Temperley, N.D., and Patton, E.E. (2010) Small molecule screening in zebrafish: an *in vivo* approach to identifying new chemical tools and drug leads. *Cell Communication and Signaling*, **8**, 11.

5 Peterson, R.T. and Fishman, M.C. (2011) Designing zebrafish chemical screens. *Methods in Cell Biology*, **105**, 525–541.

6 Chakraborty, C., Hsu, C.H., Wen, Z.H., Lin, C.S., and Agoramoorthy, G. (2009) Zebrafish: a complete animal model for *in vivo* drug discovery and development. *Current Drug Metabolism*, **10** (2), 116–124.

7 Delvecchio, C., Tiefenbach, J., and Krause, H.M. (2011) The zebrafish: a powerful platform for *in vivo*, HTS drug discovery. *Assay and Drug Development Technologies*, **9** (4), 354–361.

8 Rubinstein, A.L. (2006) Zebrafish assays for drug toxicity screening. *Expert Opinion on Drug Metabolism and Toxicology*, **2** (2), 231–240.

9 Barros, T.P., Alderton, W.K., Reynolds, H.M., Roach, A.G., and Berghmans, S. (2008) Zebrafish: an emerging technology for *in vivo* pharmacological assessment to identify potential safety liabilities in early drug discovery. *British Journal of Pharmacology*, **154** (7), 1400–1413.

10 McGrath, P. and Li, C.Q. (2008) Zebrafish: a predictive model for assessing drug-induced toxicity. *Drug Discovery Today*, **13** (9–10), 394–401.

11 Sipes, N.S., Padilla, S., and Knudsen, T.B. (2011) Zebrafish: as an integrative model for twenty-first century toxicity testing. *Birth Defects Research Part C: Embryo Today*, **93** (3), 256–267.

12 Chico, T.J., Ingham, P.W., and Crossman, D.C. (2008) Modeling cardiovascular disease in the zebrafish. *Trends in Cardiovascular Medicine*, **18** (4), 150–155.

13 He, J.H., Guo, S.Y., Zhu, F., Zhu, J.J., Chen, Y.X., Huang, C.J., Gao, J.M., Dong, Q.X., Xuan, Y.X., and Li, C.Q. (2013) A zebrafish phenotypic assay for assessing drug-induced hepatotoxicity. *Journal of Pharmacological and Toxicological Methods*, **67** (1), 25–32.

14 Selderslaghs, I.W., Hooyberghs, J., Blust, R., and Witters, H.E. (2013) Assessment of the developmental neurotoxicity of compounds by measuring locomotor activity in zebrafish embryos and larvae. *Neurotoxicology and Teratology*, **37**, 44–56.

15 Mirat, O., Sternberg, J.R., Severi, K.E., and Wyart, C. (2013) ZebraZoom: an automated program for high-throughput behavioral analysis and categorization. *Frontiers in Neural Circuits*, **7**, 107.

16 Ducharme, N.A., Peterson, L.E., Benfenati, E., Reif, D., McCollum, C.W., Gustafsson, J.A., and Bondesson, M. (2013) Meta-analysis of toxicity and teratogenicity of 133 chemicals from zebrafish developmental toxicity studies. *Reproductive Toxicology (Elmsford, NY)*, **41**, 98–108.

17 McGrath, P. and Seng, W.L. (2013) Use of zebrafish apoptosis assays for preclinical drug discovery. *Expert Opinion on Drug Discovery*, **8** (10), 1191–1202.

18 Collier, A.D. and Echevarria, D.J. (2013) The utility of the zebrafish model in conditioned place preference to assess the rewarding effects of drugs. *Behavioural Pharmacology*, **24** (5–6), 375–383.

19 Neelkantan, N., Mikhaylova, A., Stewart, A.M., Arnold, R., Gjeloshi, V., Kondaveeti, D., Poudel, M.K., and Kalueff, A.V. (2013) Perspectives on zebrafish models of hallucinogenic drugs and related psychotropic compounds. *ACS Chemical Neuroscience*, **4** (8), 1137–1150.

20 Kawahara, G. and Kunkel, L.M. (2013) Zebrafish based small molecule screens for novel DMD drugs. *Drug Discovery Today: Technologies*, **10** (1), e91–e96.

21 Jung, D.W., Oh, E.S., Park, S.H., Chang, Y.T., Kim, C.H., Choi, S.Y., and Williams, D.R. (2012) A novel zebrafish human tumor xenograft model validated for anti-cancer drug screening. *Molecular BioSystems*, **8** (7), 1930–1939.

22 Li, Y., Huang, W., Huang, S., Du, J., and Huang, C. (2012) Screening of anti-cancer agent using zebrafish: comparison with the MTT assay. *Biochemical and Biophysical Research Communications*, **422** (1), 85–90.

23 Terriente, J. and Pujades, C. (2013) Use of zebrafish embryos for small molecule screening related to cancer. *Developmental Dynamics*, **242** (2), 97–107.

24 Stewart, A.M., Cachat, J., Gaikwad, S., Robinson, K.S., Gebhardt, M., and Kalueff, A.V. (2013) Perspectives on experimental models of serotonin syndrome in zebrafish. *Neurochemistry International*, **62** (6), 893–902.

25 Mahmood, F., Mozere, M., Zdebik, A.A., Stanescu, H.C., Tobin, J., Beales, P.L., Kleta, R., Bockenhauer, D., and Russell, C. (2013) Generation and validation of a zebrafish model of EAST (epilepsy, ataxia, sensorineural deafness and tubulopathy) syndrome. *Disease Models & Mechanisms*, **6** (3), 652–660.

26 Stewart, A.M. and Kalueff, A.V. (2012) The developing utility of zebrafish models for cognitive enhancers research. *Current Neuropharmacology*, **10** (3), 263–271.

27 Ellis, L.D. and Soanes, K.H. (2012) A larval zebrafish model of bipolar disorder as a screening platform for neuro-therapeutics. *Behavioural Brain Research*, **233** (2), 450–457.

28 Stewart, A.M., Desmond, D., Kyzar, E., Gaikwad, S., Roth, A., Riehl, R., Collins, C., Monnig, L., Green, J., and Kalueff, A.V. (2012) Perspectives of zebrafish models of epilepsy: what, how and where next? *Brain Research Bulletin*, **87** (2–3), 135–143.

29 Shimada, Y., Hirano, M., Nishimura, Y., and Tanaka, T. (2012) A high-throughput fluorescence-based assay system for appetite-regulating gene and drug screening. *PLoS One*, **7** (12), e52549.

30 Wittmann, C., Reischl, M., Shah, A.H., Mikut, R., Liebel, U., and Grabher, C. (2012) Facilitating drug discovery: an automated high-content inflammation assay in zebrafish. *Journal of Visualized Experiments*, **16** (65), e4203.

31 Pfriem, A., Pylatiuk, C., Alshut, R., Ziegener, B., Schulz, S., and Bretthauer, G. (2012) A modular, low-cost robot for zebrafish handling. Conference Proceedings of the IEEE Engineering in Medicine & Biology Society, pp. 980–983.

32 Pardo-Martin, C., Allalou, A., Medina, J., Eimon, P.M., Wählby, C., and Fatih Yanik, M. (2013) High-throughput hyperdimensional vertebrate phenotyping. *Nature Communications*, **4**, 1467.

33 Rubinstein, A.L. (2003) Zebrafish: from disease modeling to drug discovery. *Current Opinion in Drug Discovery & Development*, **6** (2), 218–223.

34 Miscevic, F., Rotstein, O., and Wen, X.Y. (2012) Advances in zebrafish high content and high throughput technologies. *Combinatorial Chemistry & High Throughput Screening*, **15** (7), 515–521.

35 Gibert, Y., Trengove, M.C., and Ward, A.C. (2013) Zebrafish as a genetic model in pre-clinical drug testing and screening. *Current Medicinal Chemistry*, **20** (19), 2458–2466.

36 Lessman, C.A. (2011) The developing zebrafish (*Danio rerio*): a vertebrate model for high-throughput screening of chemical libraries. *Birth Defects Research Part C: Embryo Today*, **93** (3), 268–280.

37 Carroll, P.M., Dougherty, B., Ross-Macdonald, P., Browman, K., and FitzGerald, K. (2003) Model systems in drug discovery: chemical genetics meets genomics. *Pharmacology & Therapeutics*, **99** (2), 183–220.

38 Perrimon, N., Friedman, A., Mathey-Prevot, B., and Eggert, U.S. (2007) Drug-target identification in *Drosophila* cells: combining high-throughout RNAi and small-molecule screens. *Drug Discovery Today*, **12** (1–2), 28–33.

39 Nichols, C.D., Becnel, J., and Pandey, U.B. (2012) Methods to assay *Drosophila* behavior. *Journal of Visualized Experiments*, **61**, e3795.

40 Gladstone, M. and Su, T.T. (2011) Chemical genetics and drug screening in *Drosophila* cancer models. *Journal of Genetics and Genomics*, **38** (10), 497–504.

41 Rudrapatna, V.A., Cagan, R.L., and Das, T.K. (2012) *Drosophila* cancer models. *Developmental Dynamics*, **241** (1), 107–118.

42 Willoughby, L.F., Schlosser, T., Manning, S.A., Parisot, J.P., Street, I.P., Richardson, H.E., Humbert, P.O., and Brumby, A.M. (2013) An *in vivo* large-scale chemical screening platform using *Drosophila* for anti-cancer drug discovery. *Disease Models & Mechanisms*, **6** (2), 521–529.

43 Teleman, A.A., Ratzenböck, I., and Oldham, S. (2012) *Drosophila*: a model for understanding obesity and diabetic complications. *Experimental and Clinical Endocrinology & Diabetes*, **120** (4), 184–185.

44 Skorupa, D.A., Dervisefendic, A., Zwiener, J., and Pletcher, S.D. (2008) Dietary composition specifies consumption, obesity, and lifespan in *Drosophila melanogaster*. *Aging Cell*, **7** (4), 478–490.

45 Musselman, L.P., Fink, J.L., Narzinski, K., Ramachandran, P.V., Hathiramani, S.S., Cagan, R.L., and Baranski, T.J. (2011) A high-sugar diet produces obesity and insulin resistance in wild-type *Drosophila*. *Disease Models & Mechanisms*, **4** (6), 842–849.

46 Gasque, G., Conway, S., Huang, J., Rao, Y., and Vosshall, L.B. (2013) Small molecule drug screening in *Drosophila* identifies the 5HT2A receptor as a feeding modulation target. *Scientific Reports*, **3**, srep02120.

47 Milinkeviciute, G., Gentile, C., and Neely, G.G. (2012) *Drosophila* as a tool for studying the conserved genetics of pain. *Clinical Genetics*, **82** (4), 359–366.

48 Tracey, W.D., Jr., Wilson, R.I., Laurent, G., and Benzer, S. (2003) painless, a *Drosophila* gene essential for nociception. *Cell*, **113** (2), 261–273.

49 Neely, G.G., Hess, A., Costigan, M., Keene, A.C., Goulas, S., Langeslag, M., Griffin, R.S., Belfer, I., Dai, F., Smith, S.B., Diatchenko, L., Gupta, V., Xia, C.P., Amann, S., Kreitz, S., Heindl-Erdmann, C., Wolz, S., Ly, C.V., Arora, S., Sarangi, R., Dan, D., Novatchkova, M., Rosenzweig, M., Gibson, D.G., Truong, D., Schramek, D., Zoranovic, T., Cronin, S.J., Angjeli, B., Brune, K., Dietzl, G., Maixner, W., Meixner, A., Thomas, W., Pospisilik, J.A., Alenius, M., Kress, M., Subramaniam, S., Garrity, P.A., Bellen, H.J., Woolf, C.J., and Penninger, J.M. (2010) A genome-wide *Drosophila* screen for heat nociception identifies α2δ3 as an evolutionarily conserved pain gene. *Cell*, **143** (4), 628–638.

50 Neely, G.G., Keene, A.C., Duchek, P., Chang, E.C., Wang, Q.P., Aksoy, Y.A., Rosenzweig, M., Costigan, M., Woolf, C.J., Garrity, P.A., and Penninger, J.M. (2011) TrpA1 regulates thermal nociception in *Drosophila*. *PLoS One*, **6** (8), e24343.

51 Chattopadhyay, A., Gilstrap, A.V., and Galko, M.J. (2012) Local and global methods of assessing thermal nociception in *Drosophila* larvae. *Journal of Visualized Experiments*, **63**, e3837.

52 Sulkowski, M.J., Kurosawa, M.S., and Cox, D.N. (2011) Growing pains: development of the larval nocifensive response in *Drosophila*. *The Biological Bulletin*, **221** (3), 300–306.

53 Babcock, D.T., Shi, S., Jo, J., Shaw, M., Gutstein, H.B., and Galko, M.J. (2011) Hedgehog signaling regulates nociceptive sensitization. *Current Biology*, **21** (18), 1525–1533.

54 Manev, H. and Dimitrijevic, N. (2005) Fruit flies for anti-pain drug discovery. *Life Sciences*, **76** (21), 2403–2407.

55 van Alphen, B. and van Swinderen, B. (2013) *Drosophila* strategies to study psychiatric disorders. *Brain Research Bulletin*, **92**, 1–11.

56 Siller, S.S. and Broadie, K. (2011) Neural circuit architecture defects in a *Drosophila* model of Fragile X syndrome are alleviated by minocycline treatment and genetic removal of matrix metalloproteinase. *Disease Models & Mechanisms*, **4** (5), 673–685.

57 Schleyer, M., Saumweber, T., Nahrendorf, W., Fischer, B., von Alpen, D., Pauls, D., Thum, A., and Gerber, B. (2011) A behavior-based circuit model of how outcome expectations organize learned behavior in larval *Drosophila*. *Learning & Memory*, **18** (10), 639–653.

58 Kahsai, L. and Zars, T. (2011) Learning and memory in *Drosophila*: behavior, genetics, and neural systems. *International Review of Neurobiology*, **99**, 139–167.

59 Iijima, K. and Iijima-Ando, K. (2008) *Drosophila* models of Alzheimer's

amyloidosis: the challenge of dissecting the complex mechanisms of toxicity of amyloid-beta 42. *Journal of Alzheimer's Disease*, **15** (4), 523–540.

60 Wang, L., Chiang, H.C., Wu, W., Liang, B., Xie, Z., Yao, X., Ma, W., Du, S., and Zhong, Y. (2012) Epidermal growth factor receptor is a preferred target for treating amyloid-β-induced memory loss. *Proceedings of the National Academy of Sciences of the United States of America*, **109** (41), 16743–16748.

61 Khan, S., Jyoti, S., Naz, F., Shakya, B., Rahul, Afzal, M., and Siddique, Y.H. (2012) Effect of L-ascorbic acid on the climbing ability and protein levels in the brain of *Drosophila* model of Parkinson's disease. *The International Journal of Neuroscience*, **122** (12), 704–709.

62 Shaltiel-Karyo, R., Davidi, D., Frenkel-Pinter, M., Ovadia, M., Segal, D., and Gazit, E. (2012) Differential inhibition of α-synuclein oligomeric and fibrillar assembly in Parkinson's disease model by cinnamon extract. *Biochimica et Biophysica Acta*, **1820** (10), 1628–1635.

63 Campesan, S., Green, E.W., Breda, C., Sathyasaikumar, K.V., Muchowski, P.J., Schwarcz, R., Kyriacou, C.P., and Giorgini, F. (2011) The kynurenine pathway modulates neurodegeneration in a *Drosophila* model of Huntington's disease. *Current Biology*, **21** (11), 961–966.

64 Kaun, K.R., Devineni, A.V., and Heberlein, U. (2012) *Drosophila melanogaster* as a model to study drug addiction. *Human Genetics*, **131** (6), 959–975.

65 Heberlein, U., Tsai, L.T., Kapfhamer, D., and Lasek, A.W. (2009) *Drosophila*, a genetic model system to study cocaine-related behaviors: a review with focus on LIM-only proteins. *Neuropharmacology*, **56** (Suppl. 1), 97–106.

66 Rodan, A.R. and Rothenfluh, A. (2010) The genetics of behavioral alcohol responses in *Drosophila*. *International Review of Neurobiology*, **91**, 25–51.

67 Robinson, B.G., Khurana, S., and Atkinson, N.S. (2013) *Drosophila* larvae as a model to study physiological alcohol dependence. *Communicative & Integrative Biology*, **6** (2), e23501.

68 Lionakis, M.S. and Kontoyiannis, D.P. (2012) *Drosophila melanogaster* as a model organism for invasive aspergillosis. *Methods in Molecular Biology*, **845**, 455–468.

69 Oh, C.T., Moon, C., Choi, T.H., Kim, B.S., and Jang, J. (2012) *Mycobacterium marinum* infection in *Drosophila melanogaster* for antimycobacterial activity assessment. *The Journal of Antimicrobial Chemotherapy*, **68** (3), 601–609.

70 Arvanitis, M., Glavis-Bloom, J., and Mylonakis, E. (2013) Invertebrate models of fungal infection. *Biochimica et Biophysica Acta*, **1832** (9), 1378–1383.

71 Tzelepis, I., Kapsetaki, S.E., Panayidou, S., and Apidianakis, Y. (2013) *Drosophila melanogaster*: a first step and a stepping-stone to anti-infectives. *Current Opinion in Pharmacology*, **13** (5), 763–768.

72 Chamilos, G., Samonis, G., and Kontoyiannis, D.P. (2011) *Drosophila melanogaster* as a model host for the study of microbial pathogenicity and the discovery of novel antimicrobial compounds. *Current Pharmaceutical Design*, **17** (13), 1246–1253.

73 Tickoo, S. and Russell, S. (2002) *Drosophila melanogaster* as a model system for drug discovery and pathway screening. *Current Opinion in Pharmacology*, **2** (5), 555–560.

74 Giacomotto, J. and Ségalat, L. (2010) High-throughput screening and small animal models, where are we? *British Journal of Pharmacology*, **160** (2), 204–216.

75 Pandey, U.B. and Nichols, C.D. (2011) Human disease models in *Drosophila melanogaster* and the role of the fly in therapeutic drug discovery. *Pharmacological Reviews*, **63** (2), 411–436.

76 *C. elegans* Sequencing Consortium (1998) Genome sequence of the nematode *C. elegans*: a platform for investigating biology. *Science*, **282** (5396), 2012–2018.

77 Choy, R.K. and Thomas, J.H. (1999) Fluoxetine-resistant mutants in *C. elegans* define a novel family of transmembrane proteins. *Molecular Cell*, **4** (2), 143–152.

78 Siddiqui, S.S., Loganathan, S., Krishnaswamy, S., Faoro, L., Jagadeeswaran, R., and Salgia, R. (2008) *C. elegans* as a model organism for *in vivo* screening in cancer: effects of human c-Met in lung cancer affect *C. elegans* vulva phenotypes. *Cancer Biology & Therapy*, **7** (6), 856–863.

79 Olsen, A., Vantipalli, M.C., and Lithgow, G.J. (2006) Using *Caenorhabditis elegans* as a model for aging and age-related diseases. *Annals of the New York Academy of Sciences*, **1067**, 120–128.

80 Leung, M.C., Williams, P.L., Benedetto, A., Au, C., Helmcke, K.J., Aschner, M., and Meyer, J.N. (2008) *Caenorhabditis elegans*: an emerging model in biomedical and environmental toxicology. *Toxicological Sciences*, **106** (1), 5–28.

81 Squiban, B. and Kurz, C.L. (2011) *C. elegans*: an all in one model for antimicrobial drug discovery. *Current Drug Targets*, **12** (7), 967–977.

82 McColl, G., Roberts, B.R., Pukala, T.L., Kenche, V.B., Roberts, C.M., Link, C.D., Ryan, T.M., Masters, C.L., Barnham, K.J., Bush, A.I., and Cherny, R.A. (2012) Utility of an improved model of amyloid-beta ($A\beta_{1-42}$) toxicity in *Caenorhabditis elegans* for drug screening for Alzheimer's disease. *Molecular Neurodegeneration*, **7**, 57.

83 Lublin, A. and Link, C. (2013) Alzheimer's disease drug discovery: *in-vivo* screening using *C. elegans* as a model for β-amyloid peptide-induced toxicity. *Drug Discovery Today: Technologies*, **10** (1), e115–e119.

84 Artal-Sanz, M., de Jong, L., and Tavernarakis, N. (2006) *Caenorhabditis elegans*: a versatile platform for drug discovery. *Journal of Biotechnology*, **1** (12), 1405–1418.

85 Ségalat, L. (2006) Drug discovery: here comes the worm. *ACS Chemical Biology*, **1** (5), 277–278.

86 Silverman, G.A., Luke, C.J., Bhatia, S.R., Long, O.S., Vetica, A.C., Perlmutter, D.H., and Pak, S.C. (2009) Modeling molecular and cellular aspects of human disease using the nematode *Caenorhabditis elegans*. *Pediatric Research*, **65** (1), 10–18.

87 Leung, C.K., Wang, Y., Malany, S., Deonarine, A., Nguyen, K., Vasile, S., and Choe, K.P. (2013) An ultra high-throughput, whole-animal screen for small molecule modulators of a specific genetic pathway in *Caenorhabditis elegans*. *PLoS One*, **8** (4), e62166.

88 Coleman, R.A. (2009) Drug discovery and development tomorrow: changing the mindset. *Alternatives to Laboratory Animals*, **37** (Suppl. 1), 1–4.

89 Hillier, C. and Bunton, D. (2009) Could fresh human tissues play a key role in drug development? *Alternatives to Laboratory Animals*, **37** (Suppl. 1), 5–10.

90 Murray, R.M., Paparelli, A., Morrison, P.D., Marconi, A., and Di Forti, M. (2013) What can we learn about schizophrenia from studying the human model, drug-induced psychosis? *American Journal of Medical Genetics. Part B, Neuropsychiatric Genetics*, **162** (7), 661–670.

91 Garner, R.C. (2000) Accelerator mass spectrometry in pharmaceutical research and development: a new ultrasensitive analytical method for isotope measurement. *Current Drug Metabolism*, **1** (2), 205–213.

92 Lappin, G. and Garner, R.C. (2003) Big physics, small doses: the use of AMS and PET in human microdosing of development drugs. *Nature Reviews. Drug Discovery*, **2** (3), 233–240.

93 Combes, R.D., Berridge, T., Connelly, J., Eve, M.D., Garner, R.C., Toon, S., and Wilcox, P. (2003) Early microdose drug studies in human volunteers can minimise animal testing: proceedings of a workshop organised by Volunteers in Research and Testing. *European Journal of Pharmaceutical Sciences*, **19** (1), 1–11.

94 European Medicines Agency (2004) Position Paper on Non-Clinical Safety Studies to Support Clinical Trials with a Single Microdose. CPMP/SWP/2599/02/Rev1. Superseded by ICH M3(R2). Available at http://www.ema.europa.eu/ema/index.jsp?curl=pages/regulation/general/general_content_000400.jsp, http://www.ema.europa.eu/docs/en_GB/document_library/Scientific_guideline/2009/09/WC500002720.pdf (accessed October 27, 2013).

95 Food and Drug Administration (2006) Guidance for Industry, Investigators, and Reviewers: Exploratory IND Studies. Available at http://www.fda.gov/downloads/Drugs/GuidanceCompliance RegulatoryInformation/Guidances/UCM078933.pdf (accessed October 27, 2013).

96 Japanese Ministry of Health, Labor and Welfare (2008) Guidance for the Performing of Microdose Clinical Trials.

PFSB/ELD Notification No. 0603001 of the Evaluating and Licensing Division. Ministry of Health, Labor and Welfare, Pharmaceutical and Medical Safety Bureau, Tokyo, Japan.

97 European Medicines Agency (2009) ICH Topic M3: Note for Guidance on Non-Clinical Safety Pharmacology Studies for Human Pharmaceuticals. EMA/CPMP/ICH/286/1995. Available at http://www.ema.europa.eu/docs/en_GB/document_library/Scientific_guideline/2009/09/WC500002720.pdf (accessed October 27, 2013).

98 Lappin, G. and Garner, R.C. (2008) The utility of microdosing over the past 5 years. *Expert Opinion on Drug Metabolism and Toxicology*, **4** (12), 1499–1506.

99 Lappin, G., Noveck, R., and Burt, T. (2013) Microdosing and drug development: past, present and future. *Expert Opinion on Drug Metabolism and Toxicology*, **9** (7), 817–834.

100 Lappin, G. (2010) Microdosing: current and the future. *Bioanalysis*, **2** (3), 509–517.

101 Murgo, A.J., Kummar, S., Rubinstein, L., Gutierrez, M., Collins, J., Kinders, R., Parchment, R.E., Ji, J., Steinberg, S.M., Yang, S.X., Hollingshead, M., Chen, A., Helman, L., Wiltrout, R., Tomaszewski, J.E., and Doroshow, J.H. (2008) Designing phase 0 cancer clinical trials. *Clinical Cancer Research*, **14** (12), 3675–3682.

102 Gupta, U.C., Bhatia, S., Garg, A., Sharma, A., and Choudhary, V. (2011) Phase 0 clinical trials in oncology new drug development. *Perspectives in Clinical Research*, **2** (1), 13–22.

103 Marchetti, S. and Schellens, J.H. (2007) The impact of FDA and EMEA guidelines on drug development in relation to Phase 0 trials. *British Journal of Cancer*, **97** (5), 577–581.

104 Robinson, W.T. (2008) Innovative early development regulatory approaches: expIND, expCTA, microdosing. *Clinical Pharmacology and Therapeutics*, **83** (2), 358–360.

105 Eliopoulos, H., Giranda, V., Carr, R., Tiehen, R., Leahy, T., and Gordon, G. (2008) Phase 0 trials: an industry perspective. *Clinical Cancer Research*, **14** (12), 3683–3688.

106 Rawlins, M.D. (2004) Cutting the cost of drug development? *Nature Reviews. Drug Discovery*, **3** (4), 360–364.

107 Lappin, G., Kuhnz, W., Jochemsen, R., Kneer, J., Chaudhary, A., Oosterhuis, B., Drijfhout, W.J., Rowland, M., and Garner, R.C. (2006) Use of microdosing to predict pharmacokinetics at the therapeutic dose: experience with 5 drugs. *Clinical Pharmacology and Therapeutics*, **80** (3), 203–215.

108 Oosterhuis, B. (2010) Trends in microdosing and other exploratory human pharmacokinetic studies for early drug development. *Bioanalysis*, **2** (3), 377–379.

109 Chauhan, B.N., Modi, C.M., Mody, S.K., Patel, H.B., Dudhatra, G.B., and Kamani, D.R. (2012) Pharmaco-economics of microdosing clinical trials in drug development process. *International Journal of Analytical, Pharmaceutical and Biomedical Sciences*, **1** (3), 25–36.

110 Yamane, N., Igarashi, A., Kusama, M., Maeda, K., Ikeda, T., and Sugiyama, Y. (2013) Cost-effectiveness analysis of microdose clinical trials in drug development. *Drug Metabolism and Pharmacokinetics*, **28** (3), 187–195.

111 Sheiner, L.B. (1997) Learning versus confirming in clinical drug development. *Clinical Pharmacology and Therapeutics*, **61** (3), 275–291.

112 Patterson, S.D. (2010) Experiences with learning and confirming in drug and biological development. *Clinical Pharmacology and Therapeutics*, **88** (2), 161–163.

113 Wong, D.F., Potter, W.Z., and Brasic, J.R. (2002) Proof of concept: functional models for drug development in humans, in *Neuropsychopharmacology: The Fifth Generation of Progress* (eds K.L. Davis, D. Charney, J.T. Coyle, and N. Charles), Lippincott Williams & Wilkins, Philadelphia, PA, pp. 457–473.

114 Arendt-Nielsen, L. and Sumikura, H. (2002) From pain research to pain treatment: role of human pain models. *Journal of Nippon Medical School*, **69** (6), 514–524.

115 Wise, R.G. and Tracey, I. (2006) The role of fMRI in drug discovery. *Journal of Magnetic Resonance Imaging*, **23** (6), 862–876.

116 Arendt-Nielsen, L., Curatolo, M., and Drewes, A. (2007) Human experimental pain models in drug development: translational pain research. *Current Opinion in Investigational Drugs*, **8** (1), 41–53.

117 Olesen, A.E., Andresen, T., Staahl, C., and Drewes, A.M. (2012) Human experimental pain models for assessing the therapeutic efficacy of analgesic drugs. *Pharmacological Reviews*, **64** (3), 722–779.

118 Reddy, K.S., Naidu, M.U., Rani, P.U., and Rao, T.R. (2012) Human experimental pain models: a review of standardized methods in drug development. *Journal of Research in Medical Sciences*, **17** (6), 587–595.

119 Oertel, B.G. and Lötsch, J. (2013) Clinical pharmacology of analgesics assessed with human experimental pain models: bridging basic and clinical research. *British Journal of Pharmacology*, **168** (3), 534–553.

4
Ethical Issues and Regulations and Guidelines Concerning Animal Research

David Sabaté

4.1
Introduction

The use of animals in biomedical research has undoubtedly led to many medical advances in the past century and it continues even today, enlarging our understanding of various diseases and providing medical professionals with new safe and effective therapeutic and prophylactic tools. However, ethical issues raised by research involving animals have historically elicited an intense debate leading to a broad spectrum of public opinion.

As a result of this debate, social concerns about the protection and well-being of animals used for scientific purposes have been progressively translated into national and local laws and regulations in many countries across the world. In addition, an extensive number of guidelines, either complementing the existing regulations or offering important guidance in areas not well covered by the legal framework, have been published by government agencies and professional organizations. Given that *in vivo* animal models cannot yet be completely replaced by alternative methods, these regulations and guidelines seek to ensure that those animals that are still used in research receive the highest protection and welfare, saving them from being subjected to unnecessary pain and suffering.

The existence and regular updating of a legal framework binding researchers and institutions using *in vivo* animal models have led to a higher acceptance of their responsibility for the care and use of these animals, as well as to a progressive increase in the confidence of the society in their work.

After a short review of both the current use of animals in biomedical and pharmaceutical research and the ethical concerns and positions on it, the overall ethical principles supporting the legal obligations of humane care and use of research animals are summarized in this chapter. To conclude, an overview of the regulatory background on the protection of research animals in several countries is presented.

4.2
Current Use of Animals in Biomedical and Pharmaceutical Research

An overall consensus does exist today among the biomedical community in that all efforts should be made in order to reduce the number of animals used in research to a minimum [1,2]. The increasing adoption of modern technologies and the progressive implementation of alternative approaches to animal-based models during the last three decades have substantially helped to achieve it [3]. Nevertheless, even today the use of animals plays a pivotal role in biomedical and pharmaceutical research. Indeed, data obtained from *in vivo* animal models during drug discovery and preclinical development are crucially important to both the researchers and the regulatory authorities when deciding whether a potential medicine is effective and safe enough to be tested in clinical trials with human participants during the subsequent clinical development stages [4].

In this respect, the Declaration of Helsinki, a set of ethical principles developed by the World Medical Association regarding "human experimentation," specifically states that medical research involving human subjects must be based on adequate laboratory and, as appropriate, animal research [5]. Consequently, since its adoption in 1964, the regulatory authorities worldwide require the development of new medicinal products for human use to be supported by nonclinical data obtained with research animals prior to the start of clinical studies with human volunteers [6]. As a result, approximately one-third of all the animal research that is currently undertaken in the developed world is conducted or supported by the pharmaceutical industry [3].

Among the different stages covering the entire process of drug discovery and development, characterization of promising candidates is the one involving the highest number of animals. Indeed, 60–80% of the animals currently used by the pharmaceutical industry are used during lead identification and optimization. In contrast, relatively fewer animals are used during identification of targets and possible drugs interacting with them (5–15%) or when ensuring the safety of selected candidates (10–20%) [3].

A wide range of animal vertebrate species, including mice, rats, guinea pigs, hamsters, gerbils, rabbits, dogs, cats, and nonhuman primates, among others, are used as experimental animals in pharmaceutical research. Among them, rodents have traditionally been, and still are, the most widely used in *in vivo* animal models [7–9]. In particular, genetically modified mice are currently by far the most extensively used in biomedical research, mainly as models of human disease. This has led to a significant decrease in the use of other species of higher concern to the society, such as dogs and nonhuman primates [7,8].

From an ethical point of view, particular attention has to be paid to nonhuman primates as research animals. Because of their genetic proximity to humans and highly developed neurophysiology, they have been used for decades in drug development and safety testing. However, involvement of these animals in biomedical research has raised specific ethical questions and practical problems in terms of meeting their behavioral, environmental, and social needs in a laboratory environment [6]. Consequently, the use of nonhuman primates is being more and more restricted and controlled by the current regulations, some of them allowing it only in procedures directed to the avoidance, prevention, diagnosis, or treatment of debilitating or potentially life-threatening clinical conditions in human beings, or when there is scientific justification that the purpose of the procedure cannot be achieved by using other animal species [10].

In addition to the already mentioned species, during recent decades there has been a significant increase in the use of other vertebrates such as the zebrafish. The interest in this new experimental species is mainly based on its easy and quick reproduction in addition to its morphological and physiological similarities to mammals [11,12].

Finally, preclinical development of new veterinary medicines also requires performing studies with individuals of the intended species such as poultry, pigs, calves, horses, dogs, and cats, among others – all of them specifically bred for investigational purposes in authorized centers, like for the other traditional research species [13].

4.3
Ethical Concerns and Positions on Animal Research

Use of animals in biomedical research, including drug discovery and development, has been a subject of heated debate for many years, and still is today, with supporters and detractors arguing diametrically opposing points of view [14–17]. Among supporters, there is a strong conviction that the use of animals is necessary to improve medical and biological knowledge and to guarantee the efficacy and safety of products intended for human and animal use. In contrast, detractors argue that it is cruel, unnecessary, scientifically unreliable, and morally detestable [3].

Unfortunately, there is much confusion in our society about the use of animals in research because publicly available information is sometimes biased, albeit intentionally or unintentionally. Some animal protection groups use disturbing pictures that are not representative of the range of research that is permitted under current regulations [3]. On the other hand, some scientists and organizations representing them seek to defend animal research purely on intellectual and scientific basis, strictly focusing on the medical benefits of animal research while paying poor attention to the social concerns on the pain and suffering potentially experienced by the animals [3,14].

Historically, neither the scientific community nor society perceived the use of animals in research as an ethical issue. Indeed, the first known regulations only prohibited deliberate cruelty to animals [18–20]. In 1876, the Cruelty to Animals Act of the Parliament of the United Kingdom [21] stipulated, for the first time, that researchers would be prosecuted for cruelty, unless they conducted experiments involving infliction of pain upon animals only when "they are absolutely necessary for the due instruction of the persons to save or prolong human life."

However, it was not until the 1970s and 1980s when a growing amount of literature in moral philosophy provided a more rational approach to the ethics of animal treatment by discussing animal research from the viewpoint of moral theory [22–24]. Some authors propose the philosophical position that animals have moral value and therefore moral rights, although they still accept the existence of ethical differences between harming human and nonhuman animals, and argue that to save the former it is permissible to harm the latter [22]. In contrast, some other authors argue that benefits to human beings cannot outweigh animal suffering, and that we have no moral right to use an animal in ways that do not benefit that individual [23]. Other authors, supporters of a utilitarian ethical approach, even argue that there are no grounds to include a being's species in consideration of whether its suffering is important [24].

As described in the literature [3], these and other different approaches to the ethics of animal research have led to four main viewpoints: (i) the "anything goes" view (if humans see value in animal research, then it requires no further ethical justification); (ii) the "on balance justification" view (in moral terms, the benefits to human beings outweigh the animal research's costs to animals); (iii) the "moral dilemma" view (on the one hand, the use of animals is necessary to comply with the moral imperative to cure human disease; on the other hand, the use of animals is morally wrong by itself; therefore, either by neglecting human health or by harming animals, one always acts wrongly); and (iv) the "abolitionist" view (since any research that causes pain, suffering, or distress is wrong, there is no moral justification for harmful research on sentient animals that is not to the benefit of the individual animal). These four positions conform to a three-category spectrum constructed as follows: humans are morally required to carry out any kind of animal research they deem desirable ("anything goes" view), humans are morally permitted to carry out animal research ("on balance justification" and "moral dilemma" views), and humans are morally prohibited to carry out any type of animal research ("abolitionist" view) [3].

Notwithstanding this three-category spectrum, the currently dominant ethical position worldwide is that achievement of scientific and medical goals using animal research is desirable, so long as animal use and suffering are minimized [16]. In other words, an experiment that uses animals is justifiable only if all possible alternative methods have been explored and if it is performed in a way that causes minimal pain to the animals involved. Consequently, when using animals in their experimental models, scientists have a particular duty to avoid unnecessary cruel treatment in the way the animals are kept and handled [14].

In addition to people who are critical of the permissibility of animal research on ethical grounds, there are critics who also object to the use of animals in pharmaceutical research on scientific grounds, mainly by questioning the transferability and predictability of data obtained from animals, together with its reliability for the accurate assessment of safety of new drugs to be administered to humans [3]. Although scientific validity of most animal models currently used in pharmaceutical research is supported by cumulative successful experiences since decades, it must be accepted that, given the complexity and variability of biological systems, there are sometimes difficulties in both developing effective experimental approaches and extrapolating from model systems to humans. Consequently, the scientific community has been encouraged to accompany the use of animals in research by continuous active and critical reflection on the validity and relevance of the models and research studies, and to not overstate the predictive value and transferability of animal research to humans [3].

4.4 General Principles for the Ethical Use of Animals in Research

4.4.1 The 3Rs Principles (Replacement, Reduction, and Refinement)

The first main conceptual reference adopted by the scientific community regarding ethics in animal experimentation was proposed by Russell and Burch in the book *The Principles of Humane Experimental Technique*, published in 1959 [25]. This work established the adoption of the concepts of replacement, reduction, and refinement, referred to as the 3Rs principles, to be applied when considering the use of animals in research. Over the years, the 3Rs principles have become an internationally accepted approach for researchers working with laboratory animals. In addition to this, these principles have also been adopted by the regulatory authorities and professional organizations worldwide, so they are currently central to their regulations and corresponding guidelines.

First, according to the principle of replacement, if a viable alternative method exists that would partly or totally replace the use of animals in a given study, researchers must use it. The term includes both absolute replacement (i.e., *in vitro* techniques and computer models) and relative replacement (i.e., replacing vertebrates with animals that are lower on the phylogenetic scale) [26].

Second, according to the principle of reduction, studies must be designed to use no more than the minimum number of animals necessary to ensure scientific and statistical validity. The term involves strategies to obtain comparable levels of information from the use of fewer animals or to maximize the information obtained from a given number of animals so that less animals are needed to acquire the same scientific information (accurate design of experimental models, application of new technologies, use of appropriate statistical methods, and control of environmentally related variability in animal housing, among other strategies). However, it is widely accepted that the principle of reducing the number of animals used should never be implemented at the expense of greater pain and distress for individual animals [26].

Third, according to the principle of refinement, the whole project involving animals must be designed to avoid or minimize their pain and distress, although compatible with its scientific objective. In order to achieve this, the following must be taken into account, among other issues: the correct choice of the animal species and their adequate housing, management, care, and acclimatization, consistent with their physiological needs; the choice of appropriate experimental techniques and procedures; the use of sedatives, tranquillizers, analgesics, and anesthetics during their implementation, when needed; the design of programs for health and welfare monitoring of animals, including suitable measures for assessing pain and distress; the establishment of early intervention points and human endpoints; and the appropriate use of human methods of euthanasia [26].

Since animals cannot yet be completely replaced, it is important that researchers maximize reduction and refinement. Sometimes this can be achieved relatively easily by improving animal husbandry and housing, for example, by enriching their environment. This simple measure aims to satisfy the physiological and behavioral needs of the animals and therefore maintain their well-being [16].

In addition to the 3Rs principles, two other key principles are currently extrinsically or intrinsically considered in most regulations worldwide: justification and responsibility, the latter intrinsically including the principle of respect [10,26,27].

4.4.2
The Principle of Justification

According to the principle of justification, all projects using animals should be performed only after an accurate risk–benefit ratio analysis (potential effects on the well-being of animals versus scientific value) has been performed [26,27]. This principle is closely related to the concept of the "ethical review."

Today, it is widely agreed that if the conduct of animal experiments that have the potential to benefit humans and other animals is to be ethically defensible, an ethical review process that commands the confidence of wider society is needed. This ethical review should aim to ensure that, at all stages in the research process involving animals, there is an adequate and clearly explained ethical justification for using animals, which is subjected to ongoing, critical evaluation [28–32].

The ethical review must be a dynamic process covering the whole project from its design to the completion of the work and application of the results. During this process, every opportunity should be taken to ensure that the ethical, scientific, and practical welfare aspects are carefully considered [29,30].

Generally speaking, the ethical review should take into account (i) the balance of the predicted benefits of the work over the harms caused to the animals involved in the study (the already mentioned risk–benefit ratio analysis); (ii) the possibility that the objectives of the study might be achieved by nonanimal-based alternative means; (iii) whether and how far, given the experimental design, facilities, and expertise involved, there is reasonable expectation that the objectives of the study will be achieved in practice and the likely benefits will be maximized; and (iv) whether and how far animal suffering is minimized and animal welfare enhanced by implementation of the 3Rs, optimization of standards of animal husbandry and care, and effective training, supervision, and management of all personnel involved [28].

Many national laws currently regulate animal experiments through a system that involves some form of ethical review, although the approaches and processes vary between different countries. Some countries use local or institutional committees as ethical review committees, referred to by a variety of titles (institutional animal care and use committees, animal ethics committees, animal care committees, institutional animal ethics committees, ethics committees on the use of animals, animal research ethical committees, internal committees, or local review committees, among others). On the other hand, some countries use national ethical review processes, some use regional processes, and others work through individuals (officers, officials, inspectors, etc.) vested with the responsibility for ethical oversight. In many countries, the ethical review process involves a combination of different approaches [31]. In Europe, the current Directive does also contain specific requirement for prior ethical review of proposed projects involving animals by an Animal Welfare Body [10].

Some existing guidelines on this issue [28,33,34] have been recommended by the International Council for Laboratory Animal Science (ICLAS) Working Group on Harmonization of Guidelines on the Use of Animals in Science, to be used as international references for guidance on the ethical review of animal experiments [31].

4.4.3
The Principle of Responsibility

According to the principle of responsibility, investigators who use animals for scientific purposes have an obligation to treat them with respect and to consider their well-being as an essential factor when planning or conducting projects [26,27].

Undoubtedly, the welfare of animals used in research greatly depends on the quality and professional competence of the personnel responsible for the care and use of these animals. It is therefore essential that all personnel working on a given project involving experimental procedures with animals are fully knowledgeable about all factors that may affect the animals' well-being, and that they know the mechanisms to monitor, assess, and minimize these factors, including the appropriate actions to be taken in case adverse effects appear.

Current regulations worldwide state that institutions using animals for scientific purposes must provide adequate and continued training and support to investigators and animal care experts so that they can care for and use animals in compliance with basic principles of laboratory animal science [10,35]. However, major differences still exist between countries both in the requirements on competence and in the characteristics of teaching programs [36]. With the aim to harmonize such training, the ICLAS Working Group on Harmonization of Guidelines on the Use of Animals in Science has suggested the use of some existing guidelines as international references for guidance on education and training [37–41].

In Europe, education and training has been one of the main topics of the activities of the Federation for Laboratory Animal Science Associations (FELASA) and the area in which this organization has had the most influence [32]. The FELASA scheme of categories A (persons caring for animals), B (persons performing animal experiments), C (persons responsible for directing animal experiments), and D (laboratory animal science specialists) [39–41] has been widely recognized within the European laboratory animal science community during the last decade. With the aim to assist in the development of uniform high-quality educational programs for personnel involved in animal research, FELASA has established an accreditation system for teaching programs that follow these four categories [42]. The FELASA recommendations on this issue are currently serving as the basis for the ongoing discussions of an Expert Working Group established by the European Commission to develop an education and training framework within the European Union, which would guarantee the competence of staff caring for or using animals in procedures and facilitate the free movement of personnel [32].

4.5
Regulatory Framework for Use of Animals in Research

As previously mentioned in this chapter, an overall consensus does exist today among the regulatory authorities of most developed countries (and some emerging countries) in that all efforts should be made in order to reduce the number of animals used in experiments to a minimum and even replace them by alternative methods whenever possible. However, given that a complete phase-out of animal experimentation is not yet practically achievable, they agree that it is imperative to ensure that those animals that are still used in research for legitimate reasons receive the highest protection and welfare consistent with the aims of the experiment, avoiding them to be subjected to unnecessary pain and suffering. Still, the regulatory framework for use of animals in research varies depending on the country of origin.

A brief summary of the regulatory framework governing the protection of animals used in research in several countries across the world is presented in the following sections.

4.5.1
European Union

In the European Union, animal research is currently subjected to "Directive 2010/63/EU on the protection of animals used for experimental and other scientific purposes" [10], which came into force in 2010 and was fully implemented in January 2013. This Directive aims at ensuring a level playing field for industry and the research community, at the same time strengthening the protection of animals used in scientific procedures in line with the "EC Treaty's Protocol on Animal Welfare" [28]. Although this Directive is agreed upon at the level of the European Union, Member States still have certain flexibility to maintain national rules aimed at more extensive protection of animals, provided it does not affect the functioning of the internal market.

Prior to the current regulation, and for more than 20 years, Directive 86/609/ECC [43] and Council of Europe Convention 123 [44] were the most relevant rules in the European Union. Directive 86/609/EEC was adopted in 1986 with the aim to eliminate differences between laws, regulations, and administrative provisions of the Member States regarding the protection of experimental animals. However, although certain Member States adopted national measures ensuring a high level of protection for these animals, others only applied the minimum requirements laid down in the Directive.

The current Directive [10] provides much more detailed rules in order to reduce such disparities, including a detailed list of requirements for establishments and for the care and accommodation of animals to be strictly accomplished by all the Member States, as had previously been done by Annex A of the Council of Europe Convention 123 [44]. Furthermore, it specifies that all Member States shall ensure that each breeder, supplier, and user sets up an Animal Welfare Body and that projects are not carried out without prior authorization from the competent authority. Compared with the previous Directive, animals under protection now also include cephalopods, independently feeding larval forms, and fetal forms of mammals as from the last third of their normal development.

In addition to the regulations, a huge number of expert reports, guidelines, and recommendations focused on practical issues in laboratory animal science have been released in Europe by the FELASA [32]. FELASA represents the views and opinions of the laboratory animal science community in Europe by developing position statements on critical issues as well as by maintaining relations with both nongovernmental organizations and governmental bodies. The objective of all these documents is to advance and coordinate the development of all aspects of laboratory animal science and practice in Europe and worldwide [32].

Among all the European countries, special mention has to be made of the United Kingdom, given that it was one of the first countries to write the ethical framework concerning use of animals in research into law. Indeed, as previously mentioned, the Parliament of the United Kingdom was the first to stipulate that researchers would be prosecuted for cruelty, unless they conformed to the provisions of the Cruelty to Animals Act of 1876 [21].

Animal research in the United Kingdom is currently regulated by the Animals (Scientific Procedures) Act of 1986 [45]. The Act requires that proposals for research involving the use of animals must be fully assessed in terms of any harm to the animals and that all experiments must be regulated by three specific licenses: a license for the scientist in charge of the project, a license for the institute where the experiments will take place, and a license for each technician and scientist involved in the experiments.

In addition, the UK government introduced in 1998 the need for an Ethical Review Process to be performed at research institutions, which promote good animal welfare and humane science by ensuring that the use of animals at the designated establishment is justified [16].

4.5.2
The United States

In the United States, animal research is regulated by the Animal Welfare Act of 1966 [46]. The Act is enforced by the Animal Care Division of the Animal and Plant Health Inspection Service of the United States Department of Agriculture (USDA APHIS). It contains provisions requiring that care and welfare reach a certain standard and also requires each institution using covered species to maintain an Institutional Animal Care and Use Committee, which is responsible for local compliance with the Act. Institutions are also subject to unannounced annual inspections from USDA APHIS Veterinarian inspectors.

Another regulatory instrument in the United States is the Public Health Service Policy on Humane Care and Use of Laboratory Animals, which is enforced by the Office of Laboratory Animal Welfare (OLAW). OLAW also enforces the standards of the *Guide for the Care and Use of Laboratory Animals* published by the National Research Council's Institute for Laboratory Animal Research [35]. Compliance with the standards in this guide is intended to be guaranteed with the accreditation from the Association for Assessment and Accreditation of Laboratory Animal Care (AAALAC), a nongovernmental, nonprofit association. This accreditation is regarded by the industry as a gold standard and currently is also offered by AAALAC International to institutions worldwide.

Like the FELASA in Europe, the American Association for Laboratory Animal Science (AALAS) provides those working in laboratory animal science with additional and helpful technical information by publishing peer-reviewed journals and newsletters on practical issues.

4.5.3
Canada

In Canada, the Canadian Council on Animal Care (CCAC) was created in 1968 to ensure that optimal physical and psychological care of experimental animals in this country is implemented according to acceptable scientific standards and to promote an increased level of knowledge, awareness, and sensitivity to relevant ethical principles. In order to assist investigators to achieve this, the CCAC has published several useful guidelines [47,48]. Although the federal government does not have jurisdiction to pass laws that involve experiments on animals, the Canadian provinces have jurisdiction concerning that area and some of them even have made their own laws on animal welfare.

4.5.4
Japan

In Japan, animal research is regulated by the Law for the Humane Treatment and Management of Animals, amended in 2005 and enforced in 2006 [49]. This law only requires that researchers using animals be self-guided by the principles of the 3Rs, so that minimal distress and suffering can be achieved through monitoring and controlling the animals by the scientist themselves. In addition to this law, several guidelines on animal experimentation have also been formulated by individual scientific associations [50,51]. Although local-level inspections may be carried out, there are no governmental inspections and, unlike other countries, Japanese researchers are not required to report on the number of animals they use. Although not required by law, almost all pharmaceutical companies as well as medical schools have established an Institutional Animal Care and Use Committee [52].

4.5.5 Australia

In Australia, animal research is subjected to the *Australian Code of Practice for the Care and Use of Animals for Scientific Purposes* [27], developed in 2004 by the National Health and Medical Research Council (NHMRC). Animal Ethics Committees must also follow the Code when determining whether the use of an animal in an experimental procedure is valid or not. In order to assist investigators to achieve the goals of the Code, in 2008 the NHMRC developed and published "Guidelines to promote the well-being of animals used for scientific purposes" [26].

4.5.6 India

In India, animal research is covered by the provisions of the 1960's Prevention of Cruelty to Animals Act [53], amended in 1982, and by the Breeding of and Experiments on Animals (Control & Supervision) Rules of 1998, 2001, and 2006, framed under the Act. These provisions are enforced by the Committee for the Purpose of Control and Supervision of Experiments on Animals (CPCSEA), a statutory body under the Act. According to these provisions, the concerned establishments are required to get themselves registered with CPCSEA, to form local Institutional Animal Ethics Committees, to get their animal house facilities inspected, and to get projects involving research with animals evaluated by CPCSEA before starting the project. Breeding and trade of experimental animals are also regulated under these rules. The CPCSEA has provided several guidelines regarding the animal procurement and care and the requirements of physical facilities [54]. In 1992, the Indian National Science Academy (INSA) published the "Guidelines for Care and Use of Animals in Scientific Research," which were revised in 2000 [55].

4.5.7 China

In China, the highest policy-making body in charge of the regulation of animal research is the Administration of Laboratory Animals [56], approved in 1988 by China's State Council and enforced by the Ministry of Science and Technology (MOST). In addition, a Provincial Department of Science and Technology oversees laboratory animal administration in each province through an Administration

Office of Laboratory Animals [57]. The MOST has funded projects to study and translate animal welfare laws and guidelines from the United States, Europe, Japan, and Australia. Both the MOST's "Guideline on Humane Treatment of Laboratory Animals" [58] and the "Guideline of Beijing Municipality on Review of Welfare and Ethics of Laboratory Animals" [59] are currently offering guidance to institutions using animals for scientific purposes [57].

4.5.8
Brazil

In Brazil, animal research is subjected to a federal law on the scientific use of animals approved in 2008 [60]. This law establishes the National Council for the Control of Animal Experimentation (CONCEA) and requires institutions to constitute an Ethics Committee on the Use of Animals for day-to-day enforcement of the law and regulations [61]. In 2009, an implementing Decree defined CONCEA as a governing and advisory body, under the Ministry of Science and Technology, with the authority to provide accreditation to registered institutions and to license activities that use animals in research [61].

4.5.9
Countries without a Specific Legal Framework

To conclude, it is worth mentioning a document that provides guidance for researchers in those countries across the world where no specific legal framework on animal research exists. The Council for International Organizations of Medical Sciences (CIOMS), an international, nongovernmental, nonprofit organization established jointly by WHO and UNESCO in 1949, published, in 1985, the "International Guiding Principles for Biomedical Research Involving Animals" [62]. This document aims to provide a conceptual and ethical framework, acceptable to the international biomedical community and to moderate animal welfare groups, for whatever regulatory measure each country or scientific body chooses to adopt concerning animal research. The ICLAS Working Group on Harmonization of Guidelines on the Use of Animals in Science is currently working with the CIOMS in the revision of this document.

Acknowledgment

The author thanks Dr. Patri Vergara for her comments and advice in writing this chapter.

References

1 World Medical Association (1989) World Medical Association Statement on Animal Use in Biomedical Research (last revised in 2006). Available at http://www.wma.net/en/30publications/10policies/a18/ (accessed January 29, 2013).

2. World Veterinary Association (2001) Adopted Policy on the Use and Care of Animals Used in Testing, Research and Training. Available at http://www.worldvet.org/sites/worldvet/files/manuals/T-3-6.UseandCare.pdf (accessed January 29, 2013).

3. Nuffield Council on Bioethics (NCB) (2005) The Ethics of Research Involving Animals. Nuffield Council on Bioethics, London, UK. Available at http://www.nuffieldbioethics.org/animal-research (accessed January 31, 2013).

4. U.S. Department of Health and Human Services (2005) Guidance for Industry: Estimating the Maximum Safe Starting Dose in Initial Clinical Trials for Therapeutics in Adult Healthy Volunteers. Food and Drug Administration Center for Drug Evaluation and Research (CEDER). Available at http://www.fda.gov/downloads/Drugs/GuidanceComplianceRegulatoryInformation/Guidances/UCM078932.pdf (accessed January 30, 2013).

5. World Medical Association Declaration of Helsinki (1964) Ethical Principles for Medical Research Involving Human Subjects (last revised in 2008). Available at http://www.wma.net/en/30publications/10policies/b3/17c.pdf (accessed January 30, 2013).

6. Scientific Committee on Health and Environmental Risks (SCHER) (2009) The need for non-human primates in biomedical research, production and testing of products and devices. Available at http://ec.europa.eu/health/ph_risk/committees/04_scher/docs/scher_o_110.pdf (accessed January 31, 2013).

7. United States Department of Agriculture (USDA) (2011) Annual Report: Animal Usage by Fiscal Year. Available at http://www.aphis.usda.gov/animal_welfare/efoia/downloads/2010_Animals_Used_In_Research.pdf (accessed January 31, 2013).

8. European Commission (2010) Sixth Report on the Statistics on the Number of Animals Used for Experimental and Other Scientific Purposes in the Member States of the European Union. Report from the Commission to the Council and the European Parliament, SEC 1107. Available at http://eur-lex.europa.eu/LexUriServ/LexUriServ.do?uri=COM:2010:0511:REV1:EN:PDF (accessed January 31, 2013).

9. Home Office (2012) Statistics of Scientific Procedures on Living Animals, Great Britain. The Stationery Office, London. Available at http://www.homeoffice.gov.uk/publications/science-research-statistics/research-statistics/other-science-research/spanimals11/spanimals11?view=Binary (accessed January 31, 2013).

10. European Parliament (2010) Directive 2010/63/EU of the European Parliament and of the Council of 22 September 2010 on the protection of animals used for scientific purposes. Available at http://eurlex.europa.eu/LexUriServ/LexUriServ.do?uri=OJ:L:2010:276:0033:0079:EN:PDF (accessed January 31, 2013).

11. Rubinstein, A.L. (2003) Zebrafish: from disease modeling to drug discovery. *Current Opinion in Drug Discovery & Development*, **6** (2), 218–223.

12. Zon, L.I. and Peterson, R.T. (2005) *In vivo* drug discovery in the zebrafish. *Nature Reviews. Drug Discovery*, **4** (1), 35–44.

13. European Commission (2004) The Rules Governing Medicinal Products in the European Union, Vol. 6B. Notice to Applicants. Veterinary Medicinal Products. Directorate-General Enterprise. Pharmaceuticals: Regulatory Framework and Market Authorizations. Available at http://ec.europa.eu/health/files/eudralex/vol-6/b/vol6b_04_2004_final_en.pdf (accessed January 31, 2013).

14. Gannon, F. (2007) Animal rights, human wrongs? Introduction to the Talking Point on the use of animals in scientific research. *EMBO Reports*, **8** (6), 519–520.

15. Rollin, B.E. (2007) Animal research: a moral science. Talking Point on the use of animals in scientific research. *EMBO Reports*, **8** (6), 521–525.

16. Festing, S. and Wilkinson, R. (2007) The ethics of animal research. Talking Point on the use of animals in scientific research. *EMBO Reports*, **8** (6), 526–530.

17. Rollin, B.E. (2012) The moral status of invasive animal research. *Animals Research Ethics*, **42** (6), S4–S6.

18 Cruel Treatment of Cattle Act 1822 of the Parliament of the United Kingdom (3 Geo. IV c. 71).

19 Cruelty to Animals Act 1835 of the Parliament of the United Kingdom (citation 5 & 6 Will. 4, c. 59).

20 Cruelty to Animals Act 1849 of the Parliament of the United Kingdom (12 & 13 Vict. c. 92).

21 Cruelty to Animals Act 1876 of the Parliament of the United Kingdom (39 & 40 Vict., Public Acts, c. 77.).

22 Rollin, B.E. (1981) *Animal Rights and Human Morality*, Prometheus Books, Buffalo, NY, pp. 38–40 and 54–57.

23 Regan, T. (1983) *The Case for Animal Rights*, University of California Press, Berkeley, CA.

24 Singer, P. (1975) *Animal Liberation: A New Ethics for Our Treatment of Animals*, Random House, New York.

25 Russell, W.M.S. and Burch, R.L. (1959) *The Principles of Humane Experimental Technique*, Methuen, London, UK.

26 Expert Working Group of the Animal Welfare Committee (2008) Guidelines to promote the well-being of animals used for scientific purposes: the assessment and alleviation of pain and distress in research animals. National Health and Medical Research Council, Australian Government. Available at http://www.nhmrc.gov.au/_files_nhmrc/publications/attachments/ea18.pdf (accessed January 31, 2013).

27 National Health and Medical Research Council (NHMRC), Australian Government (2004) *Australian Code of Practice for the Care and Use of Animals for Scientific Purposes*, 7th edn. NHMRC, Australia. Available at http://www.nhmrc.gov.au/_files_nhmrc/publications/attachments/ea16.pdf (accessed January 31, 2013).

28 Smith, J.A., van den Broek, F.A., Martorell, J.C., Hackbarth, H., Ruksenas, O., and Zeller, W. (2007) Principles and practice in ethical review of animal experiments across Europe: summary of the report of a FELASA Working Group on Ethical Evaluation of Animal Experiments. *Laboratory Animals*, **41** (2), 143–160.

29 Smith, J.A. and Jennings, M. (2009) *A Resource Book for Lay Members of Ethical Review Processes*, 2nd edn. RSPCA, Horsham, UK. Available at http://www.rspca.org.uk/ethicalreview (accessed January 31, 2013).

30 Jennings, M. (ed.) (2010) *Guiding Principles on Good Practice for Ethical Review Processes*, 2nd edn. A Report by the RSPCA Research Animal Department and LASA Education, Training and Ethics Section. RSPCA, Horsham, UK. Available at http://www.rspca.org.uk/ethicalreview (accessed January 31, 2013).

31 Demers, G., Brown, M., Gauthier, C., Rozmiarek, H., Griffin, G., and Bédard, M. (2010) ICLAS International harmonization of guidance on the ethical review of proposals for the use of animals, and on the education and training of animal users in science. Available at http://iclas.org/committees/harmonization-committee (accessed January 31, 2013).

32 Guillén, J. (2012) FELASA guidelines and recommendations. *The Journal of the American Association for Laboratory Animal Science*, **51** (3), 311–21.

33 Canadian Council on Animal Care (1997) CCAC Guidelines on Animal Use Protocol Review. Available at http://www.ccac.ca/Documents/Standards/Guidelines/Protocol_Review.pdf (accessed January 31, 2013).

34 Office of Laboratory Animal Welfare (OLAW)/Applied Research Ethics National Association (ARENA) (2002) *Institutional Animal Care and Use Committee Guidebook*, 2nd edn. OLAW/ARENA. Available at http://grants.nih.gov/grants/olaw/guidebook.pdf (accessed January 31, 2013).

35 Committee for the Update of the Guide for the Care and Use of Laboratory Animals, National Research Council of the National Academies (2011) *NRC's Guide for the Care and Use of Laboratory Animals*, 8th edn. The National Academies Press, Washington, DC. Available at http://grants.nih.gov/grants/olaw/Guide-for-the-care-and-use-of-Laboratory-animals.pdf (accessed January 31, 2013).

36 Van Zutphen, B. (2007) Education and training for the care and use of laboratory animals: an overview of current practices. *The ILAR Journal*, **48** (2), 72–74.

37 Gibson, K., Bihun, C., Cavan, R., Dickson, H., Madziak, R., and Schofield, L. (1999) Canadian Council of Animal Care CCAC

Guidelines on Institutional Animal User Training with Accompanying Recommended Syllabus for an Institutional Animal User Training Program. Available at http://www.ccac.ca/Documents/Standards/Guidelines/Institutional_training.pdf (accessed January 31, 2013).

38 Medina, L.V., Hrapkiewicz, K., Tear, M., and Anderson, L.C. (2007) Fundamental training for individuals involved in the care and use of laboratory animals: a review and update of the 1991 NRC Core Training Module. *The ILAR Journal*, **48** (2), 96–108.

39 Weiss Convenor, J., Bukelskiene, V., Chambrier, P., Ferrari, L., van der Meulen, M., Moreno, M., Mulkens, F., Sigg, H., and Yates, N. (2010) FELASA recommendations for the education and training of laboratory animal technicians (category A). Report of the Federation of European Laboratory Animal Science Associations Working Group on Education of Animal Technicians (category A) accepted by the FELASA Board of Management. *Laboratory Animals*, **44** (3), 163–169.

40 Berge, E., Gallix, P., Jilge, B., Melloni, E., Thomann, P., Waynforth, B., and van Zutphen, L.F. (1999) FELASA guidelines for education of specialists in laboratory animal science (category D). Report of the Federation of Laboratory Animal Science Associations Working Group on Education of Specialists (category D) accepted by the FELASA Board of Management. *Laboratory Animals*, **33** (1), 1–15.

41 Nevalainen, T., Dontas, I., Forslid, A., Howard, B.R., Klusa, V., Käsermann, H.P., Melloni, E., Nebendahl, K., Stafleu, F.R., Vergara, P., and Verstegen, J. (2000) FELASA recommendations for the education and training of persons carrying out animal experiments (category B). Report of the Federation of European Laboratory Animal Science Associations Working Group on Education of Persons Carrying Out Animal Experiments (category B) accepted by the FELASA Board of Management. *Laboratory Animals*, **34** (3), 229–235.

42 Nevalainen, T., Blom, H.J.M., Guaitani, A., Hardy, P., Howard, B.R., and Vergara, P. (2002) FELASA recommendations for the accreditation of laboratory animal science education and training. Report of the Federation of European Laboratory Animal Science Associations Working Group on Accreditation of Laboratory Animal Science Education and Training. *Laboratory Animals*, **36** (4), 373–377.

43 European Union (1986) Council Directive 86/609/EEC of 24 November 1986 on the approximation of laws, regulations and administrative provisions of the Member States regarding the protection of animals used for experimental and other scientific purposes. Available at http://eurlex.europa.eu/LexUriServ/LexUriServ.do?uri=OJ:L:1986:358:0001:0028:EN:PDF (accessed January 31, 2013).

44 Council of Europe (2006) Appendix A of the European Convention (ETS No. 123) for the protection of vertebrate animals used for experimental and other scientific purposes. Guidelines for accommodation and care of animals (article 5 of the convention). Available at http://conventions.coe.int/Treaty/EN/Treaties/PDF/123-Arev.pdf (accessed January 31, 2013).

45 Animals (Scientific Procedures) Act 1986 (revised). Available at http://www.legislation.gov.uk/ukpga/1986/14/contents (accessed January 31, 2013).

46 The Animal Welfare Act (AWA). Public Law 89-544 (1966, amended in 1970, 1976, 1985, 1990, 2002, 2007, and 2008). Available at http://awic.nal.usda.gov/public-law-89-544-act-august-24-1966 (accessed January 31, 2013).

47 Olfert, E.D., Cross, B.M., and McWilliam, A.A. (eds) (1993) *CCAC Guide to the Care and Use of Experimental Animals*, vol. 1, 2nd edn. CCAC, Ottawa, Ontario. Available at http://www.ccac.ca/Documents/Standards/Guidelines/Experimental_Animals_Vol1.pdf (accessed January 31, 2013).

48 Canadian Council on Animal Care (1998) *CCAC Guidelines on Choosing an Appropriate Endpoint in Experiments Using Animals for Research, Teaching and Testing*. CCAC, Ottawa, Ontario. Available at http://www.ccac.ca/Documents/Standards/Guidelines/Appropriate_endpoint.pdf (accessed January 31, 2013).

49 Japanese Law for the Humane Treatment and Management of Animals – Law No. 105 (1973, revised in 2000). Available at http://

www.alive-net.net/english/en-law/L2-full-text.html (accessed January 31, 2013).
50 Ministry of Education, Culture, Sports, Science and Technology (2006) Fundamental Guidelines for Proper Conduct of Animal Experiment and Related Activities in Academic Research Institutions under the jurisdiction of the Ministry of Education, Culture, Sports, Science and Technology. Notice No. 71. Available at http://www.lifescience.mext.go.jp/policies/pdf/an_material011.pdf (accessed January 31, 2013).
51 Council of Japan (2006) Guidelines for Proper Conduct of Animal Experiments Science. Available at http://www.scj.go.jp/ja/info/kohyo/pdf/kohyo-20-k16-2e.pdf (accessed January 31, 2013).
52 Kurosawa, T.M. (2007) Japanese regulation of laboratory animal care with 3Rs. Proceedings of the 6th World Congress on Alternatives & Animal Use in the Life Sciences (AATEX 14), Special Issue, pp. 317–321.
53 The Prevention of Cruelty to Animals Act (1960, amended in 1982). Available at http://moef.nic.in/modules/rules-and-regulations/animal-welfare/ (accessed February 17, 2013).
54 Committee for the Purpose of Control and Supervision on Experiments on Animals (CPCSEA) (2005). Guidelines for Laboratory Animal Facility. Available at http://icmr.nic.in/animal_ethics.htm (accessed February 17, 2013).
55 Indian National Science Academy (INSA) (1992) Guidelines for Care and Use of Animals in Scientific Research, revised 2000. Available at http://icmr.nic.in/animal_ethics.htm (accessed February 17, 2013).
56 MOST (Ministry of Science and Technology) (1988) Statute on Administration of Laboratory Animals (2nd order). Available at http://www.most.gov.cn/zcfg/kjfg/200212/t20021217_7769.htm (accessed February 18, 2013).
57 Kong, Q. and Qin, C. (2010) Analysis of current laboratory animal science policies and administration in China. *The ILAR e-Journal*, **51**, e1–e10.
58 Ministry of Science and Technology (MOST) (2006) Guideline on Humane Treatment of Laboratory Animals. Available at http://www.most.gov.cn/zfwj/zfwj2006/200512/t20051214_54389.htm (accessed February 18, 2013).
59 Beijing Municipality Administration Office of Laboratory Animals (BAOLA) (2005) Guideline of Beijing Municipality on Review of Welfare and Ethics of Laboratory Animal. Available at http://bjxkz.lascn.com/system_manager/news_manager/UploadFile/250/250_3.doc (accessed February 18, 2013).
60 Brazilian Federal Law on Animal Experimentation (Law 11794), 2008.
61 Pinto, A.T., Saldanha, C.J., Valle, S., and Oliveira, M. (2011) The Brazilian legal framework on the scientific use of animals. *The ILAR e-Journal*, **52**, e8–e15.
62 Council for International Organizations of Medical Sciences (CIOMS) (1985) International Guiding Principles for Biomedical Research Involving Animals. Available at http://cioms.ch/publications/guidelines/1985_texts_of_guidelines.htm (accessed February 18, 2013).

5
Regulatory Issues: Safety and Toxicology Assessment
Antonio Guzmán

5.1
Introduction

Safety assessment is one of the most critical aspects of the drug discovery and development process. The primary aim of a preclinical toxicology program is to characterize the toxicological properties of the drug candidate prior to human exposure and to assess its potential to produce adverse effects in humans. The conducted toxicology studies should identify the inherent property of the test substance to produce adverse effects (hazard identification) and provide sufficient safety data for estimating risk in humans (i.e., the likelihood of a toxic effect occurring at an expected exposure level and condition).

Toxicology is a complex research field that covers a large area of drug development and several disciplines. Whereas, generally speaking, pharmacological research is focused on showing the presence of a desired pharmacological activity, toxicology focuses on the "unknown" as it aims to identify any possible, a priori unknown, undesired property. Thus, safety is studied to the greatest extent possible, assessing effects on aspects such as organ toxicity, reproductive and developmental toxicity, safety pharmacology, and genotoxicity. The further characterization of this hazard, in terms of quantification of the effect, dose dependence, relationship with exposure and reversibility, will allow assessing the potential risk that findings observed in the experimental model could also be produced in humans.

5.1.1
Animal Testing

Regulatory toxicology testing is mostly supported by *in vivo* animal studies, with some relevant exceptions for specific toxicological endpoints. Although far from being optimal, animal models are still considered the best surrogate for reproducing the plethora of complex molecular, biochemical, and physiological interactions that, as a consequence of drug exposure, can take place in humans and

In Vivo *Models for Drug Discovery*, First Edition. Edited by José M. Vela, Rafael Maldonado, and Michel Hamon.
© 2014 Wiley-VCH Verlag GmbH & Co. KGaA. Published 2014 by Wiley-VCH Verlag GmbH & Co. KGaA.

can ultimately lead to potential adverse effects. Thus, *in vivo* animal testing represents a pivotal component of the safety assessment process in drug discovery and development, and has proved to be of immensurable value in revealing human-relevant adverse effects [1].

In the context of regulatory drug development, use of *in vitro* models is limited to particular toxicological endpoints, such as cardiac channel interaction studies (e.g., hERG inhibition), genotoxicity and phototoxicity, or as part of supportive mechanistic studies. *In vitro* testing, however, plays a relevant role in the early candidate screening phases as well as in other research areas relevant for safety assessment, such as pharmacological target selectivity (on/off-target effects, interaction with drug transporters, etc.) or drug metabolism (metabolic stability or inhibition).

Although great advances have been made for *in silico* prediction of compound-related toxicities, "good predictivity" so far has only been acknowledged for toxic effects with simple underlying mechanism, such as dermal irritation and genotoxicity. *In silico* prediction models are mainly used as screening tool for rank ordering, prioritization, or screening out of drug candidates. Recently, however, *in silico* models have become part of regulatory toxicology testing, being used in the qualification of potential genotoxic impurities [2].

Altogether, animal testing will probably remain the primary tool for assessing the safety of new drug candidates in the foreseeable future. In the last decade, the advent of new technologies such as toxicogenomics, proteomics, bioinformatics, and systems biology was expected to improve the predictivity of animal testing and to favor a more prominent use of *in vitro* models. However, their inherent limitations have brought them to be regarded more as complementary tools with a relevant role in exploratory and mechanistic studies [3].

As a general rule, toxicity studies use high doses and extended treatment periods in order to increase the potential to detect adverse effects and to compensate for the relatively low number of animals treated compared with the intended target patient population. The ability to test high exposures allows to investigate dose–response relationships and to study effects that, because of practical or ethical reasons, are not possible or are difficult to study in humans, for example, tissue/organ damage through histopathological examinations, effects on embryo–fetal development, and carcinogenic potential.

For small-molecule pharmaceuticals, adverse effects can be produced by the following:

- *On-target effects*: Derived from the indented pharmacological activity of the drug.
- *Off-target effects*: Derived from promiscuity with other pharmacological targets.
- *Chemistry-related effects*: Derived from the physical and chemical properties of the drug molecule.

For biopharmaceuticals, which are characterized by exerting specific pharmacodynamic (PD) effects, treatment-related adverse effects are mostly related to their pharmacology, be it due to either exaggerated PD effects or off-site activity.

5.1.2
Regulatory Context

Because of its relevance for human safety, toxicological testing is regulated by national and international guidelines. In the international context, the most relevant regulatory guidelines are those of the International Conference on Harmonisation of Technical Requirements for Registration of Pharmaceuticals for Human Use (ICH) and the Organisation for Economic Co-operation and Development (OECD). Whereas ICH guidelines refer to general concepts of study design and program strategy to support drug development, OECD guidelines refer to specific experimental study designs for assessing the safety of chemicals, including pharmaceuticals.

ICH M3(R2) guideline plays a central role in toxicology testing, as it lists the studies generally required to assess the toxicological profile of a new drug candidate, the type of investigations and endpoints that should be assessed, and the minimum requirements for these studies to be acceptable to support the conduct of clinical studies and marketing authorization application [4]. For small-molecule drug candidates, this usually includes safety pharmacology testing, general and repeated dose toxicity studies, assessment of exposure (toxicokinetics), genotoxicity, developmental and reproduction toxicity (DART) studies, and, for drugs intended for a long duration of use (or with special cause for concern), carcinogenicity studies. For each of these areas of toxicological testing, there are specific ICH and OECD guidelines defining the minimal requirements to be fulfilled and a detailed description of study designs. ICH M3(R2) guideline further establishes when, in the context of the proposed clinical development program, these studies should be conducted. The different guidelines should, however, not be regarded as stand-alone documents but as complementary ones, to be read in conjunction with several other nonclinical and clinical guidelines. Although there are also many regional specific guidelines, these are usually based on principles of OECD and ICH guidelines.

For special types of medicinal products such as biotechnology-derived drugs [5], vaccines [6], anticancer drugs [7], and advanced therapy medicinal products (gene therapy, somatic cell therapy, and tissue engineering) [8–10], regulatory bodies have issued specific guidelines that take into consideration their particular properties.

Studies are required to be conducted under Good Laboratory Practice (GLP) conditions. When due to unique study design and practical issues this might not be feasible, it should be properly justified and studies conducted as close as possible to GLP principles in terms of data quality and integrity.

5.1.3
Clinical Context

Toxicology studies are conducted both in advance and in parallel to the clinical development program. The extent of toxicological characterization required for a particular drug candidate is conditioned by the type of product (small-molecule chemical entity or biopharmaceutical), the planned clinical studies, and the proposed clinical indication.

The traditional approach for first-in-human (FIH) clinical trials is to expose healthy volunteers to increasing single doses of the drug candidate until a maximum tolerated dose (MTD) is achieved. This type of phase I studies have no therapeutic intent, and their main objective is to assess tolerability and drug exposure (pharmacokinetics). They need to be supported by safety pharmacology, genotoxicity, and repeated dose toxicity studies (of at least 2-week duration in two animal species). An alternative approach to FIH studies is to run "exploratory clinical trials," which are not intended to examine clinical tolerability, involve limited human exposure, and can be initiated with less nonclinical support than is generally warranted for clinical development trials. Exploratory clinical studies can be used to investigate parameters such as pharmacokinetics (PK), PD, and other biomarkers in healthy individuals or selected patient populations, providing insight into human physiology/pharmacology, knowledge of drug characteristics, and therapeutic target relevance to the disease. ICH M3(R2) guideline describes five different approaches to exploratory clinical trials, ranging from the use of microdoses ($\leq 100\,\mu g$) to the use of doses in the therapeutic range, and the recommended supporting nonclinical studies.

For further clinical development, ICH M3(R2) guideline describes the nonclinical safety studies recommended to support human trials of a given scope and duration and marketing authorization. Whereas new therapeutic agents require a full study package, abbreviated packages can be suitable for generics, old compounds, drug combinations, and changes in clinical indication.

5.2
Animal Species in Toxicology Studies

The selection of animal species for toxicology testing should be primarily based on scientific criteria, in terms of animal similarity to humans with regard to physiology, PD response to the drug, PK behavior, and metabolic profile. There are, however, several practical and technical aspects that have historically contributed to establishing the usual spectrum of laboratory animals used for toxicity testing, such as cost, ease of breeding, availability, growth rate and mature size, behavior and manageability, ethics, regulatory requirements, and availability of historical data.

Animal regulatory toxicity studies are required to be conducted in mammalian species, generally rodents. For some particular toxicity studies, testing in two mammalian species is required, and for some crucial studies, such as repeated dose and embryo–fetal development toxicity, one should be a nonrodent. For some areas of toxicology testing, preferred or first choice animal species are suggested in the corresponding regulatory guidelines, because of either practical issues or historical precedence. The use of animal species for the first time for testing can cause regulatory concerns, requiring additional resources for model characterization and validation to enable acceptance of data. Hence, prior to using nonconventional animal species, it is advisable to discuss this matter with the relevant regulatory authority.

The laboratory rat is the default animal species used in most areas of toxicological testing, except in those where rodents are not considered the preferred choice (e.g., cardiovascular safety pharmacology studies) owing to their inherent limitations. Historically, dogs have been the most commonly used nonrodent species for the toxicological testing of new chemical entities (NCEs), whereas for biopharmaceuticals, the nonhuman primate (NHP) has been the species of choice owing to its inherent species-specific activity issues. In recent years, the minipig has become an alternative to dogs and primates for small molecules.

5.2.1
Rodents

Rodent regulatory toxicology studies are usually conducted in a limited number of well-characterized outbred strains, made up of genetically diverse animal lines in which maximum genetic heterozygosity is maintained by a rotational mating scheme minimizing brother–sister mating [11]. In outbred strains, each animal is a unique representative of the defined genetic pool of the population, being generally more resistant to external/environmental confounding factors and allowing an optimized detection of potential compound-related adverse effects. From a practical point of view, these strains are also cheaper to maintain. Inbred strains, made up of almost genetically identical animals produced by mating 20 or more consecutive generations of brothers and sisters, have a more restricted use in regulatory toxicology testing. Their greater phenotypic uniformity leads to more statistically powerful experiments requiring a fewer number of animals to detect a given biological effect, but the adverse consequence is that these strains are more susceptible to environmental factors (diet, bedding, temperature, etc.) [12]. Use of inbred strains for toxicology testing is generally limited to specific types of studies, as for genetically modified rodent strains used for mechanistic investigation, genotoxicity, or carcinogenicity testing.

The rat (*Rattus norvegicus*) is generally the preferred rodent species for toxicology testing, in part due to the supportive pharmacology, PK, and metabolism data generated as part of the drug discovery and development process. The two rat strains most commonly used for toxicity testing in Europe and the United States are the Sprague Dawley (SD) and the Han Wistar strains. The relevance of using adequately characterized rodent strains is exemplified by the decreased use, during the last two decades, of the Charles River SD rat in carcinogenicity testing as a consequence of the progressive decline in its life span that compromised the regulatory requirement to fulfill a 2-year treatment period for a study to be acceptable. The change in longevity was mostly attributed to a genetic change in the stock, causing excessively increased body weight and an associated higher mortality [12]. For some shorter-term toxicity studies where the availability of strain-specific historical background data is pivotal (e.g., reproductive toxicity studies), use of SD rat strain remained unchanged.

The mouse (*Mus musculus*) is the second rodent species of choice for toxicity testing, with CD-1 mouse strain being the one most commonly used in Europe and the United States. Occasionally, and in general because of metabolic profile issues, mice have been the primary rodent species for toxicology testing. Their smaller size, compared with rats, confers several advantages such as lower cost, ease of housing and handling, and lesser compound requirement. It is, however, also one of its main disadvantages, as it reduces the number of investigations and samplings that can be conducted on study animals.

5.2.2
Nonrodents

The value of nonrodent species in the development of new pharmaceuticals has been reviewed over many years, and they have been claimed to be more predictive of human toxicity than rodents. An International Life Sciences Institute (ILSI) study assessing the concordance between adverse findings observed in clinical studies and data generated in preclinical toxicology studies showed the nonrodent species (dog and primates) to have a higher frequency (63%) of positive concordance than rodents (43%) [1]. A further survey assessing the contribution of having the dog as second species showed that 63% of dog studies confirmed the results of rat studies and in 37% of dog studies new findings were seen [13].

The dog (*Canis familiaris*) is by far the most commonly used nonrodent species in toxicology studies, followed by NHPs for biologics. Because of its convenient medium size and docile nature, the Beagle dog has been used for decades in regulatory toxicology, with a prominent role in testing for repeated dose toxicity and cardiovascular (CV) safety. This breed has been thoroughly characterized and extensive information can be found in the scientific literature [14,15].

More recently, the minipig (*Sus scrofa*) has become an important model for drug safety testing in place of dogs and primates. Because of their smaller size compared with farmyard varieties, minipigs are more manageable, better adapted to laboratory housing, and require smaller amounts of compound for testing. There are numerous breeds of minipigs available, such as Minnesota, Hanford, Sinclair, and Yucatan, with Göttingen minipig being the most widely used and best characterized breed in Europe. Minipigs share many anatomical, physiological, and biochemical similarities with humans, and hence are the first choice alternative for drug classes where the dog has shown to be oversensitive to dose-limiting effects of limited human relevance, for example, gastrointestinal lesions due to nonsteroidal anti-inflammatory drugs, cardiotoxicity due to antihypertensive and sympathicomimetic drugs, and drugs causing emetic response [16–18]. The minipigs are also the species of choice for dermal studies, because of their anatomical and physiological similarities with human skin (thickness of the dermis, sparse coat of hair, rete ridge structures, and, for Göttingen minipig, slight pigmentation of skin) [16]. In terms of gastrointestinal effects, they have the same physiology of digestion as humans (both are true omnivores), are less prone to emesis than dogs, and have small intestine transit time and pH similar to humans [19]. They are also considered to have a closer anatomical structure and wound healing response of the cardiovascular system to humans, compared with dogs [19]. Adult minipigs, however, have a higher body weight than other nonrodent species, thus requiring higher amounts of test compound.

Because of their genotypic, phenotypic, and physiological similarities, non-human primates are given a high predictive value for human responses. The use of NHPs in regulatory toxicology studies requires, however, a conservative approach, being generally restricted to those conditions where other animal species are not appropriate [20]. For small molecules, this is usually a consequence of metabolic profile similarity to humans (i.e., absence of human-relevant metabolites in other animal species), whereas for biologics it is usually a consequence of species-specific pharmacological activity.

The cynomolgus monkey (*Macaca fascicularis*) is by far the most commonly used NHP in toxicology testing, followed by the rhesus monkey (*Macaca mulatta*) and the marmoset (*Callithrix jacchus*). Compared with rhesus monkeys, the cynomolgus macaques have the advantage that they are readily available and are not seasonal breeders. The significantly smaller size of the marmoset reduces compound requirement, thus being particularly relevant for expensive drug candidates. However, it also presents an important limitation: its reduced blood sampling volume that limits its use in extensive investigations. The recent implementation of sampling and analytical techniques such as dry spot analysis and microsampling, which significantly reduce sample volume requirement, might lead to increased use of marmosets in future.

The rabbit (*Oryctolagus cuniculus*) is the most common nonrodent species used for embryo–fetal development toxicity testing of small molecules, mainly because of its practicality (relatively larger litter size) and accumulated background knowledge. The most commonly used strain is the New Zealand white rabbit followed by the Himalayan rabbit, with preference mostly being driven by previous experience or available background data in the conducting research facility. Because of their medium size (2–3 kg), they do not share the blood sampling limitations of rodents.

Toxicity studies are generally required to be conducted in healthy young animals, with females being nulliparous. It is, however, not uncommon, particularly for nonrodents, to use young sexually immature animals, a factor that, in combination with study duration, can end up being a potential confounding factor in study interpretation. Due to the small group sizes used in nonrodent studies and the significant individual animal variability in sexual maturation, it is possible that by chance a higher proportion of animals in an immature state can be present in the high-dose group, which at the end of treatment could be interpreted as a treatment-related effect. A further confounding factor of using animals at an age maturing on course with the study is that attaining of sexual maturity can be compromised due to general nonspecific toxicity [21].

5.2.3
Nonconventional Animal Models

Transgenic Animal Models Genetically modified animal models have proved to be an outstanding tool in biological research, improving our understanding of mode of actions of drug-induced effects [22]. In toxicological testing, they play a relevant role in toxicity screening, and in mechanistic toxicology they are used as an investigative tool, for example, for assessing the absence of carcinogenic activity of bezo[a]pyrene in knockout mice lacking the aryl hydrocarbon receptor [23]. They are also used in regulatory toxicity testing, where transgenic animals are accepted models for assessing genotoxicity and carcinogenicity. These animal models are further described in the corresponding sections of this chapter. For an in-depth study of this topic, the reader should refer to Ref. [24].

Juvenile Animals Since the implementation of the Pediatric Regulation to facilitate the development, accessibility, and improved safe use of new medicines in children, for some drugs it is expected that pediatric clinical trials should be supported with juvenile animal studies [25]. Pediatric population refers to the population aged up to 18 years. Before including pediatric patients in clinical trials, juvenile animal studies might be warranted if safety data from previous animal and adult human experience are judged insufficient to support pediatric studies. The main objective is to assess whether juvenile animals have a different sensitivity compared with adult animals and to identify toxicity relevant for developing systems and effects on growth and/or development in the age group to be treated. Generally, juvenile animal studies should be conducted in one appropriate animal species, the first choice for repeated dose toxicity studies being rats or dogs, and the age of the animals at start of treatment and the duration of the dosing period should be adjusted to the developing organ system being assessed [26,27]. These studies are technically very challenging, as they require administration of juvenile animals (either rodent or nonrodent) within a particular age range (occasionally shortly after birth) and through the intended clinical route of administration.

5.3
Toxicology Studies

5.3.1
General Principles

Toxicology issues with drug candidates have been considered to contribute to approximately 30% of drug attrition rates [28]. As a consequence, regulatory toxicity studies are inevitably preceded by short-term or simplified exploratory toxicity studies. Their aim is to avoid development-limiting toxicity and to select compounds with better safety profiles, advancing into early development lead candidates with a better chance of successfully reaching FIH clinical trials [29].

This section describes the most relevant areas of regulatory toxicity testing required to support drug development. Although presented as individual research areas, targeting particular toxicological endpoints, they are not stand-alone disciplines but rather complementary ones. The information generated in one area of toxicity testing can complement and aid in the interpretation of others (e.g., genotoxicity study results can aid to understand the underlying mechanism of an observed carcinogenic effect). Any sign of alert should trigger follow-up studies to further evaluate the extent or relevance of the observed effect. Ultimately, it is the integrated assessment of all conducted toxicological investigations that will determine the potential toxicological risk that the exposure to a drug candidate can present to humans and also whether this risk is acceptable.

The extent and timing of the regulatory nonclinical package will depend on the design of the proposed clinical trials, with the investigator justifying the selected study design. The selected test species, dose levels, dose regimen, and route of administration should be based on the intended clinical use and available PD, PK, and toxicological information. Most regulatory toxicology studies have in common a four-animal group design:

- *Vehicle control group*: The group receiving the vehicle used for test article formulation.
- *High-dose group*: The group enabling identification of target organ(s) of toxicity, other nonspecific toxicity, and absence or presence of specific toxicological endpoint (genotoxic potential, cardiovascular safety, etc.). Ideally, the systemic exposure to the drug at this high dose level should significantly exceed the one expected or attained in the clinical setting.
- *Low-dose group*: The group ideally with a systemic exposure similar to or slightly exceeding the expected or intended clinical exposure, or producing a PD effect.
- *Intermediate-dose group*: The group that usually corresponds to the geometric mean between the high and low doses.

The use of "positive control" groups is restricted to some studies assessing specific toxicological endpoints, such as genotoxicity or safety pharmacology studies.

The classical criterion for establishing the high dose is the attainment of the MTD or the maximum feasible dose, thus increasing the potential for detecting adverse effects. However, to prevent the use of unrealistic high dosages that would not add value to predicting clinical safety, limit doses or limit of exposure (in terms of AUC) have been defined. Guidance for the different toxicology research areas can be found in the appropriate guidelines; for example, for repeated dose toxicity studies, a limit dose of 1000 mg/kg/day is considered appropriate, except when clinical dose exceeds 1 g/day, in which case the high dose should be limited by a 10-fold exposure margin or a dose of 2000 mg/kg/day, whichever is lower [4].

The three-dose level approach should allow establishing a dose–response relationship of toxicological effect, with the determination of a dose level free of adverse effects being the key issue in toxicological testing. The highest dose or exposure level at which no effects are observed, when compared with its appropriate control, is considered as the "no observed effect level" (NOEL). The highest dose or exposure level at which effects are observed, which are considered to lack toxicological relevance, is considered as the "no observed adverse effect level" (NOAEL). The NOAEL therefore takes into account the possibility that PD responses or minimum toxic effects lacking statistical or biological relevance may be observed that are not considered to endanger human health or to be precursors of adverse effects [30]. In the absence of other alerting signs, the NO(A)EL, as determined for the most sensitive and relevant animal species in the first conducted repeated dose toxicity studies, will serve as reference for estimating the starting dose and dose escalation scheme for FIH studies. NO(A)EL values obtained from longer-term studies, or from specific toxicological endpoints, will serve for determining safety margins and for risk assessment.

To establish a starting dose for FIH, the experimentally determined NO(A)EL is adjusted by allometric scaling (or on the basis of pharmacokinetics) to a human equivalent dose, which is further reduced by applying appropriate safety factors according to the toxicological properties of the compound and the proposed clinical study. A generally used default safety factor is 10, but it can be increased or decreased depending on further available information [31]. For "high-risk" medicinal products (i.e., those where there are concerns that serious adverse reactions in FIH trials may occur), the starting dose can be established based on the minimal anticipated biological effect level (MABEL) in humans, applying when appropriate an additional safety factor. When NO(A)L and MABEL calculations give different values of human starting dose, the lowest value should be applied.

Kinetics and metabolism data play an important role in the design and interpretation of preclinical safety studies, as information on systemic exposure of treated animal is essential for study interpretation and human safety assessment. Toxicokinetic investigations, assessing systemic exposure by serial blood sampling of study animals, are consequently an integral part of toxicity studies and subject of specific regulatory guidance [32]. In rodents, where blood volume can be a limiting factor, toxicokinetic sampling is usually conducted on satellite group animals. For small-molecule pharmaceuticals, metabolism can result in molecules with altered pharmacological and toxicological properties. Studies should therefore be conducted in pharmacokinetically and metabolically relevant animal species, and major metabolites achieving relevant systemic exposure in humans should be evaluated. When this is not accomplished through studies of the parent compound, specific studies with the relevant metabolites should be considered [33]. For biologics, biotransformation studies are generally less relevant, as they are metabolized to small peptides and individual amino acids lacking pharmacological or toxicological properties different from the parent compound. Some exceptions to this general rule can be, for example, oligonucleotide-based products, fusion proteins, and immunoconjugates.

5.3.2
General and Repeated Dose Toxicity Studies

The primary goal of repeated dose toxicity studies is to characterize the toxicological profile of the test compound following repeated administration, in terms of identifying target organs of toxicity, dose dependence, relationship with exposure, and, when appropriate, potential reversibility. In characterizing the toxicity of the tested compound, the study results should allow the identification of clinical symptoms, alterations in organ function and cell and tissue histology, and parameters for clinical monitoring of potential adverse effects [4]. Repeated dose toxicity studies are a pivotal component of the regulatory package and an almost inevitable part of the preclinical package supporting FIH studies, with the experimentally determined NO(A)EL playing a pivotal role in estimating a safe starting dose.

According to ICH M3(R2) guideline, repeated dose toxicity studies should be performed in two mammalian species, one being a nonrodent, unless only one species is relevant [4]. The most commonly used nonrodent for general repeated dose toxicity testing of small molecules is the dog (followed by the minipig), whereas for biologics the most common species is the NHP.

To support clinical development, the duration of the repeated dose toxicity studies conducted in two mammalian species should be equal to or exceed the duration of the proposed human clinical trial, with the exceptions that (1) a minimum duration of 2 weeks is established for animal studies, which would generally support any clinical trial of up to 2 weeks duration, and (2) clinical trials exceeding a 6-month treatment should generally be supported by 6-month rodent and 9-month (6 months in EU) nonrodent studies [4]. To support marketing authorization, the conduced repeated dose toxicity studies should exceed the intended duration of clinical treatment, as indicated in Table 5.1.

For most categories of small-molecule pharmaceuticals intended for extended use, chronic toxicity studies are expected to complete a treatment period of 6 months for rodents and 9 months for nonrodents, as indicated in Table 5.1. However, for biotechnology-derived pharmaceuticals intended for chronic use, toxicity studies of 6 months duration have generally been accepted in accordance with the ICH S6 guideline. This difference in requirements for chronic toxicity testing is based on the differences in metabolic, PK, and toxicological characteristics between small molecules and large molecular weight proteins [34,35].

For the shorter-term repeated dose toxicity studies, selected dose levels are usually on the high side as their objective is to maximize detection of "system failure," identifying a MTD. As treatment duration increases, dose levels move

Table 5.1 Recommended duration of repeated dose toxicity studies to support marketing.

Clinical treatment duration	Rodent	Nonrodent
Up to 2 weeks	1 month	1 month
>2 weeks to 1 month	3 months	3 months
>1 month to 3 months	6 months	6 months
>3 months	6 months	9 months (6 months in EU)

Taken from ICH M3(R2).

downward, with longer-term studies focusing on exploring possible effects at doses relevant to clinical exposure and occurring over longer treatment durations [35].

During the study, food intake, clinical signs, general behavior, body weight, hematology, clinical chemistry, urinalysis, electrocardiography (nonrodents only), and ophthalmology are monitored in control and drug-treated animals at relevant time points in relation to the PD or PK profile of the drug. Minimal recommendations for sampling times and clinical pathology testing (blood chemistry, hematology, and urinalysis) have been established [36], but should be modified or complemented based on species, study objective and duration, and biological activity of the test item. In general, clinical pathology samples are obtained before treatment (nonrodents only) and at the end of treatment, with some interim sampling in longer-term studies. Whereas in nonrodents examinations are conducted in all animals, in rodents, because of their limited blood volume, examinations may be performed in a subset of animals. Depending on test compound characteristics or previous observations, additional toxicological endpoints might need to be assessed as part of the study, for example, immunotoxicity [37].

All animals, dying or sacrificed during the study, are autopsied and subjected to microscopic examination. For rodents, histopathology is performed on the high-dose and the control group animals, and the examination is extended to low- and mid-dose groups for organs and tissues showing histopathological changes in the high-dose group, to clarify the exposure–response relationship. In nonrodent species, where a small number of animals are used, histopathology is conducted on all study animals. A minimum core list of tissues to be studied histologically can be found in the CHMP guideline on repeated dose toxicity [38].

When severe toxicity with potential adverse clinical impact is observed, the potential reversibility should be assessed. This can be done either through a scientific assessment of the observed effect and its recovery capacity or by inclusion of a recovery group in the study. Conditions warranting the need to include a treatment-free period in a toxicity study are described in the Questions and Answers document of ICH M3(R2) guideline [33]. However, it is not uncommon to include a recovery group in at least one of the repeated dose toxicity studies.

5.3.3
Safety Pharmacology

The objective of safety pharmacology studies is to investigate the potential for producing undesirable PD effects on physiological functions in relation to exposures in the therapeutic range and above, and their relevance to humans. Before FIH administration, small-molecule pharmaceutical should be tested in a "core battery" of safety pharmacology studies, assessing potential effects on CV, respiratory, and central nervous system (CNS) functions, which are considered acutely critical for life [39]. Assessment of other organ systems (e.g., renal, gastrointestinal, and autonomic nervous systems) will generally depend on the specific properties of each therapeutic molecule and on observations in previous studies, in which case they should be conducted before product approval. Safety pharmacology endpoints are generally assessed in dedicated single-dose studies, except when PD effects are known to occur after repeated treatment. For biotech compounds with high specific receptor targeting, no specific safety pharmacology studies are generally required, and safety pharmacology endpoints are evaluated as part of toxicology studies.

Effects on the CNS are generally studied in rodents (most commonly rats), by means of a functional observation battery [40] or modified Irwin's test [41], assessing effects on motor activity, behavior, coordination, sensory–motor reflex response, and body temperature.

CV toxicity is a leading contributor to drug withdrawal and late-stage attrition. Drug interference with cardiac repolarization and prolongation of the QT wave of the ECG is considered a particular liability, being regarded as an indicator of increased risk for development of malignant ventricular arrhythmia in humans [42]. CV safety studies should assess effects on blood pressure, heart rate, and ECG, which are generally accomplished in nonrodent species, the dog being a well-established model. Studies can be conducted either in unanesthetized freely moving telemetry-implanted animals (current gold standard) or in anesthetized animals. The drawback of having telemetry-implanted animals undergo a surgical procedure is balanced by the possibility of reusing those animals after an appropriate washout period that takes into account PK and PD effects. An alternative to surgical telemetry, compatible with integration into early toxicology studies, is to use jacketed external telemetry. Although rodents can be used for assessing effects on blood pressure and heart rate, they are not considered suitable for assessing action potential effects, as the ion channels mediating cardiac repolarization are different from those in humans. Minipigs are considered suitable and are increasingly used for CV safety pharmacology testing.

Respiratory safety pharmacology studies should assess effects on respiration rate, tidal volume and minute volume, or hemoglobin oxygen saturation. These endpoints can be assessed either in rodents, using whole-body plethysmography recording, or in nonrodents, using either intubated anesthetized animals (generally combined with CV safety testing) or unanesthetized animals with inhalation masks (less common).

5.3.4
Genotoxicity

Testing for genotoxicity aims at identifying the potential to cause DNA damage, which is considered essential for the induction of carcinogenesis and hereditary defects. Compounds that are positive for genotoxicity are considered to be potentially human carcinogens and/or mutagens. According to current regulatory requirements, and scientific recommendations, NCE pharmaceuticals are assessed for genotoxic potential by testing in a "standard battery" of *in vitro* and *in vivo* assays [43], there being two options. Option 1 requires the conduct of (1) an *in vitro* test for gene mutation in bacteria (usually the Ames test), (2) an *in vitro* mammalian cell genotoxicity test (either a cytogenetic test for chromosomal damage or a mouse lymphoma *Tk* gene mutation assay), and (3) an *in vivo* test, generally for chromosomal damage in rodent hematopoietic cells. In option 2, the *in vitro* mammalian cell assay is replaced by a second *in vivo* assay, or a second endpoint is included for assessment in the rodent micronucleus (MN) assay (typically a DNA strand breakage assay in liver).

Genetic toxicology studies are conducted early in the safety evaluation program, in a generally accepted tiered approach, with *in vitro* studies preceding *in vivo* studies. According to ICH M3(R2) guideline, a gene mutation study is required prior to single-dose phase I clinical trials, and the potential for chromosomal damage should additionally be assessed to support multiple-dose phase I studies. The complete battery should be conducted prior to phase II studies [4]. For certain exploratory clinical trials, a reduced package of genotoxicity testing might be required. *In vivo* assays are considered to play a relevant role in the overall assessment of genotoxic potential. As they fully take into account the biological processes of absorption, distribution, metabolism, and excretion of the test article, they allow assessing the biological significance of *in vitro* test result.

Testing for genotoxicity is generally not applicable for biotechnology-derived pharmaceuticals, as these substances are not expected to interact directly with DNA [5]. For this type of compounds, carcinogenic risk can be derived from the potential for selective proliferation of spontaneously mutated cells, an activity that would be linked to their pharmacological activity, which the standard battery of genotoxicity tests are not designed to detect. Testing might, however, be adequate for certain types of biotech compounds, for example, antibodies conjugated to a cytotoxin or other moiety.

In vivo genotoxicity testing is almost exclusively performed in rodents, and the rodent erythrocyte MN assay stands out as the most widely used *in vivo* assay. Micronuclei are chromosomal fragments or whole chromosomes that are left behind during the chromosomal segregation process of the dividing cell, are not incorporated into the daughter cell nucleus, and remain visible as small nuclei in the cytoplasm. The assay assesses the induction of chromosomal damage in proliferating erythroblasts by clastogenic (chromosomal damage) and aneugenic (spindle damage) agents, which will be observed as an increased frequency of recently formed erythrocytes with MN. The absence of a main nucleus in these newly formed erythrocytes makes these cells the ideal candidate for easy microscopic detection of MN. A detailed description of the erythrocyte MN test can be found in the OECD 474 guideline [44]. In the past, peripheral blood MN studies were restricted to mice, based on the fact that rat splenic function preferentially eliminates micronucleated erythrocytes from peripheral blood [45], unlike mouse in which MN erythrocytes can accumulate and reach steady state. The advent of flow cytometry techniques identifying newly formed reticulocytes by immunological labeling (e.g., CD71-expressing) has allowed the use of rat peripheral blood samples, as the large number of cells analyzed compensates for the low level of micronucleated cells. This has made the rat the preferred species, making it technically feasible to integrate the MN assay into repeated dose toxicity studies.

The rat liver is the second most used tissue for assessing MN induction *in vivo*, and because of its high metabolic capacity, it is most suitable for assessing metabolites. In the liver MN assay, hepatocyte proliferation is induced by submitting animals to partial hepatectomy [46]. More recently, the use of young rats (<4–5 weeks) has been proposed as a way to avoid the hepatic surgical procedure, by taking advantage of the developmental proliferation of hepatocytes in young rats [47]. Dogs and primates have also been claimed to be suitable for MN analysis, done generally as part of routine repeated dose toxicity studies and only rarely as stand-alone acute studies [48].

For the second *in vivo* assay, a large variety of test systems have been proposed, but only a few are in routine general use, such as the liver unscheduled DNA synthesis (UDS) assay and the Comet assay. The UDS assay assesses the induction of DNA damage in tissues with a low frequency of proliferating cells, rat liver being preferably used. The repair of test substance-induced DNA damage by the cells' excision and repair system is measured *ex vivo* by determining through autoradiography the uptake of labeled nucleosides (generally tritium-labeled thymidine) in cells that are not undergoing scheduled replicative DNA synthesis [49].

The *in vivo* alkaline single-cell gel electrophoresis assay, or Comet assay, assesses the induction of double- and single-strand breaks and alkali-labile sites in the DNA. In this assay, single-cell suspensions from the tissue of interest are layered on slides in an agarose matrix and, after lysis (to liberate DNA) and incubation under alkaline conditions (to produce single-stranded DNA), cells are submitted to electrophoresis. DNA fragments or strands migrate away from the nucleus toward the anode and, after staining with a DNA-specific dye, cells are viewed under a microscope; they appear as a comet, with the length and intensity of the tail increased with the induced DNA damage [50].

Transgenic animals are also used for genotoxicity testing, in particular for assessing *in vivo* gene mutation induction, and for follow-up testing to clarify the outcome of the initial standard battery (Table 5.2). These animals carry, integrated in their chromosomes, multiple copies of a vector carrying a reporter gene for detecting mutation. After exposure to a potential genotoxin, DNA from the tissue of interest is extracted. Gene mutation is assessed by recovering the vector either as a bacteriophage or as a plasmid (depending on the particular animal model),

Table 5.2 Transgenic animal models used in genotoxicity testing.

Model	Strain	Transgene	Reporter gene
Muta mouse	Mouse	Lambda gt10 phage shuttle vector	*lacZ* (β-galactosidase)
LacZ plasmid mouse	C57BL/6 mouse	pUR288 plasmid	*lacZ* (β-galactosidase)
Big Blue mouse	C57BL/6 and B6C3 F1 mouse	Lambda LIZα phage vector	*lacI* (β-galactosidase)
Big Blue rat	Fischer 344 rat	Lambda phage shuttle vector	*lacI* (β-galactosidase)

transfecting an appropriate bacterial host and analyzing the phenotype of the transfected cell.

A great advantage of transgenic animal models is that potentially any tissue can be sampled and assessed for gene mutation. Some drawbacks of these models are that target genes correspond to genes that are not naturally expressed; they require prolonged treatments (e.g., 28 days) to allow for mutation expression, fixation, and accumulation; and their high cost and reliance on genetically modified animals [24].

5.3.5
Development and Reproductive Toxicity Studies

The aim of DART studies is to assess any potential adverse effect of a drug candidate on mammalian reproduction and development. For this, animals are exposed by a combination of studies at all stages of development, from conception to sexual maturity [51]. For convenience of testing, the following developmental stages in the reproductive process are considered:

A) Premating to conception.
B) Conception to implantation.
C) Implantation to closure of the hard palate.
D) Closure of the hard palate to the end of pregnancy.
E) Birth to weaning.
F) Weaning to sexual maturity.

Treatment of animals during defined stages of reproduction is considered to allow more specific identification of stages at risk and to better reflect human exposure to medicinal products. The general approach for most medicinal compounds, defined as "the most probable option" in ICH S5(R2) guideline, is to assess potential DART effects by a three-study design, consisting of the following:

- Fertility and early embryonic development.
- Pre- and postnatal development, including maternal function.
- Embryo–fetal development.

Combinations of these studies or study designs might also be valid if justified by knowledge on test compound properties as determined in previously conducted studies; for example, fertility and embryo–fetal development studies might be combined if there is certainty that no effects on fertility will pose hindrance to obtaining viable litters for assessing potential embryo–fetal effects (Table 5.3).

Studies should be conducted in mammals, the preferred species being the rat mainly because of its practicality, accumulated background knowledge, and its general use in other toxicological studies providing complementary information. For embryo–fetal development toxicity studies, a second mammalian species is required, the rabbit being the preferred choice as a "nonrodent," again because of

Table 5.3 Developmental and reproductive toxicity study designs.

Treatment and covered stages	Aimed adverse effects	Assessed endpoints
Fertility and early embryonic development		
Treatment of males and females before mating, through mating, and during implantation (stages A and B)	Females: effects on estrous cycle, tubal transport, fertilization, preimplantation development of the embryo, and implantation Males: functional effects (e.g., libido, epididymal sperm maturation) that may not be detected by histological examinations	• Maturation of gametes • Mating behavior • Fertility • Preimplantation stages of the embryo • Implantation
Embryo–fetal development		
Treatment of pregnant females from implantation to closure of the hard palate (stages C and D)	Effects on the pregnant female and development of the embryo and fetus. Major organ formation, organ development, and growth	• Enhanced toxicity relative to nonpregnant females • Embryo–fetal death • Altered growth • Structural changes
Pre- and postnatal development and maternal function		
Treatment of pregnant females from implantation through weaning (stages C–F)	Effects on the pregnant/lactating female and on the development of the conceptus and the offspring. Observations continued through sexual maturity (possible delayed manifestation of induced effects)	• Enhanced toxicity relative to nonpregnant females • Pre- and postnatal death of offspring • Altered growth and development • Functional deficits in offspring, including behavior, maturation and reproduction (F1)

its practicality and accumulated background knowledge. When the rabbit is unsuitable, an alternative nonrodent or a second rodent species might be used.

Minipigs have been proposed as alternative species in DART testing when traditional species such as mice, rats, or rabbits are unsuitable, mainly because of the good availability of mature animals, relatively larger litter size, and short pregnancy period. However, methods for conducting these studies and background data are available only in a few research organizations [16], and the lack of placental transfer of macromolecules may limit the role of the minipig in reproductive testing of biotechnology products [19]. DART studies in NHP should only be conducted when they are the only relevant species. The use of NHP in reproductive toxicology studies poses several challenges: length of gestation, low conception rate, high spontaneous abortion rate (10–20%), small sample size, limited supply, high interanimal variability, and single offspring. Mating studies are not practical for NHPs, and effects on fertility are assessed by evaluating effects on the reproductive tract in repeated dose toxicity studies. Developmental toxicity studies in NHPs, due to their inherent limitations, are considered to only provide hazard identification [52].

Toxicokinetic investigations should assess exposure in pregnant animals, this being particularly relevant for rabbits where this might be the only occasion for testing in this animal species. Assessment of fetal exposure is not a routine practice, but might be required when there is special cause for concern or as a mechanistic support, although no data comparison with human is possible. The outcome of DART studies should determine whether the potential reproductive risks to humans are greater than, lesser than, or equal to those posed by other toxicological manifestations. To assess the relevance to humans, data on likely human exposures, comparative kinetics, and mechanisms of reproductive toxicity should be considered.

5.3.6
Carcinogenicity Studies

The objective of carcinogenicity testing is to identify tumorigenic potential in animals and assess relevant risk for humans. Testing for carcinogenicity is required for pharmaceuticals for which the proposed clinical use is continuously for at least 6 months or frequently in an intermittent manner [53]. A second factor that can trigger the need for carcinogenicity testing is the existence of cause of concern for carcinogenic potential, as the observation of preneoplastic lesions in previously conducted repeated dose toxicity studies or previous demonstration of carcinogenic potential in the product class considered relevant to humans. When required, carcinogenicity studies should be conducted before marketing application, unless there is special concern for the patient population, in which case they should be conducted prior to large-scale clinical trials [53].

Two studies should be conducted: (1) a long-term rodent carcinogenicity study and (2) an additional complementary rodent assay [54]. The rat is the recommended species for conducting rodent long-term carcinogenicity assays, unless there is clear evidence favoring a different species. For the second complementary assay, it is the investigator's choice to conduct either (1) a long-term carcinogenicity study in a second rodent species (generally mice) or (2) a short- or medium-term *in vivo* model, providing insight into carcinogenic endpoints and adding value to the overall weight of evidence assessment.

The traditional rodent bioassay for treatment of animals for the major part of their life span involves treatment for 2 years in rats and 1.5–2 years in mice (depending on the life span of the particular mouse strain and testing site). A detailed description of criteria for setting appropriate dose levels, and in particular the selection of the critical high dose, is presented in the ICH S1C guideline [55]. In these studies, the extent of interim investigations (e.g., clinical pathology and

Table 5.4 Transgenic animal models used in carcinogenicity testing.

Animal model	Genetic background	Testing
Tg.AC mouse	Overexpression of ras oncogene (v-Ha-ras transgene)	Genotoxic and nongenotoxic compounds
Tg.Hras2 mouse	Overexpression of ras oncogene (c-Ha-ras transgene)	Genotoxic and nongenotoxic compounds
XPA$^{-/-}$ mouse	Knockout mice; deficient in DNA nucleotide excision repair	Genotoxic compounds
p53$^{+/-}$ mouse	Knockout mice; null mutation in one allele of the p53 tumor-suppressor gene	Genotoxic compounds

exposure assessment) is more limited compared with a general repeated dose toxicity study, as the main aim is to monitor animal condition and changes of exposure in the context of geriatric animals. Another difference from rodent repeated dose toxicity studies is that histopathology is conducted on all study animals. A minimum core list of tissues to be studied histologically in carcinogenicity studies can be found in the CHMP guideline on repeated dose toxicity [38].

As an alternative to the mouse bioassay, several short- or medium-term models are cited in the ICH S1B guideline [54]. In this respect, transgenic mouse models have slowly gained acceptance as replacement for the standard lifetime mouse bioassay [56]. These animal models (see Table 5.4) were initially developed for the research on mechanisms of carcinogenesis, showing increased sensibility toward tumor development due to the presence of activated oncogenes, inactivated tumor suppressor genes, or deficient reparation systems – elements that are involved in the regulation of cell proliferation. They are claimed to have similar predictivity of human carcinogens compared to rodent bioassay and have advantages that they require shorter treatment time for tumor induction, have lower background tumors, and, as consequence, require lower animal numbers.

A positive result for carcinogenic potential can be indicated either by an increased frequency of tumors compared with vehicle control-treated animals or by the earlier appearance of tumors in treated animals, detected in-life by external palpation (testes, mammary tissues, and dermal tumors) or at necropsy after premature death or at the end of treatment (internal tumors). In this respect, knowledge of the incidence of spontaneous tumors in the used rodent strain is of relevance, as a high spontaneous rate might mask small increases in tumor incidence related to treatment.

Carcinogens operating through genotoxic mechanisms are assumed to represent carcinogenic risk for humans. However, nongenotoxic (epigenetic) carcinogens are assumed to act through mechanisms susceptible of having a threshold of effect, and exposure levels or conditions devoid of carcinogenic risk to humans can potentially be defined. There are some well-recognized tumorigenic epigenetic mechanisms operating in rodents that, because of animal-specific physiology, sensitivity, or occurrence at unrealistically high exposures (compared with clinic), are known to be either rodent specific or irrelevant for human risk assessment. Some well-known examples of rodent-specific mechanisms are (1) the induction of thyroid tumors due to enhanced clearance of thyroid hormone, (2) mammary tumors due to D_2 receptor antagonism and stimulation of prolactin secretion by hypophysis, and (3) male rat renal tumors through accumulation of $\alpha_{2\mu}$-globulin urinary protein in the renal tubules.

The current approach to carcinogenicity testing and the value of the 2-year rodent bioassays for carcinogenic risk assessment have been questioned for years, due to the high proportion of pharmaceutical compounds producing positive carcinogenicity studies, in at least one of the rodent species [56–58]. The proportion of drugs showing positive tumor outcomes in rat carcinogenicity studies has been reported to be as high as 56%, with approximately 75% of these lacking relevance for human risk assessment [56,59]. As such, there is a general consensus that the present regulatory guidance for carcinogenicity testing should be improved. In this respect, there is a growing opinion that, based on pharmacology, genotoxicity, and chronic toxicity data, the outcome of the 2-year rodent carcinogenicity studies can be anticipated, with reasonable assurance, for drugs presenting negligible risk or, conversely, likely risk of human carcinogenicity [60]. Consolidation of such an approach could eventually render the conduct of the 2-year assay unnecessary and represent a significant reduction in animal use and resources.

5.4
Translation to Clinics: Limitations and Difficulties

Despite the limited public perception on the utility of animal models in safety testing and human protection, the use of animal models has proved to be of great value in revealing human-relevant potential adverse effects. In general, animal models are considered good predictors of toxic outcomes in humans, at least from a qualitative standpoint. A survey conducted by the ILSI, assessing the concordance of animal studies for 150 compounds for which human toxicities had been reported, showed that 71% human toxicities were correctly detected by the combination of rodent and nonrodent species, with 63% alone being reported by nonrodents and 43% only by rodents [1]. Of the concordant human toxicities, 94% were predicted in studies of 1 month or less in duration. These values might, however, underestimate the real degree of concordance, as compounds showing serious adverse effects in animal studies will most probably drop off the development pipeline and never reach human clinical trials.

Concordance between animal and human toxicities varies with organs or systems, and is considered highest for hematological, gastrointestinal, and CV effects and lowest for skin, liver (idiosyncratic toxicity in particular), and immune system [61]. Potential causes for human toxicity not being observed in animals are, among others, human adverse effects that are not adequately assessed in animal studies (e.g., nausea, cognitive impairment, dizziness, and mood changes), toxic dosages not being achieved due to the presence of other dose-limiting effects, or insufficient systemic exposure. Factors contributing to interspecies differences in toxicodynamics include anatomical differences (effect occurring in an organ of questionable relevance to humans, for example, the rodent forestomach), physiological differences (e.g., different hormonal control of target organ), and biochemical differences (e.g., species differences in key biochemical component such as $\alpha_2\mu$-globulin nephropathy) [62]. For some toxicological effects, sufficient human safety data will normally be obtained in human clinical trials to supersede animal toxicity data. However, for several other endpoints, such as genotoxicity, carcinogenicity, and reproductive toxicity, for both practical and ethical reasons, the effect of drug exposure will only be investigated in nonclinical studies.

References

1 Olson, H., Betton, G., Robinson, D., Thomas, K., Monro, A., Kolaja, G., Lilly, P., Sanders, J., Sipes, G., Bracken, W., Dorato, M., Van Deun, K., Smith, P., Berger, B., and Heller, A. (2000) Concordance of the toxicity of pharmaceuticals in humans and in animals. *Regulatory Toxicology and Pharmacology*, **32**, 56–67.

2 ICH (2013) Assessment and control of DNA reactive (mutagenic) impurities in pharmaceuticals to limit potential carcinogenic risk. International Conference on Harmonisation of Technical Requirements for Registration of Pharmaceuticals for Human Use, Topic M7, Step 3 document.

3 National Research Council (2007) *Toxicity Testing in the 21st Century: A Vision and a Strategy*, The National Academies Press.

4 ICH (2008) Nonclinical Safety Studies for the Conduct of Human Clinical Trials and Marketing Authorization for Pharmaceuticals. International Conference on Harmonisation of Technical Requirements for Registration of Pharmaceuticals for Human Use, Topic M3(R2).

5 ICH (2011) Preclinical Safety Evaluation of Biotechnology-Derived Pharmaceuticals. International Conference on Harmonisation of Technical Requirements for Registration of Pharmaceuticals for Human Use, Topic S6(R1).

6 Committee for Proprietary Medicinal Products (1997) Note for Guidance on Preclinical Pharmacological and Toxicological Testing of Vaccines. EMEA/CPMP/SWP/465/95, EMA.

7 Committee for Proprietary Medicinal Products (1998) Note for Guidance on the Preclinical Evaluation of Anticancer Medicinal Products. CPMP/SWP/997/96, EMA.

8 Committee for Proprietary Medicinal Products (2001) Note for Guidance on the Quality, Preclinical and Clinical Aspects of Gene Transfer Medicinal Products. CPMP/BWP/3088/99, EMA.

9 Committee for Proprietary Medicinal Products (2008) Guideline on Human Cell-Based Medicinal Products. EMEA/CPMP/SWP/465/95, EMA.

10 Cohen-Haguenauer, O. (2013) A comprehensive resource on EU regulatory information for investigators in gene therapy clinical research and advanced therapy medicinal products. *Human Gene Therapy*, **24**, 12–18.

11 Lovell, J.A., Stuesse, S.L., Cruce, W.L., and Crisp, T. (2000) Strain differences in neuropathic hyperalgesia. *Pharmacology, Biochemistry, and Behavior*, **65**, 141–144.

12 Kacew, S. (2001) Confounding factors in toxicity testing. *Toxicology*, **160**, 87–96.

13 Broadhead, C.L., Betton, G., Combes, R., Damment, S., Everett, D., Garner, C., Godsafe, Z., Healing, G., Heywood, R., Jennings, M., Lumley, C., Oliver, G., Smith, D., Straughan, D., Topham, J., Wallis, R., Wilson, S., and Buckley, P. (2000) Prospects for reducing and refining the use of dogs in

the regulatory toxicity testing of pharmaceuticals. *Human & Experimental Toxicology*, **19**, 440–447.
14 Anderson, A.C. and Good, L.S. (eds) (1970) *The Beagle as an Experimental Dog*, Iowa State University Press, Ames, IA.
15 Gad, S.C.E. (2007) *Animal Models in Toxicology*, CRC Press.
16 Svendsen, O. (2006) The minipig in toxicology. *Experimental and Toxicologic Pathology*, **57**, 335–339.
17 Forster, R., Bode, G., Ellegaard, L., and van der Laan, J.W. (2010) The RETHINK project – minipigs as models for the toxicity testing of new medicines and chemicals: an impact assessment. *Journal of Pharmacological and Toxicological Methods*, **62**, 158–159.
18 van der Laan, J.W., Brightwell, J., McAnulty, P., Ratky, J., and Stark, C. (2010) Regulatory acceptability of the minipig in the development of pharmaceuticals, chemicals and other products. *Journal of Pharmacological and Toxicological Methods*, **62**, 184–195.
19 Bode, G., Clausing, P., Gervais, F., Loegsted, J., Luft, J., Nogues, V., and Sims, J. (2010) The utility of the minipig as an animal model in regulatory toxicology. *Journal of Pharmacological and Toxicological Methods*, **62**, 196–220.
20 European Commission (2010) Directive 2010/63/EU of the European Parliament and of the Council of 22 September 2010 and of the Council of 22 September 2010 on the protection of animals used for scientific purposes. Available at http://eurlex.europa.eu/LexUriServ/LexUriServ.do?uri=OJ:L:2010:276:0033:0079:EN:PDF (accessed 28 February 2014).
21 Creasy, D.M. (2003) Evaluation of testicular toxicology: a synopsis and discussion of the recommendations proposed by the Society of Toxicologic Pathology. *Birth Defects Research. Part B, Developmental and Reproductive Toxicology*, **68**, 408–415.
22 Bolon, B. (2004) Genetically engineered animals in drug discovery and development: a maturing resource for toxicologic research. *Basic & Clinical Pharmacology & Toxicology*, **95**, 154–161.
23 Shimizu, Y., Nakatsuru, Y., Ichinose, M., Takahashi, Y., Kume, H., Mimura, J., Fujii-Kuriyama, Y., and Ishikawa, T. (2000) Benzo[a]pyrene carcinogenicity is lost in mice lacking the aryl hydrocarbon receptor. *Proceedings of the National Academy of Sciences of the United States of America*, **97**, 779–782.
24 Boverhof, D.R., Chamberlain, M.P., Elcombe, C.R., Gonzalez, F.J., Heflich, R.H., Hernandez, L.G., Jacobs, A.C., Jacobson-Kram, D., Luijten, M., Maggi, A., Manjanatha, M.G., Benthem, J., and Gollapudi, B.B. (2011) Transgenic animal models in toxicology: historical perspectives and future outlook. *Toxicological Sciences*, **121**, 207–233.
25 EU (2006) Regulation (EC) No. 1901/2006 of the European Parliament and of the Council on medicinal products for paediatric use, amended by Regulation (EC) No. 1902/2006.
26 Committee for Human Medicinal Products (2008) Guideline on the Need for Nonclinical Testing in Juvenile Animals of Pharmaceuticals for Paediatric Indications. EMEA/CHMP/SWP/169215/2005, EMA.
27 FDA CDER (2006) Guidance for Industry: Nonclinical Safety Evaluation of Pediatric Drug Products. U.S. Department of Health and Human Services.
28 Schuster, D., Laggner, C., and Langer, T. (2005) Why drugs fail: a study on side effects in new chemical entities. *Current Pharmaceutical Design*, **11**, 3545–3559.
29 Kramer, J.A., Sagartz, J.E., and Morris, D.L. (2007) The application of discovery toxicology and pathology towards the design of safer pharmaceutical lead candidates. *Nature Reviews. Drug Discovery*, **6**, 636–649.
30 Dorato, M.A. and Engelhardt, J.A. (2005) The no-observed-adverse-effect-level in drug safety evaluations: use, issues, and definition(s). *Regulatory Toxicology and Pharmacology*, **42**, 265–274.
31 FDA CDER (2005) Guidance for Industry: Estimating the Maximum Safe Starting Dose in Initial Clinical Trials for Therapeutics in Adult Healthy Volunteers. U.S. Department of Health and Human Services.
32 ICH (1995) Toxicokinetics: A Guidance for Assessing Systemic Exposure in Toxicology Studies. International Conference on Harmonisation of Technical Requirements for Registration of Pharmaceuticals for Human Use, Topic S3A.

33 ICH (2012) Nonclinical Safety Studies for the Conduct of Human Clinical Trials and Marketing Authorization for Pharmaceuticals: Questions and Answers (R2). International Conference on Harmonisation of Technical Requirements for Registration of Pharmaceuticals for Human Use, Topic M3(R2) Q&As (R2).

34 Clarke, J., Hurst, C., Martin, P., Vahle, J., Ponce, R., Mounho, B., Heidel, S., Andrews, L., Reynolds, T., and Cavagnaro, J. (2008) Duration of chronic toxicity studies for biotechnology-derived pharmaceuticals: is 6 months still appropriate? *Regulatory Toxicology and Pharmacology*, **50**, 2–22.

35 Buckley, L.A. and Dorato, M.A. (2009) High dose selection in general toxicity studies for drug development: a pharmaceutical industry perspective. *Regulatory Toxicology and Pharmacology*, **54**, 301–307.

36 Weingand, K., Brown, G., Hall, R., Davies, D., Gossett, K., Neptun, D., Waner, T., Matsuzawa, T., Salemink, P., Froelke, W., Provost, J.P., Negro, G.D., Batchelor, J., Nomura, M., Groetsch, H., Boink, A., Kimball, J., Woodman, D., York, M., Fabianson-Johnson, E., Lupart, M., and Melloni, E. (1996) Harmonization of animal clinical pathology testing in toxicity and safety studies. *Fundamental and Applied Toxicology*, **29**, 198–201.

37 ICH (2006) Immunotoxicity Studies for Human Pharmaceuticals. International Conference on Harmonisation of Technical Requirements for Registration of Pharmaceuticals for Human Use, Topic S8.

38 Committee for Human Medicinal Products (2010) Guideline on Repeated Dose Toxicity. CPMP/SWP/1042/99 Rev 1, EMA.

39 ICH (2000) Safety Pharmacology Studies for Human Pharmaceuticals. International Conference on Harmonisation of Technical Requirements for Registration of Pharmaceuticals for Human Use, Topic S7A.

40 Mattsson, J., Spencer, P., and Albee, R. (1996) A performance standard for clinical and functional observational battery examinations of rats. *International Journal of Toxicology*, **15**, 239–254.

41 Irwin, S. (1968) Comprehensive observational assessment: Ia. A systematic, quantitative procedure for assessing the behavioral and physiologic state of the mouse. *Psychopharmacologia*, **13**, 222–257.

42 Thomas, M., Maconochie, J.G., and Fletcher, E. (1996) The dilemma of the prolonged QT interval in early drug studies. *British Journal of Clinical Pharmacology*, **41**, 77–81.

43 ICH (2011) Guidance on Genotoxicity Testing and Data Interpretation for Pharmaceuticals Intended for Human Use. International Conference on Harmonisation of Technical Requirements for Registration of Pharmaceuticals for Human Use, Topic S2(R1).

44 Organization for Economic Co-operation and Development (OECD) (1983) Genetic Toxicology: Micronucleus Test. OECD Guideline for Testing of Chemicals, No. 474.

45 Schlegel, R. and MacGregor, J.T. (1984) The persistence of micronucleated erythrocytes in the peripheral circulation of normal and splenectomized Fischer 344 rats: implications for cytogenetic screening. *Mutation Research*, **127**, 169–174.

46 Muller-Tegethoff, K., Kersten, B., Kasper, P., and Muller, L. (1997) Application of the *in vitro* rat hepatocyte micronucleus assay in genetic toxicology testing. *Mutation Research*, **392**, 125–138.

47 Suzuki, H., Takasawa, H., Kobayashi, K., Terashima, Y., Shimada, Y., Ogawa, I., Tanaka, J., Imamura, T., Miyazaki, A., and Hayashi, M. (2009) Evaluation of a liver micronucleus assay with 12 chemicals using young rats (II): a study by the Collaborative Study Group for the Micronucleus Test/Japanese Environmental Mutagen Society-Mammalian Mutagenicity Study Group. *Mutagenesis*, **24**, 9–16.

48 Rothfuss, A., Honma, M., Czich, A., Aardema, M.J., Burlinson, B., Galloway, S., Hamada, S., Kirkland, D., Heflich, R.H., Howe, J., Nakajima, M., O'Donovan, M., Plappert-Helbig, U., Priestley, C., Recio, L., Schuler, M., Uno, Y., and Martus, H.J. (2011) Improvement of *in vivo* genotoxicity assessment: combination of acute tests and integration into standard toxicity testing. *Mutation Research*, **723**, 108–120.

49 Organization for Economic Co-operation and Development (OECD) (1997) Unscheduled DNA Synthesis (UDS) Test

50 Hartmann, A., Agurell, E., Beevers, C., Brendler-Schwaab, S., Burlinson, B., Clay, P., Collins, A., Smith, A., Speit, G., Thybaud, V., and Tice, R.R. (2003) Recommendations for conducting the in vivo alkaline Comet assay. 4th International Comet Assay Workshop. *Mutagenesis*, **18**, 45–51. with Mammalian Liver Cells In Vivo. OECD Guideline for Testing of Chemicals, No. 486.

51 ICH (2006) Detection of Toxicity to Reproduction for Medicinal Products & Toxicity to Male Fertility. International Conference on Harmonisation of Technical Requirements for Registration of Pharmaceuticals for Human Use, Topic S5(R2).

52 Chellman, G.J., Bussiere, J.L., Makori, N., Martin, P.L., Ooshima, Y., and Weinbauer, G.F. (2009) Developmental and reproductive toxicology studies in nonhuman primates. *Birth Defects Research. Part B, Developmental and Reproductive Toxicology*, **86**, 446–462.

53 ICH (1996) The Need for Carcinogenicity Studies of Pharmaceuticals. International Conference on Harmonisation of Technical Requirements for Registration of Pharmaceuticals for Human Use, Topic S1A.

54 ICH (1997) Carcinogenicity: Testing for Carcinogenicity of Pharmaceuticals. International Conference on Harmonisation of Technical Requirements for Registration of Pharmaceuticals for Human Use, Topic S1B.

55 ICH (2008) Dose Selection for Carcinogenicity Studies of Pharmaceuticals. International Conference on Harmonisation of Technical Requirements for Registration of Pharmaceuticals for Human Use, Topic S1C(R2).

56 Friedrich, A. and Olejniczak, K. (2011) Evaluation of carcinogenicity studies of medicinal products for human use authorised via the European centralised procedure (1995–2009). *Regulatory Toxicology and Pharmacology*, **60**, 225–248.

57 Reddy, M.V., Sistare, F.D., Christensen, J.S., Deluca, J.G., Wollenberg, G.K., and DeGeorge, J.J. (2010) An evaluation of chronic 6- and 12-month rat toxicology studies as predictors of 2-year tumor outcome. *Veterinary Pathology*, **47**, 614–629.

58 Sistare, F.D., Morton, D., Alden, C., Christensen, J., Keller, D., Jonghe, S.D., Storer, R.D., Reddy, M.V., Kraynak, A., Trela, B., Bienvenu, J.G., Bjurstrom, S., Bosmans, V., Brewster, D., Colman, K., Dominick, M., Evans, J., Hailey, J.R., Kinter, L., Liu, M., Mahrt, C., Marien, D., Myer, J., Perry, R., Potenta, D., Roth, A., Sherratt, P., Singer, T., Slim, R., Soper, K., Fransson-Steen, R., Stoltz, J., Turner, O., Turnquist, S., van Heerden, M., Woicke, J., and DeGeorge, J.J. (2011) An analysis of pharmaceutical experience with decades of rat carcinogenicity testing: support for a proposal to modify current regulatory guidelines. *Toxicologic Pathology*, **39**, 716–744.

59 Alden, C.L., Lynn, A., Bourdeau, A., Morton, D., Sistare, F.D., Kadambi, V.J., and Silverman, L. (2011) A critical review of the effectiveness of rodent pharmaceutical carcinogenesis testing in predicting for human risk. *Veterinary Pathology*, **48**, 772–784.

60 EMA (2012) ICH Guideline S1: Regulatory Notice on Changes to Core Guideline on Rodent Carcinogenicity Testing of Pharmaceuticals. EMA/CHMP/ICH/752486/2012.

61 Greaves, P., Williams, A., and Eve, M. (2004) First dose of potential new medicines to humans: how animals help. *Nature Reviews. Drug Discovery*, **3**, 226–236.

62 Dybing, E., Doe, J., Groten, J., Kleiner, J., O'Brien, J., Renwick, A.G., Schlatter, J., Steinberg, P., Tritscher, A., Walker, R., and Younes, M. (2002) Hazard characterisation of chemicals in food and diet: dose response, mechanisms and extrapolation issues. *Food and Chemical Toxicology*, **40**, 237–282.

6
Generation and Use of Transgenic Mice in Drug Discovery

Guillaume Pavlovic, Véronique Brault, Tania Sorg, and Yann Hérault

6.1
Introduction

One of the major challenges for the pharmaceutical industry is to develop drugs for new targets in order to fulfill the yet unmet medical needs, especially in fields such as neuropharmacology and complex polygenic disorders. Defining gene function and target validation are key steps for selecting a gene sequence for drug development. With rapid advances and scale-up of DNA sequencing, ∼20 000 protein-coding genes and even more noncoding genes have been identified in humans. The question is how to assign functions to each of these genes in the context of a whole organism, in normal physiology and development, as well as the contribution of mutant alleles to inherited diseases or challenged environmental conditions.

With all the various technologies now available to manipulate the genome, the comparison of a functional and a nonfunctional (mutant) state will provide insight into the *in vivo* function of a given gene. However, understanding the pathogenicity of a given allelic variant found in the human population is still a challenge. Unlocking the functional role of the mammalian genome will have a transformative effect on biology and biotechnological innovations and also on the understanding of human diseases. It will allow the scientific community to identify and validate new candidate targets for drug development. Importantly, such approaches will also allow the assessment of the risk associated with specific target invalidation, a mandatory and key step in drug development and translational medicine.

Therefore, analysis of the function of genes, also called functional genomics or phenogenomics, constitutes a bottleneck that slows down the whole process of target and drug discovery. With its genome amenable to manipulation and its physiology and genome sequence homology close to human (99% of mouse genes have human homologs) the mouse has become the animal model of choice for deciphering gene function, identifying putative targets and pathways involved in pathogenesis and modeling human genetic diseases, and will probably stay the leading model to test new therapeutic molecules. The use of the mouse as a model

In Vivo *Models for Drug Discovery*, First Edition. Edited by José M. Vela, Rafael Maldonado, and Michel Hamon.
© 2014 Wiley-VCH Verlag GmbH & Co. KGaA. Published 2014 by Wiley-VCH Verlag GmbH & Co. KGaA.

to study biological processes relevant to human diseases was the basis of the interest for this small mammal. It started long before the creation of genetically engineered mice at the beginning of the nineteenth century with formal mouse genetics and the development of inbred strains. More than 1000 mouse models of human diseases with phenotypes closely resembling the human features have been generated. In addition to the wide variety of inbred strains and spontaneous, radiation-, or chemically induced mutations [1], mouse genetics has benefited from transgenic stem cells and homologous recombination technologies to engineer the mouse genome, allowing the generation of a variety of mutations [2]. Null or point mutations and complex chromosomal rearrangements are precisely generated to reproduce human genetic conditions [3,4]. In the last few years, it has become easier and cheaper to inactivate, overexpress, or humanize a gene. Numerous laboratories, companies or mouse clinics propose to develop genetically engineered mouse models (GEMMs) for any gene of interest within a short-term delay. As such, mouse clinics provide expertise for functional broad-based or specialized functional assessment of mouse models in a standardized and high-throughput manner. These transgenic models have proved to be relevant for the discovery and validation of new targets, for evaluation of efficacy, specificity, and safety of the compounds and for optimal human disease models [5]. In 2003, Zambrowicz and Sands [6] published a retrospective study in *Nature* of the knockout phenotypes for the 100 best-selling drugs and demonstrated that the phenotypes of the knockout model correspond well to the efficacy of the drug acting on respective target [6,7]. Replacement of the mouse gene with the human sequence or addition of the human gene allow the human condition to be mimicked on specific parameters. Mice expressing different human cytochrome P450s, enzymes involved in metabolism of xenobiotics such as many clinical drugs, demonstrated their utility for evaluation and prediction of toxicological risk [8]. Transgenic systems were also used to provide better disease models that resemble as much as possible the human physiology and pathology. Wild-type mice do not develop atherosclerosis naturally and are thus a poor model to study cholesterol-related cardiovascular disease. The numerous *ApoE* alleles mice generated develop artherosclerotic lesions similar to those found in humans and are still valuable tools in this field. Humanization of the *App* gene is a second example of a valuable model system for Alzheimer's disease (AD) research [8], even though not recapitulating all aspects of the human disease [9]. Furthermore, new techniques to phenotype this small animal enable more precise characterization, making the mouse the emerging species to study human disease. In addition, international mouse mutagenesis and phenotyping initiatives have been successfully launched to unlock the functional role of the mammalian genome [10,11]. The future knowledge that will be acquired will have a major effect on biology, accelerating the understanding of human diseases, and the biotechnological, biomedical, and pharmaceutical innovations. New candidate targets for drug development will be identified and validated. This chapter provides a summary of the recent technical developments in transgenic mouse technologies, functional evaluation, and their use as models for complex human disorders and analyzes pitfalls and opportunities for modeling of human disorders, target identification, validation, and translational research for drug discovery.

6.2 Improved Mouse Genetic Engineering

6.2.1 Recent Technical Developments

Advances in the last few years in mouse engineering leave the mouse in the position of first model for the preclinical and target discovery. A wide variety of techniques (Table 6.1) allow a large panel of modifications ranging from a single base pair (mimic human point mutation diseases) to large deletion or duplication (mimic human copy number variation (CNV)-linked diseases). Thanks to those technical advances, less time is required to obtain GEMM, almost any mouse background is accessible and combinatorial approaches are eased (Table 6.1). Tissue/cell specific inactivation allows the the effect of a target gene or of a candidate drug on a specific biological system to be evaluated (Table 6.1). Nuclease-mediated inactivations (ZFNs and TALENs) or the recent CRISPR/Cas strategies [12–14] have among other the advantage of reducing the difficulty in obtaining models for multigenic diseases (Table 6.1).

The VelocImmune mouse was created by megabase-scale humanization of the variable portion of mouse immunoglobulin (Ig) loci, that is, replacement of six megabases of mouse DNA that code for the production of immune system proteins with the corresponding human DNA. This model allows the production of human monoclonal antibodies that express human variable regions but preserve the mouse constant regions, resulting in robust immune response in the mouse (presence of mouse constant regions) with reduced immune risk for patients who will receive these antibodies as medication. This technology is thus promising to speed the generation of fully human therapeutic antibodies [15]. The Kymouse strains are based on the same approach, i.e. 2.5 megabases of human sequence is transferred to the genome of the mouse, and offer a panel of knock-in and knockout mice for human antibody generation of IgH, IgK, and IgL in the mouse [16].

6.2.2 The Advent of New Mouse Mutant Resource: One Stop Shop

In 2007, the International Knockout Mouse Consortium (IKMC) (Table 6.2), supported by three transnational programs, aimed to generate mutations in every protein-coding gene and microRNA [11,17–19]. This effort was the starting point of large standardized mutant resources in the mouse. Today, more than 22 000 mutant ES and more than 3400 mutant mouse lines are available, most of them carrying conditional mutations [11]. Two pilot programs, the European Mouse Disease Clinic (Eumodic) and the Wellcome Trust Sanger Institute Mouse Genetics

Table 6.1 Main technology for GEMMs.

Technology[a]	Main modifications for drug discovery	Advantage for drug discovery	Limitation for drug discovery
Mutagenesis by homologous recombination in ES cells	Inactivation, overexpression, humanization, small region copy number variation, large region copy number variation	• Years of experience • Panel of modifications that are possible	• Totipotent ES cells in few backgrounds are available
Integrase/recombinase-mediated transgenesis	Knockdown, overexpression, humanization	• Faster than the ES route	• Limitation to targeted transgenesis
Nuclease transgenesis (ZFNs, TALENs, CRISPR)	Inactivation, humanization	• Access to any background • Introduction of a new modification in any existing model (as a CC line)	• Efficiency of humanization
Pronuclear injection transgenesis	Knockdown, overexpression	• Panel of overexpression	• Efficiency
Cre/CreER^{T2} site-specific recombinase or other (i.e., Tet) inducible recombinase	Inactivation in specific populations	• Study the function of the gene only in the cell population of interest	• Complexity of breeding • Leakiness of the system

a) Only the most used techniques are described here. Other alternatives such as adenovirus transgenesis, SSC cells, and ICSI can be used to generate GEMMs.

Project (WTSI-MGP), demonstrated and promoted the feasibility of large-scale broad-based phenotyping effort to decipher the function of unknown genes [10]. The International Mouse Phenotyping Consortium (IMPC) project aims, in the next 10 years, to make, from this ES resource, the mouse model for virtually any of the mouse genes. The relevance of this resource for drug discovery is more than obvious.

Other large-scale programs will also be of interest for biopharmaceutical research (Table 6.2). The Cre/loxP system was developed in the early 1990s to allow the conditional inactivation of gene of interest. CreER^{T2} transgene – a ligand-activated chimeric recombinase – is an additional sophistication allowing the temporal inactivation of a gene in a tissue/cell-specific manner [20]. With such a tool to inhibit a gene in the adult mouse, it is now possible to evaluate a candidate for drug design, to restore some deficient function in the adult, and to estimate the developmental consequences. To complete the zoo, the EUCOMMTOOLS

Table 6.2 List of main large-scale mouse programs.

Program	Acronym	Objective	Web site
International Knockout Mouse Consortium	IKMC	Public resource of mouse knockout embryonic stem cells	www.mousephenotype.org/
European Mouse Disease Clinic	Eumodic	Primary phenotype assessment of knockout mouse	www.eumodic.org/
Wellcome Trust Sanger Institute Mouse Genetics Project	WTSI-MGP	Primary phenotype assessment of knockout mouse	http://www.sanger.ac.uk/mouse-portal/
International Mouse Phenotyping Consortium	IMPC	Primary phenotype assessment of knockout mouse for nearly all the protein-coding genes and miRNA	www.mousephenotype.org/
EUCOMM: Tools for Functional Annotation of the Mouse Genome	EUCOMMTOOLS	Cre driver resource and mouse knockout embryonic stem cells	www.tools.eucomm.org/
Collaborative Cross	CC	Large panel of new inbred mouse strains	http://csbio.unc.edu/CCstatus/index.py

program has developed 500 new Cre or CreER^{T2} lines targeting specific expression in a wide range of specific tissues and will generate and characterize a further 250 lines.

Other tools have been developed to increase the genetic diversity of recombinant alleles in the mouse. First, the BXD strains consist of 76 recombinant inbred strains derived from the parental strains C57BL/6J and DBA/2J [21]. Similarly, the heterogeneous stocks (HS) consist of breeding mice from very different backgrounds to generate a very large number of outbred mice. All the mice thus present different and heterogeneous genetic backgrounds and can be used to mimic the diversity of a population [22]. Furthermore, the Collaborative Cross (CC) built a panel of now more than 300 recombinant inbred mouse lines established from eight distant inbred strains of *Mus musculus*. This resource captures more than 90% of the genetic variation known in the mouse genome [23] and will thus provide high value for analysis of phenotypes caused by combinatorial allele effects [23,24]. Human genome polymorphism is a key factor explaining important variability between individuals in efficiency and adverse effects of a specific medicine. The CC resource is a promising tool to study this variability for new compounds and helps to reduce risk of combinatorial allele effects in humans. For example, this panel was very recently used to evaluate the impact of genetic variation in influenza-associated disease [25].

Overall, the genetic toolbox available so far to modify the mouse genome is still one of the most sophisticated. New tools, such as the nuclease-based technologies entering our experimental plan, will definitely benefit further combinatorial analysis to reproduce human multigenic diseases to study redundant genes and epistatic interactions [26].

6.3
Functional Evaluation and Uses of Mouse Models

To better assign the function to all genes and to better understand the pathogenicity of a given allelic variant, a number of consortia have set up initiatives to generate and phenotype mouse mutant lines with standardized functional assays (Table 6.2). At the origins, new centers, defined in the beginning of the twentieth century and named mouse clinics, with high-throughput and comprehensive physiological expertise, were designed as human clinics are and were keys to promote such efforts and to provide knowledge on the mouse mutants. Mouse clinics operated in close collaboration to make all reagents as well as the resulting phenotypic data available to the scientific community. Several points were examined: What is the genetic background that should be used? Which type of controlled environment, with basal or challenge conditions? How are the results transposable to human clinics? To what extent are the mouse models predictable for human diseases and pharmacological treatment, either at proof of concept or predictability of side effects of the molecules? Although no model can be expected to give all answers, it is important to note that the mouse is a unique specie for modeling and understanding human diseases.

6.3.1
Standardization and Harmonization

As more and more models are developed and need to be characterized, standardization of simple, validated, and reproducible assays becomes a prerequisite to obtain comparable, reliable conclusion from one phenotyping laboratory to the other. Well-known and described housing and handling procedures are a prerequisite for the standardization to take place. As shown by Champy *et al.* [27], minor changes in procedures can lead to different phenotyping results.

In parallel to the assay standardization, computational analysis had to be adapted to high-throughput phenotyping programs, recording not only the procedure variables but also the environmental conditions (e.g., the number of mice per cage, diet composition, type of bedding, fasting time, and bleeding conditions), equipment (that will never be exactly the same all over the world), and the genetic factors [28]. The ultimate goal is to have a centralized database with all mouse models' description, standardized experimental procedures, and information about the environmental conditions, while the same ontology and phenotypic vocabulary is used by all centers to have comparable data across time and phenotyping centers [10,29,30] (www.mousephenotype.org/).

Finally, Gerdin *et al.* [31] showed that routine husbandry and procedures may affect the mouse physiology and behavior, as well as the data quality. Blood glucose and core temperature measurements activate the cardiovascular system, which declines between tests but is reactivated to the same level by a subsequent measurement. They also showed that an overnight fast was associated with significant sex-specific changes in cardiovascular parameters and locomotor activities. In particular, the mechanisms underlying sex-specific differences in cardiovascular stress responses can be explained by differences in autonomic and neuroendocrine control. These findings may have important implications for the interpretation of results of phenotyping tests, since it indicates that potentially confounding effects of stress are more prevalent in female mice.

6.3.2
Genetic Background and Environmental Influences

The genetic background is certainly one of the key factors of phenotypic outcome variability. Most of the mouse models obtained by homologous recombination in ES cells were based on 129 background ES cells, and usually backcrossed on C57BL/6 mice. Although from a theoretical point of view these mice are considered as being on a C57BL/6 background, the targeted locus and its neighboring region contain 129 coding and regulatory sequences that may influence the phenotype. Even if now the main mouse mutant resources, namely, IKMC, were built using pure C57BL/6N-derived ES cells, crosses these lines with other C57BL/6 substrain such as those found between C57BL/6N and C57BL/6J [32] remain frequent and may affect the outcome of phenotyping analysis.

In addition to genetic background influence, environmental factors also have a crucial influence on the determination of complex genetic traits. For example, asthma, which can be inherited as a polygenic trait or as a monogenic, dominant trait with incomplete penetrance, is significantly influenced by environmental factors. In addition to minimizing such influence between individuals by using homogeneous housing and feeding conditions, mouse models offer a way to study environmental influence by testing different environmental conditions on genetically identical animals. Efforts to standardize test paradigms and environment across different laboratories are under way [33] and should be pursued. Those efforts will help to understand the interactions between gene and environment and, ultimately, lead to the development of more personalized therapeutic treatments of complex diseases.

6.3.3
Challenges Ahead

Similarly, there are numerous examples of transgenic models in which the baseline phenotype is unchanged or minimally changed from the wild type, only to become manifest after challenges. For example, the stress of exercise testing highlighted cardiovascular phenotypes [34]. This type of challenge allowed the cardiovascular phenotypes of several mutants to be elucidated, such as for the β-adrenergic receptor knockout mouse model [35], the phospholamban-deficient mice [36], the *mdx* murine model of muscular dystrophy [37], or the transgenic model overexpressing a mutant opioid reception (OR1) allowing increased stimulation of the inhibitory G protein in a controlled manner [38]. Similarly, challenging conditions are prone to unravel and better understand gene function, for example, in metabolic, respiratory, and immune diseases.

6.3.4
Target Identification and Translation to Humans

The major use of mouse models is to identify candidate genes for human diseases that can be studied further to better understand the pathophysiology of the diseases, the molecular and cellular pathways that are altered in an integrated biological system. In addition, the knowledge acquired will help to select biomarkers that will then be successfully used for further drug studies to validate the action on the candidate target.

Besides the genetic engineering, the main bottleneck is the capacity to translate somehow the human phenotypes to the limited mouse system. Not only appropriate functional tests should be developed, but they should also be validated and powerful enough to detect changes induced by the candidate gene. More sophisticated and robust protocols are still needed to understand the behavioral phenotypes of a mouse model and to appreciate how this translates to human clinic and diseases, such as Alzheimer's disease (AD), autism, and schizophrenia. It is sometimes necessary to go beyond the common paradigms to directly evaluate the brain functions across and to assess molecular or cellular pathways as reviewed by Hunsaker [39]. Clearly, additional paradigms are required in the behavior field, in areas such as depression and anxiety, allowing further integration and modeling of neuropsychiatric diseases and other brain illnesses [40]. At the end, several models are or will be available, but will probably not show all the criteria and symptoms observed in human diseases. However, each of these models can and will serve in the drug discovery pipeline. As reviewed by Van Dam and De Deyn [41], the various AD mouse models available up to now increase our understanding of the pathophysiological mechanisms in order to predict the efficacy of novel therapeutic molecules.

Another example comes from the diabetes area where a number of mouse models are now available through the new resources such as IKMC. McMurray *et al.* [42] illustrated such an application for four genes identified from human diabetes genome-wide association study (FTO, TCF7L2, CDKAL1, and SLC30A8). A typical example is the single-nucleotide polymorphism (SNP) in the *FTO* gene associated with an increased body mass index. Controversially, the knockout mice for this gene were lean and not affected, but the overexpression of FTO induced increase in body weight and further consequences on adipocyte function. As such, transgenic mice overexpressing FTO fed with an enriched diet displayed increased glucose tolerance showing how FTO, even if not directly involved in type 2 diabetes, could impact obesity and diabetes outcomes and how the mouse studies were valuable for further translational studies.

Although there are numerous examples in the literature showing the usefulness of knockout animals, new technologies will be needed in the future, such as cellular reprogramming leading to pluripotent, germline stem cells, plus additional techniques to work with other species, as well as RNAi to induce temporal and/or spatial gene knockdown, to resemble more closely the effect of a drug [43].

6.3.5
Use of GEMMs in Pharmaceutical Industry and Risk Assessment

Transgenic animals are widely used to have insights into the *in vivo* function of the genes and their products. They are also commonly used in the discovery research for proof of concept in pharmaceutical companies. In particular, these models help to evaluate the risk of molecules in development, their potential carcinogenesis, and the xenobiotic metabolism and/or toxicity. For example, genetically altered animals were key elements to elucidate the early onset of immune and inflammatory responses [43]. Similarly, GEMMs are useful in determining the mechanisms of toxicity and their applicability to humans. Sali *et al.* [44] showed that although the Dmd^{mdx} (*mdx*) mouse model can be used to show the benefit of a glucocorticoid treatment, it revealed some side effects [44]. Indeed, the *mdx* mice showed an early recovery and improvement in muscle strength and motor coordination but, in the long run, this benefit was lost and followed by side effects, such as loss of muscle strength and heart fibrosis.

Studies with mouse models have also shown that rimonabant, a cannabinoid CB1 receptor antagonist developed to treat obesity, induced anxiolytic effect in rodents [45]. In addition, the effects of rimonabant were the same as those observed in CB1 receptor knockout mice, but also similar to those in human patients [46]. These observations opened the way to a better understanding of the CB1 receptor blockade, dissociating the anxiety and consummator behaviors [47], with a potential development of molecules still having the anti-obesity properties, but not the adverse effects.

Another aspect is the use of the "XenoMouse," a mouse model expressing the majority of the human immunoglobulin genes [48,49]. This model is widely used for the production of humanized antibodies, with a strong affinity for their antigen, and is useful in human clinics, as its immunogenicity is very low, and if it exists, presumably not inducing hypersensitivity in patients.

Finally, mouse models are also useful in drug repositioning. For instance, it has been shown in an acute ischemic stroke model that minocycline, a broad-spectrum antibiotic, combined with tPA is beneficial for treated animals, reducing the risk of intracerebral hemorrhage [50–52] with antidepressant properties [53].

6.4
Translation to Clinics: Limitations and Difficulties

A key challenge in genetic medicine is to understand and treat complex genetic disorders. Genetic studies highlight the origin of polygenic diseases such as diabetes, obesity, cardiovascular diseases, and asthma as cumulative effects of mutations or variants, located at different loci and influenced by environmental factors. Similarly, contiguous gene syndromes (CGS) or additional structural variants have been found implicated in various human conditions and associated with complex mechanisms [54].

Manipulation of large chromosomal regions in the mouse genome using new chromosome engineering tools [10,55–57] has provided the scientific community with the opportunity to develop mouse models of CGS. Mouse models have been developed mainly for common neurodevelopmental disorders such as Down syndrome (DS; trisomy 21) and Charcot–Marie–Tooth disease type 1A [58], Prader–Willi paternal and Angelman maternal 15q11–13 deletions [59], and models of reciprocal microdeletion and microduplication for the 17q11.2 [60] and 16p11.2 [61] regions. These mouse models enabled to decipher the molecular basis of the Smith–Magenis and Potocki–Lupski syndromes for del22q11.2 (DiGeorge syndrome) [62,63] and helped to identify key dosage-sensitive genes such *Rai1* [64] and *Tbx1* [65]. Moreover, mouse models of segmental aneuploidies revealed dosage-sensitive genes that were only subsequently associated with a particular human syndrome, as was the case with the *Stat5* gene involved in immune hypersensitivity and metabolic syndrome [66]. Using models recapitulating the whole structural variation and single-gene knockout or overexpressing models allows us to both recapitulate the complexity of the syndrome and get information about the contribution of genes within the locus to molecular and cellular pathways involved in the syndrome [67]. One of the most complex viable CGS is the full autosomal trisomy 21, causing DS with at least 80 features showing variable expression. DS is the most common genetic cause of mental retardation, with deficit in learning, memory, and language, impaired motor development, and hypotonia. Associated pathologies include heart disease, immune system perturbations, and increased risks of leukemia, Alzheimer's disease, and epilepsy. A large number of mouse models have been developed to study DS [68]. These models recapitulate most of the phenotypes associated with DS [69] and have proven to be very useful tools to decipher morphological [70–72], physiological, and molecular defaults associated with the DS [73,74]. Understanding of the neurobiological defaults underlying cognitive deficits in mouse models has paved the way for therapeutic approaches that were not imaginable 10 years ago. The discovery of an imbalance of inhibitory interneurons and excitatory inputs to hippocampus provided druggable pathways to treat DS cognitive features [75]. Some drugs tested in the mouse models are now currently being tested in humans in small-scale clinical trials (http://www.clinicaltrials.gov/).

In addition to CGS, polygenic diseases such as diabetes, obesity, cardiovascular diseases, or mental disorders result from complex genetic interactions that can involve SNPs, CNVs, or DNA structural variants that, in combination, will lead to the disease phenotype or will predispose to the disease. The analysis of complex traits in mice started long before the creation of genetically engineered mice, with the development and study of inbred strains. Now more than 400 strains have hundreds of variant loci and provide ways to find out genetic region-associated specific phenotypic traits, diseases, or susceptibilities by linkage analysis. In combination with the mapping of multilocus probes, simple-sequence length polymorphisms (SSLPs), and microsatellite markers, these strains enabled the identification of a number of quantitative trait loci (QTLs) associated with human diseases [76]. However, QTLs are often large, containing many genes, and transgenic mouse models of single genes are required to investigate the implication of specific genes in the pathology. There is a plethora of monogenic mouse models that are very useful in providing insight into complex genetic diseases. For example, the use of monogenic knockout, tissue-specific knockout, and transgenic models for genes implicated in different aspects of the pathogenesis of diabetes, such as transcription factors involved in pancreas development [77] or genes of the insulin signaling pathways (coding for insulin and insulin receptors) [25,78], has provided insight into the diverse mechanisms disrupted in diabetes; even diabetes in humans is rarely caused by monogenic mutations. However, knocking out specific genes is not always informative as knockout genes do not always mimic the effect of the mutated allele in the disease, as was seen by the mouse models with the human autism allele-specific mutations for the *Nlgn3* gene that showed specific phenotypic effects different from the null allele [79]. Several examples of mouse models directly recapitulate the effects of human alleles such as the mice mutants for *Fmr1* and *MeCP2*, respectively, mutated in the fragile X mental retardation or the Rett syndrome [80,81]. Modeling human alleles is not always easy and depends on the degree of gene sequence conservation between mouse and human, especially in the case of common allelic variants leading to small effects or risk factors. In these cases, mouse models will be more effective in apprehending the function of the gene and how its perturbation will contribute to the disease rather than trying to mimic the pathological effect *per se*.

In addition to the allelic specificity, noncoding regulatory genomic regions and epigenomic environment might be different and may play a crucial role in underlying species differences in disease. To get around this problem, genetically humanized mouse models in which human genes are introduced into the mouse with their own regulatory sequences have been developed, thanks to the development of yeast artificial chromosomes (YACs) and bacterial artificial chromosomes (BACs) randomly introduced into the mouse genome by pronuclear injections. These models have already been successfully used to study common monogenic disorders such as Huntington disease and β-thalassemia and cancer susceptibility genes such as *BRCA1* and demonstrated an interspecies complementation of the human gene in the mouse null background [82–85]. Humanized mouse models harboring codon-specific mutations present in some pathology were also generated by site-specific mutagenesis techniques and enabled to analyze the implication of the mutation to the pathology [86,87]. Alternatively, human genomic regions have been introduced by specific targeting and replacement of mouse genomic loci. Targeted genomic replacement has been successfully used for studying *in vivo* human hematopoiesis and immune function [88–90]. Moreover, a humanized mouse model carrying a freely segregating human chromosome 21 has been generated using microcell-mediated chromosome transfer (MMCT) into embryonic stem cells [91] and permitted further investigation of genetic and epigenetic mechanisms, revealing that mechanisms intrinsic to the genetic sequence prevail on the epigenetic machinery and the cellular environment for directing transcriptional programs [92,93]. In addition to understand pathogenic processes, humanized mouse models offer the possibility of testing drug therapies and gene therapies in a humanized environment, avoiding species differences that limit the validation of the treatment for humans [94].

6.5 Perspectives

The mouse models are decisive in answering a large set of fundamental, biomedical, and biopharmaceutical research with an extraordinary toolbox, a short generation time, and a facility for breeding in controlled standardized conditions. Large-scale initiatives at both the genetic and the phenogenomic levels will even strengthen this position in the future with an almost complete coverage of mutations for every coding gene in the genome and a detailed annotation of the function of the genes. All this effort would have been useless if the standardization and the best practices were not defined to sustain the making and the analysis of the mutant models and captured by specific investigators and mouse clinics. It has also undeniably benefited the understanding of human disease pathophysiology and the follow-up of drug actions.

Besides a large set of evidences, the value of the mouse as a model for human disease is still debated with respect to interspecies differences. Although the relevance of the mouse in deciphering basic biological mechanisms that underlie human disease has long been demonstrated, its reliability for human medical research, particularly for preclinical trials, is still under debate [95,96]. There are many examples of treatment protocols successfully tested on mouse models that were not successful in humans [97–99]. Differences in metabolism, anatomy, and physiology such as higher blood glucose concentration [100], variation in the ability to metabolize certain chemicals leading to different magnitude of susceptibility to exposure to those products, and change in the distribution of receptors in the mouse do exist and need to be taken into account. There is therefore a real need to identify equivalent characteristics between human and rodent and to translate specific phenotypic traits into etiologically valid paradigms in order to properly evaluate and interpret results obtained from the experiments made in the mouse [101]. Such efforts to characterize phenotypes and biological mechanisms that either are conserved or diverge between human and rodent are under way [2,28,102–104] and will allow us to use the mouse as a more predictive tool in human pathological research and drug discovery.

Acknowledgments

We thank members of the ICS unit and of the EUMODIC (LSHG-CT-2006-037188), INFRAFRONTIER (FP7-INFRASTRUCTURES-2007-2.2.01/211404), INFRACOMP (FP7-INFRASTRUCTURES-2011-3.2/284501), EUCOMMTOOLS (LSHG-2011-261492), and INFRAFRONTIER I3 (FP7-INFRASTRUCTURES-2012-1.1.4/312325) consortia for their helpful comments as participants of these programs. We are grateful to all the collaborators for the useful discussion. This work was supported by the French state aid managed by the National Agency for Research under the program of future investments (PHENOMIN, ANR-10-INBS-07) and by the European funded projects listed above.

References

1. Oliver, P.L. and Davies, K.E. (2012) New insights into behaviour using mouse ENU mutagenesis. *Human Molecular Genetics*, 21, R72–R81.
2. Brown, S.D., Wurst, W., Kühn, R., and Hancock, J.M. (2009) The functional annotation of mammalian genomes: the challenge of phenotyping. *Annual Review of Genetics*, 43, 305–333.
3. Brault, V., Pereira, P., Duchon, A., and Herault, Y. (2006) Modeling chromosomes in mouse to explore the function of genes, genomic disorders, and chromosomal organization. *PLoS Genetics*, 2, e86.
4. Herault, Y., Duchon, A., Marechal, D., Raveau, M., Pereira, P.L., Dalloneau, E., and Brault, V. (2010) Controlled somatic and germline copy number variation in the mouse model. *Current Genomics*, 11, 470–780.
5. Snaith, M.R. and Tornell, J. (2002) The use of transgenic systems in pharmaceutical research. *Briefings in Functional Genomics & Proteomics*, 1, 119–130.
6. Zambrowicz, B.P. and Sands, A.T. (2003) Knockouts model the 100 best-selling drugs: will they model the next 100? *Nature Reviews. Drug Discovery*, 2, 38–51.
7. Zambrowicz, B.P., Turner, C.A., and Sands, A.T. (2003) Predicting drug efficacy: knockouts model pipeline drugs of the pharmaceutical industry. *Current Opinion in Pharmacology*, 3, 563–570.
8. Cheung, C. and Gonzalez, F.J. (2008) Humanized mouse lines and their application for prediction of human drug metabolism and toxicological risk assessment. *The Journal of Pharmacology and Experimental Therapeutics*, 327, 288–299.
9. Epis, R., Gardoni, F., Marcello, E., Genazzani, A., Canonico, P.L., and Di Luca, M. (2010) Searching for new animal models of Alzheimer's disease. *European Journal of Pharmacology*, 626, 57–63.
10. Ayadi, A. et al. (2012) Mouse large-scale phenotyping initiatives: overview of the European Mouse Disease Clinic (EUMODIC) and of the Wellcome Trust Sanger Institute Mouse Genetics Project. *Mammalian Genome*, 23, 600–610.
11. Bradley, A. et al. (2012) The mammalian gene function resource: the International Knockout Mouse Consortium. *Mammalian Genome*, 23, 580–586.
12. Carroll, D. (2011) Genome engineering with zinc-finger nucleases. *Genetics*, 188, 773–782.
13. Carlson, D.F., Fahrenkrug, S.C., and Hackett, P.B. (2012) Targeting DNA with fingers and TALENs. *Molecular Therapy. Nucleic Acids*, 1, e3.
14. Cong, L., Ran, F.A., Cox, D., Lin, S., Barretto, R., Habib, N., Hsu, P.D., Wu, X., Jiang, W., Marraffini, L.A., and Zhang, F. (2013) Multiplex genome engineering using CRISPR/Cas systems. *Science*, 339, 819–823.
15. Tkaczyk, C., Hua, L., Varkey, R., Shi, Y., Dettinger, L., Woods, R., Barnes, A., MacGill, R.S., Wilson, S., Chowdhury, P.,

Stover, C.K., and Sellman, B.R. (2012) Identification of anti-alpha toxin monoclonal antibodies that reduce the severity of *Staphylococcus aureus* dermonecrosis and exhibit a correlation between affinity and potency. *Clinical and Vaccine Immunology*, **19**, 377–385.

16 Lee, E.C. and Owen, M. (2012) The application of transgenic mice for therapeutic antibody discovery. *Methods in Molecular Biology*, **901**, 137–148.

17 Austin, C.P. *et al.* (2004) The knockout mouse project. *Nature Genetics*, **36**, 921–924.

18 Auwerx, J. *et al.* (2004) The European dimension for the mouse genome mutagenesis program. *Nature Genetics*, **36**, 925–927.

19 Skarnes, W.C., Rosen, B., West, A.P., Koutsourakis, M., Bushell, W., Iyer, V., Mujica, A.O., Thomas, M., Harrow, J., Cox, T., Jackson, D., Severin, J., Biggs, P., Fu, J., Nefedov, M., Jong, P.J.D., Stewart, A.F., and Bradley, A. (2011) A conditional knockout resource for the genome-wide study of mouse gene function. *Nature*, **474**, 337–342.

20 Birling, M.C., Gofflot, F., and Warot, X. (2009) Site-specific recombinases for manipulation of the mouse genome. *Methods in Molecular Biology*, **561**, 245–263.

21 Peirce, J.L., Lu, L., Gu, J., Silver, L.M., and Williams, R.W. (2004) A new set of BXD recombinant inbred lines from advanced intercross populations in mice. *BMC Genetics*, **5**, 7.

22 Valdar, W., Solberg, L.C., Gauguier, D., Burnett, S., Klenerman, P., Cookson, W.O., Taylor, M.S., Rawlins, J.N., Mott, R., and Flint, J. (2006) Genome-wide genetic association of complex traits in heterogeneous stock mice. *Nature Genetics*, **38**, 879–887.

23 Panthier, J.-J. and Montagutelli, X. (2012) The Collaborative Cross, a groundbreaking tool to tackle complex traits. *Médecine Sciences (Paris)*, **28**, 103–108.

24 Threadgill, D.W., Miller, D.R., Churchill, G.A., and de Villena, F.P.-M. (2011) The Collaborative Cross: a recombinant inbred mouse population for the systems genetic era. *ILAR Journal*, **52**, 24–31.

25 Ferris, M.T. *et al.* (2013) Modeling host genetic regulation of influenza pathogenesis in the Collaborative Cross. *PLoS Pathogens*, **9**, e1003196.

26 Wang, H., Yang, H., Shivalila, C.S., Dawlaty, M.M., Cheng, A.W., Zhang, F., and Jaenisch, R. (2013) One-step generation of mice carrying mutations in multiple genes by CRISPR/Cas-mediated genome engineering. *Cell*, **153**, 910–918.

27 Champy, M.F., Selloum, M., Piard, L., Zeitler, V., Caradec, C., Chambon, P., and Auwerx, J. (2004) Mouse functional genomics requires standardization of mouse handling and housing conditions. *Mammalian Genome*, **15**, 768–783.

28 Brown, S.D., Hancock, J.M., and Gates, H. (2006) Understanding mammalian genetic systems: the challenge of phenotyping in the mouse. *PLoS Genetics*, **2**, e118.

29 Morgan, H., Beck, T., Blake, A., Gates, H., Adams, N., Debouzy, G., Leblanc, S., Lengger, C., Maier, H., Melvin, D., Meziane, H., Richardson, D., Wells, S., White, J., Wood, J., de Angelis, M.H., Brown, S.D., Hancock, J.M., and Mallon, A.M. (2010) EuroPhenome: a repository for high-throughput mouse phenotyping data. *Nucleic Acids Research*, **38**, D577–D585.

30 Morgan, H., Simon, M., and Mallon, A.M. (2012) Accessing and mining data from large-scale mouse phenotyping projects. *International Review of Neurobiology*, **104**, 47–70.

31 Gerdin, A.K., Igosheva, N., Roberson, L.A., Ismail, O., Karp, N., Sanderson, M., Cambridge, E., Shannon, C., Sunter, D., Ramirez-Solis, R., Bussell, J., and White, J.K. (2012) Experimental and husbandry procedures as potential modifiers of the results of phenotyping tests. *Physiology & Behavior*, **106**, 602–611.

32 Simon, M.M., Greenaway, S., White, J.K., Fuchs, H., Gailus-Durner, V., Wells, S., Sorg, T., Wong, K., Bedu, E., Cartwright, E.J., Dacquin, R., Djebali, S., Estabel, J., Graw, J., Ingham, N.J., Jackson, I.J., Lengeling, A., Mandillo, S., Marvel, J., Meziane, H., Preitner, F., Puk, O., Roux, M., Adams, D.J., Atkins, S., Ayadi, A., Becker, J., Blake, A., Brooker, D., Cater, H., Champy, M-F., Combe, R., Danecek, P., di Fenza, A., Gates, H., Gerdin, A.K., Golini, E., Hancock, J.M., Hans, W., Hölter, S.M., Hough, T., Jurdic, P., Keane, T.M.,

Morgan, H., Müller, W., Neff, F., Nicholson, G., Pasche, B., Roberson, L.A., Rozman, J., Sanderson, M., Santos, L., Selloum, M., Shannon, C., Southwell, A., Tocchini-Valentini, G.P., Vancollie, V.E., Westerberg, H., Wurst, W., Zi, M., Yalcin, B., Ramirez-Solis, R., Steel, K.P., Mallon, A-M., de Angelis, M.H., Herault, Y., and Brown, S.D. (2013) A comparative phenotypic and genomic analysis of C57BL/6J and C57BL/6N mouse strains. *Genome Biology*, **14** (7) R82.

33 Brown, S.D., Chambon, P., and de Angelis, M.H. (2005) EMPReSS: standardized phenotype screens for functional annotation of the mouse genome. *Nature Genetics*, **37**, 1155.

34 Bernstein, D. (2003) Exercise assessment of transgenic models of human cardiovascular disease. *Physiological Genomics*, **13**, 217–226.

35 Chruscinski, A.J., Rohrer, D.K., Schauble, E., Desai, K.H., Bernstein, D., and Kobilka, B.K. (1999) Targeted disruption of the beta2 adrenergic receptor gene. *The Journal of Biological Chemistry*, **274**, 16694–16700.

36 Hoit, B.D., Khoury, S.F., Kranias, E.G., Ball, N., and Walsh, R.A. (1995) In vivo echocardiographic detection of enhanced left ventricular function in gene-targeted mice with phospholamban deficiency. *Circulation Research*, **77**, 632–637.

37 Nakamura, A., Yoshida, K., Takeda, S., Dohi, N., and Ikeda, S. (2002) Progression of dystrophic features and activation of mitogen-activated protein kinases and calcineurin by physical exercise, in hearts of mdx mice. *FEBS Letters*, **520**, 18–24.

38 Redfern, C.H., Degtyarev, M.Y., Kwa, A.T., Salomonis, N., Cotte, N., Nanevicz, T., Fidelman, N., Desai, K., Vranizan, K., Lee, E.K., Coward, P., Shah, N., Warrington, J.A., Fishman, G.I., Bernstein, D., Baker, A.J., and Conklin, B.R. (2000) Conditional expression of a Gi-coupled receptor causes ventricular conduction delay and a lethal cardiomyopathy. *Proceedings of the National Academy of Sciences of the United States of America*, **97**, 4826–4831.

39 Hunsaker, M.R. (2012) Comprehensive neurocognitive endophenotyping strategies for mouse models of genetic disorders. *Progress in Neurobiology*, **96**, 220–241.

40 Kalueff, A.V., Wheaton, M., and Murphy, D.L. (2007) What's wrong with my mouse model? Advances and strategies in animal modeling of anxiety and depression. *Behavioural Brain Research*, **179**, 1–18.

41 Van Dam, D. and De Deyn, P.P. (2011) Animal models in the drug discovery pipeline for Alzheimer's disease. *British Journal of Pharmacology*, **164**, 1285–1300.

42 McMurray, F., Moir, L., and Cox, R.D. (2012) From mice to humans. *Current Diabetes Reports*, **12**, 651–658.

43 Sacca, R., Engle, S.J., Qin, W., Stock, J.L., and McNeish, J.D. (2010) Genetically engineered mouse models in drug discovery research. *Methods in Molecular Biology*, **602**, 37–54.

44 Sali, A., Guerron, A.D., Gordish-Dressman, H., Spurney, C.F., Iantorno, M., Hoffman, E.P., and Nagaraju, K. (2012) Glucocorticoid-treated mice are an inappropriate positive control for long-term preclinical studies in the mdx mouse. *PLoS One*, **7**, e34204.

45 Griebel, G., Stemmelin, J., and Scatton, B. (2005) Effects of the cannabinoid CB1 receptor antagonist rimonabant in models of emotional reactivity in rodents. *Biological Psychiatry*, **57**, 261–267.

46 Christopoulou, F.D. and Kiortsis, D.N. (2011) An overview of the metabolic effects of rimonabant in randomized controlled trials: potential for other cannabinoid 1 receptor blockers in obesity. *Journal of Clinical Pharmacy and Therapeutics*, **36**, 10–18.

47 Gamble-George, J.C., Conger, J.R., Hartley, N.D., Gupta, P., Sumislawski, J.J., and Patel, S. (2013) Dissociable effects of CB1 receptor blockade on anxiety-like and consummatory behaviors in the novelty-induced hypophagia test in mice. *Psychopharmacology (Berlin)*, **228**, 401–409.

48 Jakobovits, A., Amado, R.G., Yang, X., Roskos, L., and Schwab, G. (2007) From XenoMouse technology to panitumumab, the first fully human antibody product from transgenic mice. *Nature Biotechnology*, **25**, 1134–1143.

49 Bellet, D., Pecking, A., and Dangles-Marie, V. (2008) XenoMouse: a feat for obtaining

human antibodies in mice. *Medical Sciences*, **24**, 903–905.
50 Murata, Y., Rosell, A., Scannevin, R.H., Rhodes, K.J., Wang, X., and Lo, E.H. (2008) Extension of the thrombolytic time window with minocycline in experimental stroke. *Stroke*, **39**, 3372–3377.
51 Machado, L.S., Sazonova, I.Y., Kozak, A., Wiley, D.C., El-Remessy, A.B., Ergul, A., Hess, D.C., Waller, J.L., and Fagan, S.C. (2009) Minocycline and tissue-type plasminogen activator for stroke: assessment of interaction potential. *Stroke*, **40**, 3028–3033.
52 Hess, D.C. and Fagan, S.C. (2010) Repurposing an old drug to improve the use and safety of tissue plasminogen activator for acute ischemic stroke: minocycline. *Pharmacotherapy*, **30**, 55S–61S.
53 Soczynska, J.K., Mansur, R.B., Brietzke, E., Swardfager, W., Kennedy, S.H., Woldeyohannes, H.O., Powell, A.M., Manierka, M.S., and McIntyre, R.S. (2012) Novel therapeutic targets in depression: minocycline as a candidate treatment. *Behavioural Brain Research*, **235**, 302–317.
54 Weischenfeldt, J., Symmons, O., Spitz, F., and Korbel, J.O. (2013) Phenotypic impact of genomic structural variation: insights from and for human disease. *Nature Reviews. Genetics*, **14**, 125–138.
55 Ramirezsolis, R., Liu, P.T., and Bradley, A. (1995) Chromosome engineering in mice. *Nature*, **378**, 720–724.
56 Vandeursen, J., Fornerod, M., Vanrees, B., and Grosveld, G. (1995) CRE-mediated site-specific translocation between nonhomologous mouse chromosomes. *Proceedings of the National Academy of Sciences of the United States of America*, **92**, 7376–7380.
57 Spitz, F., Herkenne, C., Morris, M.A., and Duboule, D. (2005) Inversion-induced disruption of the Hoxd cluster leads to the partition of regulatory landscapes. *Nature Genetics*, **37**, 889–893.
58 Lupski, J.R., Deocaluna, R.M., Slaugenhaupt, S., Pentao, L., Guzzetta, V., Trask, B.J., Saucedocardenas, O., Barker, D.F., Killian, J.M., Garcia, C.A., Chakravarti, A., and Patel, P.I. (1991) DNA duplication associated with Charcot-Marie-Tooth disease type-1A. *Cell*, **66**, 219–232.
59 Jana, N.R. (2012) Understanding the pathogenesis of Angelman syndrome through animal models. *Neural Plasticity*, **2012**, 710943.
60 Walz, K., Caratini-Rivera, S., Bi, W.M., Fonseca, P., Mansouri, D.L., Lynch, J., Vogel, H., Noebels, J.L., Bradley, A., and Lupski, J.R. (2003) Modeling del(17)(p11.2p11.2) and dup(17)(p11.2p11.2) contiguous gene syndromes by chromosome engineering in mice: phenotypic consequences of gene dosage imbalance. *Molecular and Cellular Biology*, **23**, 3646–3655.
61 Horev, G., Ellegood, J., Lerch, J.P., Son, Y.E.E., Muthuswamy, L., Vogel, H., Krieger, A.M., Buja, A., Henkelman, R.M., Wigler, M., and Mills, A.A. (2011) Dosage-dependent phenotypes in models of 16p11.2 lesions found in autism. *Proceedings of the National Academy of Sciences of the United States of America*, **108**, 17076–17081.
62 Lindsay, E.A., Botta, A., Jurecic, V., Carattini-Rivera, S., Cheah, Y.C., Rosenblatt, H.M., Bradley, A., and Baldini, A. (1999) Congenital heart disease in mice deficient for the DiGeorge syndrome region. *Nature*, **401**, 379–383.
63 Lindsay, E.A., Vitelli, F., Su, H., Morishima, M., Huynh, T., Pramparo, T., Jurecic, V., Ogunrinu, G., Sutherland, H.F., Scambler, P.J., Bradley, A., and Baldini, A. (2001) Tbx1 haploinsufficiency in the DiGeorge syndrome region causes aortic arch defects in mice. *Nature*, **410**, 97–101.
64 Walz, K., Paylor, R., Yan, J., Bi, W.M., and Lupski, J.R. (2006) Rai1 duplication causes physical and behavioral phenotypes in a mouse model of dup(17)(p11.2p11.2). *Journal of Clinical Investigation*, **116**, 3035–3041.
65 Jerome, L.A. and Papaioannou, V.E. (2001) DiGeorge syndrome phenotype in mice mutant for the T-box gene, Tbx1. *Nature Genetics*, **27**, 286–291.
66 Ermakova, O., Piszczek, L., Luciani, L., Cavalli, F.M.G., Ferreira, T., Farley, D., Rizzo, S., Paolicelli, R.C., Al-Banchaabouchi, M., Nerlov, C., Moriggl, R., Luscombe, N.M., and Gross, C. (2011) Sensitized phenotypic screening identifies gene dosage sensitive region on chromosome 11 that predisposes to disease in mice. *EMBO Molecular Medicine*, **3**, 50–66.

67 Kvajo, M., McKellar, H., and Gogos, J.A. (2012) Avoiding mouse traps in schizophrenia genetics: lessons and promises from current and emerging mouse models. *Neuroscience*, **211**, 136–164.

68 Dierssen, M., Herault, Y., and Estivill, X. (2009) Aneuploidy: from a physiological mechanism of variance to Down syndrome. *Physiological Reviews*, **89**, 887–920.

69 Herault, Y., Duchon, A., Velot, E., Marechal, D., and Brault, V. (2012) The *in vivo* Down syndrome genomic library in mouse. *Down Syndrome*, **197**, 169–197.

70 Insausti, A.M., Megias, M., Crespo, D., Cruz-Orive, L.M., Dierssen, M., Vallina, T.F., Insausti, R., and Florez, J. (1998) Hippocampal volume and neuronal number in Ts65Dn mice: a murine model of Down syndrome. *Neuroscience Letters*, **253**, 175–178.

71 Baxter, L.L., Moran, T.H., Richtsmeier, J.T., Troncoso, J., and Reeves, R.H. (2000) Discovery and genetic localization of Down syndrome cerebellar phenotypes using the Ts65Dn mouse. *Human Molecular Genetics*, **9**, 195–202.

72 Aldridge, K., Reeves, R.H., Olson, L.E., and Richtsmeier, J.T. (2007) Differential effects of trisomy on brain shape and volume in related aneuploid mouse models. *American Journal of Medical Genetics Part A*, **143A**, 1060–1070.

73 Lott, I.T. (2012) Neurological phenotypes for Down syndrome across the life span. *Down Syndrome*, **197**, 101–121.

74 Sturgeon, X., Le, T., Ahmed, M.M., and Gardiner, K.J. (2012) Pathways to cognitive deficits in Down syndrome. *Down Syndrome*, **197**, 73–100.

75 de la Torre, R. and Dierssen, M. (2012) Therapeutic approaches in the improvement of cognitive performance in Down syndrome: past, present, and future. *Down Syndrome*, **197**, 1–14.

76 Phillips, T.J., Belknap, J.K., Hitzemann, R.J., Buck, K.J., Cunningham, C.L., and Crabbe, J.C. (2002) Harnessing the mouse to unravel the genetics of human disease. *Genes Brain and Behavior*, **1**, 14–26.

77 Habener, J.F., Kemp, D.M., and Thomas, M.K. (2005) Minireview: transcriptional regulation in pancreatic development. *Endocrinology*, **146**, 1025–1034.

78 Kitamura, T., Kahn, C.R., and Accili, E. (2003) Insulin receptor knockout mice. *Annual Review of Physiology*, **65**, 313–332.

79 Tabuchi, K., Blundell, J., Etherton, M.R., Hammer, R.E., Liu, X.R., Powell, C.M., and Sudhof, T.C. (2007) Neuroligin-3 mutation implicated in autism increases inhibitory synaptic transmission in mice. *Science*, **318**, 71–76.

80 Dolen, G., Osterweil, E., Rao, B.S.S., Smith, G.B., Auerbach, B.D., Chattarji, S., and Bear, M.F. (2007) Correction of fragile X syndrome in mice. *Neuron*, **56**, 955–962.

81 Tropea, D., Giacometti, E., Wilson, N.R., Beard, C., McCurry, C., Fu, D.D., Flannery, R., Jaenisch, R., and Sur, M. (2009) Partial reversal of Rett syndrome-like symptoms in MeCP2 mutant mice. *Proceedings of the National Academy of Sciences of the United States of America*, **106**, 2029–2034.

82 Hodgson, J.G., Smith, D.J., McCutcheon, K., Koide, H.B., Nishiyama, K., Dinulos, M.B., Stevens, M.E., Bissada, N., Nasir, J., Kanazawa, I., Disteche, C.M., Rubin, E.M., and Hayden, M.R. (1996) Human huntingtin derived from YAC transgenes compensates for loss of murine huntingtin by rescue of the embryonic lethal phenotype. *Human Molecular Genetics*, **5**, 1875–1885.

83 Lane, T.F., Lin, C.W., Brown, M.A., Solomon, E., and Leder, P. (2000) Gene replacement with the human BRCA1 locus: tissue specific expression and rescue of embryonic lethality in mice. *Oncogene*, **19**, 4085–4090.

84 Chandler, J., Hohenstein, P., Swing, D.A., Tessarollo, L., and Sharan, S.K. (2001) Human BRCA1 gene rescues the embryonic lethality of Brca1 mutant mice. *Genesis*, **29**, 72–77.

85 Vadolas, J., Wardan, H., Bosmans, M., Zaibak, F., Jamsai, D., Voullaire, L., Williamson, R., and Ioannou, P.A. (2005) Transgene copy number-dependent rescue of murine beta-globin knockout mice carrying a 183 kb human beta-globin BAC genomic fragment. *Biochimica et Biophysica Acta – Gene Structure and Expression*, **1728**, 150–162.

86 Yang, Y.P., Swaminathan, S., Martin, B.K., and Sharan, S.K. (2003) Aberrant splicing induced by missense mutations

in BRCA1: clues from a humanized mouse model. *Human Molecular Genetics*, **12**, 2121–2131.
87 Jamsai, D., Zaibak, F., Khongnium, W., Vadolas, J., Voullaire, L., Fowler, K.J., Gazeas, S., Fucharoen, S., Williamson, R., and Ioannou, P.A. (2005) A humanized mouse model for a common beta(0)-thalassemia mutation. *Genomics*, **85**, 453–461.
88 Rathinam, C., Poueymirou, W.T., Rojas, J., Murphy, A.J., Valenzuela, D.M., Yancopoulos, G.D., Rongvaux, A., Eynon, E.E., Manz, M.G., and Flavell, R.A. (2011) Efficient differentiation and function of human macrophages in humanized CSF-1 mice. *Blood*, **118**, 3119–3128.
89 Rongvaux, A., Willinger, T., Takizawa, H., Rathinam, C., Auerbach, W., Murphy, A.J., Valenzuela, D.M., Yancopoulos, G.D., Eynon, E.E., Stevens, S., Manz, M.G., and Flavell, R.A. (2011) Human thrombopoietin knockin mice efficiently support human hematopoiesis *in vivo*. *Proceedings of the National Academy of Sciences of the United States of America*, **108**, 2378–2383.
90 Willinger, T., Rongvaux, A., Strowig, T., Manz, M.G., and Flavell, R.A. (2011) Improving human hemato-lymphoid-system mice by cytokine knock-in gene replacement. *Trends in Immunology*, **32**, 321–327.
91 O'Doherty, A., Ruf, S., Mulligan, C., Hildreth, V., Errington, M.L., Cooke, S., Sesay, A., Modino, S., Vanes, L., Hernandez, D., Linehan, J.M., Sharpe, P. T., Brandner, S., Bliss, T.V.P., Henderson, D.J., Nizetic, D., Tybulewicz, V.L.J., and Fisher, E.M.C. (2005) An aneuploid mouse strain carrying human chromosome 21 with Down syndrome phenotypes. *Science*, **309**, 2033–2037.
92 Wilson, M.D., Barbosa-Morais, N.L., Schmidt, D., Conboy, C.M., Vanes, L., Tybulewicz, V.L.J., Fisher, E.M.C., Tavare, S., and Odom, D.T. (2008) Species-specific transcription in mice carrying human chromosome 21. *Science*, **322**, 434–438.
93 Pope, B.D., Chandra, T., Buckley, Q., Hoare, M., Ryba, T., Wiseman, F.K., Kuta, A., Wilson, M.D., Odom, D.T., and Gilbert, D.M. (2012) Replication-timing boundaries facilitate cell-type and species-specific regulation of a rearranged human chromosome in mouse. *Human Molecular Genetics*, **21**, 4162–4170.

94 Shen, H.W., Jiang, X.L., Gonzalez, F.J., and Yu, A.M. (2011) Humanized transgenic mouse models for drug metabolism and pharmacokinetic research. *Current Drug Metabolism*, **12**, 997–1006.
95 Bolker, J. (2012) Model organisms: there's more to life than rats and flies. *Nature*, **491**, 31–33.
96 Schughart, K., Libert, C., and Kas, M.J. (2012) Human disease: strength to strength for mouse models. *Nature*, **492**, 41.
97 von Herrath, M.G. and Nepom, G.T. (2005) Lost in translation: barriers to implementing clinical immunotherapeutics for autoimmunity. *The Journal of Experimental Medicine*, **202**, 1159–1162.
98 Ostrand-Rosenberg, S. (2004) Animal models of tumor immunity, immunotherapy and cancer vaccines. *Current Opinion in Immunology*, **16**, 143–150.
99 Schnabel, J. (2008) Neuroscience: standard model. *Nature*, **454**, 682–685.
100 Daneshgari, F., Leiter, E.H., Liu, G., and Reeder, J. (2009) Animal models of diabetic uropathy. *Journal of Urology*, **182**, S8–S13.
101 Schughart, K., Libert, C., Kas, M.J., and SYSGENET Consortium (2013) Controlling complexity: the clinical relevance of mouse complex genetics. *European Journal of Human Genetics*, **21**, 1191–1196.
102 Tsaparas, P., Mariño-Ramírez, L., Bodenreider, O., Koonin, E.V., and Jordan, I.K. (2006) Global similarity and local divergence in human and mouse gene co-expression networks. *BMC Evolutionary Biology*, **6**, 70.
103 Carter, C.S. and Barch, D.M. (2007) Cognitive neuroscience-based approaches to measuring and improving treatment effects on cognition in schizophrenia: the CNTRICS initiative. *Schizophrenia Bulletin*, **33**, 1131–1137.
104 Bayés, A., Collins, M.O., Croning, M.D., van de Lagemaat, L.N., Choudhary, J.S., and Grant, S.G. (2012) Comparative study of human and mouse postsynaptic proteomes finds high compositional conservation and abundance differences for key synaptic proteins. *PLoS One*, **7**, e46683.

7
In Vivo Brain Imaging in Animal Models: A Focus on PET and MRI

Fabien Chauveau, Muthieu Verdurand, and Luc Zimmer

7.1
Introduction: Role of Animal in *In Vivo* Imaging

7.1.1
In Vivo Imaging as a Translational Approach for Basic Research

Although imaging has long been indispensable in clinical practice, *in vivo* imaging of small laboratory animals has emerged more recently as an important component of preclinical biomedical research. Small animal imaging provides a noninvasive means of exploring biological structures and functions *in vivo*, revealing qualitative and quantitative information on normal and diseased tissues in a given spatial and temporal location. Recent years have seen a large increase in the number of animal models. Rats and mice are widely used in research, and the combination of genetic manipulation (primarily in mice) and surgical and interventional models (primarily in rats) suggests an expanded role for these laboratory animals in neuroscience [1].

The success of imaging is mainly explained by its noninvasive nature, allowing longitudinal assay of animal models of human diseases, from diagnosis to progression of the pathology, and monitoring of treatment efficacy. Genetically engineered rodent models of diseases (i.e., transgenic knock-in and knockout mice) are becoming increasingly more realistic in mimicking the pathophysiology of the corresponding human disease. Importantly, and unlike alternative cell or tissue culture-based protocols, studies in intact animals, and particularly in the brain, take account of all the interacting physiological factors – neurochemical, neurophysiological, neurohormonal, nutritional, and so on – present in the complex organ *in situ*. Intact whole-animal models accessible to imaging thus facilitate investigation of systemic aspects of disease, which are almost impossible to fully replicate in *in vitro* or *ex vivo* systems.

In Vivo Models for Drug Discovery, First Edition. Edited by José M. Vela, Rafael Maldonado, and Michel Hamon.
© 2014 Wiley-VCH Verlag GmbH & Co. KGaA. Published 2014 by Wiley-VCH Verlag GmbH & Co. KGaA.

7.1.2
In Vivo Imaging in Animal Models in the Pharmaceutical Industry

In the context of drug development, many imaging studies aim to provide translatable data that will be used in the clinical development process, from preliminary proof of concept to clinical trials.

Imaging biomarkers for the development of drug therapies (pharmaco-imaging) have become more widely used in recent years. As will be described later, several characteristics of imaging biomarkers favor their use in preclinical and clinical pharmacological tests to explore the drug's binding localization and to determine its brain transport efficiency, target occupancy, or functional effect. This provides a particular advantage over the classical pharmacological approach because of the opportunity to explore brain neurochemistry *in vivo*, with shorter experimental duration, thanks to longitudinal studies. Consequently, there is increasing evidence that imaging can accelerate the drug development process from preclinical studies in animal models to clinical imaging. The largest pharmaceutical companies have bought or developed their own preclinical positron emission tomography (PET) centers, whereas others are starting to outsource their biomarker activity to platform providers or academic technology centers [2].

Despite these benefits, it should be recognized that few animals, perhaps only 1–2% of the total used in pharmaceutical drug discovery projects, ever undergo imaging. Most are assessed using other equally valid techniques such as histology, molecular biomarkers, or behavioral assessment. As yet, only certain central nervous system (CNS) drug developers systematically include molecular imaging into their early-stage clinical CNS programs whenever possible.

7.1.3
In Vivo Imaging in Animal Models and the 3R Principles

Animal models of brain pathology require information about disease impact on brain structure and/or functioning and the effects of pharmacological intervention. Such information can often only be obtained by sacrificing animals for histological and biochemical analyses. Obviously, this approach is animal consuming and precludes longitudinal studies of individual animals. One key advantage of *in vivo* imaging is the ability to perform multiple types of studies in the same animal. Because each animal can serve as its own control, the number of experimental animals required for a particular study is minimized. Imaging thus provides additional ethical benefit in reducing the number of animals; sample sizes may also be reduced because of better exclusion criteria and more reproducible endpoints [3]. In addition, imaging allows internal biological processes to be monitored, and for this to be done externally, thus reducing invasive approaches and surgery. Finally, *in vivo* imaging mainly involves acquisitions in anesthetized animals, limiting animal stress and pain.

7.2
The Choice of the Right Imaging Modality for Brain Imaging

In recent years, there has been a rapid increase in the variety of *in vivo* imaging technologies. Specialized hardware dedicated to small animal imaging has been refined to overcome the limitations of spatial resolution and sensitivity associated with clinical scanners, and new imaging techniques have also been developed for noninvasive cellular and subcellular imaging [4].

The animal models used to study the CNS have their own specificities, two of which in particular have to be taken into account when embarking on an imaging approach. The first is the complex nature of the brain. In terms of anatomy, the brain is the most complex organ in the human body. In addition to its complicated three-dimensional structure, it can be considered as containing several different organs rather than one functional entity, and the term "central nervous system" appears more appropriate than treating the brain as a single organ. The second specificity is that the brain is probably the most protected organ, first by the skull and then by the surrounding blood–brain barrier (BBB), limiting access to brain tissue for scientific, diagnostic, and therapeutic purposes.

Therefore, the advent of sophisticated technologies for imaging small animals offers an opportunity to learn to manage some of the characteristics already mentioned. Several techniques for molecular imaging are now available for animal studies, from simplistic planar imaging to isotopic imaging and nonradioactive optical imaging [5,6]. Although the recently developed bioluminescence method is more sensitive than fluorescence for small animal imaging, these techniques still represent a challenge for cerebral imaging because of heavy scattering and attenuation at the skull interface. Optical imaging of the brain is performed noninvasively in mice or rat neonates, but requires skull thinning or a cranial window in adult rats.

In contrast, computed tomography (CT) does not suffer from a lack of penetration into deep brain areas. Most X-ray techniques known from clinical medicine have been back-translated to small animal imaging, from 2D projection imaging (radiography and angiography) to the more advanced 3D computed tomography imaging techniques. Unenhanced radiography reveals skeletal anatomy, whereas contrast-enhanced imaging provides improved visualization of the vasculature and strongly vascularized areas. However, due to the poor contrast of X-rays in soft tissue, CT applications in neurology are restricted to angiography and brain infarct measurement [7].

Magnetic resonance imaging (MRI) has outstanding spatial resolution and the wide range of soft tissue contrast accounts for its widespread success in brain imaging. Complementarily, PET, developed in nuclear medicine, shows exquisite sensitivity and the ability to provide quantitative *in vivo* measurements of physiology, metabolic pathways, and molecular targets inside tissue. Small animal PET refers to imaging of animals such as rats and mice using a high-resolution PET scanner.

Because animal model-based research has in recent years driven the growth of small animal MRI and PET for brain exploration, we will focus on these two imaging approaches. We will highlight the advantages and limitations of MRI and PET in the translational use of preclinical imaging.

7.3
Small Animal Magnetic Resonance Imaging

7.3.1
Principles

Magnetic resonance imaging and magnetic resonance spectroscopy (MRS) rely on the nuclear magnetic resonance (NMR) effect. This phenomenon is found only in nuclei possessing a nonzero magnetic moment (e.g., hydrogen) in the presence of an external static magnetic field B_0, which induces coherent precession of individual magnetic moments (spins) and gives rise to net magnetization. Detecting the NMR effect requires an additional time-varying magnetic field B_1, applied perpendicularly to the static B_0 field, at the resonance condition or Larmor frequency, which is the frequency of the precession of the spins. For this, an additional radio frequency (RF) coil is used. B_1 pulses flip the *longitudinal* magnetization to an arbitrary angle with respect to the external static B_0 field. The *transverse* component of the flipped magnetization precesses around the static B_0 field at the Larmor frequency, inducing a time-varying voltage signal in the RF coil – this is the source of the NMR signal [8].

This signal is transient because relaxation processes cause a rapid decrease in the flip angle induced by the B_1 pulse. Spin–lattice relaxation describes how fast the longitudinal magnetization recovers after applying the B_1 field, and is characterized by relaxation time T_1. Spin–spin relaxation describes how fast the transverse magnetization decays, and is characterized by relaxation time T_2. In addition, B_0 field nonhomogeneities induce dephasing between the coherently precessing spins, and thus potentiate transverse magnetization decay, giving rise to T_2^* relaxation.

7.3.2
Magnetic Resonance Spectroscopy

Spins of the same isotope resonate at slightly different frequencies because of their molecular environment (i.e., chemical structure). This difference is called *chemical shift* and is commonly expressed as a relative measurement in parts per million (ppm), rendering it independent of field strength. NMR spectroscopy measures chemical shifts from a defined volume within a sample or an organ. The NMR spectrum is the Fourier transform of the acquired NMR signal. Chemical shifts allow identification of chemical substances, while the signal intensity is proportional to their concentration.

MRS provides a noninvasive window onto metabolism and can be viewed as an additional contrast besides standard anatomical MRI examination. The concentration of the following metabolites can be measured *in vivo* through a proton spectrum of the rodent brain (1H-MRS): creatine (Cr), choline (Cho), N-acetylaspartate (NAA), lactate (Lac), and *myo*-inositol (mI). The relative levels of the corresponding spectral peaks can reflect cellular homeostasis or pathological states, and can be used as biomarkers [9]. Another major application is tissue energetics with ^{31}P-NMR [10], which enables detection and quantification of adenosine triphosphate (ATP), phosphocreatine (PCr), phosphorylcholine (PC), phosphorylethanolamine (PE), glycerophosphorylcholine (GPC), glycerophosphorylethanolamine (GPE), and inorganic phosphate (Pi). ^{31}P-NMR can also provide a noninvasive estimate of tissue pH.

7.3.3
Magnetic Resonance Imaging

The formation of a stack of 2D images from individual signals of the same nuclei requires spatial coding by magnetic field gradients that vary linearly along the direction of the B_0 field. After a slice has been selected, the signal has to be spatially encoded in the two remaining dimensions. One of these directions is encoded by applying a phase-encoding gradient for a short period before signal acquisition. To achieve full spatial encoding, a number of experiments have to be carried out with stepwise variation in phase-encoding gradient. The third spatial dimension is encoded by applying a frequency-encoding gradient during data acquisition. Performing a two-dimensional Fourier transform of the acquired signal yields the position of the contributing magnetization. Different patterns of pulses produced by the three orthogonal magnetic field gradients (MRI sequences) result in various image contrasts.

Contrast in MRI derives from the complex interplay of relaxation times, proton density, and instrumental parameters. Anatomic images can be acquired as T_1-, T_2-, or T_2^*-weighted images or as proton density images. The spatial distribution of the relaxation rates can be mapped with quantitative measurements. Nonclassical (but now routine) MR techniques include the following:

- *Diffusion-weighted imaging (DWI) and diffusion tensor imaging (DTI):* These are sensitive to the microscopic diffusion of water protons, which, in disease, is affected by cytotoxic or vasogenic edema, or can be used to reconstruct CNS neuronal fiber tracts.
- *Perfusion-weighted imaging (PWI):* This enables quantification of blood flow and blood volume, with or without injection of a contrast agent (dynamic susceptibility contrast-enhanced PWI and arterial spin-labeling PWI, respectively).
- *Magnetization transfer imaging (MTI):* This uses off-resonance pulses to saturate a pool of proton spins (e.g., macromolecular) and characterizes the exchange rate between this pool and another (e.g., surrounding water).

- *Functional MRI (fMRI):* This relies on blood-oxygen-level-dependent (BOLD) contrast and highlights changes in brain activity during a task or stimulation.

The MR image contrast or sensitivity can be further modified or enhanced by a variety of MRI contrast agents: gadolinium chelates, metal-based nanoparticles, chemical exchange saturation transfer (CEST) contrast agents, and so on [11]. MRI is indeed an ideal candidate for a broad range of imaging tasks, thanks to (i) high to very high spatial resolution combined with high temporal resolution; (ii) 3D capabilities; and (iii) safety, since no harmful ionizing radiation is involved. Stroke can be cited as an example of translational success: Mismatch between perfusion and diffusion images provides a good estimate of the penumbra, which is the cerebral tissue considered amenable to treatment (Figure 7.1). PWI–DWI mismatch is now used in both experimental studies [12] and clinical trials [13] for neuroprotection.

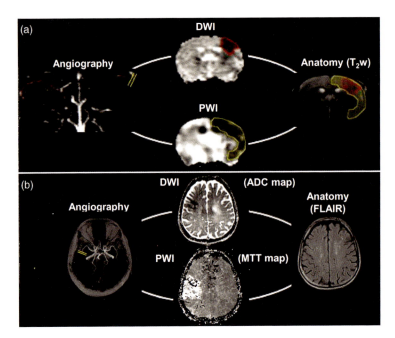

Figure 7.1 MRI translation to clinical applications: *in vivo* multimodal MRI images showing anatomy (T_2-weighted imaging, T_2w; fluid attenuation inversion recovery (FLAIR)), cytotoxic edema (diffusion-weighted imaging, with corresponding apparent diffusion coefficient map), and unilaterally affected hemodynamic status (perfusion-weighted imaging, with corresponding mean transit time map) at the acute stage of stroke in (a) a mouse and (b) a 78 year-old patient. Note that anatomical images are normal shortly after stroke onset, while DWI highlights the developing infarct within the perfusion defect shown on PWI. [Images from (a) CERMEP-Imagerie du Vivant, Lyon, France; and (b) Neurological Hospital, Hospices Civils de Lyon, France].

7.4
Positron Emission Tomography

7.4.1
Basic Principles and Instrumentation

A PET protocol relies first on the production of positron-emitting radionuclides by a biomedical cyclotron or particle accelerator. Particles (protons or deuterons) are injected near the center of the magnetic field, accelerated while passing through the electrodes, and directed toward a target containing a specific gas or fluid. Collisions of particles with the target create positron-emitting isotopes such as oxygen-15 (^{15}O), nitrogen-13 (^{13}N), carbon-11 (^{11}C) or fluorine-18 (^{18}F), with short half-lives of 2, 10, 20, and 110 min, respectively. Once produced, the radionuclide must be rapidly incorporated into a molecule to produce a radiotracer (called a *radiopharmaceutical* when injected in humans). This radiolabeling step occurs in a dedicated radiochemistry laboratory and is followed by appropriate quality controls before injection into the subject under the PET scanner.

After intravenous injection, the radioactivity emitted by the radiotracer diffusing in the subject and reaching its target provides an indirect measure of positron–electron annihilation, leading to a couple of high-energy photons traveling 180° apart. These two photons are simultaneously detected by two detectors linked in series and placed on opposite sides of a ring of scintillation crystals encircling the subject within the PET apparatus [14]. By collecting a statistically significant number of lines of response, mathematical algorithms can be used to reconstruct a three-dimensional image that reflects the distribution of the positron-emitting molecules in the body. A modern PET scanner is capable of producing images of the human brain at a resolution of 3–6 mm. Clinical PET systems are, however, inadequate for small animals such as rats or mice, where a resolution close to 1.5 mm is required [15].

The theory of PET relies on the "rule" that the injected tracer mass will cause maximal target occupancy of 5%. This is because the tracer mass injected into a small animal (tracer dose) must be sufficiently small for the natural physiological state of the animal not to be affected. Numerous PET tracers have been designed to explore a variety of biological processes and molecular targets in the brain, ranging from cerebral perfusion and substrate metabolism to receptor targets and enzyme kinetics [16,17]. PET shows exquisite sensitivity because PET tracers generally have high specific activity, defined as the ratio of the number of radioactive atoms to the total number of atoms in a given element (in a given chemical or physical form) [18]. Therefore, most PET images only require micrograms at most of the compound of interest, resulting in nanomolar or lower concentrations *in vivo*.

7.4.2
PET and Neuronal Metabolism

Neuronal metabolism is based on the brain's activity and function, and can be quantified by analyzing glucose consumption. The 2-deoxyglucose (2-DG) autoradiographic method has long been used as an *in vitro* measure of neuronal metabolism [19]. The radiotracer [^{18}F]2-fluoro-2-deoxy-D-glucose ([^{18}F]FDG) is a fluorine-18-labeled glucose analog, which is transported into the cell, phosphorylated, and trapped within the cytoplasm. Thus, changes in the rate of glucose metabolism, reflected by the [^{18}F]FDG PET signal, probably correspond to changes in neurotransmitter function [20]. Researchers have used small animal PET to investigate glucose metabolism in various rodent models (mainly in rats and, less frequently, in mice) [21] after visual activation [22], behavioral challenge [23,24], and cerebral ischemia [25] in models of epilepsy [26]. Although these examples illustrate how PET can help study neuronal activation in rats, some caveats must be mentioned. First, [^{18}F]FDG PET results in small animals are not easy to interpret alone because the radiotracer distribution is not area dependent. Second, [^{18}F]FDG kinetics has a relatively long uptake period, and therefore the neuronal activation period (e.g., prolonged seizure or iterative sensory stimulation) must also be prolonged. A process that only produces brief neuronal activity is unlikely to be visualized on [^{18}F]FDG PET, as the enhanced uptake during stimulation will be averaged with, and thus masked by, the uptake period without stimulation.

7.4.3
PET and Brain Receptors and Transporters

As previously described, PET radioligands are radiolabeled with a high specific activity that allows a very small amount to be injected. The concentration is usually far below that at which pharmacological effects might be induced. Tracers with high (subpicomolar) target affinity enable visualization and quantification of brain receptors in areas where they concentrate at picomolar levels [27]. The outcome measures of neuroreceptor imaging are (i) receptor density and (ii) the binding affinity to the receptor of interest. Using PET scan data, receptor density and binding affinity are expressed as the ratio, termed "binding potential" (BP), of receptor concentration (B_{max}) to ligand affinity (K_d). Receptor density (B_{max}) and affinity (K_d) are usually determined separately, in classical *in vitro* receptor binding studies. However, *in vivo* PET protocols can also be designed to determine these variables. The specific protocol uses a double radiotracer injection and two PET scans: the first with a high specific activity radiotracer and the second with a lower specific activity radiotracer (plus an unlabeled molecule). Receptor density (B_{max}) and affinity (K_d) can then be displayed on a Scatchard plot [28]. Various methods are used to calculate BP, such as reference tissue methods [29], graphic analysis [30–32], or a bolus plus constant infusion method [33].

Typically, brain imaging can be used to target neurotransmitters at three locations in the "neurotransmitter pathway": the presynaptic neuron, the postsynaptic neuron, and the intraneuronal metabolism [34]. In the case of the dopaminergic system, the radioligand [^{11}C]PE2I targets the dopamine transporter and provides a means to estimate its presynaptic density [35]; [^{11}C]raclopride binding to D_2 receptors allows postsynaptic imaging, and [^{18}F]fluoro-DOPA enables imaging of the dopamine metabolic pathway, essentially at presynaptic intraneuronal level [36].

Most of the PET ligands so far developed have targeted the serotoninergic and dopaminergic systems, partly because several of these two types of systems have long proved useful for treating neuropsychiatric disorders such as schizophrenia [37,38], Parkinson's disease [39], Huntington's disease [40], and depression [41]. Other neurotransmitter systems, however, are increasingly being explored, such as the cholinergic, peptidergic, and cannabinergic systems (Table 7.1).

Table 7.1 Some brain radiotracers used in small animal PET.

Biological application	Target/measured process	Radiotracer
Metabolic imaging	Glucose metabolism	[^{18}F]2-Fluoro-2-desoxyglucose (FDG)
	Cerebral blood flow	[^{15}O]H$_2$O
Monoamines	Vesicular transporter	[^{11}C]Dihydrotetrabenazine (DTBZ)
Dopaminergic system	Dopamine metabolism (DOPA decarboxylase activity)	[^{18}F]Fluoro-DOPA
	D$_1$ receptor	[^{11}C]SCH23390
	D$_2$ receptor	[^{18}F]Fallypride
		[^{11}C]FLB456
		[^{11}C]N-Methylspiperone
		[^{18}F]Spiperone
		[^{18}F]Fluoroethylspiperone
	D$_{2/3}$ receptor	[^{11}C]Raclopride
	Dopamine transporter	[^{11}C]PE2I
Noradrenergic system	Noradrenaline transporter	[^{11}C]MRB
	α2-Adrenergic receptor	[^{18}F]2-Fluoroethoxyidazoxan
Serotoninergic system	5-HT$_{1A}$ receptor	[^{18}F]MPPF
		[^{11}C]WAY100635
	5-HT$_{2A}$ receptor	[^{11}C]MDL100907
	Serotonin transporter	[^{11}C]DASB
	Serotonin storage	[^{11}C]Methyltryptophan
Cholinergic system	Muscarinic acetylcholine receptors	[^{11}C]NMPYB
		[^{11}C]Tropanylbenzylate
		[^{18}F]FP-TZTP
	Nicotinic acetylcholine receptors	[^{11}C]MPA
		[^{11}C]A-85380; [^{18}F]A-85380
	Vesicular transporter	[^{18}F]Fluoroethoxybenzovesamicol
		[^{11}C]Vesamicol
GABAergic system	GABA$_A$/benzodiazepine receptors	[^{11}C]Flumazenil

(continued)

Table 7.1 (Continued)

Biological application	Target/measured process	Radiotracer
	GABA$_A$/benzodiazepine receptors (α5-subunit)	[^{11}C]RO15-4513
Opioid system	Opioid receptors (μ, δ, κ)	[^{11}C]Diprenorphine
	Opioid receptors (μ)	[^{11}C]Carfentenil
Histaminergic system	H$_1$ receptors	[^{11}C]Dothiepin
Neuropeptides (substance P)	NK$_1$ receptors	[^{18}F]SPARQ
		[^{11}C]GR205171
Cannabinergic system	CB$_1$ receptor	[^{18}F]MK-9470
		[^{11}C]OMAR
Misfolded proteins	β-Amyloid deposits/plaques	[^{11}C]PiB
		[^{18}F]Florbetapir, [^{18}F]florbetaben [^{18}F]BF-227
(Neuro) Inflammation	Translocator protein (TSPO)	[^{11}C]PK11195

Source: Adapted from Ref. [10].

7.4.4
PET and Receptor Occupancy

Receptor occupancy refers to the percentage of a receptor population that is occupied by a drug at a specified dose or concentration in plasma [42]. PET can be used indirectly to study how drugs inhibit specific radioligand binding, by monitoring the level of binding site occupancy induced by an unlabeled drug given at varying doses. PET imaging targeting a receptor of interest can be performed before and after administration of a drug blocking the receptor (competition at the same receptor site as the radiotracer). This approach enables quantification of receptor occupancy, which may be correlated with the therapeutic effect. For example, PET enabled quantification of dopamine D$_2$ receptor blockade by using [^{11}C]raclopride [43] and serotonin 5-HT$_2$ receptor blockade using [^{11}C]N-methylspiperone [44] in the treatment of schizophrenic patients by antipsychotic drugs. The number of free receptors after cessation of drug treatment was also measured, assuming that receptor affinity remained unchanged. These studies revealed a correlation between receptor occupancy and antipsychotic or adverse effects. They also revealed that the drugs' receptor occupancy had a much longer duration than would be predicted from its plasma pharmacokinetics. This type of study is now frequently used in drug development at both preclinical and clinical stages.

7.4.5
PET and Neurotransmitter Release

Under particular conditions, PET can provide a dynamic measure of neurotransmission by measuring acute variations in synaptic neurotransmitter concentrations in the living brain. This possibility is based on the principle of competition between a radioligand and a particular neurotransmitter [45]. Changes in receptor binding parameters following pharmacological intervention may indicate a change in the number of available receptors or in receptor sensitivity. Several recent reports demonstrated that PET, using a ligand with relatively low affinity for the studied receptors, could evaluate a neurotransmitter's functional response to pharmacological manipulation as well as the interaction between neuronal systems. It has been speculated that dopamine might compete with a ligand on the same receptor binding site if the affinity of the ligand to its receptor is moderate. For instance, [^{11}C]raclopride presents higher selectivity and more moderate affinity for dopamine D_2 receptors than does dopamine. PET has been used to assess dopamine's effects on striatal [^{11}C]raclopride binding to the D_2 receptor [46], and serotonin's effects on hippocampal [^{18}F]MPPF binding to 5-HT$_{1A}$ receptor (Figure 7.2) [47]. The classical occupancy model [48] predicts an association between change in endogenous neurotransmitter levels and change in the *in vivo* binding parameters of radiotracers. However, the occupancy model does not fully explain the changes in radioligand binding observed in response to modulation of neurotransmitter release [49].

7.5
Clinical Translation: Limitations and Difficulties

Because MRI and PET are imaging technologies used in both clinical and laboratory settings, the findings of small animal imaging are readily translatable to

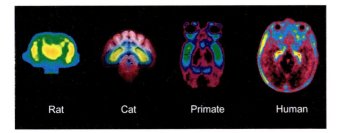

Figure 7.2 PET translation to clinical applications: *in vivo* PET images showing the distribution of [^{18}F]MPPF, a 5-HT$_{1A}$ receptor radiotracer, in rat, cat, nonhuman primate, and a healthy subject. High density [^{18}F]MPPF binding can be seen in the hippocampus, entorhinal cortex, and dorsal raphe nucleus of animal and human brains. [^{18}F]MPPF binding can be modified by extracellular 5-HT levels, internalization of 5-HT$_{1A}$, and the expression of P-glycoproteins. As the 5-HT$_{1A}$ receptor is the best-characterized subtype of currently known 5-HT receptors and is tightly implicated in the pathogenesis of depression, anxiety, epilepsy, and eating disorders, [^{18}F]MPPF represents an important tool for drug therapies targeting this receptor. [Images from CERMEP-Imagerie du Vivant, Lyon, France].

patients. Small animal imaging by MRI or PET is therefore an important preclinical component of the emerging field of "molecular imaging" (i.e., noninvasive visualization of normal as well as abnormal processes at a molecular genetic or cellular level) [50]. Despite MRI and PET being translational by definition, they nevertheless present limitations that users have to keep in mind.

7.5.1
Anesthesia

For almost all imaging techniques, subjects must be kept motionless during image acquisition, and the higher the system's resolution, the smaller the movement that can be tolerated. In the case of small animals, it is very difficult to immobilize them for such a long time or to acclimatize them to the restraint apparatus. Furthermore, the stress that these methods cause can lead to highly unusual physiological responses, which may bias experimental results [51]. Only a few animal PET studies have been carried out without anesthesia, using head fixation devices in awake animals: monkey [52], cat [53], rat [54], or mouse [55]. These limited number of publications show that very few teams have the expertise needed to condition an awake rodent to remain still in the detector ring while reducing stress. Therefore, the majority of microPET or microMRI experiments still need to be performed in anesthetized animals. Full consideration, however, must be given to the type and level of anesthetic used, since these affect both physiological and neurochemical processes and may confound the results of imaging studies. First, anesthesia causes hypothermia, so adequate warming is important during the imaging procedure [56]. Second, anesthetics have been reported to affect regional cerebral blood flow and the regional cerebral metabolism rate of oxygen and glucose, which reflects altered neuronal activity [57]. Although the mechanisms underlying the effects of anesthesia on the CNS are not yet clear, neurotransmitter systems such as the GABA and NMDA receptor systems are probably modified [58–60]. Some PET studies in animal models have demonstrated how anesthetic agents modify the binding of receptor radioligands [53,61]. In all cases, characterization of the effects of anesthesia on biological systems combined with careful anesthetic selection is required to minimize the confounding effects of anesthesia on imaging results and to allow comparison between preclinical and clinical data.

7.5.2
Spatial Resolution and Sensitivity

Two important quantities define the performance of an imaging system: (i) system resolution and (ii) sensitivity. In the case of MRI, the challenge of intrinsically low sensitivity has been continuously addressed through multiple means. First, the increased static field strength yields a theoretical increase in signal-to-noise ratio

(SNR) that can be traded against spatial or temporal resolution or a combination of the two. Most current animal MRI systems use magnetic field strengths at 4.7, 7, or 9.4 T, but systems above 10 T are also available. If higher SNR is profitable to MRS, the advantages for MRI may be hampered by larger susceptibility (T_2^*) artifacts and longer T_1 times. Increased radio frequency tissue heating may also become an issue, even in animals. Second, contrast agents act as signal amplifiers through direct detection (e.g., fluorine-containing molecules in 19F-MRI) or an indirect effect on surrounding protons (e.g., iron oxide nanoparticles), and enhance sensitivity to a specific target or mechanism. Finally, hyperpolarization provides a strong enhancement of the MR signal and allows acquisition of images from nuclei other than protons (^{3}He, ^{13}C, ^{15}N, and ^{129}Xe). Hyperpolarized molecules are themselves the source of the NMR signal, thus enabling tracer studies to be performed with MRI.

In the case of PET, the first and most obvious challenge is spatial resolution. Resolution refers to the level of details that can be distinguished in an image. Conventional PET cameras have a resolution on the order of 5 mm for whole-body human scans. In order to obtain the same image quality as conventional human scans, small animal PET systems must have volumetric spatial resolution similar to the volume of the object of interest. Since a laboratory rat weighs around 300 g and a mouse 30 g, small animal PET systems would need a reconstructed spatial resolution of less than 1 mm in all directions [62]. At present, the maximum resolution that can be achieved with high-resolution microPET imaging systems is 1.2 mm.

Another challenge to small animal PET imaging technology is the sensitivity of radioactive detection. Sensitivity refers to the number of recorded events divided by the total number of events. This parameter represents the ability of the detector ring to detect annihilation radiation. The balance between resolution and sensitivity is a major issue in PET research and development. One of the principal advantages of PET over other imaging modalities is the ability to quantify the acquired data. At present, maximum sensitivity lies in the range of 2–4% for whole-body animal scans. The highest resolution possible has not yet been reached, but some authors estimate that this will be obtained with a detector size between 0.5 and 0.75 mm for mouse imaging with fluorine-18 [63–65]. This spatial resolution will be compatible with localizing radioactivity in small rodent brain structures such as nuclei. It has to be kept in mind that alternative techniques already exist to complement much of what can be done with PET. For example, if anatomical localization is required, autoradiography may provide adequate data at considerably higher spatial resolution than can be achieved with PET.

7.5.3
The Mass Effect of Injected Tracers

In PET, the notion of a tracer dose implies that only a few receptors are occupied by the PET radiotracer. In general, to avoid physiological effects in the tracer study and to decrease the target to nontarget ratio significantly, receptor saturation should be <5% [66]. Some microPET cameras have relatively low sensitivities and require high doses of radioactivity in order to reconstruct small volumes, particularly for mouse brains. However, if a rodent receives a dose similar to that of a human PET scan, the drug concentration in the animal will be higher, potentially saturating vulnerable systems. There is, therefore, a balance to be struck between radioactivity and specific activity in order to minimize the degree of receptor occupancy and achieve maximal specific binding of the radioligand [67]. These conditions are generally achievable, since picomolar radiotracer concentrations are detectable by PET cameras. On the contrary, MRI, which has a lower detection sensitivity, requires tens to hundreds of micromoles of agent to modify the relaxivity of surrounding water molecules (e.g., Gd3+) so as to induce chemical shift (e.g., PARACEST agents) or to generate signal above background (e.g., hyperpolarized agents) [68]. It cannot therefore be ruled out that, when MRI agents are injected, they may have pharmacological or toxicological effects, sometimes limiting transfer from preclinical experiments to clinical studies.

7.5.4
Multimodal PET–MRI for Better Clinical Translation

It is clear that combining two imaging modalities can provide complementary information in terms of functional and anatomical images. Although PET and CT have already been combined in clinical and preclinical hybrid scanners, the combination has many limitations in neuroscience research. Furthermore, CT has limited soft tissue contrast and is, therefore, not ideal for brain imaging [69]. A better option would be to combine PET to MRI, which has excellent soft tissue contrast, particularly for cerebral tissue, and moreover offers the capabilities of fMRI, MRS, and perfusion measurement [70]. Unlike small animal PET–CT, all PET–MRI approaches enable simultaneous PET and MRI data acquisition without increasing anesthesia time and with the certainty that the subject remains morphologically and functionally the same, unlike in sequential acquisition. The combination of PET and MRI has many potential applications in small animal brain imaging for investigating neurotransmitters, receptor density, or metabolite concentration. In contrast, two stand-alone systems, allowing only sequential data acquisition and subsequent image fusion, cannot provide such powerful information. In the future, it seems likely that microPET scanners will always incorporate some means of acquiring an anatomical image or outline. Recently, small animal hybrid PET–MRI scanners based on a 7 T animal MRI scanner have been developed. Results on the prototypes are promising [71–74], and marketing has recently begun. At the same time, clinical PET–MRI cameras are on the market, and initial studies have demonstrated their methodological improvements and potential neurological and psychiatric applications [75]. This imaging technology, common to animal models and humans, will be beneficial for interconnecting preclinical and clinical imaging results.

References

1 Zanzonico, P. (2011) Noninvasive imaging for supporting basic research, in *Small Animal Imaging* (eds F. Kiessling and B.J. Pichler), Springer, Berlin, pp. 3–16.

2 Ricketts, S.-.A., Hockings, P.D., and Waterton, J.C. (2011) Non-invasive imaging in the pharmaceutical industry, in *Small Animal Imaging* (eds F. Kiessling and B.J. Pichler), Springer, Berlin, pp. 17–27.

3 Beckmann, N. and Maier, P. (2011) Noninvasive small rodent imaging: significance for the 3R principles, in *Small Animal Imaging* (eds F. Kiessling and B.J. Pichler), Springer, Berlin, pp. 47–57.

4 Kiessling, F., Pichler, B.J., and Hauff, P. (2011) How to choose the right imaging modality, in *Small Animal Imaging* (eds F. Kiessling and B.J. Pichler), Springer, Berlin, pp. 119–124.

5 Ustione, A. and Piston, D.W. (2011) A simple introduction to multiphoton microscopy. *Journal of Microscopy*, **243** (3), 221–226.

6 Wang, L.V. and Hu, S. (2012) Photoacoustic tomography: *in vivo* imaging from organelles to organs. *Science*, **335** (6075), 1458–1462.

7 Hayasaka, N. *et al.* (2012) *In vivo* diagnostic imaging using micro-CT: sequential and comparative evaluation of rodent models for hepatic/brain ischemia and stroke. *PLoS One*, **7** (2), e32342.

8 Schaeffter, T. and Dahnke, H. (2008) Magnetic resonance imaging and spectroscopy, in *Molecular Imaging I* (eds P. Semmler and P. Schwaiger), Springer, Berlin, pp. 75–90.

9 Rigotti, D.J. *et al.* (2012) Two-year serial whole-brain *N*-acetyl-ʟ-aspartate in patients with relapsing–remitting multiple sclerosis. *Neurology*, **78** (18), 1383–1389.

10 Chaumeil, M.M. *et al.* (2009) Multimodal neuroimaging provides a highly consistent picture of energy metabolism, validating ^{31}P MRS for measuring brain ATP synthesis. *Proceedings of the National Academy of Sciences of the United States of America*, **106** (10), 3988–3993.

11 Amanlou, M. *et al.* (2011) Magnetic resonance contrast media sensing *in vivo* molecular imaging agents: an overview. *Current Radiopharmaceuticals*, **4** (1), 31–43.

12 Cho, T.H. *et al.* (2012) Pre- and post-treatment with cyclosporine A in a rat model of transient focal cerebral ischaemia with multimodal MRI screening. *International Journal of Stroke*, **8** (8), 669–674.

13 Churilov, L. *et al.* (2013) Multiattribute selection of acute stroke imaging software platform for Extending the Time for Thrombolysis in Emergency Neurological Deficits (EXTEND) clinical trial. *International Journal of Stroke*, **8** (3), 204–210.

14 Phelps, M.E. *et al.* (1975) Application of annihilation coincidence detection to transaxial reconstruction tomography. *Journal of Nuclear Medicine*, **16** (3), 210–224.

15 Cutler, P.D. *et al.* (1992) Design features and performance of a PET system for animal research. *Journal of Nuclear Medicine*, **33** (4), 595–604.

16 Phelps, M.E. (2000) PET: the merging of biology and imaging into molecular imaging. *Journal of Nuclear Medicine*, **41** (4), 661–681.

17 Lancelot, S. and Zimmer, L. (2010) Small-animal positron emission tomography as a tool for neuropharmacology. *Trends in Pharmacological Sciences*, **31** (9), 411–417.

18 Friedlander, G. *et al.* (1981) *Nuclear and Radiochemistry*, John Wiley & Sons, Inc., New York.

19 Sokoloff, L. (1980) Regional cerebral glucose utilization measured with the 2-[^{14}C] deoxyglucose technique: its use in mapping functional activity in the nervous system. *Acta Neurologica Scandinavica. Supplementum*, **78**, 128–146.

20 Barros, L.F., Porras, O.H., and Bittner, C.X. (2005) Why glucose transport in the brain matters for PET. *Trends in Neurosciences*, **28** (3), 117–119.

21 Yu, A.S. *et al.* (2009) Quantification of cerebral glucose metabolic rate in mice using 18F-FDG and small-animal PET. *Journal of Nuclear Medicine*, **50** (6), 966–973.

22 Soto-Montenegro, M.L. *et al.* (2009) Detection of visual activation in the rat brain

using 2-deoxy-2-[^{18}F]fluoro-D: -glucose and statistical parametric mapping (SPM). *Molecular Imaging and Biology*, **11** (2), 94–99.

23 Jang, D.P. *et al.* (2009) Neural responses of rats in the forced swimming test: [F-18]FDG micro PET study. *Behavioural Brain Research*, **203** (1), 43–47.

24 Sung, K.K. *et al.* (2009) Neural responses in rat brain during acute immobilization stress: a [F-18]FDG micro PET imaging study. *NeuroImage*, **44** (3), 1074–1080.

25 Gao, F. *et al.* (2010) Protective effects of repetitive transcranial magnetic stimulation in a rat model of transient cerebral ischaemia: a microPET study. *European Journal of Nuclear Medicine and Molecular Imaging*, **37** (5), 954–961.

26 O'Brien, T.J. and Jupp, B. (2009) In-vivo imaging with small animal FDG-PET: a tool to unlock the secrets of epileptogenesis? *Experimental Neurology*, **220** (1), 1–4.

27 Boecker, H. *et al.* (2008) Positron emission tomography ligand activation studies in the sports sciences: measuring neurochemistry in vivo. *Methods (San Diego, Calif.)*, **45** (4), 307–318.

28 Litton, J.E., Hall, H., and Blomqvist, G. (1997) Improved receptor analysis in PET using *a priori* information from *in vitro* binding assays. *Physics in Medicine and Biology*, **42** (8), 1653–1660.

29 Lammertsma, A.A. and Hume, S.P. (1996) Simplified reference tissue model for PET receptor studies. *NeuroImage*, **4** (3 Part 1), 153–158.

30 Innis, R.B. and Carson, R. (2007) Consensus nomenclature: its time has come. *European Journal of Nuclear Medicine and Molecular Imaging*, **34** (8), 1239.

31 Innis, R.B. *et al.* (2007) Consensus nomenclature for *in vivo* imaging of reversibly binding radioligands. *Journal of Cerebral Blood Flow and Metabolism*, **27** (9), 1533–1539.

32 Logan, J. *et al.* (1996) Distribution volume ratios without blood sampling from graphical analysis of PET data. *Journal of Cerebral Blood Flow and Metabolism*, **16** (5), 834–840.

33 Carson, R.E. *et al.* (1993) Comparison of bolus and infusion methods for receptor quantitation: application to [^{18}F]cyclofoxy and positron emission tomography. *Journal of Cerebral Blood Flow and Metabolism*, **13** (1), 24–42.

34 Heiss, W.D. and Herholz, K. (2006) Brain receptor imaging. *Journal of Nuclear Medicine*, **47** (2), 302–312.

35 Emond, P., Guilloteau, D., and Chalon, S. (2008) PE2I: a radiopharmaceutical for *in vivo* exploration of the dopamine transporter. *CNS Neuroscience & Therapeutics*, **14** (1), 47–64.

36 Elsinga, P.H., Hatano, K., and Ishiwata, K. (2006) PET tracers for imaging of the dopaminergic system. *Current Medicinal Chemistry*, **13** (18), 2139–2153.

37 Patel, N.H. *et al.* (2010) Positron emission tomography in schizophrenia: a new perspective. *Journal of Nuclear Medicine*, **51** (4), 511–520.

38 Vyas, N.S. *et al.* (2010) Insights into schizophrenia using positron emission tomography: building the evidence and refining the focus. *The British Journal of Psychiatry*, **197** (1), 3–4.

39 Liu, L. *et al.* (2009) Evaluation of nigrostriatal damage and its change over weeks in a rat model of Parkinson's disease: small animal positron emission tomography studies with [^{11}C]beta-CFT. *Nuclear Medicine and Biology*, **36** (8), 941–947.

40 Hume, S.P. *et al.* (1996) The potential of high-resolution positron emission tomography to monitor striatal dopaminergic function in rat models of disease. *Journal of Neuroscience Methods*, **67** (2), 103–112.

41 Meyer, J.H. *et al.* (2001) Occupancy of serotonin transporters by paroxetine and citalopram during treatment of depression: a [^{11}C]DASB PET imaging study. *The American Journal of Psychiatry*, **158** (11), 1843–1849.

42 Lee, C.M. and Farde, L. (2006) Using positron emission tomography to facilitate CNS drug development. *Trends in Pharmacological Sciences*, **27** (6), 310–316.

43 Farde, L. *et al.* (1988) An open label trial of raclopride in acute schizophrenia. Confirmation of D2-dopamine receptor occupancy by PET. *Psychopharmacology*, **94** (1), 1–7.

44 Goyer, P.F. *et al.* (1996) PET measurement of neuroreceptor occupancy by typical and

atypical neuroleptics. *Journal of Nuclear Medicine*, **37** (7), 1122–1127.

45 Laruelle, M. (2000) Imaging synaptic neurotransmission with *in vivo* binding competition techniques: a critical review. *Journal of Cerebral Blood Flow and Metabolism*, **20** (3), 423–451.

46 Cumming, P. *et al.* (2002) The competition between endogenous dopamine and radioligands for specific binding to dopamine receptors. *Annals of the New York Academy of Sciences*, **965**, 440–450.

47 Zimmer, L. *et al.* (2002) Effect of endogenous serotonin on the binding of the 5-hT1A PET ligand 18F-MPPF in the rat hippocampus: kinetic beta measurements combined with microdialysis. *Journal of Neurochemistry*, **80** (2), 278–286.

48 Seeman, P., Guan, H.C., and Niznik, H.B. (1989) Endogenous dopamine lowers the dopamine D2 receptor density as measured by [3*H*]raclopride: implications for positron emission tomography of the human brain. *Synapse (New York, NY)*, **3** (1), 96–97.

49 Laruelle, M. and Huang, Y. (2001) Vulnerability of positron emission tomography radiotracers to endogenous competition: new insights. *Quarterly Journal of Nuclear Medicine*, **45** (2), 124–138.

50 Pomper, M.G. (2002) Can small animal imaging accelerate drug development? *Journal of Cellular Biochemistry. Supplement*, **39**, 211–220.

51 Lasbennes, F. *et al.* (1986) Stress and local cerebral blood flow: studies on restrained and unrestrained rats. *Experimental Brain Research*, **63** (1), 163–168.

52 Howell, L.L. *et al.* (2001) An apparatus and behavioral training protocol to conduct positron emission tomography (PET) neuroimaging in conscious rhesus monkeys. *Journal of Neuroscience Methods*, **106** (2), 161–169.

53 Hassoun, W. *et al.* (2003) PET study of the [^{11}C]raclopride binding in the striatum of the awake cat: effects of anaesthetics and role of cerebral blood flow. *European Journal of Nuclear Medicine and Molecular Imaging*, **30** (1), 141–148.

54 Hosoi, R. *et al.* (2005) MicroPET detection of enhanced 18F-FDG utilization by PKA inhibitor in awake rat brain. *Brain Research*, **1039** (1–2), 199–202.

55 Mizuma, H. *et al.* (2010) Establishment of *in vivo* brain imaging method in conscious mice. *Journal of Nuclear Medicine*, **51** (7), 1068–1075.

56 Fueger, B.J. *et al.* (2006) Impact of animal handling on the results of 18F-FDG PET studies in mice. *Journal of Nuclear Medicine*, **47** (6), 999–1006.

57 Nakao, Y. *et al.* (2001) Effects of anesthesia on functional activation of cerebral blood flow and metabolism. *Proceedings of the National Academy of Sciences of the United States of America*, **98** (13), 7593–7598.

58 Franks, N.P. and Lieb, W.R. (1994) Molecular and cellular mechanisms of general anaesthesia. *Nature*, **367** (6464), 607–614.

59 Harris, R.A. and Allan, A.M. (1985) Functional coupling of gamma-aminobutyric acid receptors to chloride channels in brain membranes. *Science*, **228** (4703), 1108–1110.

60 Thomson, A.M., West, D.C., and Lodge, D. (1985) An *N*-methylaspartate receptor-mediated synapse in rat cerebral cortex: a site of action of ketamine? *Nature*, **313** (6002), 479–481.

61 Momosaki, S. *et al.* (2004) Rat-PET study without anesthesia: anesthetics modify the dopamine D1 receptor binding in rat brain. *Synapse (New York, NY)*, **54** (4), 207–213.

62 Yao, R., Lecomte, R., and Crawford, E.S. (2012) Small-animal PET: what is it, and why do we need it? *Journal of Nuclear Medicine Technology*, **40** (3), 157–165.

63 James, S.S. *et al.* (2009) Experimental characterization and system simulations of depth of interaction PET detectors using 0.5 mm and 0.7 mm LSO arrays. *Physics in Medicine and Biology*, **54** (14), 4605–4619.

64 Stickel, J.R., Qi, J., and Cherry, S.R. (2007) Fabrication and characterization of a 0.5-mm lutetium oxyorthosilicate detector array for high-resolution PET applications. *Journal of Nuclear Medicine*, **48** (1), 115–121.

65 Yang, Y. *et al.* (2004) Optimization and performance evaluation of the microPET II scanner for *in vivo* small-animal imaging. *Physics in Medicine and Biology*, **49** (12), 2527–2545.

66 Kung, M.P. and Kung, H.F. (2005) Mass effect of injected dose in small rodent

imaging by SPECT and PET. *Nuclear Medicine and Biology*, **32** (7), 673–678.

67 Hume, S.P., Gunn, R.N., and Jones, T. (1998) Pharmacological constraints associated with positron emission tomographic scanning of small laboratory animals. *European Journal of Nuclear Medicine*, **25** (2), 173–176.

68 De Leon-Rodriguez, L.M. *et al.* (2009) Responsive MRI agents for sensing metabolism *in vivo*. *Accounts of Chemical Research*, **42** (7), 948–957.

69 Boone, J.M., Velazquez, O., and Cherry, S.R. (2004) Small-animal X-ray dose from micro-CT. *Molecular Imaging*, **3** (3), 149–158.

70 Wehrl, H.F. *et al.* (2009) Pre-clinical PET/MR: technological advances and new perspectives in biomedical research. *European Journal of Nuclear Medicine and Molecular Imaging*, **36** (Suppl. 1), S56–S58.

71 Catana, C. *et al.* (2006) Simultaneous acquisition of multislice PET and MR images: initial results with a MR-compatible PET scanner. *Journal of Nuclear Medicine*, **47** (12), 1968–1976.

72 Judenhofer, M.S. *et al.* (2007) PET/MR images acquired with a compact MR-compatible PET detector in a 7-T magnet. *Radiology*, **244** (3), 807–814.

73 Judenhofer, M.S. *et al.* (2008) Simultaneous PET-MRI: a new approach for functional and morphological imaging. *Nature Medicine*, **14** (4), 459–465.

74 Pichler, B.J. *et al.* (2006) Performance test of an LSO-APD detector in a 7-T MRI scanner for simultaneous PET/MRI. *Journal of Nuclear Medicine*, **47** (4), 639–647.

75 Catana, C. *et al.* (2012) PET/MRI for neurologic applications. *Journal of Nuclear Medicine*, **53** (12), 1916–1925.

Part II
Animal Models in Specific Disease Areas of Drug Discovery

8
Substance Abuse and Dependence
Elena Martín-García, Patricia Robledo, Javier Gutiérrez-Cuesta, and Rafael Maldonado

8.1
Introduction

Drug addiction is a chronic relapsing disorder characterized by loss of control over drug seeking and drug taking, and continuing drug use despite adverse consequences [1]. According to the main manual of psychiatry, the *Diagnostic and Statistical Manual of Mental Disorders* (DSM), the clinical definition of addiction has evolved mainly during the 1980s–1990s. In 1980, the DSM in its third edition (DSM-III) defined addiction as tolerance to the drug and/or withdrawal symptoms when drug use was stopped. This definition was drug centered and was based on the two main physical effects produced by the long-term exposure to drugs of abuse. In 1994, the DSM-IV considered that these two criteria were not necessary for the diagnosis of addiction, and this diagnosis was given only when the patient met at least three of the following seven criteria: (1) development of tolerance to a substance, (2) presence of abstinence syndrome, (3) the substance is used more times or for longer periods than intended, (4) there is a persistent desire to use the drug or unsuccessful efforts to reduce or stop drug use, (5) there is considerable time spent in obtaining the substance or using it, or recovering from its effects, (6) the important social, work, or recreational activities are neglected because of drug use, and (7) the use of the drug is continued despite knowledge of adverse consequences or exacerbation of medical or psychological problems derived from the drug use. In summary, the DSM-IV focused on five of the seven items to a loss of control over drug taking that can be collapsed into three behavioral aspects: First, items 3 and 4 indicate a difficulty to limit drug use; second, items 5 and 6 show a very strong motivation for the drug; third, item 7 refers to the fact that the patient keeps taking drug despite adverse consequences. In contrast to DSM-III, the concept of addiction in DSM-IV is considered human centered as the behavioral alteration emerges as of major importance for the transition to addiction. Therefore, addiction was initially seen as resulting from a change in drug effects, and today it is seen as a change in drug use that evolves from controlled use to loss of control over drug intake. Thus, after the initiation of use, the patient develops an occasional use followed by a regular use or even an abuse and finally addiction, which is associated with a high risk of relapse even after prolonged periods of withdrawal. However, the initiation of drug taking does not necessarily lead to addiction. Indeed, only some individuals will maintain an occasional use after initiation; some of these occasional users will develop a regular use or abuse and only some of these abusers will develop addiction. It is considered that out of 100 people initiating drug use, 15–17 will develop addiction [2]. Therefore, addiction depends on drug consumption, but also on the interaction between the drug use and a vulnerable genotype.

The fifth edition of the DSM is now complete after a decade of work and was released at the American Psychiatric Association's Annual Meeting in May 2013 [3]. Substance use disorder in DSM-5 combines the DSM-IV categories of substance abuse and substance dependence into a single disorder measured on a continuum from mild to severe. Thus, the categorical approach of DSM-IV has evolved into a dimensional approach in the DSM-5 that consists in condensing abuse and dependence as dimensions into a single manifestation of a disorder with varying levels of severity [4]. Each specific substance is addressed as a separate use disorder, but nearly all substances are diagnosed based on the same overarching criteria [3]. In contrast to addiction, a diagnosis of substance abuse previously required only 1 symptom in DSM-IV, but now mild substance use disorder in DSM-5 requires 2–3 symptoms from a list of 11. Drug craving has been added to this list, and problems with law enforcement have been eliminated because of cultural considerations that make the criteria difficult to apply internationally. DSM-5 also includes gambling disorder as the only diagnosable condition in a new category on behavioral addictions. Internet gaming disorder has not been included in DSM-5 as a behavioral addiction and it has been included in Section III of the manual because the conditions listed there require further research before their consideration as formal disorders.

8.2
Difficulties to Model Addiction in Animals

The study of drug addiction has progressed in the last years. However, the etiology and the pathophysiology of drug addiction remain largely unknown and there is a serious need for effective pharmacotherapies, in spite of almost five decades of experimental research [5]. It is now well recognized that the study of drug taking in laboratory animals cannot be considered as studying genuine addiction, characterized by loss of control over drug use [6]. The voluntary intake of drugs of abuse is a behavior largely conserved throughout phylogeny and preferences for drug-associated environments or drug-reinforced learning of tasks have been found in multiple animal species [7]. These studies on contingent drug consumption in animal models have provided important advances, such as the demonstration that drugs of abuse activate the mesolimbic system, which mediates their hedonic and motivational properties in a manner similar to natural rewards [8]. They have also contributed to the understanding of processes and neurobiological mechanisms involved in the initiation and maintenance of drug consumption [9–12]. However, mechanisms of addiction as a disease cannot be evaluated on these paradigms since drug consumption is just the first step of the complex addiction process that also involves the compulsive drug use maintained despite adverse consequences for the user and the relapse even after long periods of withdrawal [7]. Drug addiction in humans is a chronic disease that appears only in a small proportion (15–17%) of vulnerable drug users [2]. Current animal models have several limitations, since they do not allow capturing all aspects of the complexity of this pathology. Addiction is a complex psychiatric disease influenced by genetic predisposition, environmental risk factors, and the interaction between both variables [13,14]. A strong effort has been devoted to increase our knowledge about the molecular, cellular, and behavioral adaptations regulating these interactions. Although these studies have greatly enriched our understanding of the neurocircuitry mediating addictive-like behavior, the validation of the responses by means of reliable animal models has found several restrictions that had decreased the opportunity to find new treatments. Animal models for reward and reinforcement use either noncontingent forced administration of the drug or contingent self-administration in which drug taking is under the control of the animal (see Section 8.4.4). Importantly, contingent and noncontingent administration produce distinct behavioral responses that are differently reflected at the level of neuronal adaptations. The self-administration paradigm is considered the behavioral model with the highest predictive validity [15]. This model has allowed the identification of different brain circuitry mediating goal-directed activity (medial prefrontal cortex to dorsomedial striatum) and habit learning (sensory–motor cortex to the dorsolateral striatum) related to drug-reinforcing effects [16]. However, drug self-administration has the limitation of not distinguishing between two motivational states that involve positive or negative reinforcement that cause an increase of responding. Other limitations that affect certain intrinsic aspects of the model are the aversion or the anxiety produced by a novel environment or the aversion to the surgery for catheterization.

Another important concern is that most animal models do not consider the vulnerability to addiction or the interindividual differences. Piazza *et al.* were among the first authors to consider interindividual differences in drug responses and introduce the concept of vulnerability in preclinical research. They showed that vulnerability to drug use can be predicted by a behavioral trait, namely, locomotor reactivity to a novel inescapable environment that allowed to divide the population tested into low or high responders [17]. Lately, a model with great heuristic value with regard to the clinical definition of the pathology was developed and represented the first multisymptomatic model of addiction based on the DSM-IV criteria [7]. This approach consists in ranking rats for their scores for each of the three addiction-like cocaine tests – persistence in responding when the drug is no longer available (equivalent to difficulty limiting drug intake); breakpoint in a progressive ratio reinforcement schedule, in which an animal is forced to exert greater and greater effort to acquire each subsequent drug reward (equivalent to motivation to obtain the drug); and resistance to punishment (equivalent to drug use despite harmful consequences) – and to compare addict- and nonaddict-like rats. This model has allowed detecting drug-induced adaptations in the addictive phenotype and has contributed to the understanding of the neurobiological basis of the shift from controlled use to addiction [18,19]. This model has been used to demonstrate that high reactivity to novelty predict the predisposition to initiate cocaine self-administration, while high impulsivity predict the switch to compulsive cocaine taking in face of adverse consequences, which is a hallmark of addiction-like behavior [18]. The proposed neurobiological mechanism underlying this transition to addiction was the transfer of control over drug-seeking behavior from the ventral to the dorsal striatum via its regulatory dopaminergic innervation starting in the midbrain [18]. In a later study, it was revealed that animals that progressively developed the behavioral hallmarks of addiction had permanently impaired the long-term depression, an important form of synaptic plasticity in the nucleus accumbens [19]. Future steps will include developing new therapeutics to reverse the addictive-like phenotype and to predict its appearance.

8.3
Tolerance, Sensitization, and Physical Withdrawal

8.3.1
Tolerance

Drug tolerance is defined as the progressive diminution of the susceptibility of a human or an animal to the effects of a drug, resulting from its continued administration [1]. It should be differentiated from drug resistance wherein an organism, disease, or tissue fails to respond to the intended effectiveness of a chemical or drug. Tolerance occurs when a higher dose of the drug is required to achieve the same level of response achieved initially, and is the consequence of the neuroadaptive changes in the central nervous system in order to reduce the psychophysical damage induced by the repeated drug consumption. Tolerance has been included among the criteria to define drug dependence at DSM-IV, but it is not always present in the addiction process. Tolerance has been mainly studied in response to opioids, cannabinoids, and alcohol administration [20–22]. In the case of opioids, tolerance develops rapidly to the analgesic effects of the drug, which is frequently evaluated in thermal nociceptive paradigms, such as the hot plate and tail flick tests. This tolerance has been revealed in different animal species, including rodents, dogs, and monkeys. Tolerance also develops to other pharmacological responses of opioids such as those involving locomotor activity, the respiratory system, learning and memory, and the cardiovascular system [20,23]. Several studies have shown tolerance to cannabinoid effects on antinociception, locomotion, hypothermia, catalepsy, suppression of operant behavior, gastrointestinal transit, body weight, cardiovascular actions, anticonvulsant activity, ataxia, and corticosterone release. This tolerance occurs in rodents, pigeons, dogs, and monkeys [24]. Alcohol tolerance is normally assessed by monitoring body temperature and motor-impairing effects in rodents [25], since the characteristics of alcohol tolerance in mice and rats are similar to those exhibited by humans.

In addition, cross-tolerance exists between the different drugs. Δ^9-Tetrahydrocannabinol (THC) and morphine elicit cross-tolerance in mice for nociception and cardiac rhythm responses [26]. Moreover, clinical studies found evidence of cross-tolerance to ethanol among cannabis users [27,28]. In rodents, cannabinoid drugs and ethanol showed cross-tolerance for avoidance behavior and ataxia [29]. Furthermore, mice treated chronically with ethanol displayed a reduced sensitivity to cannabinoid-induced hypomotility, hypothermia, and antinociception [30]. The studies on cross-tolerance between ethanol and cannabinoids indicate that pretreatment with ethanol or THC can significantly alter the response to subsequent doses of the other compound.

8.3.2
Sensitization

Sensitization is referred to the enhanced response to a stimulus, after repeated exposure to that stimulus [31,32]. Thus, behavioral sensitization is defined by the augmented motor-stimulant response that occurs with repeated exposure to a specific drug (Figure 8.1). Several factors can affect behavioral sensitization such as number of treatments, interval between treatments, dose, sex, age, and genetics [33]. Moreover, behavioral sensitization is commonly assessed by monitoring motor activity, but can also be evaluated using conditioned place preference (CPP) or drug self-administration paradigms. To achieve the augmented motor-stimulant response after repeated drug exposure, the route of administration should have fast onset of drug effect (i.e., intraperitoneal or intravenous injection) and the drug needs to be administered intermittently [34]. In the CPP paradigm, sensitization is manifested as enhanced time spent in the drug-paired compartment [35]. Sensitization is usually determined in the drug self-administration paradigm by the ability of repeated noncontingent drug exposure to enhance the acquisition of drug self-administration or assessed by a progressive ratio schedule of reinforcement [36–38].

Behavioral sensitization has been described to occur in response to cocaine, amphetamine, morphine, ethanol, nicotine, and THC [32,39–43]. Furthermore, different studies revealed cross-sensitization between drugs. Thus, rats repeatedly exposed to THC exhibited sensitization to morphine [40], and mice repeatedly exposed to ethanol were sensitized to cocaine and vice versa [44]. This suggests that common mechanisms underlie the development of behavioral sensitization, despite the fact that different classes of drugs have distinct binding sites in the brain. Although sensitization is mostly described as a nonassociative learning process, repeated exposure to drugs of abuse causes hypersensitivity to drugs and drug-associated stimuli of the neural circuits mediating incentive salience (an increase in drug "wanting"). This *incentive sensitization* could be responsible for the dramatically exaggerated motivation for drugs displayed by addicts [45].

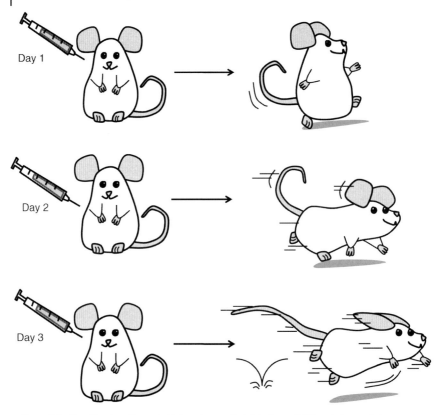

Figure 8.1 Sensitization. Repeated intermittent administration of different drugs of abuse (cocaine, D-amphetamine, and others) causes a progressive increase in drug-induced locomotor activity that is higher in magnitude compared to that induced by a single injection.

8.3.3
Physical Manifestations of Withdrawal

Physical withdrawal syndrome includes different somatic signs that occur following abrupt cessation or decrease of addictive substance use. It occurs after chronic exposure to some specific drugs with addictive potential that produces the development of a physical dependence. It is important to remark that the somatic withdrawal symptoms are usually the opposite of the acute drug effects, although they can differ significantly between individuals depending on several variables, such as the pharmacological properties of the substance consumed and the time of exposure to the drug [46]. Withdrawal symptoms in humans are described in the DSM-IV, separately for each drug of abuse. In animals, the most frequently used models of drug withdrawal are triggered by the administration of an antagonist of the addictive drug or it can be produced spontaneously by drug cessation in order to mimic human symptoms. Dramatic acute withdrawal symptoms similar to those reported can be measured in animal models in the case of depressant drugs, such as opioids, barbiturates, or alcohol. The appearance of jumping, wet dog shakes, weight loss, paw tremors, teeth chattering, abnormal posture, irritability, diarrhea, and piloerection can be measured in rodents during acute withdrawal from opioids [47]. Alcohol withdrawal in rodents includes hyperirritability upon touch, tail stiffness/rigidity, vocalizations, and abnormal posture or gait increased paw tremor, locomotor activity, seizures, and anxiety [47,48]. A high variability of the withdrawal manifestations can also be found during nicotine abstinence in rodents, which include rearing, grooming, scratching, teeth chattering, and body tremors as physical signs triggered by mecamylamine administration [49–51]. In the case of THC, several studies have reported the absence of somatic signs of spontaneous withdrawal after chronic THC treatment in rodents, pigeons, dogs, and monkeys, even after administration of high doses of THC [52]. In contrast, somatic signs of spontaneous abstinence were revealed after the abrupt interruption of chronic WIN 55,212-2 treatment [53]. In agreement, the administration of CB1 cannabinoid antagonists has been reported to precipitate somatic manifestations of withdrawal in THC-dependent rodents that include several signs such as wet dog shakes, head shakes, facial rubbing, paw tremor ataxia, hunched posture, body tremor, ptosis, piloerection, hypolocomotion, mastication, and scratching [52,54]. Interestingly, behavioral manifestations of spontaneous cannabinoid withdrawal have been reported in monkeys, during spontaneous THC abstinence, consisting in a suppression of an operant behavior maintained by food [55]. These results are in agreement with the presence of behavioral manifestations of withdrawal after discontinuing chronic marijuana use in humans [56]. Cocaine or other psychostimulants do not elicit clear physical withdrawal symptoms in animal models, and the negative emotional states that include increases in anxiety-like behavior and depression-like state are more salient. Some of these symptoms are similar to that of other psychostimulants, such as amphetamines or methamphetamine, although following a different time course. In the case of MDMA (3,4-methylenedioxy-methamphetamine, also known as ecstasy), the models of withdrawal induced by acute serotonin antagonism in chronically MDMA-maintained rodents have been shown to produce minor physical signs in comparison to other drugs. Thus, the somatic symptoms observed such as paw tremor, face rubbing, and increased locomotor activity were not accompanied by any clear aversive/dysphoric or anxiogenic-like behaviors revealing that chronic MDMA administration does not induce classical manifestations of physical dependence in mice [57].

8.3.4
Affective Manifestations of Withdrawal

Drug withdrawal is also characterized in rodents by the manifestation of affective changes similar to those observed in humans. However, the affective state produced by drug withdrawal that is probably associated with drug craving has received less attention in the literature due to methodological difficulties. Conditioned place aversion (CPA) is a behavioral model currently used to measure the affective manifestations of drug withdrawal (see Section 8.4.2). In this paradigm, the subjective aversive effects of drug withdrawal are repeatedly paired with a neutral stimulus in several conditioning cycles. When the neutral stimulus becomes a conditioned stimulus (CS), it will produce a conditioned response (CR) of avoidance. In the case of opioids, naloxone is administered in opioid-dependent animals to precipitate CPA at doses that are not aversive in naïve animals [58], from 0.1 to 1 mg/kg, s.c. [59–61]. Even lower doses of naloxone (15 μg/kg, s.c.) have been reported to produce CPA in morphine-dependent rats [62]. The previous doses of naloxone were also reported to elicit extremely persistent place aversion, 16 weeks later, in morphine-dependent rats [63]. The potency of naloxone to elicit CPA in morphine-pretreated animals also depended on the number of conditioning cycles. Then, experiments with two conditioning cycles are more potent than experiments with only one conditioning cycle in eliciting CPA [58]. The CPA paradigm has also been used to measure aversive effects induced by nicotine withdrawal. In these studies, animals typically receive chronic nicotine via osmotic pumps for 5–7 days. During conditioning, the animal receives a nicotinic receptor antagonist (such as mecamylamine) to precipitate withdrawal and is confined to one side of the apparatus. On alternate days they receive saline in the other compartment. Following conditioning, nicotine-dependent adult rats reliably display a CPA for the compartment where they experienced withdrawal [64,65]. The ability of mecamylamine to produce CPA has also been shown in nicotine-dependent mice [66,67]. With respect to alcohol, the combined stimulus properties of the GABA(A) receptor antagonist, pentylenetetrazol, together with alcohol withdrawal, facilitated the expression of CPA to alcohol withdrawal symptoms in mice [68].

Intracranial electric self-stimulation (ICSS) procedures are widely used to study the rewarding or the aversive effects of drugs of abuse (see Section 8.4.3) [69,70]. The threshold of the minimal current needed to promote ICSS is estimated and a drug that stimulates the reward circuit will decrease this threshold, whereas a drug having aversive effects or withdrawal symptoms will enhance the minimal current required to maintain the self-stimulation [71]. Thus, acute administration of all the prototypical drugs of abuse has been reported to lower intracranial self-stimulation thresholds in rats suggesting the activation of central hedonic systems [72,73]. In contrast, withdrawal from chronic treatment with different drugs of abuse can induce an opposite effect [74]. For instance, the affective properties of nicotine withdrawal have been assessed using ICSS procedures. Withdrawal from chronic nicotine produces an increase in brain reward threshold that is thought to reflect a decrease in brain reward function [51,75–77].

Other affective manifestations of drug withdrawal include anxiety and depression-like symptoms, although they are more difficult to reveal in animal models. Thus, antagonist precipitation is not usually used in the case of opioid withdrawal for these purposes, because naloxone and naltrexone are highly aversive in naïve rodents. Affective alterations due to opioid withdrawal are most frequently measured after drug cessation. The affective symptoms of opioid withdrawal include depression, anxiety, and craving and are common to other drugs of abuse such as alcohol, nicotine, cocaine, amphetamines, or MDMA [46]. Depression-like state is characterized by elevations in brain reward thresholds, dysphoric mood, fatigue, altered sleep patterns, and psychomotor agitation or retardation [78,79]. Interestingly, different studies have reported depression-like symptoms such as increased immobility time in the forced swimming test, learned helplessness, and anhedonic states (decreased experience of pleasure), as well as lethargy and fatigue due to altered sleep patterns, after withdrawal from opioids [80,81], alcohol [82], nicotine [83,84], cocaine [85,86], and MDMA [87,88]. Withdrawal depression-like behavior is associated with specific modification in dopamine and serotonergic transmission together with alterations in hypothalamic–pituitary–adrenal (HPA) axis function, as well as hippocampal neuroplasticity [46]. Withdrawal syndrome also produces craving defined as the compulsive desire to attain the drug state. This symptom is currently evaluated in animals through cue-induced craving in the intravenous self-administration paradigm and is considered closely related to the increased risk of relapse even after long periods of drug withdrawal. Recently, it has been described that BDNF levels increase in both the nucleus accumbens core and the shell during withdrawal from extended access to cocaine self-administration, but this occurs with different time courses and has different functional consequences in the two subregions [89]. The clinical implication of these results is that reducing BDNF signaling might decrease cue-induced cocaine craving at long withdrawal times and thereby help to maintain abstinence [89].

There is high comorbidity of depressive illness and anxiety with addiction in humans. It has therefore been postulated that drugs of abuse are taken acutely to alleviate psychological and psychiatric symptoms that are exacerbated during drug withdrawal. In this line, the dual deficit model postulates that the emotional manifestations of drug withdrawal are associated with drug-induced dopamine and 5-HT dysfunction with decreased synaptic dopamine underlying anhedonia and reduced synaptic 5-HT underlying depressed mood [90]. In this context, drug intake has been proposed to be considered as a method of self-medication to counteract the undesired negative emotional state [90]. Conversely, it remains unclear whether chronic use and withdrawal from drugs of abuse are the cause or the consequence of preexisting mental disorders [46].

8.4
Reward and Reinforcement

8.4.1
Drug Discrimination

The drug discrimination paradigm is used to assay the subjective effects of drugs in animals and humans [91,92]. This procedure is based on the discriminative stimulus properties of drugs, which prompt a particular response leading to the presentation of a reinforcer (reward). In animals, these experiments are typically carried out in operant boxes consisting of two levers and a device to deliver reinforcement. Subjects are usually trained on operant schedules of reinforcement to distinguish between the administration of a drug and of vehicle. During training, the animals must learn to press one lever (the drug-designated lever) following the administration of the drug, and the other lever (saline-designated lever) following vehicle administration in order to obtain a reward [93]. Most psychoactive drugs of abuse can serve as discriminative stimuli, including those with low abuse potential. Thus, this technique does not provide information about the abuse liability of drugs, but about their discriminative stimulus effects, which are thought to be associated with their positive "rewarding" properties [92–95]. Nevertheless, the abuse liability of an unknown test compound can be inferred from the similarity of its stimulus effects to those of a known prototypical abused drug [96,97]. Once discrimination training is acquired, generalization or substitution tests can be performed with a new drug, where the drug- or vehicle-appropriate responses are recorded. If a drug produces predominantly drug-appropriate response, it is said to substitute completely for the training drug and to possess discriminative stimulus properties similar to the training drug. Stimulus generalization studies are conducted to determine whether a discriminative stimulus will generalize to (substitute for) other drugs. In this procedure, an animal trained to discriminate a dose of a training drug will display stimulus generalization only to agents having a similar pharmacological effect, although not always an identical mechanism of action [92]. These experiments are influenced by behavioral and pharmacological variables, and thus they usually necessitate a full dose–response curve [91]. Cross-generalization between different types of prototypical drugs of abuse has been extensively demonstrated in several species, including rats, mice, monkeys, and humans [91].

8.4.2
Conditioned Place Preference

In the place conditioning paradigm, the animal is exposed to a drug or nondrug treatment that has appetitive or aversive properties in a previously neutral environmental context. Following several pairings of the unconditioned stimulus (US) with the distinct environmental cues (conditioned stimulus), the presence of the context alone will evoke approach or avoidance behavior (conditioned response), and it is assumed that the animal exhibits either CPP or CPA for that environment (Figure 8.2) [58,70,98,99]. The simplest version of the place conditioning apparatus consists of two compartments. During the pretest phase, animals explore freely both compartments usually in a single session. In the subsequent conditioning phase, one compartment will be repeatedly paired with the drug and the other with vehicle administration. On the test day, the animals can explore both compartments in a drug-free state, and an increase in the time spent in the drug-associated compartment is considered a measure of CPP, while a decrease indicates CPA. Two types of protocols can be used for CPP: biased and unbiased procedures. In the biased protocol, the drug is paired with the nonpreferred compartment, and CPP is measured as overcoming the initial aversion for that environment. In the nonbiased protocol, drug administration is

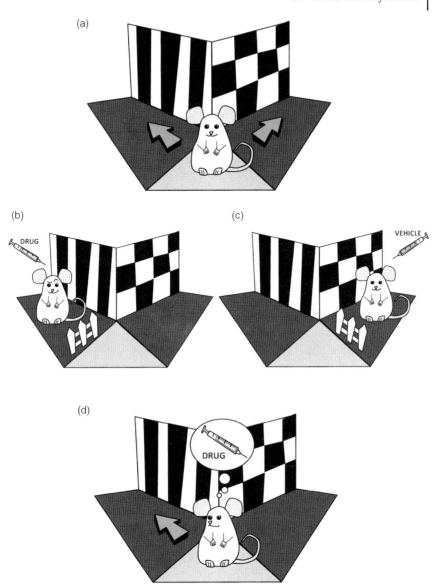

Figure 8.2 Conditioned place preference. In a conditioned place preference task, the animal learns an association between an environment with distinctive cues and a positive reinforcer. It is often used as an animal model of the subjective effects of drugs. (a) Animals are allowed to explore the apparatus for habituation. (b and c) During the conditioning phase, drug is administered noncontingently (repeated three to five times on alternate days) and the animal is confined to one compartment ("striped pattern" in this example). Drug vehicle is given to the animal confined to the other compartment (checked pattern) on alternate days from drug. (d) To test the preference, animals are placed in the neutral chamber (gray triangle) with access to both the drug- and vehicle-paired compartments. If positive conditioning occurred, the animal should spend more time in the compartment containing the drug-related cues than in the other compartment.

associated with one arbitrarily chosen compartment, which is generally counterbalanced across the subjects [58,99–101]. This model has been widely used to study the rewarding properties of drugs in animals [58,99], and recently it has been extended to humans, where subjects must rate the liking for the drug-associated room [68,102,103]. Not all drugs of abuse have a similar ability to induce CPP. Opioids and psychostimulants produce robust place preference over a wide range of experimental conditions, whereas other drugs, such as ethanol, cannabinoids, or nicotine, produce more inconsistent results. Thus, nicotine and THC tend to have aversive effects on the first exposure to this test [104,105], and priming injections before beginning the place conditioning procedure could be required for animals to surmount the initial aversion [95]. Finally, the conditioned place preference paradigm is being accepted for studying certain aspects of relapse to drug seeking. The procedure involves repeatedly pairing saline injections with both compartments until the conditioned preference is extinguished. Subsequently, reinstatement of place preference for the compartment previously paired with the drug can be obtained either by a drug priming injection, by stress, or by conditioned cues [58]. However, the operant self-administration paradigm is the most relevant and reliable reinstatement procedure in rodents, and interpretation of the results obtained when using the conditioned place preference for this purpose presents important limitations.

8.4.3
Intracranial Self-Stimulation

ICSS paradigm is a procedure where animals learn to perform an operant behavior (lever pressing or wheel turning) to deliver short electrical pulses into different brain areas comprising the brain reward circuit, such as the lateral hypothalamus, the medial forebrain bundle, and ventral tegmental area (Figure 8.3). The most commonly used ICSS techniques are the rate–frequency curve and the current–intensity threshold measures [96,106–108]. In both cases, a lowering of the stimulation threshold indicates a facilitation of brain stimulation reward, while an increase in ICSS threshold reflects less reward. The ICSS paradigm has been effectively used to study the effects of drugs of abuse on brain reward structures. Thus, it has been shown that most drugs of abuse, including cocaine, amphetamine, opioids, and nicotine, decrease this threshold, indicating reward facilitation [71,109]. In contrast to prototypical drugs of abuse, Δ^9-tetrahydrocannabinol does not exhibit reward-facilitating properties in the ICSS paradigm [109]. On the other hand, drugs that produce aversive effects or withdrawal from addictive drugs after chronic administration enhance ICSS thresholds, suggesting an anhedonic state (see Section 8.2.4) [70,71,109]. Notably, more recent data demonstrate that extended daily access to drugs of abuse, including cocaine and heroin, increases ICSS thresholds, suggesting that repeated drug exposure produces deficits in the reward systems that may contribute to compulsive drug taking [110].

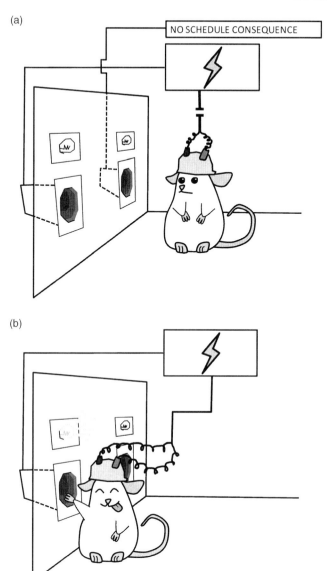

Figure 8.3 Intracranial self-stimulation. The intracranial self-stimulation procedure is a method for assessing the functional activity of the brain's reward pathways. (a) Animals are prepared with electrodes into a specific brain site that is part of the brain's reward circuit. (b) The functioning of the reward circuit is frequently assessed by measuring the minimal electrical current intensity to which the animals will make an easy response, such as nose-poke, to receive the stimulation.

8.4.4
Self-Administration

Drugs of abuse can act as reinforcers because they increase the probability of a particular response leading to the presentation of an appetitive stimulus (positive reinforcement) or to the suppression of an aversive stimulus or to a state of drug withdrawal (negative reinforcement). Thus, it has been possible to assess their abuse potential by evaluating the positive reinforcing properties of drugs of abuse in animal studies. The self-administration methods are thought to have good face and predictive validity concerning drug use in humans since they mimic drug seeking/taking, and the neurobiological substrates related to drug effects appear to be similar in humans and experimental animals [70]. Self-administration techniques can be classified according to the route of drug administration, and from a behavioral point of view, they can be either nonoperant or operant procedures. Nonoperant paradigms almost always involve oral self-administration and are common in alcohol research. Nonoperant oral ethanol self-administration can be accomplished by choice procedures where the animal has access to one bottle containing an aqueous solution of ethanol and the other containing tap water [111]. In order to train animals to drink pharmacologically relevant concentrations of ethanol (8–12%), several different paradigms have been used, including the sucrose-fading technique, the presentation of ascending concentrations of ethanol, the presentation of a sweetened solution of ethanol, or exposing the animals to a forced time period of ethanol consumption [70,112]. Some studies have also used nonoperant oral self-administration procedures to investigate the reinforcing properties of psychostimulants or opioids. However, these types of drugs show very little reinforcing efficacy in animals [113], and since they are not consumed orally by humans, the face validity of this route of administration is undermined [70].

In operant self-administration procedures, animals learn to perform an instrumental response consisting of either pressing a lever or nose-poking in order to obtain the reinforcer (Figure 8.4). A response in the active manipulandum is linked to the delivery of the drug, whereas the response in the inactive manipulandum lacks any programmed consequences, and can allow control measures of nonreinforced behavior [70,114]. The route of administration used in these operant protocols depends on the drug under study. Typically, alcohol studies use oral self-administration, whereas intravenous self-administration is widely used to determine the reinforcing properties of most drugs of abuse, including opioids, psychostimulants, cannabinoids, and nicotine. The intravenous drug self-administration model is now considered to be predictive of the abuse potential of drugs since, with a few exceptions, drugs that serve as reinforcers in animals are abused by humans [115], and it has been suggested to be used as part of a battery for the preclinical assessment of the abuse liability of new agents [96]. Indeed, most prototypical drugs of abuse, including opioids, psychostimulants, synthetic drugs, alcohol, and nicotine, are self-administered by rodents [54], except THC, which is only self-administered by monkeys [116]. Reliable operant models of acquisition

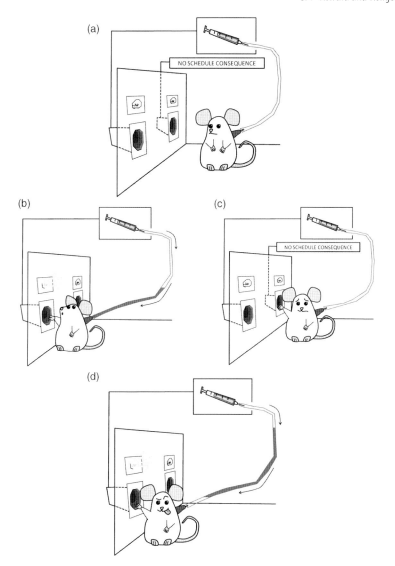

Figure 8.4 Drug self-administration. The intravenous drug self-administration procedure is a method for evaluating the positive reinforcing effects of a given compound. (a) Animals are prepared with catheters into the jugular vein. Usually two levers or nose-pokes are present in the testing chamber (nose-pokes in this representation). (b and c) Responses on the active nose-poke result in an intravenous infusion, and responses on the other nose-poke have no consequences. A light above the active nose-poke is illuminated during drug infusion and remains for a few seconds afterward to signal the drug delivery. (d) Animals should discriminate between nose-pokes, learning to nose-poke in the active hole that triggers the drug infusion delivery.

and relapse of morphine, cocaine, ecstasy, alcohol, nicotine, and synthetic cannabinoids self-administration are also now available in mice [117–119]. Application of these new models to the different lines of genetically modified mice will yield more insights into the future.

A wide variety of schedules of reinforcement are used to study drug reinforcement [120–123]. In fixed ratio schedules, the number of active responses required for drug infusion is set at a fixed number. Progressive ratio schedules are used to evaluate the reinforcing efficacy of a self-administered drug [124]. In this paradigm, the response requirements for each successive drug reinforcement are increased and the breaking point is determined, defined as the largest ratio requirement completed before the animal stops responding [125]. This value represents the maximum work a subject will perform to receive an infusion of a drug, and as such is a direct measure of its motivation to take the drug. Reinstatement of drug seeking can be modeled in rodents after drug self-administration behavior is extinguished by assessing the reinstatement of operant responding following the presentation of different triggering stimuli. In humans, stressful life events, the re-exposure to the drug itself, and the exposure to environmental stimuli previously associated with drug taking can promote relapse to drug consumption [126]. Thus, reinstatement of drug seeking has been shown to occur in animals (mice, rats, and monkeys) after a priming injection of the self-administered drug, after the presentation of the environmental stimulus associated with drug taking (light or tone), or after exposure to a stressful stimulus such as a foot-shock or a pharmacological stressor [127].

8.5
Translation to Clinics: Limitations and Difficulties

Animal paradigms of tolerance, sensitization, and physical withdrawal were of great interest to model the different aspects of drug addiction that were initially described in the drug-centered definition provided by DSM-III. These models mimic in animals the main diagnostic criteria that were recapitulated in DSM-III and have been widely used to clarify the molecular, cellular, and behavioral bases of these particular manifestations of the addictive process.

However, the relevance of these initial paradigms was very limited to mimic the main diagnostic criteria that were included in DSM-IV. Indeed, DSM-IV criteria were mainly focused on the loss of control over drug taking, which is much more difficult to model in experimental animals. The paradigms that have been developed to mimic drug subjective effects such as drug discrimination, drug rewarding effects such as CPP and ICSS, and drug reinforcing effects such as the self-administration models only mimic some specific features of the addictive process. These models have also been very useful in identifying neurobiological and behavioral bases underlying these different aspects included in the complex disease that is drug addiction. All these models are also of major interest in evaluating novel potential treatments for drug addiction and investigating the abuse liability of novel centrally acting compounds. Although these models are usually more time consuming than those initially designed to evaluate tolerance, sensitization, and physical dependence, they have been widely used for screening of new drugs and pharmacological compounds of interest. Among these models, it is important to underline the particular relevance of the operant self-administration paradigm to mimic drug consumption in humans since it requires an active operant response that results in a contingent drug administration. This paradigm directly evaluates the reinforcing properties of a drug, which cannot be evaluated when measuring the subjective effects (drug discrimination) or the rewarding aspects (CPP and ICSS).

The results obtained in the self-administration paradigm can be extrapolated to drug taking in humans. Nevertheless, only a few percentage of drug users become addicts and a behavioral model of drug taking is not a model of drug addiction. In the last decade, behavioral models that recapitulate the main DSM-IV diagnostic criteria for drug addiction have also been developed in experimental animals. These new models evaluate different aspects of the loss of control over drug taking, such as the difficulty to limit drug use, the strong motivation for the drug, and the compulsive drug intake despite the negative consequences, and can be considered the first models mimicking the main DSM-IV criteria for drug addiction. These models will now allow us to evaluate the main components of this disease and will certainly be of interest to clarify the different neurobiological mechanisms involved in drug addiction. However, the main limitation of these models of drug addiction is the enormous complexity of the behavioral paradigms. Indeed, these models were published in 2004 by two independent laboratories [18,19] using cocaine as drug of abuse, and these paradigms have not been validated as yet for other prototypical drugs of abuse. The complexity of the models also represents an important difficulty for their possible use for screening purposes.

The recent publication of DSM-5 modifies several of the diagnostic criteria for drug addiction and represents a new challenge to provide valid experimental animal models to recapitulate these novel aspects. A particular focus on drug craving has been included among the DSM-5 criteria. This new criterion can also be studied in the different models that have been previously validated using the operant self-administration paradigms.

Animal models of complex brain diseases, such as drug addiction, have always been difficult to develop. The design of these complex paradigms should be dynamic and must consider the new concepts that will be revealed when taking into account the novel aspects of the human clinical situation. These models include very complex behavioral procedures that are required to recapitulate the main aspects of the disease in a single paradigm and more simplistic models that only evaluate particular aspects of the disease. These latter models provide limited information, but can be extremely useful for screening of new potential compounds and for evaluating particular neurobiological and behavioral aspects. The use of the novel complex models of drug addiction will certainly now facilitate the understanding of the neurobiological substrate of this intricate disease.

References

1 American Psychiatric Association (2000) *Diagnostic and Statistical Manual of Mental Disorders*, 4th edn, American Psychiatric Publishing, Arlington, VA (Text revision (DSM-IV-TR).

2 Anthony, J.C., Warner, L.A., and Kessler, R.C. (1994) Comparative epidemiology of dependence on tobacco, alcohol, controlled substances and inhalants: basic findings from the National Comorbidity Survey. *Experimental and Clinical Psychopharmacology*, **2**, 244–268.

3 American Psychiatric Association (2013) *Diagnostic and Statistical Manual of Mental Disorders*, 5th edn. American Psychiatric Publishing, Arlington, VA (DSM-5).

4 Kopak, A.M., Proctor, S.L., and Hoffmann, N.G. (2012) An assessment of the compatibility of DSM-IV and proposed DSM-5 criteria in the diagnosis of cannabis use disorders. *Substance Use & Misuse*, **47** (12), 1328–1338.

5 Kreek, M.J., LaForge, K.S., and Butelman, E. (2002) Pharmacotherapy of addictions. *Nature Reviews. Drug Discovery*, **1** (9), 710–726.

6 Vanderschuren, L.J. and Ahmed, S.H. (2013) Animal studies of addictive behavior. *Cold Spring Harbor Perspectives in Medicine*, **3** (4), a011932.

7 Deroche-Gamonet, V., Belin, D., and Piazza, P.V. (2004) Evidence for addiction-like behavior in the rat. *Science*, **305** (5686), 1014–1017.

8 Volkow, N.D., Wang, G.J., Tomasi, D., and Baler, R.D. (2013) The addictive dimensionality of obesity. *Biological Psychiatry*, **73** (9), 811–818.

9 Everitt, B.J. and Wolf, M.E. (2002) Psychomotor stimulant addiction: a neural systems perspective. *The Journal of Neuroscience*, **22** (9), 3312–3320.

10 Koob, G.F. and Le Moal, M. (2005) Plasticity of reward neurocircuitry and the 'dark side' of drug addiction. *Nature Neuroscience*, **8** (11), 1442–1444.

11 Nestler, E.J. and Aghajanian, G.K. (1997) Molecular and cellular basis of addiction. *Science*, **278** (5335), 58–63.

12 Wise, R.A. (2002) Brain reward circuitry: insights from unsensed incentives. *Neuron*, **36** (2), 229–240.

13 Caspi, A. and Moffitt, T.E. (2006) Gene–environment interactions in psychiatry: joining forces with neuroscience. *Nature Reviews. Neuroscience*, **7** (7), 583–590.

14 Hamer, D. (2002) Genetics: rethinking behavior genetics. *Science*, **298** (5591), 71–72.

15 O'Connor, E.C., Chapman, K., Butler, P., and Mead, A.N. (2011) The predictive validity of the rat self-administration model for abuse liability. *Neuroscience and Biobehavioral Reviews*, **35** (3), 912–938.

16 Balleine, B.W. and O'Doherty, J.P. (2010) Human and rodent homologies in action control: corticostriatal determinants of goal-directed and habitual action. *Neuropsychopharmacology*, **35** (1), 48–69.

17 Piazza, P.V., Deminiere, J.M., Le, M.M., and Simon, H. (1989) Factors that predict individual vulnerability to amphetamine self-administration. *Science*, **245** (4925), 1511–1513.

18 Belin, D., Mar, A.C., Dalley, J.W., Robbins, T.W., and Everitt, B.J. (2008) High impulsivity predicts the switch to compulsive cocaine-taking. *Science*, **320** (5881), 1352–1355.

19 Kasanetz, F., Deroche-Gamonet, V., Berson, N., Balado, E., Lafourcade, M., Manzoni, O., and Piazza, P.V. (2010) Transition to addiction is associated with a persistent impairment in synaptic plasticity. *Science*, **328** (5986), 1709–1712.

20 Badillo-Martinez, D., Kirchgessner, A.L., Butler, P.D., and Bodnar, R.J. (1984) Monosodium glutamate and analgesia induced by morphine: test-specific effects. *Neuropharmacology*, **23** (10), 1141–1149.

21 Rodriguez de Fonseca, F. and Maldonado, R. (2002) Cannabinoid addiction: behavioral models and neural correlates. *The Journal of Neuroscience*, **22** (9), 3326–3331.

22 Tabakoff, B., Cornell, N., and Hoffman, P.L. (1986) Alcohol tolerance. *Annals of Emergency Medicine*, **15** (9), 1005–1012.

23 Holtman, J.R., Sloan, J.W., and Wala, E.P. (2004) Morphine tolerance in male and

female rats. *Pharmacology, Biochemistry, and Behavior*, **77** (3), 517–523.

24 Abood, M.E. and Martin, B.R. (1992) Neurobiology of marijuana abuse. *Trends in Pharmacological Sciences*, **13** (5), 201–206.

25 Pohorecky, L.A., Brick, J., and Carpenter, J.A. (1986) Assessment of the development of tolerance to ethanol using multiple measures. *Alcoholism, Clinical and Experimental Research*, **10** (6), 616–622.

26 Hine, B. (1985) Morphine and delta 9-tetrahydrocannabinol: two-way cross tolerance for antinociceptive and heart-rate responses in the rat. *Psychopharmacology*, **87** (1), 34–38.

27 Jones, R.T. and Stone, G.C. (1970) Psychological studies of marijuana and alcohol in man. *Psychopharmacologia*, **18** (1), 108–117.

28 Macavoy, M.G. and Marks, D.S. (1975) Divided attention performance of cannabis users and non-users following cannabis and alcohol. *Psychopharmacologia*, **44** (2), 147–152.

29 Sprague, G. and Craigmill, A. (1976) Behavioral and metabolic interaction of propylene glycol vehicle and delta-9-tetrahydrocannabinol. *Research Communications in Chemical Pathology and Pharmacology*, **14** (4), 739–742.

30 Pava, M.J. and Woodward, J.J. (2012) A review of the interactions between alcohol and the endocannabinoid system: implications for alcohol dependence and future directions for research. *Alcohol (Fayetteville, NY)*, **46** (3), 185–204.

31 Kalivas, P.W. and Stewart, J. (1991) Dopamine transmission in the initiation and expression of drug- and stress-induced sensitization of motor activity. *Brain Research. Brain Research Reviews*, **16** (3), 223–244.

32 Robinson, T.E. and Becker, J.B. (1986) Enduring changes in brain and behavior produced by chronic amphetamine administration: a review and evaluation of animal models of amphetamine psychosis. *Brain Research*, **396** (2), 157–198.

33 Post, R.M. and Contel, N.R. (1983) Human and animal studies of cocaine: implications for development of behavioral pathology, in *Stimulants: Neurochemical, Behavioral, and Clinical Perspectives* (ed. I. Creese), Raven Press, New York, pp. 169–203.

34 Samaha, A.N. and Robinson, T.E. (2005) Why does the rapid delivery of drugs to the brain promote addiction? *Trends in Pharmacological Sciences*, **26** (2), 82–87.

35 Lett, B.T. (1989) Repeated exposures intensify rather than diminish the rewarding effects of amphetamine, morphine, and cocaine. *Psychopharmacology*, **98** (3), 357–362.

36 Piazza, P.V., Deminiere, J.M., Le, M.M., and Simon, H. (1990) Stress- and pharmacologically-induced behavioral sensitization increases vulnerability to acquisition of amphetamine self-administration. *Brain Research*, **514** (1), 22–26.

37 Suto, N., Austin, J.D., Tanabe, L.M., Kramer, M.K., Wright, D.A., and Vezina, P. (2002) Previous exposure to VTA amphetamine enhances cocaine self-administration under a progressive ratio schedule in a D1 dopamine receptor dependent manner. *Neuropsychopharmacology*, **27** (6), 970–979.

38 Vezina, P. (2004) Sensitization of midbrain dopamine neuron reactivity and the self-administration of psychomotor stimulant drugs. *Neuroscience and Biobehavioral Reviews*, **27** (8), 827–839.

39 Benwell, M.E. and Balfour, D.J. (1992) The effects of acute and repeated nicotine treatment on nucleus accumbens dopamine and locomotor activity. *British Journal of Pharmacology*, **105** (4), 849–856.

40 Cadoni, C., Pisanu, A., Solinas, M., Acquas, E., and Di Chiara, G. (2001) Behavioural sensitization after repeated exposure to delta 9-tetrahydrocannabinol and cross-sensitization with morphine. *Psychopharmacology*, **158** (3), 259–266.

41 Cunningham, C.L. and Noble, D. (1992) Conditioned activation induced by ethanol: role in sensitization and conditioned place preference. *Pharmacology, Biochemistry, and Behavior*, **43** (1), 307–313.

42 Joyce, E.M. and Iversen, S.D. (1979) The effect of morphine applied locally to mesencephalic dopamine cell bodies on spontaneous motor activity in the rat. *Neuroscience Letters*, **14** (2–3), 207–212.

43 Post, R.M., Susan, R., and Weiss, B. (1992) Sensitization, kindling, and carbamazepine: an update on their implications for the course of affective illness. *Pharmacopsychiatry*, **25** (1), 41–43.

44 Itzhak, Y. and Martin, J.L. (1999) Effects of cocaine, nicotine, dizocipline and alcohol on mice locomotor activity: cocaine-alcohol cross-sensitization involves upregulation of striatal dopamine transporter binding sites. *Brain Research*, **818** (2), 204–211.

45 Robinson, T.E. and Berridge, K.C. (1993) The neural basis of drug craving: an incentive-sensitization theory of addiction. *Brain Research. Brain Research Reviews*, **18** (3), 247–291.

46 Renoir, T., Pang, T.Y., and Lanfumey, L. (2012) Drug withdrawal-induced depression: serotonergic and plasticity changes in animal models. *Neuroscience and Biobehavioral Reviews*, **36** (1), 696–726.

47 Williams, A.M., Reis, D.J., Powell, A.S., Neira, L.J., Nealey, K.A., Ziegler, C.E., Kloss, N.D., Bilimoria, J.L., Smith, C.E., and Walker, B.M. (2012) The effect of intermittent alcohol vapor or pulsatile heroin on somatic and negative affective indices during spontaneous withdrawal in Wistar rats. *Psychopharmacology*, **223** (1), 75–88.

48 Martin-Garcia, E. and Pallares, M. (2005) Effects of intrahippocampal nicotine and neurosteroid administration on withdrawal in voluntary and chronic alcohol-drinking rats. *Alcoholism, Clinical and Experimental Research*, **29** (9), 1654–1663.

49 Damaj, M.I., Kao, W., and Martin, B.R. (2003) Characterization of spontaneous and precipitated nicotine withdrawal in the mouse. *The Journal of Pharmacology and Experimental Therapeutics*, **307** (2), 526–534.

50 Plaza-Zabala, A., Flores, A., Maldonado, R., and Berrendero, F. (2012) Hypocretin/orexin signaling in the hypothalamic paraventricular nucleus is essential for the expression of nicotine withdrawal. *Biological Psychiatry*, **71** (3), 214–223.

51 Stoker, A.K., Semenova, S., and Markou, A. (2008) Affective and somatic aspects of spontaneous and precipitated nicotine withdrawal in C57BL/6J and BALB/cByJ mice. *Neuropharmacology*, **54** (8), 1223–1232.

52 Maldonado, R. (2002) Study of cannabinoid dependence in animals. *Pharmacology & Therapeutics*, **95** (2), 153–164.

53 Aceto, M.D., Scates, S.M., and Martin, B.B. (2001) Spontaneous and precipitated withdrawal with a synthetic cannabinoid, WIN 55212-2. *European Journal of Pharmacology*, **416** (1–2), 75–81.

54 Maldonado, R., Berrendero, F., Ozaita, A., and Robledo, P. (2011) Neurochemical basis of cannabis addiction. *Neuroscience*, **18**, 1–17.

55 Beardsley, P.M., Balster, R.L., and Harris, L.S. (1986) Dependence on tetrahydrocannabinol in rhesus monkeys. *The Journal of Pharmacology and Experimental Therapeutics*, **239** (2), 311–319.

56 Budney, A.J. and Hughes, J.R. (2006) The cannabis withdrawal syndrome. *Current Opinion in Psychiatry*, **19** (3), 233–238.

57 Robledo, P., Balerio, G., Berrendero, F., and Maldonado, R. (2004) Study of the behavioural responses related to the potential addictive properties of MDMA in mice. *Naunyn-Schmiedeberg's Archives of Pharmacology*, **369** (3), 338–349.

58 Tzschentke, T.M. (2007) Measuring reward with the conditioned place preference (CPP) paradigm: update of the last decade. *Addiction Biology*, **12** (3–4), 227–462.

59 Maldonado, C., Cauli, O., Rodriguez-Arias, M., Aguilar, M.A., and Minarro, J. (2003) Memantine presents different effects from MK-801 in motivational and physical signs of morphine withdrawal. *Behavioural Brain Research*, **144** (1–2), 25–35.

60 Maldonado, C., Rodriguez-Arias, M., Aguilar, M.A., and Minarro, J. (2004) GHB ameliorates naloxone-induced conditioned place aversion and physical aspects of morphine withdrawal in mice. *Psychopharmacology*, **177** (1–2), 130–140.

61 Shippenberg, T.S., Funada, M., and Schutz, C.G. (2000) Dynorphin A (2–17) attenuates the unconditioned but not the conditioned effects of opiate withdrawal in the rat. *Psychopharmacology*, **151** (4), 351–358.

62 Stinus, L., Cador, M., Zorrilla, E.P., and Koob, G.F. (2005) Buprenorphine and a

CRF1 antagonist block the acquisition of opiate withdrawal-induced conditioned place aversion in rats. *Neuropsychopharmacology*, **30** (1), 90–98.

63 Stinus, L., Caille, S., and Koob, G.F. (2000) Opiate withdrawal-induced place aversion lasts for up to 16 weeks. *Psychopharmacology*, **149** (2), 115–120.

64 O'Dell, L.E., Torres, O.V., Natividad, L.A., and Tejeda, H.A. (2007) Adolescent nicotine exposure produces less affective measures of withdrawal relative to adult nicotine exposure in male rats. *Neurotoxicology and Teratology*, **29** (1), 17–22.

65 Suzuki, T., Ise, Y., Tsuda, M., Maeda, J., and Misawa, M. (1996) Mecamylamine-precipitated nicotine-withdrawal aversion in rats. *European Journal of Pharmacology*, **314** (3), 281–284.

66 Balerio, G.N., Aso, E., Berrendero, F., Murtra, P., and Maldonado, R. (2004) Delta9-tetrahydrocannabinol decreases somatic and motivational manifestations of nicotine withdrawal in mice. *The European Journal of Neuroscience*, **20** (10), 2737–2748.

67 Jackson, K.J., Martin, B.R., Changeux, J.P., and Damaj, M.I. (2008) Differential role of nicotinic acetylcholine receptor subunits in physical and affective nicotine withdrawal signs. *The Journal of Pharmacology and Experimental Therapeutics*, **325** (1), 302–312.

68 Chester, J.A. and Coon, L.E. (2010) Pentylenetetrazol produces a state-dependent conditioned place aversion to alcohol withdrawal in mice. *Pharmacology, Biochemistry, and Behavior*, **95** (2), 258–265.

69 Olds, J. and Milner, P. (1954) Positive reinforcement produced by electrical stimulation of septal area and other regions of rat brain. *Journal of Comparative and Physiological Psychology*, **47** (6), 419–427.

70 Sanchis-Segura, C. and Spanagel, R. (2006) Behavioural assessment of drug reinforcement and addictive features in rodents: an overview. *Addiction Biology*, **11** (1), 2–38.

71 Markou, A., Weiss, F., Gold, L.H., Caine, S.B., Schulteis, G., and Koob, G.F. (1993) Animal models of drug craving. *Psychopharmacology*, **112** (2–3), 163–182.

72 Gardner, E.L., Paredes, W., Smith, D., Donner, A., Milling, C., Cohen, D., and Morrison, D. (1988) Facilitation of brain stimulation reward by delta 9-tetrahydrocannabinol. *Psychopharmacology*, **96** (1), 142–144.

73 Lepore, M., Liu, X., Savage, V., Matalon, D., and Gardner, E.L. (1996) Genetic differences in delta 9-tetrahydrocannabinol-induced facilitation of brain stimulation reward as measured by a rate-frequency curve-shift electrical brain stimulation paradigm in three different rat strains. *Life Sciences*, **58** (25), L365–L372.

74 Xi, Z.X., Spiller, K., Pak, A.C., Gilbert, J., Dillon, C., Li, X., Peng, X.Q., and Gardner, E.L. (2008) Cannabinoid CB1 receptor antagonists attenuate cocaine's rewarding effects: experiments with self-administration and brain-stimulation reward in rats. *Neuropsychopharmacology*, **33** (7), 1735–1745.

75 Epping-Jordan, M.P., Watkins, S.S., Koob, G.F., and Markou, A. (1998) Dramatic decreases in brain reward function during nicotine withdrawal. *Nature*, **393** (6680), 76–79.

76 Johnson, P.M., Hollander, J.A., and Kenny, P.J. (2008) Decreased brain reward function during nicotine withdrawal in C57BL6 mice: evidence from intracranial self-stimulation (ICSS) studies. *Pharmacology, Biochemistry, and Behavior*, **90** (3), 409–415.

77 Panagis, G., Kastellakis, A., Spyraki, C., and Nomikos, G. (2000) Effects of methyllycaconitine (MLA), an alpha 7 nicotinic receptor antagonist, on nicotine- and cocaine-induced potentiation of brain stimulation reward. *Psychopharmacology*, **149** (4), 388–396.

78 Koob, G.F. (2012) Animal models of psychiatric disorders. *Handbook of Clinical Neurology*, **106**, 137–166.

79 Weddington, W.W., Brown, B.S., Cone, E.J., Haertzen, C.A., Dax, E.M., Herning, R.I., and Michaelson, B.S. (1990) Changes in mood, craving and sleep during acute abstinence reported by male cocaine addicts. *NIDA Research Monograph*, **105**, 453–454.

80 Hodgson, S.R., Hofford, R.S., Roberts, K.W., Eitan, D., Wellman, P.J., and Eitan, S. (2010) Sex differences in affective response to opioid withdrawal during adolescence. *Journal of Psychopharmacology (Oxford, England)*, **24** (9), 1411–1417.

81 Schulteis, G., Markou, A., Gold, L.H., Stinus, L., and Koob, G.F. (1994) Relative sensitivity to naloxone of multiple indices of opiate withdrawal: a quantitative dose–response analysis. *The Journal of Pharmacology and Experimental Therapeutics*, **271** (3), 1391–1398.

82 Stevenson, J.R., Schroeder, J.P., Nixon, K., Besheer, J., Crews, F.T., and Hodge, C.W. (2009) Abstinence following alcohol drinking produces depression-like behavior and reduced hippocampal neurogenesis in mice. *Neuropsychopharmacology*, **34** (5), 1209–1222.

83 Bruijnzeel, A.W., Small, E., Pasek, T.M., and Yamada, H. (2010) Corticotropin-releasing factor mediates the dysphoria-like state associated with alcohol withdrawal in rats. *Behavioural Brain Research*, **210** (2), 288–291.

84 Zaniewska, M., McCreary, A.C., Wydra, K., and Filip, M. (2010) Effects of serotonin (5-HT)2 receptor ligands on depression-like behavior during nicotine withdrawal. *Neuropharmacology*, **58** (7), 1140–1146.

85 Markou, A. and Koob, G.F. (1992) Bromocriptine reverses the elevation in intracranial self-stimulation thresholds observed in a rat model of cocaine withdrawal. *Neuropsychopharmacology*, **7** (3), 213–224.

86 Perrine, S.A., Sheikh, I.S., Nwaneshiudu, C.A., Schroeder, J.A., and Unterwald, E.M. (2008) Withdrawal from chronic administration of cocaine decreases delta opioid receptor signaling and increases anxiety- and depression-like behaviors in the rat. *Neuropharmacology*, **54** (2), 355–364.

87 Renoir, T., Paizanis, E., El, Y.M., Saurini, F., Hanoun, N., Melfort, M., Lesch, K.P., Hamon, M., and Lanfumey, L. (2008) Differential long-term effects of MDMA on the serotoninergic system and hippocampal cell proliferation in 5-HTT knock-out vs. wild-type mice. The *International Journal of Neuropsychopharmacology*, **11** (8), 1149–1162.

88 Straiko, M.M., Gudelsky, G.A., and Coolen, L.M. (2007) Treatment with a serotonin-depleting regimen of MDMA prevents conditioned place preference to sex in male rats. *Behavioral Neuroscience*, **121** (3), 586–593.

89 Li, X., DeJoseph, M.R., Urban, J.H., Bahi, A., Dreyer, J.L., Meredith, G.E., Ford, K.A., Ferrario, C.R., Loweth, J.A., and Wolf, M.E. (2013) Different roles of BDNF in nucleus accumbens core versus shell during the incubation of cue-induced cocaine craving and its long-term maintenance. *The Journal of Neuroscience*, **33** (3), 1130–1142.

90 Rothman, R.B., Blough, B.E., and Baumann, M.H. (2008) Dual dopamine/serotonin releasers: potential treatment agents for stimulant addiction. *Experimental and Clinical Psychopharmacology*, **16** (6), 458–474.

91 Stolerman, I.P., Childs, E., Ford, M.M., and Grant, K.A. (2011) Role of training dose in drug discrimination: a review. *Behavioural Pharmacology*, **22** (5–6), 415–429.

92 Young, R. (2009) Chapter 3: Drug discrimination, in *Methods of Behavior Analysis in Neuroscience*, 2nd edn (ed. J.J. Buccafusco), CRC Press, Boca Raton, FL.

93 Colpaert, F.C. (1987) Drug discrimination in behavioral toxicology. *Zentralblatt für Bakteriologie, Mikrobiologie und Hygiene B*, **185** (1–2), 48–51.

94 Balster, R.L. (1990) Abuse potential of buspirone and related drugs. *Journal of Clinical Psychopharmacology*, **10** (3 Suppl.), 31S–37S.

95 Moser, P., Wolinsky, T., Castagne, V., and Duxon, M. (2011) Current approaches and issues in non-clinical evaluation of abuse and dependence. *Journal of Pharmacological and Toxicological Methods*, **63** (2), 160–167.

96 Koob, G.F. (1995) Animal models of drug addiction, in *Psychopharmacology: Fourth Generation in Progress* (eds F.E. Bloom and D.J. Kupfer), Raven Press, New York, pp. 759–772.

97 Preston, K.L. and Bigelow, G.E. (1991) Subjective and discriminative effects of

drugs. *Behavioural Pharmacology*, **2** (4 and 5), 293–313.
98 Mucha, R.F., van der Kooy, D., O'Shaughnessy, M., and Bucenieks, P. (1982) Drug reinforcement studied by the use of place conditioning in rat. *Brain Research*, **243** (1), 91–105.
99 Tzschentke, T.M. (1998) Measuring reward with the conditioned place preference paradigm: a comprehensive review of drug effects, recent progress and new issues. *Progress in Neurobiology*, **56** (6), 613–672.
100 Bardo, M.T., Rowlett, J.K., and Harris, M.J. (1995) Conditioned place preference using opiate and stimulant drugs: a meta-analysis. *Neuroscience and Biobehavioral Reviews*, **19** (1), 39–51.
101 Cunningham, C.L., Ferree, N.K., and Howard, M.A. (2003) Apparatus bias and place conditioning with ethanol in mice. *Psychopharmacology*, **170** (4), 409–422.
102 Childs, E. and de Wit, H. (2009) Amphetamine-induced place preference in humans. *Biological Psychiatry*, **65** (10), 900–904.
103 Napier, T.C., Herrold, A.A., and de Wit, H. (2013) Using conditioned place preference to identify relapse prevention medications. *Neuroscience and Biobehavioral Reviews*, **37** (9 Part A), 2081–2086.
104 Maldonado, R. and Rodriguez de Fonseca, F. (2002) Cannabinoid addiction: behavioral models and neural correlates. *The Journal of Neuroscience*, **22** (9), 3326–3331.
105 Shoaib, M., Stolerman, I.P., and Kumar, R.C. (1994) Nicotine-induced place preferences following prior nicotine exposure in rats. *Psychopharmacology*, **113** (3–4), 445–452.
106 Gallistel, C.R. and Davis, A.J. (1983) Affinity for the dopamine D2 receptor predicts neuroleptic potency in blocking the reinforcing effect of MFB stimulation. *Pharmacology, Biochemistry, and Behavior*, **19** (5), 867–872.
107 Kornetsky, C. and Esposito, R.U. (1979) Euphorigenic drugs: effects on the reward pathways of the brain. *Federation Proceedings*, **38** (11), 2473–2476.
108 Miliaressis, E., Rompre, P.P., Laviolette, P., Philippe, L., and Coulombe, D. (1986) The curve-shift paradigm in self-stimulation. *Physiology & Behavior*, **37** (1), 85–91.
109 Vlachou, S., Paterson, N.E., Guery, S., Kaupmann, K., Froestl, W., Banerjee, D., Finn, M.G., and Markou, A. (2011) Both GABA(B) receptor activation and blockade exacerbated anhedonic aspects of nicotine withdrawal in rats. *European Journal of Pharmacology*, **655** (1–3), 52–58.
110 Kenny, P.J. (2007) Brain reward systems and compulsive drug use. *Trends in Pharmacological Sciences*, **28** (3), 135–141.
111 Samson, H.H., Czachowski, C.L., and Slawecki, C.J. (2000) A new assessment of the ability of oral ethanol to function as a reinforcing stimulus. *Alcoholism, Clinical and Experimental Research*, **24** (6), 766–773.
112 Boyle, A.E., Smith, B.R., Spivak, K., and Amit, Z. (1994) Voluntary ethanol consumption in rats: the importance of the exposure paradigm in determining final intake outcome. *Behavioural Pharmacology*, **5** (4 and 5), 502–512.
113 Meisch, R.A. (2001) Oral drug self-administration: an overview of laboratory animal studies. *Alcohol (Fayetteville, NY)*, **24** (2), 117–128.
114 Thomsen, M. and Caine, S.B. (2007) Intravenous drug self-administration in mice: practical considerations. *Behavior Genetics*, **37** (1), 101–118.
115 Schuster, C.R. and Thompson, T. (1969) Self administration of and behavioral dependence on drugs. *Annual Review of Pharmacology*, **9**, 483–502.
116 Tanda, G., Munzar, P., and Goldberg, S.R. (2000) Self-administration behavior is maintained by the psychoactive ingredient of marijuana in squirrel monkeys. *Nature Neuroscience*, **3** (11), 1073–1074.
117 Martin-Garcia, E., Barbano, M.F., Galeote, L., and Maldonado, R. (2009) New operant model of nicotine-seeking behaviour in mice. *The International Journal of Neuropsychopharmacology*, **12** (3), 343–356.
118 Mendizabal, V., Zimmer, A., and Maldonado, R. (2006) Involvement of kappa/dynorphin system in WIN 55,212-2 self-administration in mice. *Neuropsychopharmacology*, **31** (9), 1957–1966.
119 Soria, G., Barbano, M.F., Maldonado, R., and Valverde, O. (2008) A reliable method

to study cue-, priming-, and stress-induced reinstatement of cocaine self-administration in mice. *Psychopharmacology*, **199** (4), 593–603.
120 Johanson, C.E. (1978) Effects of intravenous cocaine, diethylpropion, d-amphetamine and perphenazine on responding maintained by food delivery and shock avoidance in rhesus monkeys. *The Journal of Pharmacology and Experimental Therapeutics*, **204** (1), 118–129.
121 Katz, J.L. (1989) Interactions of clonidine and naloxone on schedule-controlled behavior in opioid-naive mice. *Psychopharmacology*, **98** (4), 445–447.
122 Spealman, R.D. and Goldberg, S.R. (1978) Drug self-administration by laboratory animals: control by schedules of reinforcement. *Annual Review of Pharmacology and Toxicology*, **18**, 313–339.
123 Young, R. and Herning, S. (1986) Drugs as reinforcers: studies in laboratory animals, in *Behavioral Analysis of Drug Dependence* (eds S.R. Goldberg and I.P. Stolerman), Academic Press, Orlando, FL, pp. 9–67.
124 Shippenberg, T.S. and Koob, G.F. (2002) Recent advances in animal models of drug addiction and alcoholism, in *Neuropsychopharmacology: The Fifth Generation of Progress* (eds K.L. Davis, D. Charney, J.T. Oyle, and C. Emeroff), Lippincott Williams and Wilkins, Philadelphia, pp. 1381–1397.
125 Stafford, D. and Branch, M.N. (1998) Effects of step size and break-point criterion on progressive-ratio performance. *Journal of the Experimental Analysis of Behavior*, **70** (2), 123–138.
126 O'Brien, C.P. and Gardner, E.L. (2005) Critical assessment of how to study addiction and its treatment: human and non-human animal models. *Pharmacology & Therapeutics*, **108** (1), 18–58.
127 Yan, Y. and Nabeshima, T. (2009) Mouse model of relapse to the abuse of drugs: procedural considerations and characterizations. *Behavioural Brain Research*, **196** (1), 1–10.

9
Mood and Anxiety Disorders
Guy Griebel and Sandra Beeské

9.1
Introduction

Mood and anxiety disorders are chronic, disabling conditions that impose enormous costs on both individuals and society at large [1–5]. These disorders are the most frequent diagnosed neuropsychiatric diseases in Western countries. According to a recent 3-year multimethod study covering 30 European countries and a population of 514 million people, anxiety and mood disorders had the highest 12-month prevalence estimates (total 14 and 6.9%, respectively) compared with all other psychiatric conditions [2]. Although there are many treatment options available for these disorders, drug discovery research in this area is still very active, with the objective of finding alternative, better tolerated, and more effective pharmacological treatments for anxiety and mood disorders.

The reliance on animal models of these conditions is crucial to find new treatments. Preclinical research has devised numerous ways to test for anxiety and mood, with well over 100 tests and models by recent counts [6]. The specifics of these tests have been described in many comprehensive reviews on this topic [6–9] and we will only briefly introduce the most frequently used ones here to illustrate the strengths and weaknesses of current approaches in general. One general consideration from the outset is validity. The validity of a test for anxiety/mood in an animal rests on three criteria: face validity (Does it measure something analogous to one or more human anxiety/mood symptoms?), predictive validity (Is it reliably sensitive to clinically efficacious anxiolytics/antidepressants?), and construct validity (Does it involve some of the same pathophysiological mechanisms found in human anxiety/mood disorders?) [10]. None of the available tests or models of anxiety or mood can be said to unequivocally meet these criteria.

9.2
Animal Models of Anxiety Disorders

9.2.1
Preclinical Measures of Anxiety

A group of tests that have been a mainstay of preclinical anxiety research for many years [11] assay anxiety-like behavior by generating a conflict between a drive to approach novel areas and simultaneously avoid potential threat therein (Figure 9.1). These simple tests that include the open-field, elevated plus maze, and light–dark exploration tests were developed in the 1980s to exploit the natural tendency of mainly rats [12] and mice [13,14], but also guinea pigs [15] and gerbils [16] to prefer enclosed areas over exposed/elevated places. They have been used in nearly 10 000 drug discovery-related experiments and continue to be very popular. More than half of the rodent-based experiments on anxiety-related drugs have employed one or more of these tests, and among them, by far the most commonly used has been the elevated plus maze.

While the approach–avoidance tests generate a conflict, the term "conflict-based test" has often been used to describe measures of the suppression of a behavior by mild electric shock. This group includes the Vogel conflict [17] and Geller–Seifter

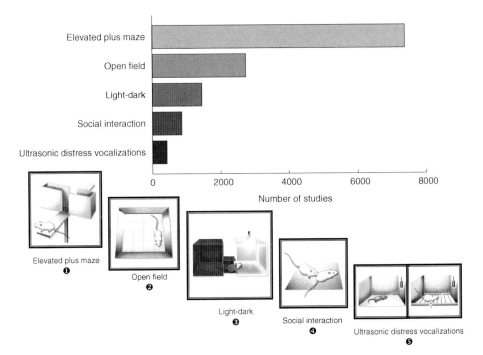

Figure 9.1 The five most commonly used tests in anxiolytic drug discovery. Values represent the number of experiments performed with each test as of 2012 (*Sources:* HCAPLUS, Medline, Embase, and Biosis.)

[18] tests, which measure anxiolytic-like activity as the maintenance of a behavioral response (licking and bar pressing) despite receipt of shock. These tests were part of many drug discovery programs in the 1980s and 1990s, but have fallen out of favor perhaps because they require animals to be trained over multiple days and are more labor intensive and time consuming than the approach–avoidance tasks.

Some anxiety tests have been designed to tap into fundamental defensive responses shown by animals in the face of immediate danger. Such defensive or "fear" behaviors can be conceptually distinguished from the anxiety states produced by less imminent, more ambiguous threats [11], and may be most relevant to anxiety disorders, such as panic disorder (PD) and posttraumatic stress disorder (PTSD). The mouse defense test battery (MDTB) was designed to provide multiple measures related to fear and anxiety, based on observations of how wild rodents respond to danger [19]. In this task, mice are placed in an oval runway and tested for responses (fight, flight, freeze, vocalize, scan, etc.) to an approaching anesthetized rat (a natural predator). Interestingly, specific behavioral measures in this test are sensitive to specific classes of anxiolytic medication, with, for example, benzodiazepines (BZ) that are effective in generalized anxiety disorder (GAD) reducing risk assessment and serotonergic agents that are efficacious in PD and PTSD, attenuating fight and flight behaviors [20]. In spite of these promising results, however, the task has not been widely adopted, again likely due to the training and technical demands involved. As a compromise, some researchers incorporated measures derived from the analysis of defensive behavior into the simpler anxiety-related assays such as the elevated plus maze, in some cases improving the sensitivity to certain anxiolytic classes [21].

Another set of fear-based tests involve variations on classical Pavlovian conditioning. Here, the animal learns to associate a context or specific environmental stimulus (e.g., a light or a sound) with electric shock to produce a conditioned fear response that can be quantified in various ways (freezing, escape, avoidance, startle, etc.). Studies of Pavlovian fear have contributed greatly to the understanding of the basic neural and molecular mechanisms of memory, but have not been traditionally considered tests for use in anxiolytic drug discovery. This may be changing, however, with the recent focus on devising ways to pharmacologically attenuate fearful memories through the process of reconsolidation or extinction [22] and, more generally, by a growing appreciation of abnormal learning and cognition in anxiety.

9.2.2
Preclinical Anxiety Models and Endophenotypes

Tests for anxiety, in which the animal is placed in an experimental situation to evoke an acute anxiety-like response, can be distinguished from models of anxiety, where the animal has been manipulated in some way to produce a more lasting increase in anxiety. The goal of anxiety models is to produce a form of abnormally elevated anxiety that more closely approximates to the pathology of an anxiety disorder (Table 9.1). This can be achieved, for example, by acutely or chronically subjecting animals to stressors prior to testing [23,24]. Another approach involves

Table 9.1 Modeling symptoms of anxiety disorders in rodents.

Symptom	Assay	Situation
Avoidance of places from which escape could be difficult	Exploration of exposed and well-lit spaces in the elevated plus maze and light–dark box	Acute avoidable
Anxiety provoked by situations for which opposing impulses lead to decisional uncertainty	Increase in punished responding in the punished drinking and four-plate tests	Acute avoidable
Anxiety provoking obsessions/impulsive behavior	Marble burying	Acute nonavoidable
Difficulty in concentrating	Cognitive impairment due to predator stress	Acute nonavoidable
Worry/difficult to control the worry	Risk assessment in the defense battery	Acute nonavoidable
Irritability/aggressivity	Defensive aggression in the defense battery, human threat	Acute nonavoidable
Sudden onset of intense fearfulness	Flight in the defense battery	Acute nonavoidable
Autonomic hyperarousal	Stress-induced hyperthermia	Acute nonavoidable
Difficulty in concentrating, hyperarousal (PTSD)	Trauma-induced long-term cognitive or adaptive deficits	Chronic nonavoidable

identifying genetic populations or engineering animals that are inherently anxiety prone. Examples of the former are inbred mouse strains, such as BALB/cJ, and selectively bred "high-anxiety behavior" rat and mouse lines [25,26]. Illustrative of the latter are the plethora of transgenic and gene knockout mice that have been generated and tested for anxiety-like phenotypes. These mutant mice have been valuable as models to screen for novel anxiolytics [27–29].

The term endophenotype describes a symptomatic feature or premorbid risk factor of an anxiety disorder that can be more readily quantifiable than the disease as a whole. Certain rodent behavioral measures can also be considered endophenotypes of specific anxiety symptoms: risk assessment and flight in the MDTB, for example, can be related to threat hypervigilance and threat avoidance in GAD and PD, respectively [19]. Moreover, assessing the extinction of fearful memories has become a popular measure in anxiety research because the procedures, as well as the underlying neurobiology, closely overlap in animals and humans, and extinction has a close therapeutic analog in the form of exposure therapy. The objective of many preclinical extinction studies is to screen for drugs that can be administered as adjuncts during exposure to strengthen the formation of extinction memories and thereby reduce the future recurrence of anxiety symptoms [30,31]. There have been some successes in developing clinically efficacious anxiolytics (e.g., D-cycloserine) based upon predictions from studies of fear extinction in rodents [32], and this is currently an active approach for further drug discovery.

9.3 Animal Models of Mood Disorders

9.3.1 Major Depressive Disorder

Given the subjective and heterogeneous nature of most of the core symptoms of major depressive disorder (MDD) and the lack of valid state markers, modeling this condition poses a number of substantial challenges. Further complication derives from the observation that current antidepressants, which all target monoaminergic neurotransmission, have inconsistent effects in the clinic (about 50% of patients will not respond to a first-line treatment). This has important implications for modeling as it limits the use of reference drugs as a validation criterion for novel drug effect. Despite these issues, there are several animal procedures that are claimed to model certain aspects of depressive symptoms and that are used extensively in antidepressant drug discovery (Figure 9.2).

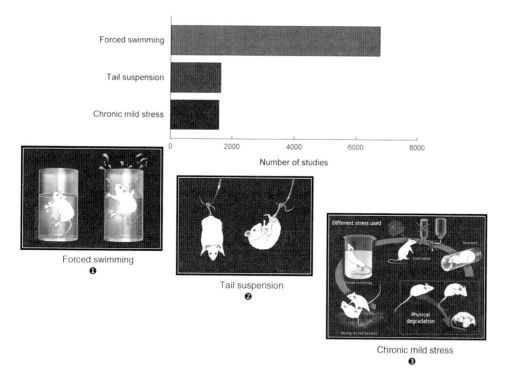

Figure 9.2 The three most commonly used tests in antidepressant drug discovery. Values represent the number of experiments performed with each test as of 2012 (*Sources:* HCAPLUS, Medline, Embase, and Biosis.)

9.3.1.1 Preclinical Measures of Depression

These models are based on epidemiological evidence that stress and adverse psychosocial experiences often precede the onset, or predict the recurrence, of depressive episodes. They can be subdivided into several categories based on the behavioral endpoint related to the depressive symptoms [33].

Negative Affect This refers to a form of behavioral passivity and quiescence, often referred to as "despair," occurring in many species upon exposure to uncontrollable stress. This increase in inactivity can be delayed or normalized by antidepressants. Tests that measure this activity or escape deficit include either simple behavioral procedures (e.g., forced swimming [34] and tail suspension [35]) or more elaborate paradigms (e.g., learned helplessness [36]). By far the most widely utilized is the forced swimming test, which can be used with rats and mice. The common application of this test is linked directly to the robust and reproducible effects of monoamine reuptake inhibitors.

Positive Affect or Hedonia This refers to the ability to experience pleasure. Reduction in this behavior, often referred to as anhedonia, is commonly observed in MDD and represents a hallmark endophenotype of this condition [37]. Common behavioral tests used to quantify anhedonia in rodents are the sucrose preference test, intracranial self-stimulation (ICSS), and sexual behavior [38–40]. The sucrose preference test is based on the idea that repeated mild unpredictable stressors will lead to a reduction of sucrose consumption. The test is normally run under conditions of free access to sucrose and water, and anhedonia is quantified based on the ratio of sucrose to water consumption over that time. ICSS behavior allows a direct evaluation of the sensitivity to reward in animals. Several approaches, including electrical stimulation of basal forebrain [41] and ventral tegmental area [40], have been used. In this procedure, rats are allowed to electrically self-stimulate the targeted brain area. Following repeated exposure to a variety of stressors, stimulation threshold is generally increased in stressed rats, suggesting a decrease in the rewarding properties of brain stimulation (i.e., a correlate of anhedonia). Sexual behaviors have also been used to quantify anhedonia [42,43]. Pharmacological studies using antidepressants have shown that these deficits in hedonic behaviors can be normalized following chronic treatment of these agents.

Socioaffective Function Socioaffective alterations are another important feature of MDD symptoms [37]. Studies in primates and rats have demonstrated the occurrence of deficits in social behaviors upon repeated exposure to stressors, such as maternal separation or social defeat. The most salient aspects of socioaffective alterations are expression of a stereotypical prostrated and socially unresponsive posture (in primates), the exacerbation of socially submissive behaviors, and social avoidance (in primates and rats). Despite the strong face validity, primate models of socioaffective deficits have been rarely used in antidepressant drug discovery because of obvious technical and ethical limitations [44]. Rodent social stress models such as the social defeat paradigm [45] and tests of dominant–submissive behavior such as the visible burrow system procedure [46,47] provide a number of valid alternatives to examine antidepressant drug effects.

Cognition According to the cognitive model of depression described by Aaron Beck ~40 years ago, biased acquisition and processing of information have a primary role in the development and maintenance of depression [48]. This model derives from the observation that MDD patients overemphasize negatively valenced information, resulting in difficulties in redirecting their attention or thoughts away from negative beliefs. Although pessimistic decision biases *per se* cannot be modeled in animals, there are several behavioral tasks of attention and executive function (e.g., CANTAB battery [49]) in rodents and primates that could serve to measure cognitive deficits in MDD models. Unfortunately, these tests are technically challenging and not necessarily suitable for drug testing.

9.3.1.2 Endophenotype Models of Depression

The last two decades have seen the emergence of endophenotype models of depression, with the engineering of animals that are inherently depression prone. For example, animals carrying mutations replicating naturally occurring single-nucleotide polymorphisms that alter the function or candidate genes for MDD, such as *BDNF* [50], *TPH2* [51], *5-HTT* [52], *DISC1* [53], or *CRHR1* [54], have been reported to display depression-like phenotypes. However, the lack of a highly penetrant mutation associated with MDD, along with the unclear epidemiological evidence that these genetic variants significantly increase the MDD risk, seriously questions the idea that these mutants represent valid models of depression. Another approach involves the identification of animal populations that display inherently depression-like behaviors. Examples are inbred rat strains, such as Flinders sensitive line (FSL) [55] and Wistar Kyoto (WKY) [56], and selectively bred, "high reaction to stress test" (HR) [57], "swim low-active" (SwLo) [58], or "inbred learned helpless" (cLH) [59] rat and mouse lines. These animals have been valuable as models to screen for novel anxiolytics.

9.3.2
Bipolar Disorder

Bipolar disorder (BPD) is phenotypically a very complex disease, characterized by vulnerability to episodic depression and mania and spontaneous cycling. Because of its heterogeneous clinical phenotype, along with the relative lack of knowledge about its underlying pathophysiology, the development of animal models for BPD has been difficult [60,61]. One approach for the development of appropriate tests has been to model separately a number of its critical behavioral aspects. For example, the most widely used test that has been validated in the context of mania includes psychostimulant-induced hyperactivity [62]. This test was developed on the basis of the observation that psychostimulants, such as amphetamine, induce mania in susceptible individuals and that mood stabilizers can prevent these effects. There have been attempts to model other components of the manic pole of

BPD in mice, such as reward seeking (using the sweet solution preference test), intrusive or aggressive behavior (using the resident–intruder paradigm), and increased vigor and resilience to despair (using a variation of the forced swim test). It has been suggested that these tests could be integrated into a coherent and continuous test battery [60].

Large-scale candidate and genome-wide association studies have generated a rapidly growing list of risk genes for BPD. Despite the uncertainty as to whether, and to what extent, risk variance causes gene dysfunction and whether risk genes are causally linked to behavioral abnormalities in BPD, there is a plethora of mutant rodent strains that have been generated using genetic (e.g., gene transgenic, knockout, or mutation knock-in manipulation) or other biological means (e.g., viral vector-based gene overexpression or knockdown), which show behavioral clusters or activity patterns reminiscent of mood syndromes [63]. These include mCLOCK [64], glutamate receptor 6 (GluR6)$^{-/-}$ [65], extracellular signal-regulated kinase-1 (ERK1)$^{-/-}$ [66], opioid receptor, and glycogen synthase kinase-3 (GSK-3)$^{-/-}$ [67]. This so-called reverse translation model animal approach has so far been used to analyze the causal relationship between biological abnormalities resulting from genetic BPD risk variants, early-life environmental factors, and behavioral manifestations of BPD, but it will certainly be essential for the development of true novel drug therapies.

9.4
Translation to Clinics: Limitations and Difficulties

Most of the tests described were developed 30 years ago and have been used since then with little modifications. Because of the failure of virtually all anxiolytic and antidepressant drug development programs during the past decades, the capability of current models to detect new molecules with mechanisms of action different from the prototypical BZs and monoamine-interacting drugs has been repeatedly questioned. Several comprehensive reviews have been published in recent years discussing the pros and cons of each model and proposing guidelines for their improvement, with a strong consensus on the need to better incorporate etiological factors in the design of novel paradigms [33,68,69]. We summarize herein some of the potential solutions for how preclinical research in this area can be improved.

Classical conflict or despair tests, such as the elevated plus maze or forced swimming, have proven to be of limited utility for detecting non-BZ anxiolytic or nonmonoaminergic antidepressant activity, respectively, and should only be employed with this caveat in mind. On the other hand, their throughput is high and they can be used as first-line screening assays when performing selection from large libraries of compounds. As many anxiety and depression tests are highly sensitive to procedural variables and environment factors, the tests should be validated in-house and methods fully reported. Integrating results from multiple preclinical tests and developing tests that assess multiple symptom-related

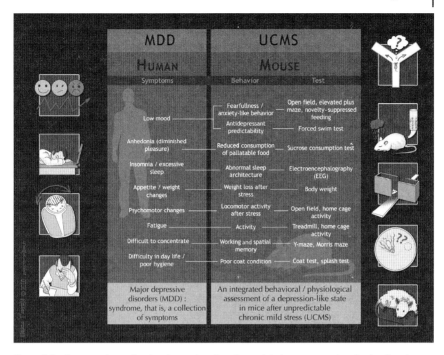

Figure 9.3 State markers of major depressive disorder and their mouse analogs in the chronic mild stress model.

behaviors (e.g., MDTB, chronic mild stress) (Figure 9.3) will increase confidence in the potential of a novel target. Anxiety tests and models that are based on abnormal learning and cognitive processes in anxiety disorders (e.g., fear generalization and impaired fear extinction) may offer a tractable and translatable approach. Anxiety or depression models that generate excessive levels of anxiety- or despair-like behavior (e.g., by chronic stress exposure, gene mutation, or selected breeding) may be closer to the clinical situation and thereby have better predictive power than simple assays. Because rodent strains vary greatly in anxiety- or depression-like behavior and response to known drugs, genetic background must be a principal consideration in choosing subjects and interpreting results.

Clearly, the growing burden of anxiety and mood disorders requires better treatment options. Future research advances in both biological information and behavioral methodology will be essential for the rapid development of true novel drug treatments for relieving anxiety and mood symptoms.

Acknowledgment

We thank Dr. Andrew Holmes (National Institute on Alcohol Abuse and Alcoholism, National Institutes of Health) for his helpful comments on this chapter.

References

1. Kessler, R.C. (2007) The global burden of anxiety and mood disorders: putting the European Study of the Epidemiology of Mental Disorders (ESEMeD) findings into perspective. *Journal of Clinical Psychiatry*, **68** (Suppl. 2), 10–19.
2. Wittchen, H.U., Jacobi, F., Rehm, J., Gustavsson, A., Svensson, M., Jonsson, B., Olesen, J., Allgulander, C., Alonso, J., Faravelli, C., Fratiglioni, L., Jennum, P., Lieb, R., Maercker, A., van, O.J., Preisig, M., Salvador-Carulla, L., Simon, R., and Steinhausen, H.C. (2011) The size and burden of mental disorders and other disorders of the brain in Europe 2010. *European Neuropsychopharmacology*, **21**, 655–679.
3. Kessler, R.C., Ormel, J., Petukhova, M., McLaughlin, K.A., Green, J.G., Russo, L.J., Stein, D.J., Zaslavsky, A.M., Aguilar-Gaxiola, S., Alonso, J., Andrade, L., Benjet, C., de Girolamo, G., de Graaf, R., Demyttenaere, K., Fayyad, J., Haro, J.M., Hu, C., Karam, A., Lee, S., Lepine, J.P., Matchsinger, H., Mihaescu-Pintia, C., Posada-Villa, J., Sagar, R., and Ustun, T.B. (2011) Development of lifetime comorbidity in the World Health Organization world mental health surveys. *Archives of General Psychiatry*, **68**, 90–100.
4. Kessler, R.C., Aguilar-Gaxiola, S., Alonso, J., Chatterji, S., Lee, S., and Ustun, T.B. (2009) The WHO World Mental Health (WMH) surveys. *Psychiatrie (Stuttgart, Germany)*, **6**, 5–9.
5. Ormel, J., Petukhova, M., Chatterji, S., Aguilar-Gaxiola, S., Alonso, J., Angermeyer, M.C., Bromet, E.J., Burger, H., Demyttenaere, K., de Girolamo G., Haro, J.M., Hwang, I., Karam, E., Kawakami, N., Lepine, J.P., Medina-Mora, M.E., Posada-Villa, J., Sampson, N., Scott, K., Ustun, T.B., Von, K.M., Williams, D.R., Zhang, M., and Kessler, R.C. (2008) Disability and treatment of specific mental and physical disorders across the world. *British Journal of Psychiatry*, **192**, 368–375.
6. Haller, J., Aliczki, M., and Gyimesine, P.K. (2012) Classical and novel approaches to the preclinical testing of anxiolytics: a critical evaluation. *Neuroscience & Biobehavioral Reviews*, **37**, 2318–2330.
7. Belzung, C. and Lemoine, M. (2011) Criteria of validity for animal models of psychiatric disorders: focus on anxiety disorders and depression. *Biology of Mood & Anxiety Disorders*, **1**, 9–14.
8. Cryan, J.F. and Holmes, A. (2005) The ascent of mouse: advances in modelling human depression and anxiety. *Nature Reviews. Drug Discovery*, **4**, 775–790.
9. Griebel, G. and Holmes, A. (2013) 50 years of hope and hurdles in anxiolytic drug discovery. *Nature Reviews. Drug Discovery*, **12**, 667–687.
10. McKinney, W.T., Jr. and Bunney, W.E., Jr. (1969) Animal model of depression. I. Review of evidence: implications for research. *Archives of General Psychiatry*, **21**, 240–248.
11. Hall, C.S. (1934) Emotional behavior in the rat. I: defecation and urination as measures of individual differences in emotionality. *Journal of Comparative Psychology*, **18**, 385–403.
12. Handley, S.L. and Mithani, S. (1984) Effects of alpha-adrenoceptor agonists and antagonists in a maze-exploration model of "fear"-motivated behaviour. *Naunyn-Schmiedeberg's Archives of Pharmacology*, **327**, 1–5.
13. Crawley, J.N. (1981) Neuropharmacologic specificity of a simple animal model for the behavioral actions of benzodiazepines. *Pharmacology, Biochemistry, and Behavior*, **15**, 695–699.
14. Lister, R.G. (1987) The use of a plus-maze to measure anxiety in the mouse. *Psychopharmacology*, **92**, 180–185.
15. Rex, A., Fink, H., Skingle, M., and Marsden, C.A. (1996) Involvement of 5-HT1D receptors in cortical extracellular 5-HT release in guinea-pigs on exposure to the elevated plus maze. *Journal of Psychopharmacology*, **10**, 219–224.
16. Varty, G.B., Morgan, C.A., Cohen-Williams, M.E., Coffin, V.L., and Carey, G.J. (2002) The gerbil elevated plus-maze I: behavioral characterization and pharmacological validation. *Neuropsychopharmacology*, **27**, 357–370.

17. Vogel, J.R., Beer, B., and Clody, D.E. (1971) A simple and reliable conflict procedure for testing anti-anxiety agents. *Psychopharmacologia*, **21**, 1–7.
18. Geller, I., Kulak, J.T., and Seifter, J. (1962) The effects of chlordiazepoxide and chlorpromazine on a punishment discrimination. *Psychopharmacologia*, **3**, 374–385.
19. Griebel, G. and Beeské, S. (2011) The mouse defense test battery: a model measuring different facets of anxiety-related behaviors, in *Mood and Anxiety Related Phenotypes in Mice* (ed. T.D. Gould), Springer Science+Business Media, pp. 97–106.
20. Blanchard, D.C., Griebel, G., and Blanchard, R.J. (2003) The Mouse Defense Test Battery: pharmacological and behavioral assays for anxiety and panic. *European Journal of Pharmacology*, **463**, 97–116.
21. Rodgers, R.J., Cao, B.J., Dalvi, A., and Holmes, A. (1997) Animal models of anxiety: an ethological perspective. *Brazilian Journal of Medical and Biological Research*, **30**, 289–304.
22. Steckler, T. and Risbrough, V. (2012) Pharmacological treatment of PTSD: established and new approaches. *Neuropharmacology*, **62**, 617–627.
23. Mozhui, K., Karlsson, R.M., Kash, T.L., Ihne, J., Norcross, M., Patel, S., Farrell, M.R., Hill, E.E., Graybeal, C., Martin, K.P., Camp, M., Fitzgerald, P.J., Ciobanu, D.C., Sprengel, R., Mishina, M., Wellman, C.L., Winder, D.G., Williams, R.W., and Holmes, A. (2010) Strain differences in stress responsivity are associated with divergent amygdala gene expression and glutamate-mediated neuronal excitability. *Journal of Neuroscience*, **30**, 5357–5367.
24. Belzung, C., El Hage, W., Moindrot, N., and Griebel, G. (2001) Behavioral and neurochemical changes following predatory stress in mice. *Neuropharmacology*, **41**, 400–408.
25. Muigg, P., Scheiber, S., Salchner, P., Bunck, M., Landgraf, R., and Singewald, N. (2009) Differential stress-induced neuronal activation patterns in mouse lines selectively bred for high, normal or low anxiety. *PLoS One*, **4**, e5346.
26. Holmes, A. and Singewald, N. (2013) Individual differences in recovery from traumatic fear. *Trends in Neurosciences*, **36**, 23–31.
27. Holmes, A. (2008) Genetic variation in cortico-amygdala serotonin function and risk for stress-related disease. *Neuroscience & Biobehavioral Reviews*, **32**, 1293–1314.
28. Holmes, A.J., Lee, P.H., Hollinshead, M.O., Bakst, L., Roffman, J.L., Smoller, J.W., and Buckner, R.L. (2012) Individual differences in amygdala-medial prefrontal anatomy link negative affect, impaired social functioning, and polygenic depression risk. *Journal of Neuroscience*, **32**, 18087–18100.
29. Donaldson, Z.R., Nautiyal, K.M., Ahmari, S.E., and Hen, R. (2013) Genetic approaches for understanding the role of serotonin receptors in mood and behavior. *Current Opinion in Neurobiology*, **23**, 399–406.
30. Holmes, A. and Quirk, G.J. (2010) Pharmacological facilitation of fear extinction and the search for adjunct treatments for anxiety disorders: the case of yohimbine. *Trends in Pharmacological Sciences*, **31**, 2–7.
31. Myers, K.M. and Davis, M. (2007) Mechanisms of fear extinction. *Molecular Psychiatry*, **12**, 120–150.
32. Richardson, R., Ledgerwood, L., and Cranney, J. (2004) Facilitation of fear extinction by D-cycloserine: theoretical and clinical implications. *Learning & Memory*, **11**, 510–516.
33. Berton, O., Hahn, C.G., and Thase, M.E. (2012) Are we getting closer to valid translational models for major depression? *Science*, **338**, 75–79.
34. Porsolt, R.D., Le Pichon, M., and Jalfre, M. (1977) Depression: a new animal model sensitive to antidepressant treatments. *Nature*, **266**, 730–732.
35. Steru, L., Chermat, R., Thierry, B., and Simon, P. (1985) The tail suspension test: a new method for screening antidepressants in mice. *Psychopharmacology*, **85**, 367–370.
36. Maier, S.F. (1984) Learned helplessness and animal models of depression. *Progress in Neuro-Psychopharmacology & Biological Psychiatry*, **8**, 435–446.
37. American Psychiatric Association (2000) *Diagnostic and Statistical Manual of Mental*

38 Strekalova, T., Couch, Y., Kholod, N., Boyks, M., Malin, D., Leprince, P., and Steinbusch, H.M. (2011) Update in the methodology of the chronic stress paradigm: internal control matters. *Behavioral and Brain Functions*, **7**, 9.

39 Papp, M., Willner, P., and Muscat, R. (1991) An animal model of anhedonia: attenuation of sucrose consumption and place preference conditioning by chronic unpredictable mild stress. *Psychopharmacology*, **104**, 255–259.

40 Moreau, J.L., Jenck, F., Martin, J.R., Mortas, P., and Haefely, W.E. (1992) Antidepressant treatment prevents chronic unpredictable mild stress-induced anhedonia as assessed by ventral tegmentum self-stimulation behavior in rats. *European Neuropsychopharmacology*, **2**, 43–49.

41 Carlezon, W.A., Jr. and Chartoff, E.H. (2007) Intracranial self-stimulation (ICSS) in rodents to study the neurobiology of motivation. *Nature Protocols*, **2**, 2987–2995.

42 Barrot, M., Wallace, D.L., Bolanos, C.A., Graham, D.L., Perrotti, L.I., Neve, R.L., Chambliss, H., Yin, J.C., and Nestler, E.J. (2005) Regulation of anxiety and initiation of sexual behavior by CREB in the nucleus accumbens. *Proceedings of the National Academy of Sciences of the United States of America*, **102**, 8357–8362.

43 Fawcett, J., Clark, D.C., Scheftner, W.A., and Hedeker, D. (1983) Differences between anhedonic and normally hedonic depressive states. *American Journal of Psychiatry*, **140**, 1027–1030.

44 Ferdowsian, H.R., Durham, D.L., Kimwele, C., Kranendonk, G., Otali, E., Akugizibwe, T., Mulcahy, J.B., Ajarova, L., and Johnson, C.M. (2011) Signs of mood and anxiety disorders in chimpanzees. *PLoS One*, **6**, e19855.

45 Berton, O., McClung, C.A., DiLeone, R.J., Krishnan, V., Renthal, W., Russo, S.J., Graham, D., Tsankova, N.M., Bolanos, C.A., Rios, M., Monteggia, L.M., Self, D.W., and Nestler, E.J. (2006) Essential role of BDNF in the mesolimbic dopamine pathway in social defeat stress. *Science*, **311**, 864–868.

46 Blanchard, D.C. and Blanchard, R.J. (1990) Behavioral correlates of chronic dominance–subordination relationships of male rats in a seminatural situation. *Neuroscience and Biobehavioral Reviews*, **14**, 455–462.

47 Blanchard, D.C., Sakai, R.R., McEwen, B., Weiss, S.M., and Blanchard, R.J. (1993) Subordination stress: behavioral, brain, and neuroendocrine correlates. *Behavioural Brain Research*, **58**, 113–121.

48 Disner, S.G., Beevers, C.G., Haigh, E.A., and Beck, A.T. (2011) Neural mechanisms of the cognitive model of depression. *Nature Reviews. Neuroscience*, **12**, 467–477.

49 Fray, P.J. and Robbins, T.W. (1996) CANTAB battery: proposed utility in neurotoxicology. *Neurotoxicology and Teratology*, **18**, 499–504.

50 Yu, H., Wang, D.D., Wang, Y., Liu, T., Lee, F.S., and Chen, Z.Y. (2012) Variant brain-derived neurotrophic factor Val66Met polymorphism alters vulnerability to stress and response to antidepressants. *Journal of Neuroscience*, **32**, 4092–4101.

51 Beaulieu, J.M., Zhang, X., Rodriguiz, R.M., Sotnikova, T.D., Cools, M.J., Wetsel, W.C., Gainetdinov, R.R., and Caron, M.G. (2008) Role of GSK3 beta in behavioral abnormalities induced by serotonin deficiency. *Proceedings of the National Academy of Sciences of the United States of America*, **105**, 1333–1338.

52 Carneiro, A.M., Airey, D.C., Thompson, B., Zhu, C.B., Lu, L., Chesler, E.J., Erikson, K.M., and Blakely, R.D. (2009) Functional coding variation in recombinant inbred mouse lines reveals multiple serotonin transporter-associated phenotypes. *Proceedings of the National Academy of Sciences of the United States of America*, **106**, 2047–2052.

53 Porteous, D.J., Millar, J.K., Brandon, N.J., and Sawa, A. (2011) DISC1 at 10: connecting psychiatric genetics and neuroscience. *Trends in Molecular Medicine*, **17**, 699–706.

54 Refojo, D., Schweizer, M., Kuehne, C., Ehrenberg, S., Thoeringer, C., Vogl, A.M., Dedic, N., Schumacher, M., von, W.G., Avrabos, C., Touma, C., Engblom, D., Schutz, G., Nave, K.A., Eder, M., Wotjak, C.T., Sillaber, I., Holsboer, F., Wurst, W., and Deussing, J.M. (2011) Glutamatergic and dopaminergic neurons mediate anxiogenic

and anxiolytic effects of CRHR1. *Science*, **333**, 1903–1907.

55 Overstreet, D.H. and Wegener, G. (2013) The Flinders sensitive line rat model of depression: 25 years and still producing. *Pharmacological Reviews*, **65**, 143–155.

56 Will, C.C., Aird, F., and Redei, E.E. (2003) Selectively bred Wistar–Kyoto rats: an animal model of depression and hyper-responsiveness to antidepressants. *Molecular Psychiatry*, **8**, 925–932.

57 Touma, C., Bunck, M., Glasl, L., Nussbaumer, M., Palme, R., Stein, H., Wolferstatter, M., Zeh, R., Zimbelmann, M., Holsboer, F., and Landgraf, R. (2008) Mice selected for high versus low stress reactivity: a new animal model for affective disorders. *Psychoneuroendocrinology*, **33**, 839–862.

58 Weiss, J.M., Cierpial, M.A., and West, C.H.K. (1998) Selective breeding of rats for high and low motor activity in a swim test: toward a new animal model of depression. *Pharmacology, Biochemistry, and Behavior*, **61**, 49–66.

59 Vollmayr, B. and Henn, F.A. (2001) Learned helplessness in the rat: improvements in validity and reliability. *Brain Research. Brain Research Protocols*, **8**, 1–7.

60 Flaisher-Grinberg, S. and Einat, H. (2009) Mice models for the manic pole of bipolar disorder, in *Mood and Anxiety Related Phenotypes in Mice* (ed. T.D. Gould), Humana Press, pp. 297–326.

61 Gould, T.D. and Einat, H. (2007) Animal models of bipolar disorder and mood stabilizer efficacy: a critical need for improvement. *Neuroscience and Biobehavioral Reviews*, **31**, 825–831.

62 Borison, R.L., Sabelli, H.C., Maple, P.J., Havdala, H.S., and Diamond, B.I. (1978) Lithium prevention of amphetamine-induced 'manic' excitement and of reserpine-induced 'depression' in mice: possible role of 2-phenylethylamine. *Psychopharmacology*, **59**, 259–262.

63 Chen, G., Henter, I.D., and Manji, H.K. (2010) Translational research in bipolar disorder: emerging insights from genetically based models. *Molecular Psychiatry*, **15**, 883–895.

64 Roybal, K., Theobold, D., Graham, A., DiNieri, J.A., Russo, S.J., Krishnan, V., Chakravarty, S., Peevey, J., Oehrlein, N., Birnbaum, S., Vitaterna, M.H., Orsulak, P., Takahashi, J.S., Nestler, E.J., Carlezon, W.A., Jr., and McClung, C.A. (2007) Mania-like behavior induced by disruption of CLOCK. *Proceedings of the National Academy of Sciences of the United States of America*, **104**, 6406–6411.

65 Shaltiel, G., Maeng, S., Malkesman, O., Pearson, B., Schloesser, R.J., Tragon, T., Rogawski, M., Gasior, M., Luckenbaugh, D., Chen, G., and Manji, H.K. (2008) Evidence for the involvement of the kainate receptor subunit GluR6 (GRIK2) in mediating behavioral displays related to behavioral symptoms of mania. *Molecular Psychiatry*, **13**, 858–872.

66 Creson, T.K., Hao, Y., Engel, S., Shen, Y., Hamidi, A., Zhuo, M., Manji, H.K., and Chen, G. (2009) The anterior cingulate ERK pathway contributes to regulation of behavioral excitement and hedonic activity. *Bipolar Disorders*, **11**, 339–350.

67 Prickaerts, J., Moechars, D., Cryns, K., Lenaerts, I., Van, C.H., Goris, I., Daneels, G., Bouwknecht, J.A., and Steckler, T. (2006) Transgenic mice overexpressing glycogen synthase kinase 3beta: a putative model of hyperactivity and mania. *Journal of Neuroscience*, **26**, 9022–9029.

68 Nestler, E.J. and Hyman, S.E. (2010) Animal models of neuropsychiatric disorders. *Nature Neuroscience*, **13**, 1161–1169.

69 Griebel, G. and Holsboer, F. (2012) Neuropeptide receptor ligands as drugs for psychiatric diseases: the end of the beginning? *Nature Reviews. Drug Discovery*, **11**, 462–478.

10
Schizophrenia
Ronan Depoortère and Paul Moser

10.1
Introduction

Schizophrenia is characterized by positive symptoms (thought disorder, delusion, hallucination, and agitation) and negative symptoms (flattening of affect, poverty of speech, social dysfunction, and/or withdrawal) as well as by cognitive deficits (impaired attention and learning and memory problems) [1]. Not only does this disease impose a great toll on the patients and their families but it also stigmatizes patients, further impeding their social insertion. With a prevalence of around 1%, schizophrenia remains a major public health issue. Early attempts at treating this disease included rather esoteric and dangerous approaches, such as extraction of the "stone of madness" by trepanation (immortalized by Hieronymus Bosch in one of his paintings) or brain surgery (cortical lobotomies). These were followed/accompanied by more medically acceptable methods such as sismotherapy and insulin shock.

Nowadays, pharmacotherapy constitutes the mainstay of treatment of this pathology. Although *Rauvolfia serpentina*, a plant that contains the alkaloid reserpine, has been used for centuries in India as the "herb of insanity" to calm down patients, it took until the mid-twentieth century for the synthesis of the first true antipsychotic drug (APD). With the invention of chlorpromazine, by Laborit and Deniker in the early 1950s, the treatment of schizophrenia was revolutionized. Chlorpromazine was followed by a series of APDs, the best known being haloperidol. Elucidation of the mechanism of action of chlorpromazine started in the early 1960s with the hypothesis that it might block noradrenaline, dopamine, and serotonin receptors [2]. However, it was only a decade later that the role of the dopamine (DA) D_2 subtype of receptor in the therapeutic activity of APDs was demonstrated [3].

Despite these early advances, some 60 years after the introduction of chlorpromazine, there still remains a clear need for better compounds in terms of efficacy (around two-third of patients are not satisfactorily treated, especially for negative symptoms and cognitive deficits) and incidence of side effects (mainly extrapyramidal symptoms, such as akathisia, dystonia, and tardive dyskinesia for the first-generation compounds; metabolic disturbances for the newer ones).

Discovery of new APDs is a slow and painstaking process – largely a target-based approach. As such, new chemical entities go through a series of *in vitro* assays to verify that they interact with the target of interest (mainly receptors or enzymes) using affinity and/or pharmacological activity assays. Interesting hits then proceed to the next step of the flowchart: determination of *in vivo* pharmacodynamic effects, in a model(s) considered to be "therapeutically relevant." This step constitutes a pivotal element, but the choice of the model(s) remains problematic. This is particularly true of novel targets for which there is no clinically active compound for pharmacological validation.

Designing an animal model for any psychiatric disease poses a formidable challenge to the scientific community, and schizophrenia is no exception to this rule. Ideally, an animal model should fulfill the criteria of the "holy trilogy," that is, have construct, face, and predictive validity, a task considered totally illusive by some authors [4]. Indeed, considering that we still do not understand the etiology of schizophrenia, there are clearly going to be major difficulties reproducing the mechanisms that trigger this pathology in animals (construct validity).

Similarly, schizophrenia affects to a great extent the cognitive sphere of an individual, a sphere that presents some difficulties to study in the laboratory (e.g., how to model delusions in animals?). The non-pathognomonic nature of the disease adds an extra layer of difficulty: schizophrenic patients can be quite heterogeneous in terms of signs and symptoms. Even for a given patient, these can fluctuate in nature with time. For these various reasons, satisfying the second criterion, face validity, stands as a daunting task.

The final element of the triplet, predictive validity, presents moderate grounds for optimism. Indeed, some preclinical models (mainly those based on the use of DA receptor agonists) have been useful in bringing to fruition "me-too" or "me-also" compounds. There is now a flurry of marketed APDs, their purported primary mechanism of action being blockade of DA D_2 receptors, which were almost exclusively selected based on their activity in this type of model. However, recent failures, exemplified by the lack of efficacy of the mGlu2/3 receptor agonist pomaglumetad in schizophrenia patients [5], despite activity in several relevant preclinical models of LY404 039 (of which pomaglumetad is a prodrug) [6], are here to remind us that the translational value of our models is suboptimal.

Last, but not least, there are time, cost, expertise, and logistic considerations that impose great constraints on the choice of animal models in drug discovery. Setting up an apomorphine-induced climbing assay in mice is much more convenient, faster, and cheaper, and requires less expertise and training than implementing a chronic phencyclidine (PCP)-induced deficit in a touch screen-based cognitive task in monkeys.

This chapter attempts to provide an overview of the *in vivo* models that can be used in the process of APD drug discovery. Emphasis has been laid on models that are most commonly used in drug development processes, but reference to less common ones (mostly because of time and money constraints) is also made.

10.2
Models Amenable to Use in Screening

This section will deal with models whose format and ease of implementation make them amenable to use in screening in the context of drug discovery. For these reasons, such models are almost exclusively implemented in rodents – rats and mice in most cases – under acute conditions of administration. The first cluster of models uses pharmacological agents to induce neurochemical states purported to reproduce those present in schizophrenia (mainly hyperdopaminergia and hypoglutamatergia). The second cluster concerns models that resort to nonpharmacologically induced behaviors.

10.2.1
Models Based on the Use of Pharmacological Agents

This section will describe the most common types of assays used in screening for APDs. The philosophy here is to inject the subjects with a pharmacological compound (i.p., s.c., or p.o., less frequently i.v. or i.c.v.), to produce a distinct behavior and to assess the potential of investigational compounds (almost exclusively injected i.p., s.c., or p.o.) to block this specific behavior.

10.2.1.1 Dopaminergic Agonists

The use of dopaminergic agonists is based on the hypothesis that positive symptoms of schizophrenia arise from a hyperdopaminergic state (see Section 10.1). These models constitute the most commonly used pharmacological models and rely on the administration of either indirect or direct DA receptor agonists: D-amphetamine and apomorphine being the prototypical representatives of the former and latter types, respectively.

Hyperlocomotor Activity Administration of dopaminergic agonists produces a general state of arousal and behavioral activation, which is expressed as enhanced motor activity (horizontal displacement and rearing) at lower doses and stereotypies (head bobbing, gnawing, sniffing, and licking) at higher doses. It has been suggested that these two effects represent activation of limbic and nigrostriatal dopaminergic systems, respectively. Antagonism of hyperlocomotion is thought to indicate potential antipsychotic effects, whereas antagonism of stereotypies may be related to the propensity to induce extrapyramidal side effects (EPS) [7].

D-Amphetamine (1–2 mg/kg i.p. or s.c.) is the most widely used substance to produce hyperlocomotion for screening APDs. Briefly, rats are injected with D-amphetamine and, usually, placed 15–30 min later in activity meters for recording of motor activity for periods varying from 30 min to several hours. The most common method of motor activity detection is by breaking infrared beams that cross the arena in one or two directions perpendicular to each other at a height suitable for the species being studied (e.g., 1 cm for mice and 2 cm for rats).

Apomorphine (or other DA receptor agonists selective for the D_2 and/or D_3 subtypes such as 7-OH-DPAT, PD 128907, or quinpirole) is less widely used and requires a different methodological approach. Thus, contrary to D-amphetamine, which has a much larger magnitude of effect, a period of habituation to the activity meter (usually 15–30 min) is required for observation of enhanced locomotor activity (i.e., to allow basal activity to fall to sufficiently low levels to be able to observe the effects of apomorphine).

Some activity meters also comprise an array of infrared cells placed higher up (around 10–15 cm above the ground) to allow measurement of rearing. Other technologies have been developed to quantify motor activity, the two most common being based on force transducers and on video tracking. In the former, movements of the subject are detected by transducers (strain gauge or piezoelectric accelerometers) placed underneath the activity meter floor. Video tracking procedures (in which the position is determined either by contrast between the animal and the background or by changes in pixel intensity between frames) in particular can offer finer analysis of motor behavior, for example, by computing the average speed or maximal speed of displacement, the amount of time spent in the middle of the activity meter or near its perimeter.

Stereotypies As already mentioned, higher doses of DA receptor agonists produce stereotypies and diminish locomotor activity by means of a behavioral competition phenomenon. Here, the method of scoring is usually manual, and consists in recording the frequency and duration of specific behaviors (e.g., sniffing, licking, biting, etc.). In rats, dopaminergic agents most frequently used are D-amphetamine and apomorphine and, more rarely, methylphenidate. Stereotypies are usually recorded 15–30 min postinjection of the DAergic agent.

In mice, the most common model is apomorphine climbing. Mice are placed in a cylinder whose wall is lined with a wire mesh: apomorphine produces stereotyped climbing behavior (the mouse climbs the mesh and clings to it) [8]. Time spent climbing is usually recorded for a short period (1–2 min). This model presents the advantage of using mice (lower cost and maintenance), short periods of scoring (allowing for greater throughput than locomotor activity or stereotypy assays), simplicity, low cost, and small size of apparatus (Plexiglas or glass cylinder with mesh walls), as well as use of small quantities of pharmacological compounds (particularly advantageous in the context of early-stage screening campaigns for putative APDs).

DA-induced hyperlocomotion, stereotypies, and climbing are sensitive to a whole range of APDs that incorporate DA D_2 receptor antagonist or partial agonist activity in their pharmacological spectrum [9,10].

Prepulse Inhibition of the Startle Reflex Deficits Prepulse inhibition (PPI) of the startle reflex is a phenomenon where the strength of the startle response, elicited by a startling pulse (usually white noise, 110–120 dB, of 30–50 ms duration, alternatively an air puff or light flash), is attenuated by a preceding stimulus of milder amplitude (the prepulse, that is, 70–80 dB, of 10–30 ms duration, delivered around 100 ms before the startling pulse). This model of preattentional sensorimotor gating processes has gained popularity over the years for screening of antipsychotic-like activity. This is based on the fact that psychiatric patients, including schizophrenics, present deficits of PPI [11]. The fact that it can be easily measured in both patients and laboratory animals renders this assay attractive as a tool in translational (bench to bedside) drug development research.

In the laboratory, PPI deficits can be induced by direct (i.e., apomorphine) and indirect (i.e., D-amphetamine) dopaminergic agonists (see Ref. [12]). Of note, there seems to be a difference between rats and mice in their sensitivity to direct dopaminergic D_2/D_3 agonists (which do not produce deficits in the latter species) [13]. In rats, apomorphine-induced PPI disruption is reversed by established APDs whereas some putative APDs (particularly those with substantial agonist activity at serotonergic 5-HT_{1A} receptors) reverse poorly, if at all, these deficits [14].

10.2.1.2 NMDA/Glutamate Receptor Antagonists

The hyperdopaminergic hypothesis of schizophrenia (see above) has been more recently complemented by the hypoglutamatergic hypothesis, considered as being more appropriate to explain some aspects of schizophrenia (such as negative symptoms and cognitive deficits) that could not be accounted for by the hyperdopaminergic hypothesis [15,16]. The most robust argument in favor of the hypoglutamatergic hypothesis is the observation that compounds of the phencyclidine family can induce psychoses in human volunteers [17] and precipitate psychotic episodes in stabilized schizophrenic patients [18,19]. Phencyclidine-like compounds are known to bind to a site localized inside the ionophore of the N-methyl-D-aspartate (NMDA) receptor complex [15], and as such reduce NMDA receptor-mediated glutamatergic transmission.

The two most widely used antiglutamatergic compounds in animal studies are phencyclidine and MK-801 (dizocilpine). Ketamine, possibly because of its very short half-life, is less commonly used in the laboratory, although it is by far the most commonly used in human clinical studies.

Hyperlocomotor Activity Basic principles for measuring this type of behavior are similar to those described for indirect DA agonists. For example, this model has been used to detect activity of DA D_3 receptor antagonists as potential APDs [20]. A recent in-depth analysis of the activity of established and novel putative APDs in the MK-801-induced hyperlocomotor activity model in mice has led the authors to conclude that such a model could be useful in detecting antipsychotic-like activity for compounds acting at $M_{1/4}$ and $mGluR_{2/3}$ receptors [21]. Similarly, ketamine-induced hyperlocomotion in rats is sensitive to a wide range of established and putative APDs [10]. To our knowledge, there appears to be only one comparative study that highlights that some, but not all, APDs could reduce PCP-induced hyperlocomotion [22]. However, having been conducted some 30 years ago, newer APDs are missing from this comparative analysis.

Prepulse Inhibition of the Startle Reflex Deficits As with DAergic agents that increase central DA neurotransmission, NMDA glutamatergic antagonists produce robust deficits in PPI. The first demonstration was made with PCP, the prototypical NMDA glutamatergic noncompetitive antagonist [23]. In addition, disruption of PPI is also seen with competitive antagonists at the glutamate binding site and some antagonists at the associated glycine B site [24]. This type of PPI deficit is usually reported to be sensitive to compounds such as clozapine, but not haloperidol [12]. However, the apparent absence of reduction of PPI with ketamine in humans [25,26] suggests some caution concerning the translational value of this model. This might be a methodological issue as using a brain electromagnetic activity imaging system, Boeijinga *et al.* [27] demonstrated that ketamine could blunt inhibition of the response to a tone burst produced by a preceding click stimulus.

10.2.1.3 Other Pharmacological Agents Used to Induce Behavioural Changes

The following sections concern the use of pharmacological agents that have been more sporadically used in models for detection of antipsychotic activity. Their use is based on the assumption that neurochemical systems other than the dopaminergic and NMDA glutamatergic systems are perturbed in schizophrenia.

10.2.1.4 5-HT$_{2A}$ Receptor Agonists

5-HT$_{2A}$ receptors have been implicated in the etiology of schizophrenia: agonists such as psilocybin and (+)-lysergic acid diethylamide (LSD) produce in humans a psychosis-like state mainly characterized by halucinations [28]. Indeed, risperidone was the first 5-HT$_{2A}$/DA D$_2$ antagonist on the market, with its 5-HT$_{2A}$ component proposed to be responsible for its lower propensity to induce EPS [29]. Additionally, the 5-HT$_{2A}$ inverse agonist pimavanserin (ACP-103) has recently shown activity against psychosis in parkinsonian patients [30]. The two most widely used models with 5-HT$_{2A}$ receptor agonists (mainly 2,5-dimethoxy-4-iodophenyl)-2-aminopropane: DOI) are the deficits in PPI (mostly in rats) and head twitches in mice. More detailed description of the effects of APDs on these two models, as well as the extent of their translational values, is given in Ref. [31].

10.2.1.5 Cannabinoid Receptor Agonists

Recognition that psychosis is associated with the use of hashish is more than a century old [32]. Confirmation of this association has been buttressed by more recent epidemiological, animal, and human psychopharmacological studies [33]. One key finding is that exposure to cannabis during adolescence exposes individuals to an increased risk of developing schizophrenia later on [34]. Although cannabis contains several psychoactive substances, its potency in inducing psychoactive effects seems to depend on its Δ^9-THC content. Based on these epidemiological findings, several studies have investigated the impact of exposing adolescent rats to various cannabinoid agonists. When tested at the adult age, these rats present deficits in PPI and in various cognition models (reviewed in Ref. [35]).

10.2.1.6 Muscarinic Receptor Antagonists

Several lines of evidence implicate the cholinergic system in schizophrenia, and muscarinic receptor antagonists such as scopolamine or atropine can evoke a psychotic state known as "antimuscarinic psychosis," which resembles endogenous schizophrenia [36]. As a consequence, there has been a renewed interest in the use of M_1 and M_4 muscarinic (see Ref. [37]) or $\alpha_4\beta_2$ and α_7 nicotinic (reviewed in Ref. [38]) agonists for schizophrenia.

The scopolamine-induced "antimuscarinic psychosis" has captured the attention of some preclinical scientists. It has been shown that scopolamine, through an increase in striatal DA, produces hyperlocomotion and stereotypies and induces latent inhibition and PPI deficits (reviewed in Ref. [39]). However, the bulk of studies with scopolamine and mecamylamine have focused on impairments produced in models of cognition and memory [39], with few studies investigating the effects of (putative) APDs on these impairments [40–42].

10.2.1.7 Glycine B Receptor Antagonists

The last one, a rather discreet newcomer, has been recently resurrected in the context of the preclinical pharmacological characterization of inhibitors of the glycine transporter type 1 (GLYT1). L-687,414, a NMDA/glycine site (aka glycine B receptor) antagonist, was shown back in 1994 to produce hyperlocomotion in mice by Tricklebank *et al.* [43]. More recently, this model has been pharmacologically explored by Roche scientists, who reported that L-687,414-induced hyperlocomotion in mice is attenuated by several GLYT1 inhibitors, as well as typical and atypical established APDs [44,45]. Depending on the final clinical results with bitopertin (RO-4917838, RG1678), currently completing several phase 3 studies after an initial POC [46] and in the event of its registration, this type of model might occupy a more central position in the years to come.

10.2.2
Models Not Based on the Use of Pharmacological Agents

10.2.2.1 Conditioned Avoidance Response

This is probably one of the most popular models used: the subject is trained to avoid the delivery of a mild electric shock (called the unconditioned stimulus (UCS), usually delivered to the paw by an electrified grid floor) by previous presentation of a cue stimulus (called the conditioned stimulus (CS), usually a tone or a light stimulus). The CS and UCS are separated by 10–20 s in order to allow the animal to respond appropriately to avoid the UCS. Earliest studies used the pole version, where the subject was required to cling to a safety pole in order to avoid or to escape from the shock [47]. Alternative methods have used operant conditioning techniques such as pressing a lever or pulling a chain, and the more common "shuttle box," where the subject is required to travel from one side to the other side of a rectangular box in order to avoid the UCS.

APDs are reported to interfere with the avoidance response, with minimal or lesser effect on the escape response [10] (reviewed in Ref. [48]). Of note, the latency time to escape from the shock is usually taken as a surrogate marker for sedation or motor-interfering effects.

10.2.2.2 Potentiation of PPI of the Startle Reflex

The PPI of the startle reflex model has been quasi-exclusively used in the variants where APDs are tested for their ability to reverse pharmacologically induced PPI deficits. However, there have been several instances where APDs have been reported to enhance basal PPI (listed in Refs [49–51]). It is of interest that potentiation of PPI has been observed with putative APDs with novel mechanism of action: for example, GLYT1 inhibitors have been shown to enhance PPI in DBA2 or C57BL mice [52–54]. If GLYT1 inhibitors prove their utility in the clinic as APDs, this model might represent a fairly straightforward tool to screen for APDs with new mechanisms of action.

10.2.3 Models More Time Consuming and/or Difficult to Implement

The complexity and chronicity of schizophrenia have led to a search for animal models that might better reflect these aspects of the disease as demonstrated by the Measurement and Treatment Research to Improve Cognition in Schizophrenia (MATRICS) and NEWMEDS initiatives [55,56]. Although the acute models discussed earlier remain useful for drug screening and have shown reasonably good pharmacological validity, it would be naïve to think that they are capable of reproducing schizophrenia. In fact, it is naïve to think that *any* procedure would be capable of reproducing schizophrenia in an animal. However, that does not preclude attempts to reproduce processes that may be important in the etiology of schizophrenia. The development of more complex models of schizophrenia has focused around three more or less independent themes, which are often combined. These are (1) attempts to model some of the more complex signs/symptoms of schizophrenia in animals; (2) reproduction of the chronic nature of the disease; and (3) mimicking of the perinatal insults that are thought to be among the risk factors for schizophrenia.

10.2.3.1 Models Aimed at Reproducing More Complex Symptoms of Schizophrenia

Measurement of social interaction and cognitive performance has dominated this area as the animal tests are well established and these symptom domains represent two major areas of unmet need in the treatment of schizophrenia. However, these tests are often time consuming and are not usually suitable for primary drug screening. Social interaction and cognitive deficits are not unique to schizophrenia and so these tests are often combined with a means to induce the deficit, which is usually the same as those already discussed for primary screening, that is, PCP or amphetamine. It would be nice to think that the reversal of a PCP-induced deficit in social interaction would be a better model than reversal of PCP-induced hyperactivity or PPI deficit, but we are not aware of any major differences in the pharmacology of these two approaches. However, by studying behaviors more closely related to the specific symptoms of schizophrenia, it is hoped that drug effects on those behaviors will better translate to therapeutic efficacy as the underlying neuronal systems are often similar. Thus, although the use of these complex behavioral tests is in many ways a simple extension of the use of screening tests such as locomotor activity, it is an attempt to at least study neuronal systems more pertinent to the therapeutic needs of schizophrenics. Indeed, the areas studied with these models, such as social interaction, cognitive impairment, and anhedonia, are all considered to be more pertinent to the negative signs and symptoms of schizophrenia, a major area of unmet therapeutic need.

Models of Social Interaction Deficits Social interaction is typically assessed between two animals in an open field that is often $50 \times 50\,\text{cm}^2$ for rats and $25 \times 25\,\text{cm}^2$ for mice. The exact conditions of testing vary but are important considerations, as the test was originally described as a model for anxiety [57]. Thus, factors such as familiarity and lighting intensity that can affect anxiety levels need to be chosen with care: It appears that low light and familiar conditions should be used to minimize the role that anxiety plays in this test. Social interaction is a complex behavior and it is often valuable to separate different elements such as approach/avoidance behavior, active versus passive social interaction, aggressive versus nonaggressive interaction, nose–nose or nose–anogenital contact, and so on. Additionally, although not very practical, these behaviors should be scored separately for each animal.

Both acute and repeated administration of NMDA antagonists have been reported to decrease social investigation [58–60] and this is the most widely used approach to inducing a deficit in this model. In general, typical antipsychotics such as haloperidol do not acutely reverse these deficits [58,61,62]. Conflicting data exist for clozapine with some authors finding it inactive [61] and others active [58]. Comparable effects of acute administration of PCP and MK-801 occur in the mouse [63,64], although aggression is often more prevalent in this species. Ideally, we are trying to model social withdrawal, which is more prevalent in schizophrenia than is aggression.

Repeated administration of PCP or MK-801 also decreases social investigation in the rat [65], an effect that persists on discontinuation of PCP [66], an approach referred to as subchronic administration (see later). Acute treatment with the atypical agents, ziprasidone and aripiprazole, has been reported to reverse subchronic PCP-induced deficits in social investigation in the rat, whereas similar treatment with haloperidol or clozapine was without effect [67,68]. In the mouse, deficits in social investigation induced by subchronic PCP treatment have been reversed by clozapine but not haloperidol [69].

Overall, these studies suggest that so-called atypical APDs such as clozapine and aripiprazole may be more effective in reversing NMDA antagonist-induced deficits in social interaction in the rat or the mouse than are typical APDs such as haloperidol.

Models of Cognitive Dysfunction Schizophrenic patients have cognitive deficits across a broad range of cognitive domains and these remain one of the least well-treated aspects of the disorder. A concerted effort to develop this field was made in the early 2000s with the MATRICS initiative [70] and the Cognitive Neuroscience Approaches to the Treatment of Impaired Cognition in Schizophrenia (CNTRICS). As far as preclinical models are concerned, there is still not a clear consensus on what might be the appropriate models (see Ref. [71] for a recent review). Among the most commonly used tests are the Morris water maze for spatial memory, object recognition for recognition memory, and 5-choice serial reaction time task (5-CSRTT) for attention/vigilance. Other tests such as latent inhibition have been evaluated to more specifically address the deficits of executive functioning in schizophrenia [72], but these are not used widely.

One recent development is to try and reproduce tests that have analogous procedures in both animals and humans. The 5-CSRTT and related tests are such procedures [73], as are tests using touch screens [74].

10.2.3.2 Models Aimed at Reproducing the Chronic Nature of Schizophrenia

Typically, this approach has used chronic administration of NMDA antagonists such as PCP. In these models, there is an attempt to incorporate adaptive changes that occur in response to the chronic hypoglutamatergic state. One advantage of this approach, compared with studying the acute effects of PCP or MK-801, is that the more dominant acute behavioral changes (such as hyperlocomotion) are attenuated, and thus allow the study of other behaviors without this confounding effect. The duration of PCP treatment typically ranges from 3 to 14 days [60,67,75] with the shorter durations being referred to as "subchronic." More recently, the subchronic approach has become more popular and has been employed in numerous laboratories. What is particularly interesting in this approach is that several behavioral changes, including social interaction deficits, novel object exploration deficits, and so on, have been reported following a 1-week washout period after the final PCP administration [67,76], demonstrating that this approach should be considered to be very different from the use of acute PCP in screening models where the effects are evaluated within 1 or 2 h after administration.

Developmental Models of Schizophrenia The third approach has been to try and reproduce developmental insults that have been identified as contributing to the risk of developing schizophrenia in epidemiological studies. There is a broad consensus that schizophrenia has a neurodevelopmental component [77–79]. The exact nature of the insult that results in these developmental changes does not seem to be particularly specific, with clinical data suggesting that prenatal malnutrition, maternal infection during pregnancy, birth complications, and so on all lead to a small but measurable increase in the incidence of schizophrenia in later life. Few data are available to determine if these various insults all impact a common mechanism, but with such a weight of evidence in favor of the neurodevelopmental hypothesis of schizophrenia, and in the absence of other models with compelling construct validity, it is natural that researchers have tried to reproduce some of these findings in animals. The objective is to understand further how these early insults can affect brain development and the appearance of schizophrenia-like symptoms, and also to serve as a model for testing putative antipsychotic treatments.

Maternal Infection/Immune Challenge   Maternal viral, bacterial, or parasitic infections during pregnancy are associated with an increased risk of schizophrenia in the offspring (reviewed in Ref. [80]). Although much of the evidence has revolved around influenza, many types of infections have been implicated, suggesting that it is activation of the immune system rather than a particular pathogen that is responsible for the increased risk. This has led to the development of models where immune system activation is obtained using, for example, the influenza virus, the parasite *Toxoplasma gondii*, the bacterial endotoxin lipopolysaccharide (LPS), the viral mimic polyriboinosinic–polyribocytidylic acid (polyI:C), or the proinflammatory cytokine interleukin-6 [81,82]. The mid-phase of gestation is typically targeted with these interventions and both rats and mice have been used successfully [82]. Of particular interest for this model is the observation that behavioral abnormalities appear only at late adolescence.

These models have been extensively studied in tests pertaining to schizophrenia such as locomotor activity, sensitivity to psychostimulants, sensorimotor gating (PPI), vigilance, and cognitive deficits (for review, see Ref. [83]). The deficits observed in these models have also been extended to tests pertinent to negative symptoms where both the polyI:C and influenza virus models have demonstrated a deficit in social interaction [84,85].

Ventral Hippocampal Lesion   First described in Ref. [86], this model has been the subject of several recent reviews [87,88]. Essentially, the model consists of an excitotoxic lesion of the ventral hippocampus around postnatal day 7 using ibotenic acid. Behavioral testing of neonatally lesioned rats is typically undertaken from around postnatal day 30, that is, after weaning and usually after puberty.

Numerous studies in different laboratories have demonstrated effects in a wide range of tests pertinent to schizophrenia, including deficits in social interaction, anhedonia, increased reactivity to stimulants, and deficits in PPI [89–94], suggesting that the effects of these lesions are robust.

Drug effects have been extensively evaluated against these deficits, and in general the results show that those behavioral changes thought to be more related to the positive symptoms (hyperactivity, PPI deficits, etc.) are reversed by current APDs, in contrast to deficits in social interaction, more pertinent to negative symptomatology, that are not reversed [92].

Very recently, Naert *et al.* [95] have applied the neonatal ventral hippocampus lesion to mice. Using an electrolytic lesion on postnatal day 6 they reproduced many of the effects seen in the rat model, including hyperactivity and hypersensitivity to amphetamine, as well as cognitive deficits.

10.2.3.3 Models Based on Genetic Manipulations

Schizophrenia has a major genetic component [96], although the gene(s) implicated have not yet been clearly identified. Numerous putative genetic risk factors have been identified through linkage studies, and there has been substantial work exploring the consequences of modifying these genes in transgenic rodents. This work has primarily been concerned with identifying the phenotypical effects of various genetic modifications rather than being used to provide models for testing putative APDs. However, despite a wider availability of knockout (KO) mice, this approach has gained only modest momentum over the years, for obvious reasons of complexity and cost of carrying behavioral and pharmacological studies with KO mice. Nonetheless, we think this approach will probably gain a more privileged status in future APD drug discovery strategies.

Mice Genetically Modified for Susceptibility Genes There have been numerous genes associated with putative pathophysiological mechanisms of, and candidate risk genes for, schizophrenia: these have formed the basis for the generation of a dozen or so transgenic lines. The main genes to have been investigated are Disc1 and NRG1, with additional ones such as ERBB4, dysbindin, and reelin. Studies covering these genes are reviewed in Refs [97,98].

Dopamine Transporter (DAT) Knockout Mice The use of this type of KO mouse is justified by the fact that they present an augmented dopaminergic tone. Indeed, as a result, DAT KO mice display hyperlocomotor activity and stereotypies in a novel environment, and PPI deficits. These can be normalized by APDs such as haloperidol, raclopride, and clozapine (reviewed in Ref. [99]).

Glutamatergic System Genetically Modified Mice As a mirror image to the use of DAT in the context of the hyperdopaminergic hypothesis, several transgenic rodents with a hypoglutamatergic status have been generated. Thus, mice with NMDA type 1 receptor expression reduced by 95% display behaviors related to schizophrenia such as hyperactivity and social interaction deficits [100]. Likewise, Grin1(D481N) mutant mice, with reduced occupancy of the glycine/NMDA binding site, present hyperactivity and increased stereotypies [101].

10.2.4
Models for Side Effects

Like most, if not all, medicines, APDs can display a broad array of side effects, including EPS, weight gain, metabolic and endocrine disturbances, autonomic dysfunctions (orthostatic hypotension, dry mouth, and blurred vision), cardiovascular impact (tachycardia and QT interval prolongation), and sexual dysfunction, to cite the main ones. One aspect of APD development that has gained momentum recently is the study of potential side effects of putative APDs. Whereas the search for a procataleptogenic potential or a cardiovascular impact has been customary for decades, with the advent of new-generation APDs, less inclined to produce EPS but more prone to metabolic side effects, there has been an effort at setting up preclinical models addressing the latter. In the following section, we have briefly addressed the more serious side effects that have been associated with APDs.

10.2.4.1 Models for Motor Side Effects

Dopamine is a neurotransmitter that plays a central role in the initiation and control of motor output. Whereas hyperdopaminergic states provoke hyperlocomotion and stereotypies (see above), hypodopaminergia, consecutive to blockade of DA D_2 receptors or neurodegeneration of dopaminergic neurons (as in Parkinson's disease), produces motor impairment. Thus, APDs, especially those from the first generation (i.e., chlorpromazine, fluphenazine, and haloperidol), are prone to produce EPS. The latter can take the form of dystonia (abnormal posture and slow movements), parkinsonism (hypokinesia, rigidity, and resting tremor), akathisia (motor restlessness), and dyskinesia (abnormal movements). Although second-generation APDs are less prone to produce EPS, the possibility of evoking these motor side effects with putative APDs is of concern, and necessitates testing them in models with predictive validity.

Catalepsy in Rodents Catalepsy (the inability to move from an awkward and uncomfortable position) is considered to have validity in predicting potential to produce EPS and is fairly straightforward to measure in rodents. There are three main techniques: the bar, the crossed legs, and the four platforms tests. In the first one, the forelimbs are placed on a horizontal, cylindrical bar (around 1 cm diameter, 10 cm above the bench surface for a rat). In the second test, each hind limb is placed over its ipsilateral forelimb. In the final test, each paw is positioned on a wooden platform ($\sim 1\,\text{cm}^2$, 8–10 and 12–15 cm between contralateral and ipsilateral platforms, respectively). For all three variants, the time spent in these constrained positions is recorded, with a time-out limit usually around 30–60 s. An extensive comparative study of the cataleptogenic potential of APDs has been published by Bardin *et al.* [10].

Paw Test in Rodents This model was originally described in Ref. [102]. It consists in placing a rat on a platform fitted with four holes appropriately spaced apart to comfortably accommodate all four paws, and a groove for the tail. The experimenter then records the latency time before the subject retracts its forelimbs and hind limbs, following pretreatment with an APD. The paw test is considered to discriminate between first-generation APDs, which are equipotent in prolonging both the forelimb and hindlimb retraction time, and atypical APDs, which are much more potent in prolonging hindlimb than forelimb retraction time. This test, easy and quite fast to implement, has been explored pharmacologically by other teams [103–108].

Catalepsy-Associated Behavior and Haloperidol Sensitization in Monkeys Catalepsy-associated behavior (CAB) is considered to represent a better model of EPS in humans than catalepsy in rodents [109]. In effect, nonhuman primates, following administration of an APD such as haloperidol, display a wider array of abnormal motor postures (crouching, decreased head movements, static posture, abnormal positions, etc.) than rodents (catalepsy). As such, this model is considered to allow for a more refined analysis of the potential of APDs to produce EPS in humans. Indeed, it can differentiate between some partial agonists and antagonists at DA D_2 receptors, with only the latter producing CAB [110]. In contrast, neither type produces catalepsy in rodents [10]. The main and most obvious drawbacks of this model are that it necessitates having access to a colony of monkeys, and that periods of washout are necessary between two successive administrations of APDs.

10.2.4.2 Hyperprolactinemia

Increased circulating level of prolactin is considered to be the consequence of the blocking of DA D_2 receptors located on lactotroph neurons in the pituitary gland. Although considered central, these receptors lie outside the blood–brain barrier, so that APDs with low central bioavailability (i.e., risperidone, sulpiride, etc.) are prone to this type of side effect. In addition to sexual dysfunction, galactorrhea, and gynecomastia, long-term hyperprolactinemia can lead to breast and prostate cancer [111]. Testing of prolactinemic effects of APDs is straightforward, and requires blood sampling with subsequent determination of plasma levels of prolactin with a commercially available kit. There are notable differences in the efficacy and potency of classical and newer APDs to produce hyperprolactinemia [112], with partial agonists at DA D_2 receptors having a lower propensity to do so.

10.2.4.3 Sedation and Motor Incoordination

Locomotor activity and rotarod are used to assess sedation and motor coordination, respectively, albeit only rarely for the latter [113]. In general, the intrinsic effects of APDs on spontaneous locomotor activity are recorded in parallel with those on hyperlocomotion induced by a DA agonist or NMDA glutamatergic antagonist. Care should be taken to record effects over comparable time windows to avoid possible pharmacokinetic concerns. It is generally considered that the wider the potency difference between inhibition of hyperlocomotion and effects on spontaneous locomotion, the better.

10.2.4.4 Models for Cognitive Side Effects

Some of the models described earlier to assess the ability of APDs to attenuate cognitive deficits can also be used to evaluate the potential negative impact of APDs themselves on the cognitive sphere. In effect, patients frequently present cognitive deficits, so that it appears justified to assess the negative impact of APDs on preclinical models of cognition/memory.

10.2.4.5 Metabolic Disorders Models

Considering the mounting problem of metabolic syndrome observed with newer APDs, most notably clozapine and olanzapine, several studies have looked at the impact of protracted administration of APDs on various measures such as weight gain, adiposity, lipidemia, and glucose tolerance (for a list of studies on weight gain, see Ref. [114]).

10.2.4.6 Models for Cardiovascular Effects

Long-term use of APDs is associated with increased mortality from cardiovascular events [115]. Thus, the impact of experimental APDs on the cardiovascular system has become the object of close scrutiny. Some APDs inhibit the delayed potassium rectifier channel in cardiac tissue (coded by the human ether-a-go-go-related gene (hERG)), causing prolongation of the QT interval. This undesirable property has led to the temporary withdrawal of sertindole from the market. Prolongation of the QT interval can trigger ventricular tachycardia with "torsade de pointes," possibly leading to sudden cardiac death [116]. Thus, binding to hERG channel or recording of hERG channel currents with the patch-clamp technique constitutes the front-line approach for evaluating potential cardiovascular adverse effects of ADs. This is complemented by assessment of changes in the action potential in isolated rabbit or dog Purkinje fibers, and ECG recording in anaesthetized or awake rats, dogs, or monkeys [117].

10.3
Translation to the Clinic: Limitations and Difficulties

As alluded to above, schizophrenia is one of the most complex pathologies affecting the most complex organ (brain) and functions (cognition and memory) of the most complex species (humans). As a consequence, the use of animals (mostly rodents) with simpler neuroanatomical characteristics and cognitive capacities far more limited than those of humans presents a major reductionist drawback. There seems to be little that can be done to change this. Current animal models of schizophrenia present other weak points, which could be – at least partially – addressed, some of which are briefly discussed in the following sections.

10.3.1
Use of "Standard Subjects"

Fortunately, schizophrenia affects only a few percent of the human population. This consideration is seldom, if ever, integrated in the "required technical specifications" of an animal model of this disease. APDs, whether those clinically used or at the investigational level, are in most cases tested in a cohort of "standard" animal subjects. There appears to have been very few attempts at circumventing or at least addressing this confounding effect. One such instance is where rats were first screened for their high response to novelty or their sensitivity to the effects of the direct DAergic agent apomorphine, giving rise after successive generational breeding to a colony of "Apo-susceptible" rats [118]. This approach could be considered akin to that mentioned earlier of using genetically modified animals.

Another tactic to answer the critique of using "standard" subjects would be to preselect subjects based on neurochemical or behavioral characteristics. Indeed, one of the present authors (R.D.) attempted to select rats based on their basal level of PPI. Whereas the group means (i.e., low versus high PPI values) clearly separated session after session, there were enough intraindividual variations from one session to the next within the same group to cast doubts about the utility of this approach (unpublished data).

10.3.2
From Here to . . . ?

Perhaps experimental models combining several possible etiologic factors for schizophrenia will help shed light on the underlying pathological process and assist in the search for better pharmacotherapy. One such combination includes susceptibility genes and manipulations that impair neurodevelopment. For example, recent studies have combined neonatal immune activation with polyI:C (see above) in inducible human dominant-negative form of DISC1 genetically manipulated mice. These mice exhibited impaired object recognition, social recognition and interaction, and augmented susceptibility to MK-801-induced hyperactivity [119]. Of interest, it was subsequently reported that both clozapine (3 mg/kg) and haloperidol (1 mg/kg) administered once a day p.o. 1 week before behavioral testing suppressed the augmentation of MK-801-induced hyperactivity, but only the former improved the deficit in the novel object recognition task [120]. Other examples are detailed in Ref. [121]. However, such sophisticated models cannot constitute first-line elements in a drug discovery program, and can only be reserved for selected drug candidates. On the other hand, we should perhaps expect that modeling a complex disorder such as schizophrenia will require model systems that have a suitable level of complexity. Perhaps the difficulty of finding novel APDs over the last half-century is a reflection of the fact that we have clung on for too long to the idea that we can manage with the simple screening models described in the first part of this chapter: To take the next leap, it is likely that the more complex models described here will need to become the norm. Indeed, it also seems likely that we will need to combine several of these approaches (e.g., a neurodevelopmental insult on a specific genetic background followed by assessment in a complex behavioral task related to specific symptom domains) in order to identify truly novel therapeutic agents for this disorder.

References

1 Andreasen, N.C., Flaum, M., Swayze, V.W., Tyrrell, G., and Arndt, S. (1990) Positive and negative symptoms in schizophrenia. A critical reappraisal. *Archives of General Psychiatry*, **47**, 615–621.

2 Carlsson, A. and Lindqvist, M. (1963) Effect of chlorpromazine or haloperidol on formation of 3-methoxytyramine and normetanephrine in mouse brain. *Acta Pharmacologica et Toxicologica*, **20**, 140–144.

3 Seeman, P., Chau-Wong, M., Tedesco, J., and Wong, K. (1975) Brain receptors for antipsychotic drugs and dopamine: direct binding assays. *Proceedings of the National Academy of Sciences of the United States of America*, **72**, 4376–4380.

4 Willner, P. (1984) The validity of animal models of depression. *Psychopharmacology*, **83** (1), 1–16.

5 Eli-Lilly (2012) Lilly stops Phase III development of pomaglumetad methionil for the treatment of schizophrenia based on efficacy results. Eli-Lilly press release. Available at http://lilly.mediaroom.com/index.php?s=9042&item=132278 (accessed August 29, 2012).

6 Rorick-Kehn, L.M., Johnson, B.G., Burkey, J.L., Wright, R.A., Calligaro, D.O., Marek, G.J., Nisenbaum, E.S., Catlow, J.T., Kingston, A.E., Giera, D.D., Herin, M.F., Monn, J.A., McKinzie, D.L., and Schoepp, D.D. (2007) Pharmacological and pharmacokinetic properties of a structurally novel, potent, and selective metabotropic glutamate 2/3 receptor agonist: *in vitro* characterization of agonist (−)-(1R,4S,5S,6S)-4-amino-2-sulfonylbicyclo[3.1.0]-hexane-4, 6-dicarboxylic acid (LY404039). *The Journal of Pharmacology and Experimental Therapeutics*, **321** (1), 308–317.

7 Costall, B., Domeney, A.M., and Naylor, R.J. (1982) Behavioural and biochemical consequences of persistent overstimulation of mesolimbic dopamine systems in the rat. *Neuropharmacology*, **21** (4), 327–335.

8 Protais, P., Costentin, J., and Schwartz, J.C. (1976) Climbing behavior induced by apomorphine in mice: a simple test for the study of dopamine receptors in striatum. *Psychopharmacology*, **50** (1), 1–6.

9 Bardin, L., Kleven, M.S., Barret-Grévoz, C., Depoortère, R., and Newman-Tancredi, A. (2006) Antipsychotic-like vs cataleptogenic actions in mice of novel antipsychotics having D2 antagonist and 5-HT$_{1A}$ agonist properties. *Neuropsychopharmacology*, **31** (9), 1869–1879.

10 Bardin, L., Auclair, A., Kleven, M.S., Prinssen, E.P., Koek, W., Newman-Tancredi, A., and Depoortère, R. (2007) Pharmacological profiles in rats of novel antipsychotics with combined dopamine D$_2$/serotonin 5-HT$_{1A}$ activity: comparison with typical and atypical conventional antipsychotics. *Behavioural Pharmacology*, **18** (2), 103–118.

11 Braff, D., Stone, C., Callaway, E., Geyer, M., Glick, I., and Bali, L. (1978) Prestimulus effects on human startle reflex in normals and schizophrenics. *Psychophysiology*, **15** (4), 339–343.

12 Geyer, M.A., Krebs-Thomson, K., Braff, D.L., and Swerdlow, N.R. (2001) Pharmacological studies of prepulse inhibition models of sensorimotor gating deficits in schizophrenia: a decade in review. *Psychopharmacology*, **156** (2–3), 117–154.

13 Ralph-Williams, R.J., Lehmann-Masten, V., and Geyer, M.A. (2003) Dopamine D$_1$ rather than D$_2$ receptor agonists disrupt prepulse inhibition of startle in mice. *Neuropsychopharmacology*, **28** (1), 108–118.

14 Auclair, A.L., Kleven, M.S., Besnard, J., Depoortère, R., and Newman-Tancredi, A. (2006) Actions of novel antipsychotic agents on apomorphine-induced PPI disruption: influence of combined serotonin 5-HT$_{1A}$ receptor activation and dopamine D$_2$ receptor blockade. *Neuropsychopharmacology*, **31** (9), 1900–1909.

15 Javitt, D.C. and Zukin, S.R. (1991) Recent advances in the phencyclidine model of schizophrenia. *The American Journal of Psychiatry*, **148**, 1301–1308.

16 Olney, J.W. and Farber, N.B. (1995) Glutamate receptor dysfunction and

17. Allen, R.M. and Young, S.J. (1978) Phencyclidine-induced psychosis. *The American Journal of Psychiatry*, **135**, 1081–1084.
18. Lahti, A.C., Koffel, B., LaPorte, D., and Tamminga, C.A. (1995) Subanesthetic doses of ketamine stimulate psychosis in schizophrenia. *Neuropsychopharmacology*, **13**, 9–19.
19. Tamminga, C.A., Holcomb, H.H., Gao, X.M., and Lahti, A.C. (1995) Glutamate pharmacology and the treatment of schizophrenia: current status and future directions. *International Clinical Psychopharmacology*, **10** (Suppl. 3), 29–37.
20. Leriche, L., Schwartz, J.C., and Sokoloff, P. (2003) The dopamine D_3 receptor mediates locomotor hyperactivity induced by NMDA receptor blockade. *Neuropharmacology*, **45** (2), 174–181.
21. Bradford, A.M., Savage, K.M., Jones, D.N., and Kalinichev, M. (2010) Validation and pharmacological characterisation of MK-801-induced locomotor hyperactivity in BALB/C mice as an assay for detection of novel antipsychotics. *Psychopharmacology*, **212** (2), 155–170.
22. Freed, W.J., Bing, L.A., and Wyatt, R.J. (1984) Effects of neuroleptics on phencyclidine (PCP)-induced locomotor stimulation in mice. *Neuropharmacology*, **23** (2A), 175–181.
23. Mansbach, R.S. and Geyer, M.A. (1989) Effects of phencyclidine and phencyclidine biologs on sensorimotor gating in the rat. *Neuropsychopharmacology*, **2** (4), 299–308.
24. Depoortere, R., Perrault, G., and Sanger, D.J. (1999) Prepulse inhibition of the startle reflex in rats: effects of compounds acting at various sites on the NMDA receptor complex. *Behavioural Pharmacology*, **10** (1), 51–62.
25. Abel, K.M., Allin, M.P., Hemsley, D.R., and Geyer, M.A. (2003) Low dose ketamine increases prepulse inhibition in healthy men. *Neuropharmacology*, **44** (6), 729–737.
26. Heekeren, K., Neukirch, A., Daumann, J., Stoll, M., Obradovic, M., Kovar, K.A., Geyer, M.A., and Gouzoulis-Mayfrank, E. (2007) Prepulse inhibition of the startle reflex and its attentional modulation in the human S-ketamine and N,N-dimethyltryptamine (DMT) models of psychosis. *Journal of Psychopharmacology (Oxford, England)*, **21** (3), 312–320.
27. Boeijinga, P.H., Soufflet, L., Santoro, F., and Luthringer, R. (2007) Ketamine effects on CNS responses assessed with MEG/EEG in a passive auditory sensory-gating paradigm: an attempt for modelling some symptoms of psychosis in man. *Journal of Psychopharmacology (Oxford, England)*, **21** (3), 321–337.
28. Nichols, D.E. (2004) Hallucinogens. *Pharmacology & Therapeutics*, **101** (2), 131–181.
29. Meltzer, H.Y. (1995) Role of serotonin in the action of atypical antipsychotic drugs. *Clinical Neuroscience*, **3** (2), 64–75.
30. ACADIA (2012) ACADIA announces pimavanserin meets primary and key secondary endpoints in pivotal Phase III Parkinson's disease psychosis trial. ACADIA press release. Available at http://ir.acadia-pharm.com/phoenix.zhtml?c=125180&p=irol-newsArticle&ID=1761922&highlight= (accessed November 27, 2012).
31. Halberstadt, A.L. and Geyer, M.A. (2013) Serotonergic hallucinogens as translational models relevant to schizophrenia. *The International Journal of Neuropsychopharmacology*, **13**, 1–16.
32. Warnock, J. (1903) Insanity from hasheesh. *Journal of Mental Science*, **49**, 96–110.
33. D'Souza, D.C., Sewell, R.A., and Ranganathan, M. (2009) Cannabis and psychosis/schizophrenia: human studies. *European Archives of Psychiatry and Clinical Neuroscience*, **259** (7), 413–431.
34. Andreasson, S., Allebeck, P., Engstrom, A., and Rydberg, U. (1987) Cannabis and schizophrenia. A longitudinal study of Swedish conscripts. *Lancet*, **2**, 1483–1486.
35. Malone, D.T., Hill, M.N., and Rubino, T. (2010) Adolescent cannabis use and psychosis: epidemiology and neurodevelopmental models. *British Journal of Pharmacology*, **160** (3), 511–522.
36. Terry, A.V. Jr. (2008) Role of the central cholinergic system in the therapeutics of

37 Money, T.T., Scarr, E., Udawela, M., Gibbons, A.S., Jeon, W.J., Seo, M.S., and Dean, B. (2010) Treating schizophrenia: novel targets for the cholinergic system. *CNS & Neurological Disorders – Drug Targets*, **9** (2), 241–256.

38 Haydar, S.N. and Dunlop, J. (2010) Neuronal nicotinic acetylcholine receptors: targets for the development of drugs to treat cognitive impairment associated with schizophrenia and Alzheimer's disease. *Current Topics in Medicinal Chemistry*, **10** (2), 144–152.

39 Barak, S. (2009) Modeling cholinergic aspects of schizophrenia: focus on the antimuscarinic syndrome. *Behavioural Brain Research*, **204** (2), 335–351.

40 Depoortere, R., Auclair, A.L., Bardin, L., Bruins Slot, L., Kleven, M.S., Colpaert, F. et al. (2007) F15063, a compound with D_2/D_3 antagonist, $5\text{-}HT_{1A}$ agonist and D_4 partial agonist properties. III. Activity in models of cognition and negative symptoms. *British Journal of Pharmacology*, **151** (2), 266–277.

41 Millan, M.J., Loiseau, F., Dekeyne, A., Gobert, A., Flik, G., Cremers, T.I. et al. (2008) S33138 (N-[4-[2-[(3aS,9bR)-8-cyano-1,3a,4,9b-tetrahydro[1] benzopyrano[3,4-c] pyrrol-2(3H)-yl]-ethyl]phenyl-acetamide), a preferential dopamine D_3 versus D_2 receptor antagonist and potential antipsychotic agent. III. Actions in models of therapeutic activity and induction of side effects. *The Journal of Pharmacology and Experimental Therapeutics*, **324** (3), 1212–1226.

42 Barak, S. and Weiner, I. (2011) The M1/M4 preferring agonist xanomeline reverses amphetamine-, MK801- and scopolamine-induced abnormalities of latent inhibition: putative efficacy against positive, negative and cognitive symptoms in schizophrenia. *The International Journal of Neuropsychopharmacology*, **14** (9), 1233–1246.

43 Tricklebank, M.D., Bristow, L.J., Hutson, P.H., Leeson, P.D., Rowley, M., Saywell, K., Singh, L., Tattersall, F.D., Thorn, L., and Williams, B.J. (1994) The anticonvulsant and behavioural profile of L-687,414, a partial agonist acting at the glycine modulatory site on the N-methyl-D-aspartate (NMDA) receptor complex. *British Journal of Pharmacology*, **113** (3), 729–736.

44 Alberati, D., Moreau, J.L., Mory, R., Pinard, E., and Wettstein, J.G. (2010) Pharmacological evaluation of a novel assay for detecting glycine transporter 1 inhibitors and their antipsychotic potential. *Pharmacology, Biochemistry, and Behavior*, **97** (2), 185–191.

45 Alberati, D., Moreau, J.L., Lengyel, J., Hauser, N., Mory, R., Borroni, E., Pinard, E., Knoflach, F., Schlotterbeck, G., Hainzl, D., and Wettstein, J.G. (2012) Glycine reuptake inhibitor RG1678: a pharmacologic characterization of an investigational agent for the treatment of schizophrenia. *Neuropharmacology*, **62** (2), 1152–1161.

46 Umbricht, D., Martin-Facklam, M., Pizzagalli, F. et al. (2012) Glycine transporter type 1 (GlyT1) inhibitor RG1678: results of the proof-of-concept study for the treatment of negative symptoms in schizophrenia. 28th CINP World Congress of Neuropsychopharmacology, The International College of Neuropsychopharmacology (CINP), No. S28.

47 Cook, L. and Weidley, E. (1957) Behavioral effects of some psychopharmacological agents. *Annals of the New York Academy of Sciences*, **66** (3), 740–752.

48 Wadenberg, ML. (2010) Conditioned avoidance response in the development of new antipsychotics. *Current Pharmaceutical Design*, **16** (3), 358–370.

49 Depoortere, R., Perrault, G., and Sanger, D.J. (1997) Potentiation of prepulse inhibition of the startle reflex in rats: pharmacological evaluation of the procedure as a model for detecting antipsychotic activity. *Psychopharmacology*, **132** (4), 366–374.

50 Depoortere, R., Perrault, G., and Sanger, D.J. (1997) Some, but not all, antipsychotic drugs potentiate a low level of prepulse inhibition shown by rats of the Wistar strain. *Behavioural Pharmacology*, **8** (4), 364–372.

51 Ouagazzal, A.M., Jenck, F., and Moreau, J.L. (2001) Drug-induced potentiation of prepulse inhibition of acoustic startle reflex in mice: a model for detecting antipsychotic activity? *Psychopharmacology*, **156** (2–3), 273–283.

52 Depoortère, R., Dargazanli, G., Estenne-Bouhtou, G., Coste, A., Lanneau, C., Desvignes, C., Poncelet, M., Heaulme, M., Santucci, V., Decobert, M., Cudennec, A., Voltz, C., Boulay, D., Terranova, J.P., Stemmelin, J., Roger, P., Marabout, B., Sevrin, M., Vigé, X., Biton, B., Steinberg, R., Françon, D., Alonso, R., Avenet, P., Oury-Donat, F., Perrault, G., Griebel, G., George, P., Soubrié, P., and Scatton, B. (2005) Neurochemical, electrophysiological and pharmacological profiles of the selective inhibitor of the glycine transporter-1 SSR504734, a potential new type of antipsychotic. *Neuropsychopharmacology*, **30** (11), 1963–1985.

53 Kopec, K., Flood, D.G., Gasior, M., McKenna, B.A., Zuvich, E., Schreiber, J., Salvino, J.M., Durkin, J.T., Ator, M.A., and Marino, M.J. (2010) Glycine transporter (GlyT1) inhibitors with reduced residence time increase prepulse inhibition without inducing hyperlocomotion in DBA/2 mice. *Biochemical Pharmacology*, **80** (9), 1407–1417.

54 Singer, P., Zhang, W., and Yee, BK. (2013) SSR504734 enhances basal expression of prepulse inhibition but exacerbates the disruption of prepulse inhibition by apomorphine. *Psychopharmacology*, **230** (2), 309–317.

55 Hughes, B. (2009) Novel consortium to address shortfall in innovative medicines for psychiatric disorders. *Nature Reviews. Drug Discovery*, **8**, 523–524.

56 Lustig, C., Kozak, R., Sarter, M., Young, J.W., and Robbins, T.W. (2013) CNTRICS final animal model task selection: control of attention. *Neuroscience and Biobehavioral Reviews*, **37**, 2099–2110.

57 File, S.E., Ouagazzal, A.M., Gonzalez, L.E., and Overstreet, D.H. (1999) Chronic fluoxetine in tests of anxiety in rat lines selectively bred for differential 5-HT$_{1A}$ receptor function. *Pharmacology, Biochemistry, and Behavior*, **62**, 695–701.

58 Becker, A. and Grecksch, G. (2004) Ketamine-induced changes in rat behaviour: a possible animal model of schizophrenia. Test of predictive validity. *Progress in Neuro-Psychopharmacology and Biological Psychiatry*, **28**, 1267–1277.

59 Rung, J.P., Carlsson, A., Ryden, M.K., and Carlsson, M.L. (2005) (+)-MK-801 induced social withdrawal in rats: a model for negative symptoms of schizophrenia. *Progress in Neuro-Psychopharmacology and Biological Psychiatry*, **29**, 827–832.

60 Sams-Dodd, F. (1999) Phencyclidine in the social interaction test: an animal model of schizophrenia with face and predictive validity. *Reviews in the Neurosciences*, **10**, 59–90.

61 Boulay, D., Depoortere, R., Louis, C., Perrault, G., Griebel, G., and Soubrie, P. (2004) SSR181507, a putative atypical antipsychotic with dopamine D$_2$ antagonist and 5-HT$_{1A}$ agonist activities: improvement of social interaction deficits induced by phencyclidine in rats. *Neuropharmacology*, **46**, 1121–1129.

62 Rung, J.P., Carlsson, A., Markinhuhta, K.R., and Carlsson, M.L. (2005) The dopaminergic stabilizers (−)-OSU6162 and ACR16 reverse (+)-MK-801-induced social withdrawal in rats. *Progress in Neuro-Psychopharmacology and Biological Psychiatry*, **29**, 833–839.

63 Olszewski, R.T., Wegorzewska, M.M., Monteiro, A.C., Krolikowski, K.A., Zhou, J., Kozikowski, A.P., Long, K., Mastropaolo, J., Deutsch, S.I., and Neale, J.H. (2008) Phencyclidine and dizocilpine induced behaviors reduced by N-acetylaspartylglutamate peptidase inhibition via metabotropic glutamate receptors. *Biological Psychiatry*, **63**, 86–91.

64 Zou, H., Zhang, C., Xie, Q., Zhang, M., Shi, J., Jin, M., and Yu, L. (2008) Low dose MK-801 reduces social investigation in mice. *Pharmacology, Biochemistry, and Behavior*, **90**, 753–757.

65 Geyer, M.A. and Ellenbroek, B. (2003) Animal behavior models of the mechanisms underlying antipsychotic atypicality. *Progress in Neuro-Psychopharmacology and Biological Psychiatry*, **27**, 1071–1079.

66 Tanaka, K., Suzuki, M., Sumiyoshi, T., Murata, M., Tsunoda, M., and Kurachi, M. (2003) Subchronic phencyclidine administration alters central vasopressin receptor binding and social interaction in the rat. *Brain Research*, **992**, 239–245.

67 Snigdha, S. and Neill, J.C. (2008) Efficacy of antipsychotics to reverse phencyclidine-induced social interaction deficits in female rats: a preliminary investigation. *Behavioural Brain Research*, **187**, 489–494.

68 Snigdha, S. and Neill, J.C. (2008) Improvement of phencyclidine-induced social behaviour deficits in rats: involvement of 5-HT$_{1A}$ receptors. *Behavioural Brain Research*, **191**, 26–31.

69 Qiao, H., Noda, Y., Kamei, H., Nagai, T., Furukawa, H., Miura, H., Kayukawa, Y., Ohta, T., and Nabeshima, T. (2001) Clozapine, but not haloperidol, reverses social behavior deficit in mice during withdrawal from chronic phencyclidine treatment. *Neuroreport*, **12**, 11–15.

70 Marder, S.R. and Fenton, W. (2004) Measurement and Treatment Research to Improve Cognition in Schizophrenia: NIMH MATRICS initiative to support the development of agents for improving cognition in schizophrenia. *Schizophrenia Research*, **72** (1), 5–9.

71 Young, J.W., Powell, S.B., and Geyer, M.A. (2012) Mouse pharmacological models of cognitive disruption relevant to schizophrenia. *Neuropharmacology*, **62**, 1381–1390.

72 Moser, P.C., Hitchcock, J.M., Lister, S., and Moran, P.M. (2000) The pharmacology of latent inhibition as an animal model of schizophrenia. *Brain Research. Brain Research Reviews*, **33** (2–3), 275–307.

73 Lustig, C.1., Kozak, R., Sarter, M., Young, J.W. and Robbins, T.W. (2013) CNTRICS final animal model task selection: control of attention. *Neuroscience & Biobehavioral Reviews*, **37** (9 Pt B), 2099–2110.

74 Bussey, T.J., Holmes, A., Lyon, L., Mar, A. C., McAllister, K.A.L., Nithianantharajah, J., Oomen, C.J., and Saksida, L.M. (2012) New translational assays for preclinical modelling of cognition in schizophrenia: the touch screen testing method for mice and rats. *Neuropharmacology*, **62**, 1191–1203.

75 Lee, P.R., Brady, D.L., Shapiro, R.A., Dorsa, D.M., and Koenig, J.I. (2005) Social interaction deficits caused by chronic phencyclidine administration are reversed by oxytocin. *Neuropsychopharmacology*, **30**, 1883–1894.

76 Snigdha, S., Idris, N., Grayson, B., Shahid, M., and Neill, J.C. (2011) Asenapine improves phencyclidine-induced object recognition deficits in the rat: evidence for engagement of a dopamine D$_1$ receptor mechanism. *Psychopharmacology*, **214**, 843–853.

77 Fatemi, S.H. and Folsom, T.D. (2009) The neurodevelopmental hypothesis of schizophrenia, revisited. *Schizophrenia Bulletin*, **35**, 528–548.

78 Murray, R.M., Lappin, J., and Di Forti, M. (2008) Schizophrenia: from developmental deviance to dopamine dysregulation. *European Neuropsychopharmacology*, **18**, S129–S134.

79 Rapoport, J.L., Giedd, J.N., and Gogtay, N. (2012) Neurodevelopmental model of schizophrenia: update 2012. *Molecular Psychiatry*, **17**, 1228–1238.

80 Patterson, P.H. (2009) Immune involvement in schizophrenia and autism: etiology, pathology and animal models. *Behavioural Brain Research*, **204** (2), 313–321.

81 Meyer, U. and Feldon, J. (2010) Epidemiology-driven neurodevelopmental animal models of schizophrenia. *Progress in Neurobiology*, **90**, 285–326.

82 Meyer, U. (2013) Prenatal poly(I:C) exposure and other developmental immune activation models in rodent systems. *Biological Psychiatry*. doi: 10.1016/j.biopsych.2013.07.011.

83 Meyer, U., Feldon, J., and Fatemi, S.H. (2009) *In-vivo* rodent models for the experimental investigation of prenatal immune activation effects in neurodevelopmental brain disorders. *Neuroscience and Biobehavioral Reviews*, **33**, 1061–1079.

84 Shi, L., Fatemi, S.H., Sidwell, R.W., and Patterson, P.H. (2003) Maternal influenza infection causes marked behavioural and pharmacological changes in the offspring. *The Journal of Neuroscience*, **23**, 297–302.

85 Smith, S.E.P., Li, J., Garbett, K., Mirnics, K., and Patterson, P.H. (2007) Maternal immune activation alters fetal brain development through interleukin-6. *The Journal of Neuroscience*, **27**, 10695–10702.

86 Lipska, B.K. and Weinberger, D.R. (1993) Delayed effects of neonatal hippocampal damage on haloperidol-induced catalepsy and apomorphine induced stereotypic behaviors in the rat. *Brain Research. Developmental Brain Research*, **75**, 213–222.

87 Tseng, K.Y., Chambers, R.A., and Lipska, B.K. (2009) The neonatal ventral hippocampal lesion as a heuristic neurodevelopmental model of schizophrenia. *Behavioural Brain Research*, **204**, 295–305.

88 O'Donnell, P. (2012) Cortical disinhibition in the neonatal ventral hippocampal lesion model of schizophrenia: new vistas on possible therapeutic approaches. *Pharmacology & Therapeutics*, **133**, 19–25.

89 Sams-Dodd, F., Lipska, B.K., and Weinberger, D.R. (1997) Neonatal lesions of the ventral hippocampus result in hyperlocomotion and deficits in social behaviour in adulthood. *Psychopharmacology*, **132**, 303–310.

90 Becker, A., Greksch, G., Bernstein, H.-G., Höllt, V., and Bogerts, B. (1999) Social behaviour in rats lesioned with ibotenic acid in the hippocampus: quantitative and qualitative analysis. *Psychopharmacology*, **144**, 333–338.

91 Blas-Valdivia, V., Cano-Europa, E., Hernandez-Garcia, A., and Ortiz-Butron, R. (2009) Neonatal bilateral lidocaine administration into the ventral hippocampus caused postpubertal behavioral changes: an animal model of neurodevelopmental psychopathological disorders. *Neuropsychiatric Disease and Treatment*, **5**, 15–22.

92 Rueter, L.E., Ballard, M.E., Gallagher, K.B., Basso, A.M., Curzon, P., and Kohlhass, K.L. (2004) Chronic low dose risperidone and clozapine alleviate positive but not negative symptoms in the rat neonatal ventral hippocampal lesion model of schizophrenia. *Psychopharmacology*, **176**, 312–319.

93 Le Pen, G., Gaudet, L., Mortas, P., Mory, L., and Moreau, J.-L. (2002) Deficits in reward sensitivity in a neurodevelopmental rat model of schizophrenia. *Psychopharmacology*, **161**, 434–441.

94 Wan, R.Q., Giovanni, A., Kafka, S.H., and Corbett, R. (1996) Neonatal ventral hippocampal lesions induced hyperresponsiveness to amphetamine: behavioural and *in vivo* microdialysis studies. *Behavioural Brain Research*, **78**, 211–223.

95 Naert, A., Gantois, I., Laeremans, A., Vreysen, S., Van den Bergh, G., Arckens, L., Callaerts-Vegh, Z., and D'Hooge, R. (2013) Behavioural alterations relevant to developmental brain disorders in mice with neonatally induced ventral hippocampal lesions. *Brain Research Bulletin*, **94**, 71–81.

96 Allen, N.C., Bagade, S., McQueen, M.B., Ioannidis, J.P., Kavvoura, F.K., Khoury, M.J., Tanzi, R.E., and Bertram, L. (2008) Systematic meta-analyses and field synopsis of genetic association studies in schizophrenia: the SzGene database. *Nature*, **40**, 827–834.

97 Kirby, B., Waddington, J.L., and O'Tuathaigh, C.M.P. (2010) Advancing a functional genomics for schizophrenia: psychopathological and cognitive phenotypes in mutants with gene disruption. *Brain Research Bulletin*, **83** (3–4), 162–176.

98 van den Buuse, M. (2010) Modeling the positive symptoms of schizophrenia in genetically modified mice: pharmacology and methodology aspects. *Schizophrenia Bulletin*, **36** (2), 246–270.

99 Gainetdinov, R.R. (2008) Dopamine transporter mutant mice in experimental neuropharmacology. *Naunyn-Schmiedeberg's Archives of Pharmacology*, **377** (4–6), 301–313.

100 Mohn, A.R., Gainetdinov, R.R., Caron, M.G., and Koller, B.H. (1999) Mice with reduced NMDA receptor expression display behaviors related to schizophrenia. *Cell*, **98**, 427–436.

101 Labrie, V., Lipina, T., and Roder, J.C. (2008) Mice with reduced NMDA receptor glycine

affinity model some of the negative and cognitive symptoms of schizophrenia. *Psychopharmacology*, **200** (2), 217–230.

102. Ellenbroek, B.A., Peeters, B.W., Honig, W.M., and Cools, A.R. (1987) The paw test: a behavioural paradigm for differentiating between classical and atypical neuroleptic drugs. *Psychopharmacology*, **93** (3), 343–348.

103. Prinssen, E.P., Kleven, M.S., and Koek, W. (1999) Interactions between neuroleptics and 5-HT$_{1A}$ ligands in preclinical behavioral models for antipsychotic and extrapyramidal effects. *Psychopharmacology*, **144** (1), 20–29.

104. Guan, H.J., Dai, J., and Zhu, X.Z. (2000) Atypical antipsychotic effects of quetiapine fumarate in animal models. *Acta Pharmacologica Sinica*, **21** (3), 205–210.

105. Patel, S., Chavhan, S., Soni, H., Babbar, A.K., Mathur, R., Mishra, A.K., and Sawant, K. (2011) Brain targeting of risperidone-loaded solid lipid nanoparticles by intranasal route. *Journal of Drug Targeting*, **19** (6), 468–474.

106. Pereira, M., Siba, I.P., Chioca, L.R., Correia, D., Vital, M.A., Pizzolatti, M.G., Santos, A.R., and Andreatini, R. (2011) Myricitrin, a nitric oxide and protein kinase C inhibitor, exerts antipsychotic-like effects in animal models. *Progress in Neuro-Psychopharmacology & Biological Psychiatry*, **35** (7), 1636–1644.

107. Morais, L.H., Lima, M.M., Martynhak, B.J., Santiago, R., Takahashi, T.T., Ariza, D., Barbiero, J.K., Andreatini, R., and Vital, M.A. (2012) Characterization of motor, depressive-like and neurochemical alterations induced by a short-term rotenone administration. *Pharmacological Reports*, **64** (5), 1081–1090.

108. Baptista, P.P., de Senna, P.N., Paim, M.F., Saur, L., Blank, M., do Nascimento, P., Ilha, J., Vianna, M.R., Mestriner, R.G., Achaval, M., and Xavier, L.L. (2013) Physical exercise down-regulated locomotor side effects induced by haloperidol treatment in Wistar rats. *Pharmacology, Biochemistry, and Behavior*, **104**, 113–118.

109. Casey, D.E. (1991) Extrapyramidal syndromes in nonhuman primates: typical and atypical neuroleptics. *Psychopharmacology Bulletin*, **27** (1), 47–50.

110. Auclair, A.L., Kleven, M.S., Barret-Grévoz, C., Barreto, M., Newman-Tancredi, A., and Depoortère, R. (2009) Differences among conventional, atypical and novel putative D$_2$/5-HT$_{1A}$ antipsychotics on catalepsy-associated behaviour in cynomolgus monkeys. *Behavioural Brain Research*, **203** (2), 288–295.

111. Cookson, J., Hodgson, R., and Wildgust, H.J. (2012) Prolactin, hyperprolactinaemia and antipsychotic treatment: a review and lessons for treatment of early psychosis. *Journal of Psychopharmacology (Oxford, England)*, **26** (5 Suppl.), 42–51.

112. Cosi, C., Carilla-Durand, E., Assié, M.B., Ormiere, A.M., Maraval, M., Leduc, N., and Newman-Tancredi, A. (2006) Partial agonist properties of the antipsychotics SSR181507, aripiprazole and bifeprunox at dopamine D$_2$ receptors: G protein activation and prolactin release. *European Journal of Pharmacology*, **535** (1–3), 135–144.

113. Park, W.K., Jeong, D., Cho, H., Lee, S.J., Cha, M.Y., Pae, A.N., Choi, K.I., Koh, H.Y., and Kong, J.Y. (2005) KKHA-761, a potent D$_3$ receptor antagonist with high 5-HT$_{1A}$ receptor affinity, exhibits antipsychotic properties in animal models of schizophrenia. *Pharmacology, Biochemistry, and Behavior*, **82** (2), 361–372.

114. Mann, S., Chintoh, A., Giacca, A., Fletcher, P., Nobrega, J., Hahn, M., and Remington, G. (2013) Chronic olanzapine administration in rats: effect of route of administration on weight, food intake and body composition. *Pharmacology, Biochemistry, and Behavior*, **103** (4), 717–722.

115. Raedler, T.J. (2010) Cardiovascular aspects of antipsychotics. *Current Opinion in Psychiatry*, **23** (6), 574–581.

116. Nielsen, J., Graff, C., Kanters, J.K., Toft, E., Taylor, D., and Meyer, J.M. (2011) Assessing QT interval prolongation and its associated risks with antipsychotics. *CNS Drugs*, **25** (6), 473–490.

117. Pollard, C.E., Abi Gerges, N., Bridgland-Taylor, M.H., Easter, A., Hammond, T.G., and Valentin, J.P. (2010) An introduction to QT interval prolongation and non-clinical approaches to assessing and

reducing risk. *British Journal of Pharmacology*, **159** (1), 12–21.

118 Cools, A.R., Brachten, R., Heeren, D., Willemen, A., and Ellenbroek, B. (1990) Search after neurobiological profile of individual-specific features of Wistar rats. *Brain Research Bulletin*, **24** (1), 49–69.

119 Ibi, D., Nagai, T., Koike, H., Kitahara, Y., Mizoguchi, H., Niwa, M., Jaaro-Peled, H., Nitta, A., Yoneda, Y., Nabeshima, T., Sawa, A., and Yamada, K. (2010) Combined effect of neonatal immune activation and mutant DISC1 on phenotypic changes in adulthood. *Behavioural Brain Research*, **206** (1), 32–37.

120 Nagai, T., Kitahara, Y., Ibi, D., Nabeshima, T., Sawa, A., and Yamada, K. (2011) Effects of antipsychotics on the behavioral deficits in human dominant-negative DISC1 transgenic mice with neonatal poly I:C treatment. *Behavioural Brain Research*, **225** (1), 305–310.

121 Hida, H., Mouri, A., and Noda, Y. (2013) Behavioral phenotypes in schizophrenic animal models with multiple combinations of genetic and environmental factors. *Journal of Pharmacological Sciences*, **121** (3), 185–191.

11
Migraine and Other Headaches
Inger Jansen-Olesen, Sarah Louise T. Christensen, and Jes Olesen

11.1
Introduction

Migraine is number seven in WHO's list of all diseases causing disability [1] and it is the third most costly neurological disorder [2]. Even though the triptans revolutionized the acute treatment of migraine, a huge unmet need for better or different acute treatments exists [3].

There is a general agreement that migraine pain is a result of activation of the trigeminovascular system, which comprises the intracranial blood vessels, nerve fibers around the arteries, and their central projection via the trigeminal ganglion to the trigeminal nucleus caudalis(TNC) (Figure 11.1). Animal experimental studies of migraine in general focus on this system and also on cortical spreading depression(CSD), which occurs in migraine with aura. In this chapter, we outline the most commonly used animal models for migraine research and some of the relevant results achieved using each method. We describe models studying peripheral events that can initiate a pain response as well as cortical spreading depression and electrical recordings from the intracranial pain structures. Furthermore, models for provocation of migraine, transgenic models, and behavioral responses will be described. Finally, we discuss about the validity of these models for translating these results into clinical use.

11.2
Vascular Models

Dilatation of extra- and intracranial arteries has for decades been suggested to be involved in migraine pathogenesis [5]. When large blood vessels in the dura mater and pia mater are stimulated in neurosurgical patients, they experience a throbbing unilateral migraine-like pain [6], indicating that these structures are involved in migraine headache. The cranial arteries are innervated by sympathetic, parasympathetic, and sensory nerve fibers containing signaling substances with contractile or relaxant effect on the arteries. Different vascular models that have

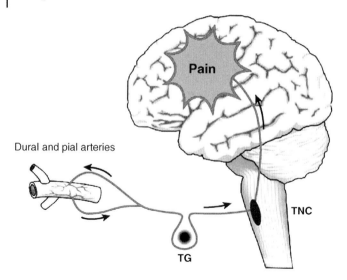

Figure 11.1 Schematic illustration demonstrating the central role of the trigeminovascular system, bridging from intracranial arteries and veins to the trigeminocervical complex with, for example, TNC. Intracranial blood vessels are invested with mechano and sensory Aδ and C fibers containing, for example, CGRP, substance P, PACAP, and nociceptin *inter alia*. Tracing studies have shown that the thin C fibers end in lamina I, whereas the Aδ fibers end up in lamina IV of the brainstem. From these synapses, the pain signaling carries up to higher levels and involves, for example, PAG thalamus and cortex. (Reprinted from Ref. [4].)

been used to characterize the effect of these signaling substances on cranial arteries are described below.

Triptans, a group of 5-hydroxytryptamine $(5\text{-HT})_{1B/D/F}$ receptor agonists that are effective in the acute treatment of migraine, were developed from the concept that if vasodilatation induces a migraine attack then substances causing constriction of cranial arteries would abort an attack [7]. Thus, initially, vascular models were used in the development of the first triptans.

11.2.1
In Vitro

In vitro classification of cerebrovascular receptors has been successfully performed on isolated arterial segments from animals [8–12] and humans [13–18]. Most commonly, the wire myograph system is used in which circular segments of an artery are mounted in a tissue bath on two wires, one of which is connected to a force displacement transducer and the other to a movable unit for adjusting the resting tension of the artery. Contractions are studied by adding the substance of interest to the artery in increasing concentrations. The same is done for vasodilatation studies; however, in this case, the artery must be precontracted. The experiments can be performed in the presence of pharmacological receptor antagonists or blockers of second messenger systems. Using this method in arteries of animals and humans, several studies related to migraine have been performed. The vascular effect of 5-HT receptor activating and blocking drugs has been characterized and triptans have been shown to act on $5\text{-}HT_{1B}$ receptors on human cranial arteries [14,19]. Also, the potent relaxant effect of the sensory peptide calcitonin gene-related peptide (CGRP) was characterized by this method in humans [16,20] and guinea pigs [8,21]. The method can also be used for investigating contraction of peripheral arteries as an adverse effect [22].

In another vascular *in vitro* model, the pressure myograph system, the arteries are mounted on two capillaries allowing a pressurized flow through the lumen. For the purpose of migraine research, this method has mostly been used to study the effect of intraluminal application of pharmacological substances [23]. The information acquired can tell us whether a substance acts via the endothelium or if it has the ability to pass the blood–brain barrier.

11.2.2
In Vivo

Currently, the most popular model for studying craniovascular effects of a drug is the genuine closed cranial window technique [24,25]. This model has the advantage over the formerly used open cranial window that the skull has not been removed but is only thinned with the help of a dental drill. Furthermore, the dura mater is intact and responses of dural arteries can be studied. Drugs can be administered by an intravenous or intracarotid arterial infusion. The advantage of the latter is that the drug is administered directly into the intracranial arteries before reaching the peripheral circulation. Thus, autoregulatory effects of pial arteries due to a fall in blood pressure are avoided [25]. Using this method, the effects of several migraine provoking substances on rat dural and pial arteries have been studied [26–30]. Relaxant effects on a pial artery without a concomitant fall in blood pressure indicate that the drug is able to pass the blood–brain barrier or is acting via endothelial receptors. The method has also the advantage that it permits the direct study of neurogenic release of vasoactive signaling substances from the peripheral branch of the trigeminovascular system. Electrical stimulation causes a reproducible increase in arterial diameter due to the release of CGRP [30,31]. Sumatriptan and other mixed $5\text{-}HT_{1B/D}$ agonists inhibit this effect, whereas a $5\text{-}HT_{1F}$ receptor agonist does not [32,33]. Among substances with known antimigraine effect, it can be mentioned that the nonspecific nitric oxide synthase inhibitor L-nitroarginine methyl ester (L-NAME) [31], the nonsteroidal anti-inflammatory drug (NSAID) indomethacin [34], and topiramate [35] were effective in inhibiting the dilatation of meningeal arteries due to electrical stimulation. Furthermore, the NK1 receptor antagonist RP67580 that was not effective in the acute treatment of migraine was also not effective in inhibiting the release of CGRP from sensory afferents [36].

11.3
Neurogenic Inflammation

In the 1980s, Moskowitz *et al.* suggested that migraine was due to neurogenic inflammation of dura mater [37,38]. It was suggested that dilation of dural arteries increases vascular permeability, subsequently activating perivascular sensory nerve fibers and mast cells causing inflammatory responses. Models mimicking these circumstances were among the first animal models of migraine [38]. In this model, neurogenic inflammatory responses are induced by applying a strong electrical stimulation (0.6–3.0 mA with square pulses of 5 ms duration for 5 min) to the trigeminal ganglion or by i.v. infusion of inflammatory substances such as substance P (0.3–1 nmol/kg) [38–40], bradykinin (0.1 µmol/kg) [40], or capsaicin (1 µmol/kg) [40]. The amount of neurogenic inflammation was determined by measuring the amount of [^{125}I]BSA or Evans blue leaking into dura mater. The markers were administered i.v. 5 min before stimulation. Initially, it was found that all known substances with efficacy in migraine also inhibited dural plasma protein extravasation and the model seemed extremely promising to predict the effectiveness of a substance in migraine treatment. During the end of 1980s and 1990s, several different substances were investigated for an inhibitory effect on plasma protein extravasation (see Table 11.1) and thus possible antimigraine effect. However, the NK1 receptor antagonists GR205171 and L-758,298 as well as the endothelin receptor antagonist bosentan, which were effective inhibitors of plasma protein extravasation, failed in clinical trials for acute or prophylactic migraine treatment [41–45].

11.4
Nociceptive Activation of the Trigeminovascular System

Sensory nerve fibers exhibit at least two functions: first, transmit painful stimulation from peripheral tissue to the brainstem, mainly represented by the TNC; and second, promote a sterile neurogenic inflammatory response in the target tissue by the release of sensory peptides causing vasodilation and increased vascular permeability. Such nociceptive activation can be initiated in animal models by using several methods of noxious stimulation of peripheral tissues innervated by the trigeminal system. These methods include electrical stimulation of the superior sagittal sinus (SSS) [56], an inflammatory cocktail or capsaicin on dura mater [57], and electrical stimulation of dura mater [58] or trigeminal ganglion [56,59]. Also mechanical stimulation of dura mater by von Frey hair has been used alone or in combination with various chemical stimuli [60,61]. The nociceptive output is then measured by release of sensory neuropeptides or by direct electrophysiological recordings from sensory neurons in the trigeminal ganglia [62] or TNC [60,63–66].

Table 11.1 Neurogenic inflammation model: effect of different inhibitors on dural plasma protein extravasation [46].

	Treatment	Dose (i.v.)	Inhibition of dural plasma protein extravasation	Reference
Electrical stimulation (1.2 mA)	Indomethacin	1 mg/kg	++	[39]
		2 mg/kg	++	
		10 mg/kg	+	
	Acetylsalicylic acid	50 mg/kg	++	
	Dexamethasone	1 mg/kg	+	
Electrical stimulation (1.2 mA)	Sumatriptan	30 µg/kg	−	[40]
		100 µg/kg	+++	
		300 µg/kg	+	
Electrical stimulation (1.2 mA)	α-Methylhistamine	5 µmol/kg	−	[47]
		15 µmol/kg	+++	
	SMS 2111-905 (somatostatin agonist)	0.1 µmol/kg	−	
		0.3 µmol/kg	−	
		1 µmol/kg	+++	
	UK-14,304 (α_2 receptor agonist)	34 nmol/kg	−	
		100 nmol/kg	+	
		340 nmol/kg	++	
Electrical stimulation (1.2 mA)	Sodium valproate	3 mg/kg	+	[48]
		10 mg/kg	++	
		30 mg/kg	++	
		100 mg/kg	++	
Electrical stimulation (1.2 mA)	Muscimol	10 µg/kg	+	[48]
		100 µg/kg	++	
		1000 µg/kg	++	
	Baclofen	10 µg/kg	−	
		100 µg/kg	−	
		1 mg/kg	−	
		10 mg/kg	−	
Electrical stimulation (1.2 mA)	GR82334 (NK1 receptor antagonist)	0.02 mg/kg	+	[49]
		0.2 mg/kg	+	
	SR 48968 (NK2 receptor antagonist)	1 mg/kg	−	
			+	
	CGRP(8–37)	0.1 mg/kg	−	
Electrical stimulation (1.2 mA)	Bosentan (mixed ET receptor antagonist)	10 mg/kg	++	[50]
		30 mg/kg	++	
	BQ-123 (ET_A receptor antagonist)	10 mg/kg	−	
	Ro-46-8443 (ET_B receptor antagonist)	10 mg/kg	+++	

(continued)

Table 11.1 (Continued)

	Treatment	Dose (i.v.)	Inhibition of dural plasma protein extravasation	Reference
Electrical stimulation (1.2 mA)	Sumatriptan	1 μg/kg	−	[32]
		10 μg/kg	−	
		100 μg/kg	+	
		1 mg/kg	+	
	CP 122,288	1 pg/kg	−	
		10 pg/kg	−	
		100 pg/kg	+	
	CP 93, 129	10 μg/kg	−	
		100 μg/kg	−	
		1 mg/kg	+	
		3 mg/kg	+	
Electrical stimulation (1.2 mA)	100% Oxygen	200 mmHg	+	[51]
		300 mmHg	++	
		400 mmHg	++	
Electrical stimulation (0.6 mA)	CP 99,994 (NK1 receptor antagonist)	10 μg/kg	−	[52]
		100 μg/kg	+	
		1 mg/kg	+	
		3 mg/kg	+	
	Sumatriptan	10 μg/kg	−	
		100 μg/kg	+	
		1 mg/kg	+	
Electrical stimulation (0.6 mA)	Rizatriptan	1 μg/kg	−	[53]
		10 μg/kg	−	
		100 μg/kg	+	
		1000 μg/kg	+	
Electrical stimulation (1.2 mA) (guinea pig)	SMS 2111-905 (somatostatin agonist)	0.1 μmol/kg	−	[47]
		0.3 μmol/kg	+	
		1 μmol/kg	+++	
Electrical stimulation (1.5 mA) (guinea pig)	GR82 334 (NK1 receptor ant)	0.02 mg/kg	−	[49]
		0.2 mg/kg	+	
	CGRP(8–37)	0.1 mg/kg	+	
Electrical stimulation (1.5 mA) (guinea pig)	PNU 10 929 (5-HT$_{1D}$ agonist)	0.24 nmol/kg	−	[54]
		2.4 nmol/kg	++	
		7.3 nmol/kg	++	
		24.4 nmol/kg	++	
		73.3 nmol/kg	++	
Substance P (1 nmol/kg)	Indomethacin	2 mg/kg	−	[39]
		10 mg/kg	+	
	Acetylsalicylic acid	10 mg/kg	−	
		50 mg/kg	+	
	Dexamethasone	1 mg/kg	−	

Substance P (1 nmol/kg)	Sodium valproate	3 mg/kg	+	[48]
		10 mg/kg	+	
		30 mg/kg	+	
		100 mg/kg	+	
	Muscimol	0.3 mg/kg	+	
		1 mg/kg	+	
		30 mg/kg	+	
Substance P (1 nmol/kg)	Sumatriptan	100 µg/kg	−	[40]
Substance P (0.3 nmol/kg)	Sumatriptan	100 µg/kg	−	[40]
		300 µg/kg	−	
Bradykinin (0.1 µmol/kg)	Sumatriptan	10 µg/kg	−	[40]
		30 µg/kg	+	
		100 µg/kg	+	
Capsaicin (1 µmol/kg)	Sumatriptan	30 µg/kg	−	[40]
		100 µg/kg	+	
Capsaicin (0.5 µmol/kg) (guinea pig)	Sumatriptan	10 µg/kg	−	[40]
		30 µg/kg	+	
Capsaicin (1 µmol/kg)	α-Methylhistamine	15 µmol/kg	++	[47]
	SMS 2111-905	1 µmol/kg	+++	
	UK-14,304	100 nmol/kg	++	
Capsaicin (0.37 mg/kg)	Bosentan (mixed ET receptor antagonist)	3 mg/kg	−	[50]
		10 mg/kg	++	
		30 mg/kg	++	
Capsaicin (0.37 mg/kg)	Sumatriptan	300 µg/kg	++	[50]
Substance P (1 nmol/kg)	α-Methylhistamine	15 µmol/kg	−	[47]
	SMS 2111-905	1 µmol/kg	−	
	UK-14,304	100 nmol/kg	−	
GTN (60 µg/kg i.v.)	L-NMMA	20 mg/kg i.v.	+	[55]
	L-NIL (iNOS)	4 mg/kg i.p.	+	

Significant effect: (+) $p < 0.05$; (++) $p < 0.01$; (+++) $p < 0.001$.

Migraine has also been suggested to involve peripheral and central sensitization, which can be distinguished by electrical recording from either the trigeminal ganglion (peripheral) or the TNC (central) [67]. Combining these two methods, the antimigraine action of sumatriptan was examined (Figure 11.2). The study showed that sumatriptan inhibited spontaneous firing after inflammatory soup in central neurons but not in peripheral neurons [67].

11.4.1
Electrophysiological Recordings on Primary Dural Afferents in Trigeminal Ganglion

Only few studies have been published due to complicated technical matters [68]. The trigeminal ganglion is only accessible for microelectrode recordings by insertion of the electrode through the cerebral cortex. Stimulation of the

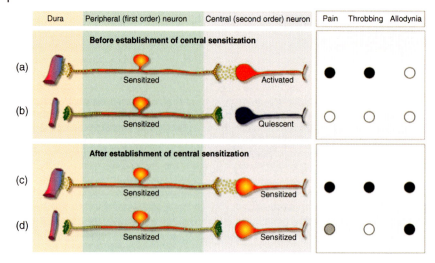

Figure 11.2 Proposed mechanism of action for 5-HT$_{1B/1D}$ agonists during migraine. (a) Minutes after the onset of migraine, activated meningeal nociceptors enter a new physiological state, denoted peripheral sensitization, and release a host of neuropeptides such as CGRP, substance P, and neurokinin A (yellow circles), which promote local vasodilatation and plasma extravasation (i.e., neurogenic inflammation) through their peripheral branch in the meninges and activation of central trigeminovascular neurons through their central branch in the dorsal horn. After peripheral sensitization sets in, rhythmic pulsation of the meninges generates bursts of action potentials that activate the central trigeminovascular neuron (shown in red) and the pain (●) begins to throb (●). (b) Systemically administered triptan molecules (green circles) bind to presynaptic 5-HT$_{1B/1D}$ receptors on terminals of both the peripheral and central branches of the meningeal nociceptor, resulting in blockade of neuropeptide release. At this stage, blockade of neuropeptide release from the peripheral terminal has no effect on the hyperexcitability of the meningeal nociceptor. However, blockade of neuropeptide release from the central terminal of meningeal nociceptor renders the central trigeminovascular neuron inactive (shown in blue), resulting in termination of pain (○) and throbbing (○). (c) After the establishment of central sensitization, the pain continues to throb (●) and the skin becomes allodynic (●). (d) At this stage, blockade of neuropeptide release from the central terminals of the meningeal nociceptor cannot reverse the hyperexcitability of the central trigeminovascular neuron because its activity no longer depends on input from the meningeal nociceptor. In the face of the autonomous activity of the central trigeminovascular neuron, this blockade of synaptic transmission provides only partial pain relief (◐), terminates the throbbing (○), but does not resolve the allodynia (●). From Ref. [67].

nasociliary nerve is used because it is at a sufficient distance from the recording site in the trigeminal ganglion [68]; however, it supplies only a small area of the dura mater around the frontal part of the superior sagittal sinus [69]. Recordings of neurons in the trigeminal ganglion that received afferent information from dura mater responded to mechanical and heat stimuli [69]. Chemosensitive afferents reacted to application of capsaicin, bradykinin, and an inflammatory soup. Almost all receptors responded to mechanical, thermal, and chemical agents and can be regarded as polymodal receptors. Dural application of inflammatory soup, low pH, and capsaicin cause a direct excitation of the neurons and an enhancement of their mechanical sensitivity (peripheral sensitization) [62].

11.4.2
Electrophysiological Recordings in Trigeminal Nucleus Caudalis

Primary afferent trigeminal nerve fibers from the trigeminal ganglion enter the brainstem at the level of pons and project from there to the trigeminal nucleus caudalis [70]. In the study of Schepelmann *et al.* [57], neurons with input from the dura mater were located at two distinct sites in the ipsilateral trigeminal nucleus, one at the level of the obex and the other about 2 mm caudal to this level. The first site corresponds to the transition zone of subnuclei interpolaris and caudalis, and the second to the caudal subnucleus caudalis of the spinal trigeminal nucleus. Most of the neurons were located in deep layers of the trigeminal nucleus (III–IV). In laminae I and II, no units with meningeal input were found [57]. The neurons could be activated by mechanical stimulation (by von Frey hair) to the meningeal receptive fields causing activation of the central trigeminal neurons. The dural receptive fields were mostly located at or in close proximity to the middle meningeal artery. Only rarely was the receptive field located at the superior sagittal sinus or the posterior meningeal artery [57]. In another study, the receptive field was found in the transverse sinus [71], most probably due to a different location of the cranial window. A large number of known antimigraine drugs for acute [63,72–75], prophylactic [76], and potential [77–80] treatments have been examined in this model. In short, drugs with an acute antimigraine effect seemed to act on second-order neurons to inhibit neuronal activation in TNC [63,72–75]. The acute administration of the prophylactic drug topiramate was effective only when given in high doses or by iontophoretic application to the trigeminothalamic pathway [76,81]. Among the potential antimigraine drugs with effect in this model are adenosine A_1 receptor agonists [78], the noncompetitive *N*-methyl-D-aspartate (NMDA) receptor channel blocker memantine [82], and AMPA/kainite antagonists [77]. However, the known inhibitory effect of memantine after microiontophoretic application in the trigeminocervical complex (TCC) was not reproduced with intravenous administration [83].

11.4.3
Histological Markers after Nociceptive Stimulation of the Trigeminovascular System

One of the most widely used markers for pain signaling is Fos, which initially was reported to be expressed in TNC and spinal cord dorsal horn following peripheral noxious and nonnoxious stimulation [84]. The expression of c-fos to trace the neuronal circuits for nociception is consistent with the pathways mapped by electrophysiological and other tracing methods [85]. The majority of studies in the field of migraine have employed this technique to map neuronal activation in response to intracranial dural stimulation. In these studies, Fos-positive cells were reported within a subpopulation of TNC in response to the injection of autologous blood into the subarachnoid space of the rat [86,87] or after cortical spreading depression [88]. Noxious dural stimulation resulted in the labeling of Fos immunoreactive cells to lamina I, whereas facial stimulation labeled both laminae I and II [89]. The labeling was most dense in the venterolateral segment of the dorsal horn and also lightly extended to the dorsolateral segment, which is roughly comparable to the locations of the referred pain produced by electrical stimulation of dural arteries in humans [6]. One of the confounding factors when using Fos as a pain marker is the effect of surgery [90] and anesthesia on c-fos expression [91]. Furthermore, it should be noted that fos is not expressed in all the activated neurons and that it requires a strong consistent stimulation to activate c-fos [92,93]. Thus, pain activation might happen without an increase in c-fos expression. This is as an example of the enigma that electrophysical signals in TNC after noxious stimulation of dura mater are mostly detectable in the deeper (laminae III and IV) layers of TNC, whereas c-fos expression activated by a similar type of stimulation is seen in TNC laminae I and II.

11.5
Cortical Spreading Depression

The most common aura symptom is scintillating scotomas, which propagate from the center to the periphery of the visual field. Lashley analyzed his own visual scotoma and calculated the speed of the advancing process to be about 3 mm/min [94]. Leão later described a transient cortical depression of neuronal activity that moved at a velocity of 5 mm/min. He proposed that this CSD was the cause of migraine with aura [95]. The hypothesis was forgotten but resurrected by the findings that both the aura in humans and CSD in animals are associated with a reduction of regional cerebral blood flow [96]. CSD can be induced in animals by local mechanical stimulation, depolarization initiated by raising the extracellular K^+ concentrations above a certain threshold, or electrical stimulation [97]. Also hypoosmotic medium, metabolic inhibitors, glutamate receptor agonists, ouabain, and endothelin have been shown to trigger CSD [98]. Further details on the methods to trigger CSD can be found in Ref. [99]. CSD can be measured by electrophysiological recording of extracellular negative slow potential shift, diffusion-weighted magnetic resonance imaging, laser Doppler flow recordings, and optical intrinsic signal imaging. CSD is accompanied by temporary changes in the intra- and extracellular neurophysiological environment. These changes include changes in pH, the release and diffusion of several chemical mediators, such as excitatory amino acids, neurokinin, calcitonin gene-related peptide, serotonin, and brain-derived neurotrophic factor into the interstitial space, which may change the receptor affinities and subsequently alter the neuronal network activities [100], and ionic shifts accompanied by cellular swelling [101].

Glutamate is believed to play a key role in the initiation and propagation of CSD. It is released during CSD *in vitro* and *in vivo* [102,103] and CSD can be inhibited by NMDA receptor antagonists [104,105].

CSD has been shown to involve several variants of ion channels and pumps [106]. CSD is inhibited by P/Q channel blockers [107] and openers of KCNQ (Kv7) potassium channels [108]. The sodium channel blocker TTX has been shown to inhibit the cerebral blood flow response during CSD induced by mechanical stimulation [109] but it does not inhibit CSD evoked by several other stimuli. Other ion channels have been shown to be able to evoke CSD; among these are inhibitors of Kv1.1 and Kv1.2 potassium channels (dendrotoxin and tityustoxin) that have been shown to activate SD in cerebellum [110] and the Na^+/K^+ ATPase inhibitor ouabain that evokes CSD in brain slice preparations [111,112].

A drug developed for its ability to inhibit cortical spreading depression, tonabersat [113], has prophylactic efficacy against migraine with aura [114], but not in migraine without aura [115]. Taken together with extensive human brain blood flow studies, it seems overwhelmingly likely that cortical spreading depression in animals is a valid model for the testing of prophylactic drugs against migraine with aura [114,116]. The number of patients suffering from a high frequency of attacks of migraine with aura is, however, limited. Probably, the small market size for this indication is the reason why the pharma industry has made little use of the cortical spreading depression model for drug development. Whether this model might also be relevant to migraine without aura is debatable. From human brain blood flow studies, there is no indication of CSD in migraine without aura [117,118], but prophylactic migraine drugs seem to inhibit CSD in rats when dosed for 2 weeks or more [119,120]. Thus, CSD models may perhaps predict efficacy of prophylactic drugs not only for migraine with aura but also for migraine without aura.

11.6
Human Experimental Migraine Provoking Models

It has been known for more than 100 years that glyceryl trinitrate (GTN) induces headache [121] and its headache-inducing effect was demonstrated in provocation experiments [122]. GTN is highly lipid soluble and easily penetrates membranes including the blood–brain barrier. It can therefore deliver NO to extracerebral as well as intracerebral compartments. It was first shown that GTN induces headache in normal volunteers in a dose-dependent fashion with a ceiling effect at a relatively modest dose [122]. In a series of studies [122–125], this model was refined and an infusion model using 0.5 mg/kg/min for 20 min was validated. In migraine patients compared with normal subjects, infusion of GTN causes a more intense immediate headache during the infusion and, more importantly, it also leads to a delayed headache that is maximal around 6–7 h after the infusion [126]. This delayed headache has the characteristics of typical attacks of migraine without aura. Likewise, patients themselves find that the provoked attacks are identical to their spontaneous attacks. In normal subjects, delayed headache is largely absent. A nonselective nitric oxide synthase (NOS) inhibitor, N^G-monomethyl-L-arginine (L-NMMA), was effective in treating spontaneous migraine attacks [127], which confirmed that NO is an important offending molecule throughout the duration of a migraine attack. Other substances that induce more headaches in migraine sufferers than in nonsufferers and a delayed headache that is identical to the spontaneous migraine attacks of the patients are histamine [128], sildenafil [129], dipyridamole [130], CGRP [131], PACAP [132,133], prostaglandin E_2 [134], and prostaglandin I_2 [135].

Specific inhibitors of the migraine-inducing substances are thus likely to be useful in the treatment of spontaneous migraine attacks. This is also true for NOS inhibitors [127] and CGRP antagonists [136,137], but not for antihistamines [138]. Blockers of the other migraine-inducing substances have so far not been examined in the treatment of spontaneous migraine attacks. Pretreatment with the histamine H_1 antagonist mepyramine was shown to cure immediate headache as well as delayed migraine attacks induced by histamine [128]. However, mepyramine did not inhibit GTN-induced headache and arterial dilatation [139]. The GTN model has been used to test acute and preventive drugs. The specific antimigraine drug sumatriptan reduced GTN-induced immediate headache and increased temporal, middle, and radial artery diameters as compared with placebo [140]. Administration of aspirin, zolmitriptan, and the CGRP antagonist olcegepant after GTN infusion had no effect on GTN-induced headache or migraine [141,142]. This suggests that the active drug must be given as a pretreatment before the administration of GTN. The efficacy of the prophylactic drug valproate [143] and the lack of effect of propranolol on GTN-induced headache suggest that the efficacy of future prophylactic drugs in the GTN model depends on their mechanisms of action.

11.7
Animal Experimental Migraine Provoking Models

In relation to animal models, it may be an advantage to mimic human experimental models. A number of naturally occurring signaling substances or drugs interacting with known pathological pathways are able to induce headache in normal volunteers and migraine attacks in migraine sufferers [122,126,128–133,144–146]. The most extensively studied of these models is the GTN model (Table 11.2) [122,126,146]. It has been mimicked in numerous animal experimental studies. In rats, it is believed that increase in Fos expression within the dorsolateral laminae I and II of the caudal region of the TNC may indicate activation of the trigeminal vascular system [147,148]. A dose approximately 1000 times the human dose has unfortunately been used in most animal studies [149–156]. It lowers blood pressure and activates c-fos also in areas of the brain that are not related to pain [150,151]. Other variations of this model have used anesthetized animals [55,157–160]. However, anesthesia and surgery by themselves affect the expression of c-fos

Table 11.2 Glyceryl trinitrate infusion studies: effects observed after infusion of GTN and the effect of different treatments on these effects [46].

	Effect observed	Treatment	Inhibition of effect studied by treatment	Reference
GTN 0.25 μg/kg/min i.v. (cat); anesthetized	Increase in pial artery diameter Increase in rCBF Increase in NO concentration			[159]
GTN 60 μg/kg over 30 min i.v., anesthetized	Increase in NO concentration	Sumatriptan	+	[158]
	Decrease in superoxide concentration	Sumatriptan	+	
	Increase in rCBF	Sumatriptan	+	
GTN 10 mg/kg s.c.	Increase in TNC c-fos expression Increase in TNC nNOS expression			[154]
GTN 10 mg/kg s.c.	Decrease in TNC CGRP-IR expression Increase in TNC 5-HT-IR expression			[164]
GTN 10 mg/kg s.c.	Increase in CamKII-IR in TNC		−	[165]
GTN 10 mg/kg i.p.	Increase in TNC c-fos expression	Kynurenine (450 mg/kg) and probenecid (200 mg/kg)	+	[166]
GTN 10 mg/kg i.p.	Increase in TNC c-fos expression	Kynurenic acid (1 mmol/kg i.p.)	+++	[167]
		SZR-72 (kynurenate analog) (1 mmol/kg i.p.)	+++	
GTN 10 mg/kg i.p.	Increase in c-fos expression in TNC and 10 other brain nuclei			[162]
GTN 10 mg/kg i.p.	Increase in c-fos expression	L-NAME (50 mg/kg i.p.)	+	[152]
		7-NI (20 mg/kg i.p.)	+	
		Ephedrine (25 mg/kg i.p.)	+	
		Indomethacin (5 mg/kg i.p.)	+	
		Capsaicin depletion	+	
GTN 10 mg/kg i.p.	Increase in cGMP in TNC lamina I/II			[168]

(continued)

Table 11.2 (Continued)

	Effect observed	Treatment	Inhibition of effect studied by treatment	Reference
GTN 10 mg/kg i.p.	Increase in c-fos expression	Parthenolide (15 mg/kg for 6 days)	+	[169]
GTN 10 mg/kg i.p.	Increase in c-fos expression	Anandamide (20 mg/kg i.p.)	+	[170]
GTN 10 mg/kg s.c.	Increase in CamKII expression in TNC	NS398 (COX-2 inhibitor)		[171]
		1 mg/kg	−	
		3 mg/kg	+	
		5 mg/kg	++	
		SC 560 (COX-1 inhibitor)		
		1 mg/kg	−	
		3 mg/kg	−	
		5 mg/kg	−	
GTN 80 μg/kg over 20 min i.v.; awake rats	Increase in c-fos expression	Sumatriptan (1.8 mg/kg i.v.)	+	[163]
GTN 80 μg/kg over 20 min i.v.; awake rats	Increase in c-fos expression	L-NAME (40 mg/kg i.v.)	+	[172]
		Olcegepant (1 mg/kg i.v.)	+	
		L-733 060 (NK1 receptor antagonist) (1 mg/kg i.v.)	+	
GTN 80 μg/kg over 20 min i.v.; awake rats	Increase in c-fos expression in TNC Increase in pERK in dura mater, TG, TNC Increase in CamKII in TNC Increase in ATF1 in TNC Increase in pCREB in TNC			[173]
GTN 10 μg/kg i.v. over 20 min; anesthetized	No effect on c-fos expression in TNC			[174]
GTN 10 mg/kg s.c. (mice)	Increase in c-fos expression in TNC Induces thermal allodynia	Sumatriptan		[156]
		intrathecal 0.06 μg	+	
		i.p. 300 μg/kg	−	
		i.p. 600 μg/kg	+	
	Induces mechanical allodynia No effect on CSD threshold	Sumatriptan		
		intrathecal 0.06 μg	+	
		i.p. 300 μg/kg	−	
		i.p. 600 μg/kg	−	

GTN 60 μg/kg i.v.; anesthetized	Increase in IL-1β expression in dura mater Increase in iNOS expression in dura mater Increase in mast cell degranulation	[55]

Significant effect: (+) p < 0.05; (++) p < 0.01; (+++) p < 0.001.

[90,161]. In anaesthetized rats, GTN-induced hypotension by itself causes c-fos expression [162]. Therefore, c-fos expression has been confounded by a number of unspecific factors, which indicate a major deviation from studies in awake human subjects. A more naturalistic model in the rat has recently been presented (Figure 11.3) [163]. GTN was administered to awake, freely moving rats in a dose (4 μg/kg/min for 20 min) eight times the human dose, probably the equivalent of the human dose in rats. A significant increase in c-fos mRNA expression was observed in the trigeminal nucleus caudalis at 30 min and 2 h that was followed by an increase in Fos protein in the trigeminal nucleus caudalis at 2 and 4 h after GTN infusion. Treatment with sumatriptan and nonselective NOS inhibitor L-NAME as well as pretreatment with the CGRP receptor antagonist olcegepant attenuated the activation of c-fos at 4 h. However, a NK1 receptor antagonist that has no efficacy in migraine also attenuated c-fos expression [163]. Other migraine provoking agents such as CGRP, PACAP, histamine, prostanoids, and phosphodiesterase (PDE) inhibitors have received limited or no study in this model. Finally, it may be considered whether animals should be sensitized in some way.

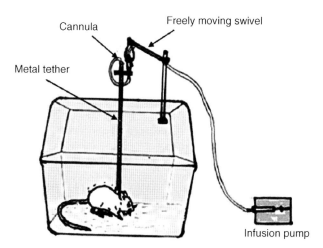

Figure 11.3 The setup used in the naturalistic GTN infusion model to awake rats. The indwelling catheter in the femoral artery is connected through a metal tether at the nape of the neck and the rats are allowed to move freely in the cage. GTN is infused intravenously after recovery from surgery. No anesthesia is used.

11.8
Transgenic Models

Three genes have been identified for familial hemiplegic migraine (FHM), a rare autosomal dominant subtype of migraine with aura that is characterized by transient hemiparesis during the aura phase of an attack. The genes are CACNA1A (FHM1) [175], ATP1A2 (FHM2) [176], and SCN1A (FHM3) [177]. Knock-in (KI) mouse models have been developed where the human pathogenic mutations are introduced. Two KI models for the CACNA1A gene mutations have so far been developed [178,179]. The R192Q mutation of the CACNA1A causes a mild form of FHM1, whereas the S218 L mutation is more severe and often lethal. These models have been used in several physiological and behavioral experiments with considerable success [180]. In R192Q mutant mice, a reduced threshold and an increased velocity of CSD have been found [179]. Furthermore, the model shows enhanced synaptic acetylcholine release under conditions in which the synaptic Ca^{2+} sensors are not saturated [179]. It also seems that the R192Q mutation has an effect on the trigeminal system, as CGRP immunoreactivity was decreased in thoracic ganglia and in the superficial lamina of the trigeminocervical complex in R192Q knock-in mice [181]. A major problem with the CACNA1A knock-in mice seems to be the validity of these animals for the prevalent types of migraine, migraine without aura (MO) and migraine with typical aura (MA). In humans, it has been shown that FHM differs from MA and MO not only in genetics but also in the response to migraine provoking agents [182–184]. Perhaps the FHM mice are not useful for the prevalent types of migraine. CGRP release from the trigeminal ganglion was increased in R192Q knock-in mice as compared with wild-type mice [185]. No change in CGRP release was found in dura mater between mutant and wild-type mice [185]. During restrain these animals seem to spontaneously express changes in facial expression that were reversed by rizatriptan [186]. Another type of genetically modified mice has elevated expression of human receptor activity-modifying protein 1 (hRAMP1), a subunit of the CGRP receptor [187]. Experiments using these models are further described in the following section.

11.9
Behavioral Models

Studying behavior makes it possible to use the animals over and over again. This has some major advantages as compared with lethal studies in terms of experimental design (crossover placebo-controlled trials), thereby reducing the number of animals needed to perform experiments. With this in mind, many obstacles need to be overcome in developing behavioral models that close the gap between preclinical and clinical testing of drugs. The behaviors tested should be spontaneous rather than evoked, as the major clinical symptom of migraine is spontaneous pain rather than evoked hyperalgesia [188–191]. Currently, no generally accepted behavioral migraine models exist, but several groups are working on different approaches to provide a clinically relevant rodent model. Migraine is diagnosed using a set of clinical criteria established by the International Headache Society [192]. The most common migraine symptoms are unilateral headache, nausea, hypersensitivity to light and sound, and decreased daily routine activity. A behavioral model of migraine should measure some of these manifestations. The models that have so far been employed show a great diversity of headache-inducing protocols and different behaviors as output.

11.9.1
Allodynia or Hyperalgesia

Facial and peripheral allodynia or hyperalgesia are symptoms occurring in up to 79% of migraine patients during an attack [193], probably due to central sensitization [194]. However, it is not a diagnostic symptom of migraine in the International Headache Classification [192]. As a behavioral parameter, it is evoked rather than spontaneous, but it is nevertheless one of the most tested behaviors in animal models of headache and facial pain due to its simplicity and ease of quantification using von Frey filaments, different temperatures, or irritants to test for mechanical, thermal, or chemical allodynia, respectively [156,195–201].

The two most promising models utilizing hyperalgesia as behavioral output are the well-established nitroglycerin-induced migraine model and a novel spontaneous trigeminal allodynia (STA) rat model.

Animals treated with nitroglycerin show hyperalgesia [156,202]. The GTN-induced hypersensitivity is reduced by sumatriptan [156], suggesting migraine specificity. The model mimics the very common human nitroglycerin infusion model [203] and also shows other migraine-related behaviors (see later sections) and upregulation of pain markers in the trigeminal system [156,204].

A novel migraine model in rats has been presented as the STA rat model of primary headache. Accordingly, STA rats have five features in common with migraineurs: (1) episodically changing trigeminal thresholds to von Frey filaments, possibly reflecting trigeminal hypersensitivity, (2) the STA trait is inherited, (3) the STA rats have increased sensitivity to sound as compared with normal rats, (4) increased sensitivity to the headache triggers GTN and CGRP, and (5) the STA rats respond to commonly used acute and preventive migraine therapeutics [199]. The model is interesting in the sense that it is spontaneous rather than provoked and does not need any manipulations in order to show the desired phenotype. To further validate and increase face and construct validities of the STA model, it must be shown that it is in fact having episodes of spontaneous migraine and not just allodynia. This can be done through testing of spontaneous behaviors detecting clinical manifestations of headache. One major disadvantage of using a spontaneous model like this compared with a provocation model is the episodic nature of the disease presence. Planning and performing experiments will be challenged by the fact that the animals need to be tested every day in order to determine whether they have headache or not.

11.9.2
Face Grooming

Models based on face grooming behavior utilize the fact that rats are known to exhibit short episodes of grooming directed specifically toward an area of irritation, compared with the more prolonged general grooming behavior performed to maintain the pelage [205,206]. This behavior has proved to be relevant for pain induced by formalin in the orofacial region [207,208]. Intuitively, this spontaneous behavior has high validity, as it is oriented directly toward the affected area. In spite of these findings, very few studies within headache research report the use of facial grooming as behavioral output.

Face grooming behavior has been used to detect trigeminal neuropathic pain in the chronic constriction injury model [200,209]. Also, rats infused with capsaicin in the cisterna magna show increased head grooming and scratching [210]. Within the migraine field, the behavior has been employed in detecting the presence of migraine in CGRP (1 μg/kg i.p.)-treated rats sensitized with GTN (10 mg/kg i.p.) prior to CGRP administration [211]. Additionally, this was reversed by sumatriptan, suggesting predictive validity of the model. Interestingly, GTN itself, though given in a dose that induces c-fos expression in the trigeminal nucleus caudalis, does not induce increased face grooming in these experiments unless a late effect is seen, which is hidden by the administration of CGRP. In order to become a major model in migraine research, the GTN/CGRP rat model needs further validation in terms of both testing other behaviors relevant to migraine and response to other treatments. Furthermore, it should be kept in mind that the GTN dose is equal to the high dose discussed in 11.7.

11.9.3
Photophobia

Photophobia is a common symptom associated with migraine [192] and it seems obvious to evaluate this behavior in animal models as it is easily quantified in a light–dark box setup.

Andrew Russo's group from the University of Iowa has extensively studied the effect of CGRP on light-aversive behavior in first genetically engineered *nestin/hRAMP1* mice that are sensitized to CGRP [212] and later wild-type mice using a light–dark box setup. The rationale of this model is based on the sensitivity of migraineurs to CGRP and the assumption that light aversion as detected in the light–dark box is a surrogate marker of photophobia. Generally, the results show that 2 μl of 0.5 nmol CGRP injected intracerebroventricularly is capable of inducing light-aversive behavior, although the wild-type mice need much stronger stimuli (in terms of much brighter light and habituation to the test chamber) to make the light aversion evident compared with the *nestin/hRAMP1* mice. Light-aversive behavior was observed in CGRP-treated animals spending significantly less time in the light zone compared with vehicle-treated controls. Treatment with the CGRP receptor antagonist olcegepant inhibits this effect, which validates that the light aversion demonstrated is indeed mediated by the CGRP receptor. Additionally, the light aversion is reversed by rizatriptan – a drug commonly used to treat migraine.

The model has been thoroughly validated to test for confounding parameters. It was shown that the aversion toward the light compartment is due to the light and not due to learning, nor due to the light zone being uncovered. If both compartments are dark, animals show no preference for either of them. The role of CGRP-induced anxiety was tested in an open field and no difference between vehicle and treatment groups was found [187,213–215].

11.9.4
Various Behaviors

Another genetically modified mouse has been recently proposed as a relevant migraine model [191]. Here, a transgenic knock-in mouse carrying the missense mutation for familial hemiplegic migraine is used that exhibits several migraine symptoms: photophobia, increased and lateralized head grooming, and abnormal eye closures. They were sex and stress dependent and specific antimigraine agents could reverse the symptoms. Some variability in the test group is expected because some animals will not have the attack at the specific time of testing. This was the case in all tested behaviors, but proved most problematic in the photophobia testing. Therefore, very large group sizes were required. However, this model must be considered one of the most promising behavioral models of familial hemiplegic migraine, as it has construct validity (the genetic components involved are identical), face validity (the model show relevant symptoms), and predictive validity (responds to commonly known therapeutics).

The effect of CSD on rat behavior has been studied in a panel of tests. CSD was introduced by NMDA topically applied to the dura mater through a catheter in freely moving rats. These rats showed changes in freezing behavior and a number of wet dog shakes in the first hour after provocation of CSD. Grooming, locomotion, circling, rearing, eating, and drinking behavior were not altered. Neither were the ultrasonic vocalizations compatible with pain calls [216]. These data suggest that CSD does not induce severe pain in rats.

11.10
Translation to Clinics: Limitations and Difficulties

In general, animal models are often of uncertain validity in predicting efficacy of new drugs. Multiple models of stroke in rodents, which seemingly mimic the human conditions exactly, have, for example, shown efficacy of new drugs, but this was not translated into efficacy in patients [217–219]. Many other disappointments can be mentioned, but the fact remains that the pharmaceutical industry normally requires positive effects in animal models before moving novel chemical entities into clinical trials. Migraine drug development is currently severely hampered by a lack of generally accepted animal models with ability to predict efficacy of antimigraine drugs.

We have described a number of animal models that are most commonly used in migraine research. However, the final proof of the pudding is whether models respond to specific acute antimigraine drugs. Fortunately, there are now several drugs with efficacy in migraine and no efficacy in any other painful condition. This pertains to the 5-$HT_{1B/D}$ receptor agonists, CGRP receptor antagonists, and 5-HT_{1F} receptor agonists. Because of their extreme receptor specificity, these drugs provide excellent validation of acute migraine models [220]. NSAIDs not only are effective in migraine [221], but also have efficacy in all other painful conditions and are thus not suitable for validating a migraine model. A valid animal model should be sensitive and specific. As with diagnostic criteria for diseases, too rigorous criteria result in very low sensitivity but high specificity. As a best compromise, we suggest that a useful model should respond to at least two of the three classes of specific antimigraine drugs. Whether the bar should be higher is, however, debatable. One might require that all specific drugs should work in the model and no unspecific drugs should work. This would be a very strict requirement and it seems unlikely that any animal model would be able to deliver such results. It is more likely that a model would respond to one or two of the specific drugs but not to the others and that a number of different models must be used to test future antimigraine drugs. Depending on the type of new drug, one model might respond and another not. The existence of a number of such models would allow a relatively precise estimation of new drugs for the acute treatment of migraine.

References

1 Steiner, T.J. et al. (2013) Migraine: the seventh disabler. *The Journal of Headache and Pain*, **14**, 1.

2 Olesen, J. et al. (2012) The economic cost of brain disorders in Europe. *European Journal of Neurology*, **19**, 155–162.

3 Tfelt-Hansen, P. and Olesen, J. (2012) Taking the negative view of current migraine treatments. *CNS Drugs*, **26**, 375–382.

4 Edvinsson, L. and Uddman, R. (2005) Neurobiology in primary headaches. *Brain Research. Brain Research Reviews*, **48**, 438–456.

5 Wolff, H.G. (1963) *Headache and Other Head Pain*, Oxford University Press.

6 Ray, B.S. and Wolff, H.G. (1940) Experimental studies on headache: pain-sensitive structures of the head and their significance in headache. *Archives of Surgery*, **41**, 813.

7 Humphrey, P.P. (2007) The discovery of a new drug class for the acute treatment of migraine. *Headache*, **47** (Suppl. 1), S10–S19.

8 Jansen-Olesen, I. et al. (2001) Characterization of CGRP1 receptors in the guinea pig basilar artery. *European Journal of Pharmacology*, **414**, 249–258.

9 Edvinsson, L. et al. (1990) Cerebrovascular responses to capsaicin *in vitro* and *in situ*. *British Journal of Pharmacology*, **100**, 312–318.

10 Edvinsson, L. and Jansen, I. (1987) Characterization of tachykinin receptors in isolated basilar arteries of guinea-pig. *British Journal of Pharmacology*, **90**, 553–559.

11 Uddman, R. et al. (1999) Helospectin-like peptides: immunochemical localization and effects on isolated cerebral arteries and on local cerebral blood flow in the cat.

Journal of Cerebral Blood Flow and Metabolism, **19**, 61–67.

12. Jansen-Olesen, I. et al. (1994) Vasoactive intestinal peptide (VIP) like peptides in the cerebral circulation of the cat. *Journal of the Autonomic Nervous System*, **49**, 97–103.

13. Edvinsson, L. et al. (1991) Analysis of the vasoconstrictor effects of sumatriptan on human cranial arteries. *Cephalalgia*, **11**, 210–211.

14. Nilsson, T. et al. (1999) Contractile 5-HT$_{1B}$ receptors in human cerebral arteries: pharmacological characterization and localization with immunocytochemistry. *British Journal of Pharmacology*, **128**, 1133–1140.

15. Adner, M. et al. (1994) Endothelin-A receptors mediate contraction in human cerebral, meningeal and temporal arteries. *Journal of the Autonomic Nervous System*, **49**, 117–121.

16. Jansen-Olesen, I. et al. (2003) In-depth characterization of CGRP receptors in human intracranial arteries. *European Journal of Pharmacology*, **481**, 207–216.

17. Jansen-Olesen, I. et al. (2004) Peptidergic and non-peptidergic innervation and vasomotor responses of human lenticulostriate and posterior cerebral arteries. *Peptides*, **25**, 2105–2114.

18. Jansen-Olesen, I. et al. (1997) Role of endothelium and nitric oxide in histamine-induced responses in human cranial arteries and detection of mRNA encoding H$_1$- and H$_2$-receptors by RT-PCR. *British Journal of Pharmacology*, **121**, 41–48.

19. Edvinsson, L. and Jansen, I. (1989) Characterization of 5-HT receptors mediating contraction of human cerebral, meningeal and temporal arteries: target for GR 43175 in acute treatment of migraine. *Cephalalgia*, **9**, 39–40.

20. Jansen, I. et al. (1992) Characterization of calcitonin gene-related peptide receptors in human cerebral vessels. *Annals of the New York Academy of Sciences*, **657**, 435–440.

21. Sams, A. et al. (1999) Equipotent *in vitro* actions of α- and β-CGRP on guinea pig basilar artery are likely to be mediated via CRLR derived CGRP receptors. *Regulatory Peptides*, **85**, 67–75.

22. Ferro, A. et al. (1995) A comparison of the contractile effects of 5-hydroxytryptamine, sumatriptan and MK-462 on human coronary artery *in vitro*. *British Journal of Clinical Pharmacology*, **40**, 245–251.

23. Edvinsson, L. et al. (2007) Inhibitory effect of BIBN4096BS, CGRP(8–37), a CGRP antibody and an RNA-Spiegelmer on CGRP induced vasodilatation in the perfused and non-perfused rat middle cerebral artery. *British Journal of Pharmacology*, **150**, 633–640.

24. Williamson, D. et al. (1997) Intravital microscope studies on the effects of neurokinin agonists and calcitonin gene-related peptide on dural vessel diameter in the anaesthetized rat. *Cephalalgia*, **17**, 518–524.

25. Gupta, S. et al. (2010) Improvement of the closed cranial window model in rats by intracarotid infusion of signalling molecules implicated in migraine. *Cephalalgia*, **30**, 27–36.

26. Juhl, L. et al. (2007) Effect of two novel CGRP-binding compounds in a closed cranial window rat model. *European Journal of Pharmacology*, **567**, 117–124.

27. Gozalov, A. et al. (2005) Role of KATP channels in the regulation of rat dura and pia artery diameter. *Cephalalgia*, **25**, 249–260.

28. Gozalov, A. et al. (2007) Role of BKCa channels in cephalic vasodilation induced by CGRP, NO and transcranial electrical stimulation in the rat. *Cephalalgia*, **27**, 1120–1127.

29. Boni, L.J. et al. (2009) The *in vivo* effect of VIP, PACAP-38 and PACAP-27 and mRNA expression of their receptors in rat middle meningeal artery. *Cephalalgia*, **29**, 837–847.

30. Petersen, K. et al. (2004) Inhibitory effect of BIBN4096BS on cephalic vasodilatation induced by CGRP or transcranial electrical stimulation in the rat. *British Journal of Pharmacology*, **143**, 697–704.

31. Akerman, S. et al. (2002) Nitric oxide synthase inhibitors can antagonize neurogenic and calcitonin gene-related peptide induced dilation of dural

meningeal vessels. *British Journal of Pharmacology*, **137**, 62–68.

32 Shepherd, S. *et al.* (1997) Differential effects of 5-HT$_{1B/1D}$ receptor agonists on neurogenic dural plasma extravasation and vasodilation in anaesthetized rats. *Neuropharmacology*, **36**, 525–533.

33 Shepheard, S. *et al.* (1999) Possible antimigraine mechanisms of action of the 5HT$_{1F}$ receptor agonist LY334370. *Cephalalgia*, **19**, 851–858.

34 Akerman, S. *et al.* (2002) The effect of anti-migraine compounds on nitric oxide-induced dilation of dural meningeal vessels. *European Journal of Pharmacology*, **452**, 223–228.

35 Akerman, S. and Goadsby, P.J. (2005) Topiramate inhibits trigeminovascular activation: an intravital microscopy study. *British Journal of Pharmacology*, **146**, 7–14.

36 Williamson, D. *et al.* (1997) Sumatriptan inhibits neurogenic vasodilation of dural blood vessels in the anaesthetized rat-intravital microscope studies. *Cephalalgia*, **17**, 525–531.

37 Moskowitz, M.A. (1984) The neurobiology of vascular head pain. *Annals of Neurology*, **16**, 157–168.

38 Markowitz, S. *et al.* (1987) Neurogenically mediated leakage of plasma protein occurs from blood vessels in dura mater but not brain. *Journal of Neuroscience*, **7**, 4129–4136.

39 Gabriella Buzzi, M. *et al.* (1989) Indomethacin and acetylsalicylic acid block neurogenic plasma protein extravasation in rat dura mater. *European Journal of Pharmacology*, **165**, 251–258.

40 Buzzi, M.G. and Moskowitz, M.A. (1990) The antimigraine drug, sumatriptan (GR43175), selectively blocks neurogenic plasma extravasation from blood vessels in dura mater. *British Journal of Pharmacology*, **99**, 202–206.

41 Connor, H. *et al.* (1998) Clinical evaluation of a novel, potent, CNS penetrating NK1 receptor antagonist in the acute treatment of migraine. *Cephalalgia*, **18**, 392.

42 Goldstein, D. *et al.* (1997) Ineffectiveness of neurokinin-1 antagonist in acute migraine: a crossover study. *Cephalalgia*, **17**, 785–790.

43 Norman, B. *et al.* (1998) To explore the preliminary safety and efficacy of intravenous L-758,298 (a prodrug of the NK1 receptor antagonist L-754,030) in the acute treatment of migraine. *Cephalalgia*, **18**, 1092–1093.

44 May, A. *et al.* (1996) Endothelin antagonist bosentan blocks neurogenic inflammation, but is not effective in aborting migraine attacks. *Pain*, **67**, 375–378.

45 Goldstein, D. *et al.* (2001) Lanepitant, an NK-1 antagonist, in migraine prevention. *Cephalalgia*, **21**, 102–106.

46 Jansen-Olesen, I. *et al.* (2013) Animal migraine models for drug development: status and future perspectives. *CNS Drugs*, **27**, 1049–1068.

47 Matsubara, T. *et al.* (1992) UK-14,304, *R*(−)-α-methyl-histamine and SMS 201-995 block plasma protein leakage within dura mater by prejunctional mechanisms. *European Journal of Pharmacology*, **224**, 145–150.

48 Lee, W.S. *et al.* (1995) Peripheral GABAA receptor-mediated effects of sodium valproate on dural plasma protein extravasation to substance P and trigeminal stimulation. *British Journal of Pharmacology*, **116**, 1661–1667.

49 O'Shaughnessy, C.T. and Connor, H.E. (1994) Investigation of the role of tachykinin NK1, NK2 receptors and CGRP receptors in neurogenic plasma protein extravasation in dura mater. *European Journal of Pharmacology*, **263**, 193–198.

50 Brändli, P. *et al.* (1996) Role of endothelin in mediating neurogenic plasma extravasation in rat dura mater. *Pain*, **64**, 315–322.

51 Schuh-Hofer, S. *et al.* (2006) Effect of hyperoxia on neurogenic plasma protein extravasation in the rat dura mater. *Headache*, **46**, 1545–1551.

52 Shepheard, S.L. *et al.* (1995) Comparison of the effects of sumatriptan and the NK1 antagonist CP-99,994 on plasma extravasation in dura mater and c-fos mRNA expression in trigeminal nucleus caudalis of rats. *Neuropharmacology*, **34**, 255–261.

53 Williamson, D.J. *et al.* (1997) The novel anti-migraine agent rizatriptan inhibits neurogenic dural vasodilation and

extravasation. *European Journal of Pharmacology*, **328**, 61–64.

54 Cutrer, F.M. et al. (1999) Effects of PNU-109,291, a selective 5-HT$_{1D}$ receptor agonist, on electrically induced dural plasma extravasation and capsaicin-evoked c-fos immunoreactivity within trigeminal nucleus caudalis. *Neuropharmacology*, **38**, 1043–1053.

55 Reuter, U. et al. (2001) Delayed inflammation in rat meninges: implications for migraine pathophysiology. *Brain*, **124**, 2490–2502.

56 Lambert, G.A. et al. (1988) Comparative effects of stimulation of the trigeminal ganglion and the superior sagittal sinus on cerebral blood flow and evoked potentials in the cat. *Brain Research*, **453**, 143–149.

57 Schepelmann, K. et al. (1999) Response properties of trigeminal brain stem neurons with input from dura mater encephali in the rat. *Neuroscience*, **90**, 543–554.

58 Ebersberger, A. et al. (1999) Release of substance P, calcitonin gene-related peptide and prostaglandin E2 from rat dura mater encephali following electrical and chemical stimulation *in vitro*. *Neuroscience*, **89**, 901–907.

59 Goadsby, P.J. et al. (1988) Release of vasoactive peptides in the extracerebral circulation of humans and the cat during activation of the trigeminovascular system. *Annals of Neurology*, **23**, 193–196.

60 Burstein, R. et al. (1998) Chemical stimulation of the intracranial dura induces enhanced responses to facial stimulation in brain stem trigeminal neurons. *Journal of Neurophysiology*, **79**, 964–982.

61 Ellrich, J. et al. (1999) Acetylsalicylic acid inhibits meningeal nociception in rat. *Pain*, **81**, 7–14.

62 Strassman, A.M. et al. (1996) Sensitization of meningeal sensory neurons and the origin of headaches. *Nature*, **384**, 560–564.

63 Fischer, M.J.M. et al. (2005) The nonpeptide calcitonin gene-related peptide receptor antagonist BIBN4096BS lowers the activity of neurons with meningeal input in the rat spinal trigeminal nucleus. *The Journal of Neuroscience*, **25**, 5877–5883.

64 Goadsby, P.J. and Hoskin, K.L. (1996) Inhibition of trigeminal neurons by intravenous administration of the serotonin (5HT)$_{1B/D}$ receptor agonist zolmitriptan (311C90): are brain stem sites therapeutic target in migraine? *Pain*, **67**, 355–359.

65 Koulchitsky, S. et al. (2004) Biphasic response to nitric oxide of spinal trigeminal neurons with meningeal input in rat: possible implications for the pathophysiology of headaches. *Journal of Neurophysiology*, **92**, 1320–1328.

66 Levy, D. et al. (2005) Calcitonin gene-related peptide does not excite or sensitize meningeal nociceptors: implications for the pathophysiology of migraine. *Annals of Neurology*, **58**, 698–705.

67 Levy, D. et al. (2004) Disruption of communication between peripheral and central trigeminovascular neurons mediates the antimigraine action of 5HT$_{1B/1D}$ receptor agonists. *Proceedings of the National Academy of Sciences of the United States of America*, **101**, 4274–4279.

68 Messlinger, K. and Ellrich, J. (2001) Meningeal nociception: electrophysiological studies related to headache and referred pain. *Microscopy Research and Technique*, **53**, 129–137.

69 Bove, G.M. and Moskowitz, M.A. (1997) Primary afferent neurons innervating guinea pig dura. *Journal of Neurophysiology*, **77**, 299–308.

70 Marfurt, C.F. (1981) The central projections of trigeminal primary afferent neurons in the cat as determined by the tranganglionic transport of horseradish peroxidase. *The Journal of Comparative Neurology*, **203**, 785–798.

71 Burstein, R. et al. (1998) Chemical stimulation of the intracranial dura induces enhanced responses to facial stimulation in brain stem trigeminal neurons. *Journal of Neurophysiology*, **79**, 964–982.

72 Hoskin, K.L. et al. (1996) Central activation of the trigeminovascular pathway in the cat

is inhibited by dihydroergotamine. *Brain*, **119**, 249–256.

73 Cumberbatch, M.J. *et al.* (1998) The effects of 5-HT$_{1A}$, 5-HT$_{1B}$ and 5-HT$_{1D}$ receptor agonists on trigeminal nociceptive neurotransmission in anaesthetized rats. *European Journal of Pharmacology*, **362**, 43–46.

74 Cumberbatch, M.J. *et al.* (1997) Rizatriptan has central antinociceptive effects against durally evoked responses. *European Journal of Pharmacology*, **328**, 37–40.

75 Cumberbatch, M.J. *et al.* (1999) Dural vasodilation causes a sensitization of rat caudal trigeminal neurones *in vivo* that is blocked by a 5-HT$_{1B/1D}$ agonist. *British Journal of Pharmacology*, **126**, 1478–1486.

76 Storer, R.J. and Goadsby, P.J. (2004) Topiramate inhibits trigeminovascular neurons in the cat. *Cephalalgia*, **24**, 1049–1056.

77 Andreou, A.P. and Goadsby, P.J. (2009) Therapeutic potential of novel glutamate receptor antagonists in migraine. *Expert Opinion on Investigational Drugs*, **18**, 789–803.

78 Goadsby, P.J. (2002) Adenosine A$_1$ receptor agonists inhibit trigeminovascular nociceptive transmission. *Brain*, **125**, 1392–1401.

79 Holland, P.R. *et al.* (2006) Modulation of nociceptive dural input to the trigeminal nucleus caudalis via activation of the orexin 1 receptor in the rat. *The European Journal of Neuroscience*, **24**, 2825–2833.

80 Charbit, A.R. *et al.* (2009) Comparison of the effects of central and peripheral dopamine receptor activation on evoked firing in the trigeminocervical complex. *The Journal of Pharmacology and Experimental Therapeutics*, **331**, 752–763.

81 Andreou, A.P. and Goadsby, P.J. (2011) Topiramate in the treatment of migraine: a kainate (glutamate) receptor antagonist within the trigeminothalamic pathway. *Cephalalgia*, **31**, 1343–1358.

82 Storer, R. and Goadsby, P. (2009) *N*-Methyl-D-aspartate receptor channel complex blockers including memantine and magnesium inhibit nociceptive traffic in the trigeminocervical complex of the rat. *Cephalalgia*, **29**, 135–1135.

83 Hoffmann, J. *et al.* (2013) Magnesium and memantine do not inhibit nociceptive neuronal activity in the trigeminocervical complex of the rat. *The Journal of Headache and Pain*, **1**, P71.

84 Hunt, S.P. *et al.* (1987) Induction of c-fos-like protein in spinal cord neurons following sensory stimulation. *Nature*, **328**, 632–634.

85 Willis, W. (1989) The origin and destination of pathways involved in pain transmission, in *Textbook of Pain*, Churchill Livingstone, pp. 112–127.

86 Nozaki, K. *et al.* (1992) CP-93,129, sumatriptan, dihydroergotamine block c-fos expression within rat trigeminal nucleus caudalis caused by chemical stimulation of the meninges. *British Journal of Pharmacology*, **106**, 409–415.

87 Nozaki, K. *et al.* (1992) Expression of c-fos-like immunoreactivity in brainstem after meningeal irritation by blood in the subarachnoid space. *Neuroscience*, **49**, 669–680.

88 Moskowitz, M. *et al.* (1993) Neocortical spreading depression provokes the expression of c-fos protein-like immunoreactivity within trigeminal nucleus caudalis via trigeminovascular mechanisms. *Journal of Neuroscience*, **13**, 1167–1177.

89 Strassman, A. *et al.* (1994) Distribution of fos-like immunoreactivity in the medullary and upper cervical dorsal horn produced by stimulation of dural blood vessels in the rat. *Journal of Neuroscience*, **14**, 3725–3735.

90 Stenberg, C. *et al.* (2005) Effect of local anaesthesia on neuronal c-fos expression in the spinal dorsal horn and hypothalamic paraventricular nucleus after surgery in rats. *Basic & Clinical Pharmacology & Toxicology*, **96**, 381–386.

91 Takayama, K. *et al.* (1994) The comparison of effects of various anesthetics on expression of Fos protein in the rat brain. *Neuroscience Letters*, **176**, 59–62.

92 Lima, D. *et al.* (1993) Differential activation of c-fos in spinal neurones by distinct classes of noxious stimuli. *Neuroreport*, **4**, 747–750.

93 Bullitt, E. (1989) Induction of c-fos-like protein within the lumbar spinal cord and

thalamus of the rat following peripheral stimulation. *Brain Research*, **493**, 391–397.

94 Lashley, K.S. (1941) Patterns of cerebral integration indicated by the scotomas of migraine. *Archives of Neurology and Psychiatry*, **46**, 331.

95 Leão, A.A.P. (1944) Spreading depression of activity in the cerebral cortex. *Journal of Neurophysiology*, **7**, 359–390.

96 Lauritzen, M. (1985) On the possible relation of spreading cortical depression to classical migraine. *Cephalalgia*, **5** (Suppl. 2), 47–51.

97 Lauritzen, M. (1994) Pathophysiology of the migraine aura. *Brain*, **117**, 199–210.

98 Charles, A. and Brennan, K. (2009) Cortical spreading depression: new insights and persistent questions. *Cephalalgia*, **29**, 1115–1124.

99 Ayata, C. (2013) Pearls and pitfalls in experimental models of spreading depression. *Cephalalgia*, **33**, 604–613.

100 Haghir, H. *et al.* (2009) Patterns of neurotransmitter receptor distributions following cortical spreading depression. *Neuroscience*, **163**, 1340–1352.

101 Andreou, A.P. *et al.* (2010) Animal models of headache: from bedside to bench and back to bedside. *Expert Review of Neurotherapeutics*, **10**, 389–411.

102 Basarsky, T.A. *et al.* (1999) Glutamate release through volume-activated channels during spreading depression. *Journal of Neuroscience*, **19**, 6439–6445.

103 Fabricius, M. *et al.* (1993) Microdialysis of interstitial amino acids during spreading depression and anoxic depolarization in rat neocortex. *Brain Research*, **612**, 61–69.

104 Peeters, M. *et al.* (2007) Effects of pan- and subtype-selective *N*-methyl-d-aspartate receptor antagonists on cortical spreading depression in the rat: therapeutic potential for migraine. *The Journal of Pharmacology and Experimental Therapeutics*, **321**, 564–572.

105 Lauritzen, M. and Hansen, A.J. (1992) The effect of glutamate receptor blockade on anoxic depolarization and cortical spreading depression. *Journal of Cerebral Blood Flow and Metabolism*, **12**, 223–229.

106 Somjen, G.G. (2001) Mechanisms of spreading depression and hypoxic spreading depression-like depolarization. *Physiological Reviews*, **81**, 1065–1096.

107 Kunkler, P.E. and Kraig, R.P. (2004) P/Q Ca^{2+} channel blockade stops spreading depression and related pyramidal neuronal Ca^{2+} rise in hippocampal organ culture. *Hippocampus*, **14**, 356–367.

108 Wu, Y.-J. *et al.* (2003) (*S*)-*N*-[1-(3-Morpholin-4-ylphenyl)ethyl]-3-phenylacrylamide: an orally bioavailable KCNQ2 opener with significant activity in a cortical spreading depression model of migraine. *Journal of Medicinal Chemistry*, **46**, 3197–3200.

109 Akerman, S. *et al.* (2008) Mechanically-induced cortical spreading depression associated regional cerebral blood flow changes are blocked by Na^+ ion channel blockade. *Brain Research*, **1229**, 27–36.

110 Chen, G. *et al.* (2005) Involvement of Kv1 potassium channels in spreading acidification and depression in the cerebellar cortex. *Journal of Neurophysiology*, **94**, 1287–1298.

111 Dietz, R.M. *et al.* (2008) Zn^{2+} influx is critical for some forms of spreading depression in brain slices. *The Journal of Neuroscience*, **28**, 8014–8024.

112 Basarsky, T.A. *et al.* (1998) Imaging spreading depression and associated intracellular calcium waves in brain slices. *Journal of Neuroscience*, **18**, 7189–7199.

113 Chan, W.N. *et al.* (1999) Identification of (−)-*cis*-6-acetyl-4*S*-(3-chloro-4-fluoro-benzoylamino)-3,4-dihydro-2,2-dimethyl-2*H*-benzo[*b*]pyran-3*S*-ol as a potential antimigraine agent. *Bioorganic & Medicinal Chemistry Letters*, **9**, 285–290.

114 Hauge, A.W. *et al.* (2009) Effects of tonabersat on migraine with aura: a randomised, double-blind, placebo-controlled crossover study. *Lancet Neurology*, **8**, 718–723.

115 Goadsby, P.J. *et al.* (2009) Randomized, double-blind, placebo-controlled, proof-of-concept study of the cortical spreading depression inhibiting agent tonabersat in migraine prophylaxis. *Cephalalgia*, **29**, 742–750.

116 Parsons, A.A. (2004) Cortical spreading depression: its role in migraine pathogenesis and possible therapeutic intervention strategies. *Current Pain and Headache Reports*, **8**, 410–416.

117 Afridi, S.K. et al. (2005) A PET study exploring the laterality of brainstem activation in migraine using glyceryl trinitrate. Brain, 128, 932–939.

118 Weiller, C. et al. (1995) Brain stem activation in spontaneous human migraine attacks. Nature Medicine, 1, 658–660.

119 Ayata, C. et al. (2006) Suppression of cortical spreading depression in migraine prophylaxis. Annals of Neurology, 59, 652–661.

120 Bogdanov, V.B. et al. (2011) Migraine preventive drugs differentially affect cortical spreading depression in rat. Neurobiology of Disease, 41, 430–435.

121 Tfelt-Hansen, P.C. and Tfelt-Hansen, J. (2009) Nitroglycerin headache and nitroglycerin-induced primary headaches from 1846 and onwards: a historical overview and an update. Headache, 49, 445–456.

122 Iversen, H.K. et al. (1989) Intravenous nitroglycerin as an experimental model of vascular headache. Basic characteristics. Pain, 38, 17–24.

123 Iversen, H. et al. (1989) Headache and changes in the diameter of the radial artery during 7 hours intravenous nitroglycerin infusion. Cephalalgia, 9, 82–83.

124 Iversen, H.K. et al. (1992) Dose-dependent headache response and dilatation of limb and extracranial arteries after three doses of 5-isosorbide-mononitrate. European Journal of Clinical Pharmacology, 42, 31–35.

125 Iversen, H.K. et al. (1993) Lack of tolerance of headache and radial artery diameter during a 7 hour intravenous infusion of nitroglycerin. European Journal of Clinical Pharmacology, 44, 47–50.

126 Thomsen, L.L. et al. (1994) A nitric oxide donor (nitroglycerin) triggers genuine migraine attacks. European Journal of Neurology, 1, 73–80.

127 Lassen, L.H. et al. (1998) Nitric oxide synthase inhibition: a new principle in the treatment of migraine attacks. Cephalalgia, 18, 27–32.

128 Lassen, L.H. et al. (1995) Histamine induces migraine via the H_1-receptor. Support for the NO hypothesis of migraine. Neuroreport, 6, 1475–1479.

129 Kruuse, C. et al. (2003) Migraine can be induced by sildenafil without changes in middle cerebral artery diameter. Brain, 126, 241–247.

130 Kruuse, C. et al. (2006) Dipyridamole may induce migraine in patients with migraine without aura. Cephalalgia, 26, 925–933.

131 Lassen, L.H. et al. (2002) CGRP may play a causative role in migraine. Cephalalgia, 22, 54–61.

132 Schytz, H.W. et al. (2009) PACAP38 induces migraine-like attacks in patients with migraine without aura. Brain, 132, 16–25.

133 Schytz, H.W. et al. (2010) The PACAP receptor: a novel target for migraine treatment. Neurotherapeutics, 7, 191–196.

134 Antonova, M. et al. (2012) Prostaglandin E_2 induces immediate migraine-like attack in migraine patients without aura. Cephalalgia, 32, 822–833.

135 Wienecke, T. et al. (2010) Prostaglandin I_2 (epoprostenol) triggers migraine-like attacks in migraineurs. Cephalalgia, 30, 179–190.

136 Olesen, J. et al. (2004) Calcitonin gene-related peptide receptor antagonist BIBN 4096 BS for the acute treatment of migraine. The New England Journal of Medicine, 350, 1104–1110.

137 Ho, T.W. et al. (2008) Efficacy and tolerability of MK-0974 (telcagepant), a new oral antagonist of calcitonin gene-related peptide receptor, compared with zolmitriptan for acute migraine: a randomised, placebo-controlled, parallel-treatment trial. Lancet, 372, 2115–2123.

138 Anthony, M. et al. (1978) Controlled trials of cimetidine in migraine and cluster headache. Headache, 18, 261–264.

139 Lassen, L.H. et al. (1996) Histamine-1 receptor blockade does not prevent nitroglycerin induced migraine. European Journal of Clinical Pharmacology, 49, 335–339.

140 Iversen, H. and Olesen, J. (1996) Headache induced by a nitric oxide donor (nitroglycerin) responds to sumatriptan. A human model for development of migraine drugs. Cephalalgia, 16, 412–418.

141 Tvedskov, J.F. et al. (2010) CGRP receptor antagonist olcegepant (BIBN4096BS) does

not prevent glyceryl trinitrate-induced migraine. *Cephalalgia*, **30**, 1346–1353.
142. Tvedskov, J.F. et al. (2010) Nitroglycerin provocation in normal subjects is not a useful human migraine model? *Cephalalgia*, **30**, 928–932.
143. Tvedskov, J.F. et al. (2004) The prophylactic effect of valproate on glyceryltrinitrate induced migraine. *Cephalalgia*, **24**, 576–585.
144. Krabbe, A.A. and Olesen, J. (1980) Headache provocation by continuous intravenous infusion of histamine. Clinical results and receptor mechanisms. *Pain*, **8**, 253–259.
145. Kruuse, C. et al. (2002) The phosphodiesterase 5 inhibitor sildenafil has no effect on cerebral blood flow or blood velocity, but nevertheless induces headache in healthy subjects. *Journal of Cerebral Blood Flow and Metabolism*, **22**, 1124–1131.
146. Christiansen, I. et al. (1999) Glyceryl trinitrate induces attacks of migraine without aura in sufferers of migraine with aura. *Cephalalgia*, **19**, 660–667.
147. Meng, I.D. and Bereiter, D.A. (1996) Differential distribution of fos-like immunoreactivity in the spinal trigeminal nucleus after noxious and innocuous thermal and chemical stimulation of rat cornea. *Neuroscience*, **72**, 243–254.
148. Sugiyo, S. et al. (2009) Effects of systemic bicuculline or morphine on formalin-evoked pain-related behaviour and c-fos expression in trigeminal nuclei after formalin injection into the lip or tongue in rats. *Experimental Brain Research*, **196**, 229–237.
149. Tassorelli, C. et al. (1996) Central effects of nitroglycerin in the rat: new perspectives in migraine research. *Functional Neurology*, **11**, 219–235.
150. Tassorelli, C. and Joseph, S. (1995) NADPH-diaphorase activity and Fos expression in brain nuclei following nitroglycerin administration. *Brain Research*, **695**, 37–44.
151. Tassorelli, C. et al. (1999) The effects on the central nervous system of nitroglycerin: putative mechanisms and mediators. *Progress in Neurobiology*, **57**, 607–624.
152. Tassorelli, C. et al. (2000) Effect of nitric oxide donors on the central nervous system: nitroglycerin studies in the rat. *Functional Neurology*, **15**, 19–27.
153. Tassorelli, C. et al. (2002) Nitroglycerin-induced activation of monoaminergic transmission in the rat. *Cephalalgia*, **22**, 226–232.
154. Pardutz, A. et al. (2000) Systemic nitroglycerin increases nNOS levels in rat trigeminal nucleus caudalis. *Neuroreport*, **11**, 3071–3075.
155. Knyihár-Csillik, E. and Vécsei, L. (1999) Effect of a nitric oxide donor on nitroxergic nerve fibers in the rat dura mater. *Neuroscience Letters*, **260**, 97–100.
156. Bates, E.A. et al. (2010) Sumatriptan alleviates nitroglycerin-induced mechanical and thermal allodynia in mice. *Cephalalgia*, **30**, 170–178.
157. Offenhauser, N. et al. (2005) CGRP release and c-fos expression within trigeminal nucleus caudalis of the rat following glyceryltrinitrate infusion. *Cephalalgia*, **25**, 225–236.
158. Read, S.J. et al. (1999) Effects of sumatriptan on nitric oxide and superoxide balance during glyceryl trinitrate infusion in the rat. Implications for antimigraine mechanisms. *Brain Research*, **847**, 1–8.
159. Read, S. et al. (1997) Enhanced nitric oxide release during cortical spreading depression following infusion of glyceryl trinitrate in the anaesthetized cat. *Cephalalgia*, **17**, 159–165.
160. Zhang, X. et al. (2013) Vascular ERK mediates migraine-related sensitization of meningeal nociceptors. *Annals of Neurology*, **73**, 741–750.
161. Sommers, M.G. et al. (2008) Suppression of noxious-induced c-fos expression in the rat lumbar spinal cord by isoflurane alone or combined with fentanyl. *Anesthesia and Analgesia*, **106**, 1303–1308.
162. Tassorelli, C. and Joseph, S.A. (1995) Systemic nitroglycerin induces Fos immunoreactivity in brainstem and forebrain structures of the rat. *Brain Research*, **682**, 167–181.

163 Ramachandran, R. et al. (2012) A naturalistic glyceryl trinitrate infusion migraine model in the rat. *Cephalalgia*, **32**, 73–84.

164 Pardutz, A. et al. (2002) Effect of systemic nitroglycerin on CGRP and 5-HT afferents to rat caudal spinal trigeminal nucleus and its modulation by estrogen. *The European Journal of Neuroscience*, **15**, 1803–1809.

165 Pardutz, A. et al. (2007) Oestrogen-modulated increase of calmodulin-dependent protein kinase II (CamKII) in rat spinal trigeminal nucleus after systemic nitroglycerin. *Cephalalgia*, **27**, 46–53.

166 Knyihár-Csillik, E. et al. (2007) Kynurenine in combination with probenecid mitigates the stimulation-induced increase of c-fos immunoreactivity of the rat caudal trigeminal nucleus in an experimental migraine model. *Journal of Neural Transmission*, **114**, 417–421.

167 Knyihar-Csillik, E. et al. (2008) The kynurenate analog SZR-72 prevents the nitroglycerol-induced increase of c-fos immunoreactivity in the rat caudal trigeminal nucleus: comparative studies of the effects of SZR-72 and kynurenic acid. *Neuroscience Research*, **61**, 429–432.

168 Tassorelli, C. et al. (2004) Nitroglycerin enhances cGMP expression in specific neuronal and cerebrovascular structures of the rat brain. *Journal of Chemical Neuroanatomy*, **27**, 23–32.

169 Tassorelli, C. et al. (2005) Parthenolide is the component of *Tanacetum parthenium* that inhibits nitroglycerin-induced Fos activation: studies in an animal model of migraine. *Cephalalgia*, **25**, 612–621.

170 Greco, R. et al. (2010) Alterations of the endocannabinoid system in an animal model of migraine: evaluation in cerebral areas of rat. *Cephalalgia*, **30**, 296–302.

171 Varga, H. et al. (2009) Selective inhibition of cyclooxygenase-2 attenuates nitroglycerin-induced calmodulin-dependent protein kinase II alpha in rat trigeminal nucleus caudalis. *Neuroscience Letters*, **451**, 170–173.

172 Ramachandran, R. et al. (2013) Nitric oxide synthase, calcitonin gene-related peptide and NK-1 receptor mechanisms are involved in GTN induced neuronal activation. *Cephalalgia*, **34**, 136–147.

173 Ramachandran, R. et al. (2013) Downstream signalling mechanisms in the trigeminal vascular system of awake rats after glyceryl trinitrate (GTN) infusion. Available at http://journals.lww.com/neuroreport/Abstract/1997/03240/Trigeminovascular_stimulation_in_conscious_rats.12.aspx (accessed July 9, 2013).

174 Martin, R.S. and Martin, G.R. (2001) Investigations into migraine pathogenesis: time course for effects of *m*-CPP, BW723C86 or glyceryl trinitrate on appearance of Fos-like immunoreactivity in rat trigeminal nucleus caudalis (TNC). *Cephalalgia*, **21**, 46–52.

175 Ophoff, R.A. et al. (1996) Familial hemiplegic migraine and episodic ataxia type-2 are caused by mutations in the Ca^{2+} channel gene CACNL1A4. *Cell*, **87**, 543–552.

176 De Fusco, M. et al. (2003) Haploinsufficiency of ATP1A2 encoding the Na^+/K^+ pump alpha2 subunit associated with familial hemiplegic migraine type 2. *Nature Genetics*, **33**, 192–196.

177 Dichgans, M. et al. (2005) Mutation in the neuronal voltage-gated sodium channel SCN1A in familial hemiplegic migraine. *Lancet*, **366**, 371–377.

178 Tottene, A. et al. (2005) Specific kinetic alterations of human $Ca_V2.1$ calcium channels produced by mutation S218L causing familial hemiplegic migraine and delayed cerebral edema and coma after minor head trauma. *The Journal of Biological Chemistry*, **280**, 17678–17686.

179 Van den Maagdenberg, A.M.J. et al. (2004) A Cacna1a knockin migraine mouse model with increased susceptibility to cortical spreading depression. *Neuron*, **41**, 701–710.

180 Tottene, A. et al. (2002) Familial hemiplegic migraine mutations increase Ca^{2+} influx through single human $Ca_V2.1$ channels and decrease maximal $Ca_V2.1$ current density in neurons. *Proceedings of the*

National Academy of Sciences of the United States of America, **99**, 13284–13289.
181 Mathew, R. *et al.* (2011) Immunohistochemical characterization of calcitonin gene-related peptide in the trigeminal system of the familial hemiplegic migraine 1 knock-in mouse. *Cephalalgia*, **31**, 1368–1380.
182 Hansen, J.M. *et al.* (2008) Calcitonin gene-related peptide does not cause the familial hemiplegic migraine phenotype. *Neurology*, **71**, 841–847.
183 Hansen, J.M. *et al.* (2008) Familial hemiplegic migraine type 1 shows no hypersensitivity to nitric oxide. *Cephalalgia*, **28**, 496–505.
184 Hansen, J.M. *et al.* (2008) Familial hemiplegic migraine type 2 does not share hypersensitivity to nitric oxide with common types of migraine. *Cephalalgia*, **28**, 367–375.
185 Fioretti, B. *et al.* (2011) Trigeminal ganglion neuron subtype-specific alterations of $Ca_V2.1$ calcium current and excitability in a Cacna1a mouse model of migraine. *The Journal of Physiology*, **589**, 5879–5895.
186 Langford, D.J. *et al.* (2010) Coding of facial expressions of pain in the laboratory mouse. *Nature Methods*, **7**, 447–449.
187 Russo, A.F. *et al.* (2009) A potential preclinical migraine model: CGRP-sensitized mice. *Molecular and Cellular Pharmacology*, **1**, 264–270.
188 Mogil, J.S. and Crager, S.E. (2004) What should we be measuring in behavioral studies of chronic pain in animals? *Pain*, **112**, 12–15.
189 Blackburn-Munro, G. (2004) Pain-like behaviours in animals: how human are they? *Trends in Pharmacological Sciences*, **25**, 299–305.
190 Mogil, J.S. (2009) Animal models of pain: progress and challenges. *Nature Reviews. Neuroscience*, **10**, 283–294.
191 Chanda, M.L. *et al.* (2013) Behavioral evidence for photophobia and stress-related ipsilateral head pain in transgenic Cacna1a mutant mice. *Pain*, **154**, 1254–1262.
192 Olesen, J. (2008) The international classification of headache disorders. *Headache*, **48**, 691–693.
193 Burstein, R. *et al.* (2000) An association between migraine and cutaneous allodynia. *Annals of Neurology*, **47**, 614–624.
194 Burstein, R. (2000) The development of cutaneous allodynia during a migraine attack: clinical evidence for the sequential recruitment of spinal and supraspinal nociceptive neurons in migraine. *Brain*, **123**, 1703–1709.
195 Wieseler, J. *et al.* (2012) Indwelling supradural catheters for induction of facial allodynia: surgical procedures, application of inflammatory stimuli, and behavioral testing. *Methods in Molecular Biology*, **851**, 99–107.
196 Edelmayer, R.M. *et al.* (2012) Activation of TRPA1 on dural afferents: a potential mechanism of headache pain. *Pain*, **153**, 1949–1958.
197 Stucky, N.L. *et al.* (2011) Sex differences in behavior and expression of CGRP-related genes in a rodent model of chronic migraine. *Headache*, **51**, 674–692.
198 Oshinsky, M.L. and Gomonchareonsiri, S. (2007) Episodic dural stimulation in awake rats: a model for recurrent headache. *Headache*, **47**, 1026–1036.
199 Oshinsky, M.L. *et al.* (2012) Spontaneous trigeminal allodynia in rats: a model of primary headache. *Headache*, **52**, 1336–1349.
200 Vos, B. *et al.* (1994) Behavioral evidence of trigeminal neuropathic pain following chronic constriction injury to the rat's infraorbital nerve. *Journal of Neuroscience*, **14**, 2708–2723.
201 Wei, X. *et al.* (2011) Activation of TRPV4 on dural afferents produces headache-related behavior in a preclinical rat model. *Cephalalgia*, **31**, 1595–1600.
202 Tassorelli, C. *et al.* (2003) Nitroglycerin induces hyperalgesia in rats: a time-course study. *European Journal of Pharmacology*, **464**, 159–162.
203 Olesen, J. *et al.* (1995) The nitric oxide hypothesis of migraine and other vascular headaches. *Cephalalgia*, **15**, 94–100.
204 Greco, R. *et al.* (2013) Effect of sex and estrogens on neuronal activation in an animal model of migraine. *Headache*, **53**, 288–296.
205 Griswold, J.G. *et al.* (1977) Condition of the pelage regulates sandbathing and

206 Cohen, J.A. and Price, E.O. (1979) Grooming in the Norway rat: displacement activity or "boundary-shift"? *Behavioral and Neural Biology*, **26**, 177–188.

207 Clavelou, P. *et al.* (1989) Application of the formalin test to the study of orofacial pain in the rat. *Neuroscience Letters*, **103**, 349–353.

208 Vos, B.P. *et al.* (1998) Behavioral assessment of facial pain in rats: face grooming patterns after painful and non-painful sensory disturbances in the territory of the rat's infraorbital nerve. *Pain*, **76**, 173–178.

209 Deseure, K.R. and Adriaensen, H.F. (2002) Comparison between two types of behavioral variables of non-evoked facial pain after chronic constriction injury to the rat infraorbital nerve. *Comparative Medicine*, **52**, 6.

210 Kemper, R.H. *et al.* (1997) Trigeminovascular stimulation in conscious rats. *Neuroreport*, **8**, 1123–1126.

211 Yao, D. and Sessle, B.J. (2008) Nitroglycerin facilitates calcitonin gene-related peptide-induced behavior. *Neuroreport*, **19**, 1307–1311.

212 Zhang, Z. *et al.* (2007) Sensitization of calcitonin gene-related peptide receptors by receptor activity-modifying protein-1 in the trigeminal ganglion. *The Journal of Neuroscience*, **27**, 2693–2703.

213 Kaiser, E.A. *et al.* (2012) Modulation of CGRP-induced light aversion in wild-type mice by a 5-HT$_{1B/D}$ agonist. *The Journal of Neuroscience*, **32**, 15439–15449.

214 Recober, A. *et al.* (2009) Role of calcitonin gene-related peptide in light-aversive behavior: implications for migraine. *The Journal of Neuroscience*, **29**, 8798–8804.

215 Recober, A. *et al.* (2010) Induction of multiple photophobic behaviors in a transgenic mouse sensitized to CGRP. *Neuropharmacology*, **58**, 156–165.

216 Akcali, D. *et al.* (2010) Does single cortical spreading depression elicit pain behaviour in freely moving rats? *Cephalalgia*, **30**, 1195–1206.

217 Gladstone, D.J. (2002) Toward wisdom from failure: lessons from neuroprotective stroke trials and new therapeutic directions. *Stroke*, **33**, 2123–2136.

218 Cook, D.J. and Tymianski, M. (2011) Translating promising preclinical neuroprotective therapies to human stroke trials. *Expert Review of Cardiovascular Therapy*, **9**, 433–449.

219 Mergenthaler, P. and Meisel, A. (2012) Do stroke models model stroke? *Disease Models & Mechanisms*, **5**, 718–725.

220 Hirsch, S. *et al.* (2013) The CGRP receptor antagonist BIBN4096BS peripherally alleviates inflammatory pain in rats. *Pain*, **154**, 700–707.

221 Tfelt-Hansen, P. and Rolan, P. (2006) Nonsteroidal inflammatory drugs in the acute treatment of migraine, in *The Headaches*, 3rd edn (eds J. Olesen, P.J. Goadsby, N.M. Ramadan, P. Tfelt-Hansen, and K.M.A. Welch), Lippincott, Williams & Wilkins, Philadelphia, pp. 449–457.

12
Nociceptive, Visceral, and Cancer Pain

Christophe Mallet, Denis Ardid, and David Balayssac

12.1
Introduction

This chapter describes, in three separate parts, classical animal tests or models used to study acute pain, cancer pain, and visceral pain. The first part briefly describes acute pain tests performed in the early steps of drug development in a rapid and less extensive way. In the second part, most of the visceral pain models used in preclinical studies are described. The last part describes animal models developed for cancer pain studies. Pain originating from metastatic cancer is the most important and requires strong analgesic treatment.

12.2
Acute Pain Tests

12.2.1
Introduction

The nociceptive pain tests can be divided into the following:

- *Phasic pain tests*: These tests include the tail flick test and the hot plate test. A brief noxious stimulus is applied to produce a pain-like state in the animal. The endpoint is the latency of the animal's response in escaping the pain source. The threshold is thus the latency of the response or the intensity of the stimulus needed to induce such a response. The main advantage of this kind of tests is that they are efficient. Only a few seconds are needed to apply the stimulus and the response of the animal appears usually less than 1 min after application.
- *Tonic pain tests*: These tests involve the injection of a noxious substance (formalin, acetic acid, mustard oil, capsaicin, or bee venom). The measure can be quantitative (time spent in the nociceptive behavior) or qualitative (score of the behavior) of a nociceptive behavior induced. Despite the fact that these tests are time consuming,

the clinical relevance is high because animals cannot escape the stimulus and have to cope with pain, similar to a human being in pain.

Typically, acute nociceptive tests are classified based on the nature of the stimulus used to evoke a pain response. Table 12.1 briefly describes all acute pain tests.

Table 12.1 Overview and description of acute pain tests.

Stimulus	Test	Principle	Endpoint	References
Mechanical	Paw pressure test	An increasing pressure is applied to the hind paw of the animal	Pressure required to elicit withdrawal of the hind paw	[1]
	Tail pressure test	An increasing pressure is applied at ~3 cm from the base of the tail	Latency of the first motor response of struggling or withdrawal of the tail due to the pressure	[2,3]
	Tail clip test	A clip is applied at ~1 cm from the base of the tail	Latency to bite or grasp the clip	[4,5]
	von Frey filaments (mice)	Calibrated von Frey filaments were applied to the plantar surface of a hind paw	Threshold force required to elicit withdrawal of the hind paw	[6]
Thermal (warm)	Tail/paw immersion	The paw or the distal half of the tail is dipped into a bath of noxious warm water thermostatically controlled	Latency to withdraw the tail/hind paw from the bath	[7]
	Radiant heat source test	A radiant heat source (focused high-intensity projector lamp beam) is focused on the plantar surface of the hind paw	Latency to withdraw paw from the stimulus	[8–10]
	Hot plate test	Animals are placed on a metal surface maintained at a noxious warm temperature	Latency to respond with a hind paw lick or shake/flutter	[11,12]
	Dynamic hot plate	The plate temperature increases up from non-noxious to noxious at a rate of 1 °C/min	Number of escape behaviors (jumps) in mice; number of paw licking and paw withdrawal in rat	[13,14]
	Escape test	Quantification of learned operant and innate reflex responses to a thermal stimulus (heat)	Latency and duration of escape from a compartment where the floor is heated	[15]

Thermal (cold)	Cold plate	Animals are placed on a metal surface maintained at a noxious cold temperature	Latency to respond with a hind paw lick or shake/flutter	[16,17]
	Tail/paw immersion	The paw or the distal half of the tail is dipped into a bath of noxious cold water thermostatically controlled	Latency to withdraw the tail/hind paw from the bath	[18]
	Dynamic cold plate	The plate temperature decreases down from 20 to 1 °C for mice and 5 °C for rats at a rate of 1 °C/min	Number of escape behaviors (jumps) in mice; number of paw licking and paw withdrawal in rats	[14]
	Escape test	Quantification of learned operant and innate reflex responses to a thermal stimulus (cold)	Latency and duration of escape from a compartment where the floor is cooled	[15]
Electrical	Grid shock test or shock titration test	Electrical stimulus induced by electrodes (implanted in tail, muscle, tooth pulp, etc.) or a grid (foot shock)	Latency or threshold stimulus intensity for evoking a withdrawal response. Responses can also be scored on a predicted scale of behaviors (e.g., crouch, jump, run, etc.)	[19–21]
Chemical	Writhing test	Intraperitoneal injection of acetic acid, phenyl benzoquinone, magnesium sulfate, and so on.	Number of abdominal contractions "writhes"	[22,23]
	Formalin test	Subcutaneous injection of diluted formalin into the plantar surface of a hind paw	Number or duration of nociceptive response (paw lifting, licking/biting, and flinching)	[24–27]
	Capsaicin test	Subcutaneous injection of diluted capsaicin into the hind paw or the face	Number or duration of nociceptive response (paw lifting, licking/biting, and flinching) during 5 min	[28]
	Bee venom test	Subcutaneous injection of honey bee venom into the hind paw	Number of paw flinches occurring during 5 min intervals	[29,30]

12.2.2
Electrical Stimulus

In contrast to other nociceptive stimuli that first activate nociceptors (end of the C fibers) and thus nerves, electrical stimulation directly activates primary afferents in a nonspecific manner, that is, fibers involved in pain or not. This nonnatural stimulus can be performed in different parts of the animal: tail, dental pulp, and limbs. Nowadays, this kind of stimulus is rarely used except in inducing stress, aversive/conditioning context, and so on. Variations of the electrode impedance can induce variation in results [31].

12.2.3
Thermal Stimulus

At first sight, thermal tests seem similar, for instance, tail flick and tail immersion tests, which consist of a thermal stimulation of the tail. However, they have to be distinguished in terms of physics (speed of cutaneous temperature variation is not the same for both the focused thermal stimulus and the immersion-induced stimulus), surface area [31], and site of stimulation on the organ [32].

Historically, tail flick, hot plate, and immersion tests were used for screening full opioids. Indeed, they were efficient for such drugs but not efficient for partial opioids or nonopioid analgesics. Moreover, they are prone to provoke an all-or-none response toward full opioids [31], which is clinically not relevant [33]. However, tests were adapted, for example, to a warm noxious context: tail flick or tail immersion tests used with lower temperatures [34] or with a linear increasing temperature [35] conferred a better efficiency for screening nonopioid analgesics or partial opioids. In an analogous manner, it is also the case for cold water tail flick test: used at 0 °C, kappa agonists produced poor antinociceptive effects [36], but at −10 °C, a variety of kappa agonists are efficient in producing antinociception [37].

Immersion tests require the animals to be restrained, which can induce stress and anxiety [38] and an experimenter bias [39], and thus difference in pain threshold. On the contrary, hot or cold plate tests have the advantage of allowing the animal to be free to move, thus allowing observation of spontaneous behaviors with less stress. However, these kinds of tests have the following disadvantages: (1) they present a huge variability of results even in the same laboratory [31,33]; (2) they promote habituation: repeated testing in this assay leads to marked latency changes [40,41]; and (3) they trigger diffuse inhibitory controls because all paws and/or the tail are stimulated simultaneously [42].

The main problem with these thermal tests resides in animal's thermoregulation. First, pharmacological compounds decreasing or increasing cutaneous blood flux can either decrease or increase the latency of animal's response [43]. Second, results will also depend on ambient temperature. Finally, Le Bars' team demonstrated that spontaneous variations of the temperature of the tail up to 8 °C can be produced and influence results [44,45]. This demonstration highlights that a careful control of the ambient temperature is needed.

12.2.4
Mechanical Stimulus

Mechanical stimulus has been used earlier as a noxious stimulation in clinical pain research. Devices used by Randall and Sellito (modified and called analgesy-meter) apply a known progressive pressure on the paw of the animal placed between a flat surface and a blunt pointer. Restraining the animal in a vertical position can induce a stress that can interfere with pain evaluation. Another drawback of this technique is the touch sensation (when the probe first touches the foot) that can be thought of as a conditional stimulus.

Another way to evaluate pain induced by a mechanical stimulus is through a calibrated von Frey filament. This test is almost always used to assess allodynia or hyperalgesia in chronic pain models, but can be used in naïve mice (not rat) to induce a noxious stimulus [46]. Currently, it is being assessed whether von Frey stimulation evokes nociception or "tickle" to the mice [47]. Limitations of this test remain on the precision of the threshold, which can be affected by the opposing force performed by the animal limb on the filament and/or by the logarithmic scale of the measure. Bias can also be introduced by the experimenter who manually determines the load rate, decides how long to apply the stimulus, and subjectively determines what constitutes the withdrawal.

Other devices based on these two tests have been proposed: "automated" von Frey, calibrated forceps, force transducer mounted on a unit fitted to the operator's thumb, and so on.

12.2.5
Chemical Stimulus

Nociceptive tests described up to this point are evoked pain tests. Patients suffering from chronic pain complain more about spontaneous or ongoing pain than evoked pain [48–50]. Pain tests using chemical stimulation, especially the formalin test, can partially model spontaneous pain, which is an advantage. Except for the first phase of the formalin test and contrary to the phasic pain tests, tonic pain tests present an inflammatory component. Indeed, only these latter phases are sensible to COX inhibitors.

The writhing test is largely used to screen analgesics because of its high sensibility and, hence, is used in preliminary screening phases. However, it is not predictive of analgesic effect because many compounds (not commonly considered to be analgesics) protect against writhing [51].

Contrary to this test, some authors declare that the formalin test (especially the second phase) can reflect a neuropathic pain [52,53]. This test is a time-consuming task, which is a serious disadvantage. Several systems have been employed to automate the formalin test [54,55].

12.3
Visceral Pain Models

12.3.1
Introduction

Visceral disorders constitute a significant socioeconomic burden worldwide. They are characterized by pain and discomfort. Visceral pains consist in diffuse and irradiant painful sensation. They are linked with hypersensitivity phenomenon, motor impairment, and influenced by psychological state of the patient. They can arise from three main body regions: chest, abdomen, and pelvic regions. These pains can be subdivided into functional bowel disorders, chronic pelvic pain with or without identifiable origins, and chronic inflammatory visceral pain due to organ inflammation (e.g., cystitis, pancreatitis, and inflammatory bowel diseases (IBDs)). Visceral pains share many characteristics with somatic pain, but differ in some ways: they are diffuse in terms of location and timing, lead to poorly defined sensations and referred phenomena, and are accompanied by strong autonomic reflexes. The origin of pain at the peripheral level can be due to visceral sensitization induced by low- or strong-grade inflammation or by unexplained phenomena that lead to an increase in excitability of primary afferent fibers. At the central level, that is, spinal cord or central nervous system, they share many sensitization mechanisms that can be found in somatic pain. The study of the mechanisms involved in these visceral pains is made difficult by the accessibility to visceral structures and the poor knowledge of their pathophysiology. Treating visceral pain is a real challenge, especially when there is no known pathophysiological basis like functional gastrointestinal disorders (FGIDs). Relief from visceral pain is based on antispasmodic drugs for the low painful forms to antidepressants for the severe forms. The management of these visceral pains needs improvement that depends on better understanding of the pathophysiological mechanisms. For this purpose, animal models are important because they allow fundamental mechanisms involved in several pathological contexts to be studied and could lead to exploration of new targets. In this section, we address the question of the validity of the model developed and their relationship with human disorders. We will first describe methods used to determine pain in animal models of visceral pain, and then focus on the different models developed according to the concerned physiological system.

12.3.2
Pain Achievement Test

Pain exploration in visceral models is based on several endpoints. Contrary to somatic pain that used many reflex responses to determine a threshold or a delay after applied pain stimulation, most of the tests used in the visceral field measured an integrated response. Among them, the contraction of the abdominal muscle is commonly used. Electrodes are implanted in the abdominal muscles and the visceral motor reflex (VMR) is generally quantified by measuring the amplitude of the electromyographic response to abdominal or pelvic organ distension [56] following externalization of the electrodes or using radiotelemetric implants. This technique is mainly used in abdominal and pelvic area stimulation, but it can also be used in other visceral stimulations as done by Rouzade *et al.* [57] in measuring electromyographic response of neck muscle to gastric distension. Some other techniques were developed to avoid the surgical procedure of the implantation of the electrodes. Some papers relate the use of a manometric recording of the intracolonic pressure during distension. Comparison of results from this method with those from the VMR method showed a good correlation, which validates this technique [58]. Other paradigms are based on the observation of the animal behavior during distension to determine the threshold of visceral sensitivity [59] or to quantify the painful reaction [60]. Pseudoaffective response is also evaluated by measuring the variation in blood pressure and heart rate. This response can be different in vigil and anesthetized animals and according to the anesthetic used [56]. Visceral sensitivity can also be determined by measuring neuronal activity. Evaluation can be performed either directly by using electrophysiological techniques recording neuronal activity in anesthetized animals or indirectly by measuring the expression of immediate early gene transcription factors such as c-Fos in spinal cord layers. Another indirect measurement of visceral hypersensitivity can be done using the evaluation of referred allodynia. It was first demonstrated by Giamberardino *et al.* [61] using electrical muscle stimulation and vocalization recording, but some techniques are less invasive by using von Frey hair applications at the referred somatic area [59].

12.3.3
Animal Models

Modeling chronic visceral pain is a real challenge because of the difficulty in reaching the organ and because, for most of the pathologies, mechanisms involved in visceral hypersensitivity are unknown. Most of the models used to study visceral hypersensitivity were developed in the colon. This organ is indeed the most easy to reach to perform distension in awake animals. However, other studies were performed in other chronic visceral pain contexts such as endometriosis, pancreatitis, gall bladder, and dyspepsia.

Ureter In 1988, Giamberardino *et al.* [62] described a new model of referral hypersensitivity measured by electromyographic recording of the dorsal muscle in response to an electrical stimulation of ureter. However, their paper describes a complex technique with a nonphysiological stimulation of the organ. The same team has developed a ureteral calculosis pain model consisting in the implantation of a dental cement stone in the ureter [63]. Hypersensitivity was determined using an electrical or manual stimulation of the obliquus externus muscle or the c-Fos expression at the spinal cord level. In the same manner, Matsumoto *et al.* [64] demonstrated that electrical stimulation of the ureter induced an increase in the medullary c-Fos expression associated with an increase in the arterial blood pressure. Roza and Laird [65] have developed a distension test of the ureter in an anesthetized animal by measuring the increase in arterial blood pressure. The same team has also shown that there are several plasticity phenomena at the spinal cord level (increase in basal neuronal activity, recruitment of primary afferent fibers, and decrease in convergent neuronal excitability threshold) leading to referral hyperalgesia phenomenon [66].

Female Reproductive Organs The distension test is mostly used in the study of pain in female reproductive organs. Guilbaud *et al.* [67] described the overactivation of thalamic neurons in response to sensitized uterus and vagina distension. Bradshaw et al. [68] showed a modification of behavioral response (escape response) to uterus or vagina distension. Wesselmann and Lai [69] have developed a model of uterine horn sensitization induced by local mustard oil with analysis of pain behaviors. Sandner-Kiesling et al. [70] described a distension test of the uterine cervix with an electromyographic recording of the abdominal writhes in which the C fibers are involved.

There are several models of endometriosis in primates, but also in rats and mice. Some of these models have demonstrated an increase in the uterine or vaginal sensitivity.

Bladder Most of the published works on bladder and pain were performed in sensitized models by instillation of algogenic compounds or after systemic injection of cystitis-induced compounds. However, some works have been performed in healthy conditions. For example, Vizzard [71] described an increase in the medullar c-Fos expression following distension of the bladder using saline. Ness et al. [72] have developed a bladder distension test in anesthetized male and female rats with determination of the variation of blood pressure and electromyographic recording of abdominal writhes. Concerning cystitis, a spontaneous model of cystitis exists in cats with clear related human symptoms [73]. The most used model is the cyclophosphamide-induced cystitis. Well known from the early 1970s, several studies were performed. In this model, cyclophosphamide metabolite, acrolein, synthesized at the bladder level damages the interstitial cells [74]. This model is used by Boucher et al. [75] who measured the visceral pain by determining a behavioral score. This model was adapted in mice, in which painful behavioral phases [76] and referral pain (assessed through an abdominal von Frey score) [77] were observed. Other algogenic compounds were used to induce cystitis. For example, xylene instillation in the bladder induced painful behavioral responses [78]. McMahon and Abel [79] used several proinflammatory substances intravesically administered in decerebrated rats and showed a hypersensitivity to bladder distension associated with referred hyperalgesia. Terebentin oil bladder inflammation is associated with a somatic hyperalgesia measured by the decrease in withdrawal threshold in the hind paw pressure test [80]. The intravesical injection of NGF induced inflammation, bladder hyperreflexia, and increased expression of the c-Fos in the spinal cord [81]. Ribeiro et al. [82] demonstrated the involvement of nitric oxide (NO) in a model of hemorrhagic cystitis induced by ifosfamide. In a model of cystitis induced by acetic acid instillation, Cruz and Downie [83] showed an increase in abdominal visceromotor reflex during urination or bladder distension. Zymosan can also be used to induce bladder hypersensitivity [84].

Prostate Several models (spontaneous, infectious, immune, hormonal, or induced by stress or chemical irritants) of prostatitis in animals are described by Vykhovanets et al. [85] in their review. However, pain has been rarely explored, and when it was, it was done with von Frey hair application to the abdominal area [86].

Colon Colon has been extensively studied in the context of visceral pain because of its accessibility. Two different colonic pain models exist: the first type of model is induced by inflammation of the gut wall as observed in IBD in humans, and the second type of model is developed to mimic colonic hypersensitivity of irritable bowel syndrome (IBS). IBD models consist in several acute and chronic modes of induction of mucosal inflammation. In his exhaustive review, Mizoguchi [87] describes 66 models of IBD in several species. Most of them consist in genetically engineered mice models, chemically induced mice models, and other models (spontaneous, using cell transfer, and congeneic models). The genetic models are conventional or conditional knockout (KO) focusing on cytokine production, whereas oldest models consist in chemically induced inflammation in rats and mice. Among the chemically induced colonic inflammation models, the well-known model of trinitrobenzene sulfonic acid (TNBS), first described by Morris *et al.* [88], has been extensively used. Instillation of zymosan [89] and dextran sodium sulfate in drinking water [90] induced slight inflammation compared with TNBS. The face validity of these models is limited by the fact that these models develop a sustained inflammation different from IBD pathologies characterized by inflammation spurts. IBS models were developed according to epidemiological and pathophysiological clinical data. They can be divided into two classes according to their induction procedure: models involving stimulations of the CNS and models involving peripheral stimulations. CNS stimulation models are based on stress-induced colonic hypersensitivity and include acute stress, chronic mild stress, neonatal maternal separation stress, genetic model of chronic stress, and posttraumatic stress disorder models (see references in Ref. [91]). Concerning peripheral stimulations, some models are based on intestinal homeostasis perturbation of newborns, including painful stimulation or irritation [60]. Regarding human IBS etiology, other models are based on postinfectious or postinflammatory origins. Bacteria and parasite infections induced long-lasting colonic hypersensitivity that is longer than those obtained with chemical irritants such as TNBS [92]. Recent interesting approaches utilized supernatants from human biopsies or fecal sample from IBS or IBD patients to induce animal colonic hypersensitivity [93,94].

12.3.4
Pathophysiology and Pharmacology

Animal models of visceral pain are based on the induction of a visceral hypersensitivity of an organ. This hypersensitivity can involve different mechanisms at peripheral and central levels. In fact, sensitization of viscera can be obtained following inflammatory mediators released from inflammatory or immune cells, from tissue, from nerve endings, or from blood vessels. As for somatic pain, the inflammatory mixture can sensitize nociceptors and lead to an increase in their excitability. This contributes to some phenomena such as the decrease in the activation threshold, overresponse to a supraliminal stimulation, spatial summation of the responses, and waking of silent nociceptors. At the central level, the spinal cord plays an important role. At this level, neuronal plasticity contributes to the hyperexcitability of convergent neurons and to the modification of the descending control. The spinal cord is also involved in the viscerosomatic convergences responsible for referred allodynia to cutaneous fields and the viscerovisceral hypersensitivity by which the hypersensitivity of a viscus could lead to the hypersensitivity of another. Finally, at the central level, the brain is also mainly involved. It is well documented that anxiety, stress, and depression modulate visceral sensitivity and that several brain regions are able to modify the pain experience arising from viscera. Many animal models, more and more sophisticated, were developed for modeling this hypersensitivity, but new innovative treatments are still lacking in clinical practice.

12.4
Cancer Pain Models

12.4.1
Introduction

More than 10 million people are diagnosed with cancer every year. Pain is the first symptom of cancer in 20–50% of all patients with cancer, and 30–50% of these patients have moderate to severe pain [95]. Frequency and intensity of cancer pain increase with advancing stages of disease, and 75–90% of patients with metastatic or advanced stage cancer experience cancer pain [96]. Cancer pain can be due to a direct tumor infiltration or due to iatrogenic effects of diagnostic and therapeutic support (surgery, radiotherapy, and anticancer drugs) [96]. In most cases, cancer pain prevalence, *stricto sensu*, originated more from cancer metastases than from primary tumors such as sarcoma. Tumor-induced bone pain is the most common pain in patients with advanced cancer and the most common presenting symptom indicating metastases [96]. Bone marrow, mineralized bone, and periosteum are highly innervated with sensory and sympathetic nerves [96]. Pain treatment from bone metastases involves the use of various complementary approaches, including radiotherapy, chemotherapy, and treatment with bisphosphonates and analgesics [96]. However, cancer-induced pain, and particularly bone cancer pain, is difficult to manage. The main analgesic drug used (e.g., NSAIDs and opioids) can be limited by adverse reactions [96]. In this context, numerous animal models of cancer-induced pain have been developed in order to understand the specificity of cancer pain and to improve therapeutic strategies.

12.4.2
Pain Assessment in Animal Models of Cancer Pain

As the majority of pain models tried to reproduce bone metastases in hind limbs, nociceptive disorders in these animal models are assessed with mechanical or thermal stimuli applied to the hind paw. The main pain symptom assessed is the mechanical allodynia or hyperalgesia with the von Frey hair test or the Randall–Selitto test [95]. The hot thermal hyperalgesia/allodynia was assessed with the Hargreaves' test [97] or the hot plate test [98]. Nocifensive behaviors (e.g., guarding, fighting, and vocalization) were also recorded following the palpation of animals [99,100]. Spontaneous behaviors of animals were also evaluated, such as licking, grooming, guarding, flinching, or hunching [95,98,100–104].

12.4.3
Animal Models

Various animal models of cancer pain have been performed by using the graft of cancer cells [105] or using transgenic mice developing spontaneous cancer [100]. Many of these animal models result from the injection of cancer cells mimicking a metastatic encroachment [105] such as bone metastasis [96]. Models were developed in both mice and rats. Murine models offer the possibility to use athymic mice, which can receive allograft of cancer cells from other species (e.g., human cancer cells) [105]. The main sites of cell injection remained hind limb bones [106], but more rarely other injection sites could also be used such as near the sciatic nerve [107] or orofacial areas [108,109].

Bone Cancer Pain Animal models of bone pain were developed by the injection of cancer cells into osseous cavities (e.g., femur and tibia) [99,106] or near the bones (e.g., plantar hind paw, upper part of the thigh, and calcaneus) [95,110,111]. Injected cancer cells were from various origins such as human tongue squamous cell carcinoma [105], mice fibrosarcoma cells (NCTC 2472) [101], and rat mammary gland carcinoma cells (MRMT-1) [102]. Cancer cell growth and encroachment were responsible for edema and osteolysis, which was validated with radiography or tomodensitometry [99].

Bone cancer pain remains a very good approach. In the United States, prostate cancer is the most commonly diagnosed cancer in males and the second leading cause of death from cancer in men [112]. Bone is by far the most common site for prostate cancer metastasis, since $\sim 90\%$ of patients suffering from a metastatic prostate cancer presented spine metastases [113] at autopsy.

Visceral Cancer Pain Few animal models explore visceral cancer pain. A model of spontaneous pancreatic cancer has been developed using transgenic mice expressing the N-terminal 127 amino acids of simian virus 40 large T antigen, under the control of the rat elastase-1 promoter [100]. Animals displayed spontaneous pain behaviors (hunching) and palpation-induced vocalization [100]. Another model of rat bladder cancer was developed by the injection of a rat bladder cancer cell line into the left lateral wall of the bladder [114].

Orofacial Cancer Pain Animal models of orofacial cancer pain have been developed by the injection of cancer cell lines into the vibrissal pad (Walker carcinosarcoma 256/B cells) and the gingiva (squamous cell carcinoma SCC-158 cells) of rats [108,109]. These models provided interesting information similar to orofacial cancer patients, involving trigeminal nerve area, with mechanical allodynia, thermal hyperalgesia, and feeding disorders [108].

12.4.4
Pathophysiology and Pharmacology

These animal models offer a deeper insight into cancer pain pathophysiology. Osteolysis observed in bone cancer is directly responsible for pain (for review and discussion, see Ref. [115]). Tumors and osteoclasts promoted a local acidosis that would stimulate acid-sensing ion channels expressed by nociceptors (e.g., transient receptor potential vanilloid 1 and acid-sensing ion channel-3) [115]. According to this pathway, the bisphosphonate ibandronate was able to attenuate bone cancer pain in a bone cancer pain murine model preventing bone destruction, inducing tumor cell necrosis, and preventing neuronal sensitization in the spinal cord [116]. This therapeutic approach is particularly interesting since ibandronate may represent a good strategy for patients suffering from bone cancer pain [117].

Besides osteolysis, the nervous system can be sensitized by the cancer cells and their microenvironment with the production of algogens (e.g., prostaglandin, bradykinin, nerve growth factor (NGF), and endothelin-1) [96]. Endothelins are small peptides mainly secreted by endothelial cells, cardiomyocytes, and leukocytes with vascular and nonvascular effects mediated by the protein kinase C pathway. Multiple cancers produced endothelin-1 (e.g., prostate, breast, colon, pancreatic, hepatocellular, endometrial, lung, and oral squamous cell carcinoma) [118]. Recent works suggested that endothelin-1 was involved in the pathogenesis of pain (for review, see Ref. [118]). Endothelin-A receptor antagonism attenuates cancer pain in a mice model of plantar cancer cell injection (human tongue squamous cell carcinoma) [105]. More interestingly, this analgesic effect of endothelin-A receptor antagonism is mediated through endogenous opioids [105]. Recent work has suggested that the NGF pathway could represent an interesting strategy. In a mouse model of bone metastasis, after femoral injection of canine prostate carcinoma cells, anti-NGF therapy reduced nociceptive behaviors, sensory and sympathetic nerve sprouting, and neuroma formation associated with cancer cells [119]. In March 2012, the FDA renewed its interest in the development of anti-NGF products as part of the analgesic armamentarium and notably for cancer pain.

12.4.5
Conclusions

These animal models represent a very good base to mimic cancer pain induced by bone metastasis, with the inoculation of cancer cells into long bones. However, it is to be noted that metastases occur generally in the spinal bones.

These animal models offer a good response to a majority of analgesics (e.g., opioids, cannabinoids, and NSAIDs) and also offer the opportunity of innovative strategies such as endothelin-1 inhibitor or anti-NGF.

12.5
Translation to Clinics: Difficulties and Limitations

Pain is a symptom occurring from different and multiple disorders. Etiology and pathophysiology of many such disorders are unknown. This is one reason (among many others) that makes validation of animal pain models and translation to clinics challenging and suboptimal.

12.5.1
Acute Pain Tests

These classical nociceptive tests are routinely used in naïve animals as preclinical screens for novel analgesics. Interestingly, many acute animal pain tests were based on clinical pain tests performed in healthy patients. However, in both cases (healthy animal or volunteers), dysfunctional or modified neuronal mechanisms did not appear in healthy but in pathophysiological context. Efficiency of a new analgesic can thus be masked because target of the therapeutic compound cannot be entirely apparent in a naïve condition, but be expressed in pain condition (inflammation, neuropathy, etc.). These tests can be performed in animal pain models (inflammatory, neuropathic, cancer pain models, etc.) to reveal hyperalgesia (an increased response to a stimulus that is normally painful). However, even in this context, they only reflect the sensory-discriminative dimension of pain (stimulus localization, intensity, and modality). These tests did not provide information concerning the affective-motivational (unpleasantness, fear, distress, arousal, etc.) and cognitive (attention, memory, etc.) processing of pain. This bias can be reduced by using different paradigms (elevated plus maze, social and spatial recognition memory tests, Morris water maze, open field tests, forced swim test, sucrose preference test, etc.) that assess motor activity, coordination, anxiety- and depression-related behavior, learning, and memory in pain animal models. The other solution, complementary to the latter, would be to develop assays measuring the affective-motivational aspect of pain (drug-induced reward-related behavior, escape/avoidance paradigm, activity in home cage, conditioned place preference/aversion, etc.). Some of these tests attempt to measure spontaneous pain. New approaches to measuring spontaneous pain evolve in that way as the grimace scale, the catwalk, and so on. An evolution of the classical nociceptive tests toward more clinically relevant pain states is needed to better characterize the global impact of pain. It would also improve the evaluation of the new analgesics and the predictive validity and, thus, the translation of novel treatments into successful patient pain management.

12.5.2
Visceral Pain Models

The advantage of the visceral animal models developed consists in the exploration of fundamental mechanisms of visceral hypersensitivity. But several questions remain unanswered and the validity of these models is thus questionable. Strong construct validity is difficult to obtain as it is a matter of fact that in many cases the human etiology is unknown and several specificities of the visceral field are still ignored. For example, although many visceral pains affect particularly women as per IBS pathology, most of the studies are performed with males. The face validity of these models is mainly based on the apparition of a visceral hypersensitivity not always described in human pathologies or far from the described clinical pain and associated symptoms as, for example, in IBS. This face validity will be increased if other behavioral parameters are measured as spontaneous pain (locomotion, food intake, conditioned place preference, etc.) or cognitive and emotional impairments induced by pain. The predictive validity is still questionable because there is no recognized analgesic compound effective in human pathologies. However, all these models represent good tools to study mechanisms involved in the sensitization phenomena that we can suspect in chronic visceral pain and identified new pharmacological targets.

12.5.3
Cancer Pain Models

Even if these animal models are very interesting, we can underline some misleading approaches.

The majority of cancer pain models were developed to mimic bone metastases. Bone metastases were reproduced with the injection of cancer cells into hind limb bones, whereas in clinical practice, bone metastases can affect numerous different bones (e.g., vertebra, hip, or rib bones). One can suppose that the site of bone metastasis can influence the level of pain perception. Besides bone pain, the bone metastases can also be responsible for bone fractures and spinal cord compression resulting in complications (e.g., numbness or urination difficulties), which are rarely or never assessed in animal models. Also, the normal evolution and dissemination of cancer in patients with bone metastases is not yet reproduced with the radical etiology of these animal models by injecting cancer cells. Another misleading concept is that models of bone cancer pain are mainly performed with young adult and healthy animals, whereas the median age at diagnosis for cancer of all sites corresponds to senior citizens aged 66 years (National Cancer Institute), and frequently suffering from comorbidities.

Finally, getting closer to the clinical setting, the next step could be the assessment of cancer pain and chemotherapy-induced peripheral neuropathy in one animal model, since aside from cancer pain, iatrogenic pain induced by chemotherapy regimens still represents an important issue in patient care [120].

12.5.4
Conclusions

Even though animal models are improving, tests performed on them represent only some symptoms found in clinics: the evoked pain. However, patients complain more about spontaneous pain than evoked pain. Evolution is needed and has started in some laboratories with the detection of not only one symptom but a cluster of symptoms attempting to evaluate cognitive and affective dimensions of pain.

Each animal model has got its advantages and disadvantages. We thus think that novel therapies should be evaluated in multiple complementary models attempting to mirror a variety of clinical researches.

Finally, a general limitation of the translational research is the differences between the cultures of preclinical and clinical research [121]. For us, a solution to improve the quality of translational medicine is to improve and facilitate the communication between preclinical research and clinical development through translational projects.

References

1 Randall, L.O. and Selitto, J.J. (1957) A method for measurement of analgesic activity on inflamed tissue. *Archives Internationales de Pharmacodynamie et de Therapie*, **111**, 409–419.

2 Chiba, S., Nishiyama, T., Yoshikawa, M. and Yamada, Y. (2009) The antinociceptive effects of midazolam on three different types of nociception in mice. *Journal of Pharmacological Sciences*, **109**, 71–77.

3 Green, A.F. and Young, P.A. (1951) A comparison of heat and pressure analgesiometric methods in rats. *British Journal of Pharmacological and Chemotherapy*, **6**, 572–585.

4 Bianchi, C. and Franceschini, J. (1954) Experimental observations on Haffner's method for testing analgesic drugs. *British Journal of Pharmacology and Chemotherapy*, **9**, 280–284.

5 Takagi, H., Inukai, T., and Nakama, M. (1966) A modification of Haffner's method for testing analgesics. *Japanese Journal of Pharmacology*, **16**, 287–294.

6 Chaplan, S.R., Bach, F.W., Pogrel, J.W., Chung, J.M., and Yaksh, T.L. (1994) Quantitative assessment of tactile allodynia in the rat paw. *Journal of Neuroscience Methods*, **53**, 55–63.

7 D'Amour, F.E. and Smith, D.L. (1941) A method for determining loss of pain sensation. *The Journal of Pharmacology and Experimental Therapeutics*, **72**, 74–79.

8 Hardy, J.D., Jacobs, I., and Meixner, M.D. (1953) Thresholds of pain and reflex contraction as related to noxious stimulation. *Journal of Applied Physiology*, **5**, 725–739.

9 Hardy, J.D., Stoll, A.M., Cunningham, D., Benson, W.M., and Greene, L. (1957) Responses of the rat to thermal radiation. *American Journal of Physiology*, **189**, 1–5.

10 Hargreaves, K., Dubner, R., Brown, F., Flores, C., and Joris, J. (1988) A new and sensitive method for measuring thermal nociception in cutaneous hyperalgesia. *Pain*, **32**, 77–88.

11 O'Callaghan, J.P. and Holtzman, S.G. (1975) Quantification of the analgesic activity of narcotic antagonists by a modified hot-plate procedure. *The Journal of Pharmacology and Experimental Therapeutics*, **192**, 497–505.

12 Woolfe, G. and McDonald, A.L. (1944) The evaluation of the analgesic action of

pethidine hydrochloride. *The Journal of Pharmacology and Experimental Therapeutics*, **80**, 300–307.

13 Hunskaar, S., Berge, O.G., and Hole, K. (1986) Dissociation between antinociceptive and anti-inflammatory effects of acetylsalicylic acid and indomethacin in the formalin test. *Pain*, **25**, 125–132.

14 Yalcin, I., Charlet, A., Freund-Mercier, M.-J., Barrot, M., and Poisbeau, P. (2009) Differentiating thermal allodynia and hyperalgesia using dynamic hot and cold plate in rodents. *Journal of Pain*, **10**, 767–773.

15 Mauderli, A.P., Acosta-Rua, A., and Vierck, C.J. (2000) An operant assay of thermal pain in conscious, unrestrained rats. *Journal of Neuroscience Methods*, **97**, 19–29.

16 Allchorne, A.J., Broom, D.C., and Woolf, C.J. (2005) Detection of cold pain, cold allodynia and cold hyperalgesia in freely behaving rats. *Molecular Pain*, **1**, 36.

17 Bennett, G.J. and Xie, Y.K. (1988) A peripheral mononeuropathy in rat that produces disorders of pain sensation like those seen in man. *Pain*, **33**, 87–107.

18 Pizziketti, R.J., Pressman, N.S., Geller, E.B., Cowan, A., and Adler, M.W. (1985) Rat cold water tail-flick: a novel analgesic test that distinguishes opioid agonists from mixed agonist-antagonists. *European Journal of Pharmacology*, **119**, 23–29.

19 Charpentier, J. (1964) Comparative results of pain induced by trigeminal and cutaneous stimulations. *Journal of Physiology (Paris)*, **56**, 317–318.

20 Evans, W.O. (1961) A technique for the investigation of some effects of psychotropic and analgesic drugs on reflexive behavior in the rat. *Reports of the US Army Medicinal Research Laboratory*, **476**, 1–9.

21 Neil, A. and Terenius, L. (1982) An improved foot-shock titration procedure in rats for centrally acting analgesics. *Acta Pharmacologica et Toxicologica (Copenhagen)*, **50**, 93–99.

22 Koster, R., Anderson, M., and De Beer, J. (1959) Acetic acid for analgesic screening. *Federal Proceeding*, **18**, 412–417.

23 Siegmund, E., Cadmus, R., and Lu, G. (1957) A method for evaluating both non-narcotic and narcotic analgesics. *Proceedings of the Society for Experimental Biology and Medicine*, **95**, 729–731.

24 Dubuisson, D. and Dennis, S.G. (1977) The formalin test: a quantitative study of the analgesic effects of morphine, meperidine, and brain stem stimulation in rats and cats. *Pain*, **4**, 161–174.

25 Saddi, G. and Abbott, F.V. (2000) The formalin test in the mouse: a parametric analysis of scoring properties. *Pain*, **89**, 53–63.

26 Shibata, M., Ohkubo, T., Takahashi, H., and Inoki, R. (1989) Modified formalin test: characteristic biphasic pain response. *Pain*, **38**, 347–352.

27 Wheeler-Aceto, H., Porreca, F., and Cowan, A. (1990) The rat paw formalin test: comparison of noxious agents. *Pain*, **40**, 229–238.

28 Pelissier, T., Pajot, J., and Dallel, R. (2002) The orofacial capsaicin test in rats: effects of different capsaicin concentrations and morphine. *Pain*, **96**, 81–87.

29 Chen, J., Luo, C., Li, H., and Chen, H. (1999) Primary hyperalgesia to mechanical and heat stimuli following subcutaneous bee venom injection into the plantar surface of hindpaw in the conscious rat: a comparative study with the formalin test. *Pain*, **83**, 67–76.

30 Lariviere, W.R. and Melzack, R. (1996) The bee venom test: a new tonic-pain test. *Pain*, **66**, 271–277.

31 Le Bars, D., Gozariu, M., and Cadden, S.W. (2001) Animal models of nociception. *Pharmacological Reviews*, **53**, 597–652.

32 Leem, J.W., Willis, W.D., and Chung, J.M. (1993) Cutaneous sensory receptors in the rat foot. *Journal of Neurophysiology*, **69**, 1684–1699.

33 Miller, L.C. (1948) A critique of analgesic testing methods. *Annals of the New York Academy of Sciences*, **51**, 34–50.

34 Ankier, S.I. (1974) New hot plate tests to quantify antinociceptive and narcotic antagonist activities. *European Journal of Pharmacology*, **27**, 1–4.

35 Hunskaar, S., Berge, O.G., and Hole, K. (1986) A modified hot-plate test sensitive to mild analgesics. *Behavioral Brain Research*, **21**, 101–108.

36 Adams, J.U., Chen, X., DeRiel, J.K., Adler, M.W., and Liu-Chen, L.Y. (1994) Intracerebroventricular treatment with an antisense oligodeoxynucleotide to kappa-opioid receptors inhibited kappa-agonist-induced analgesia in rats. *Brain Research*, **667**, 129–132.

37 Briggs, S.L., Rech, R.H., and Sawyer, D.C. (1998) Kappa antinociceptive activity of spiradoline in the cold-water tail-flick assay in rats. *Pharmacology, Biochemistry, and Behavior*, **60**, 467–472.

38 Gamaro, G.D., Xavier, M.H., Denardin, J.D., Pilger, J.A., Ely, D.R., Ferreira, M.B. et al. (1998) The effects of acute and repeated restraint stress on the nociceptive response in rats. *Physiology & Behavior*, **63**, 693–697.

39 Chesler, E.J., Wilson, S.G., Lariviere, W.R., Rodriguez-Zas, S.L., and Mogil, J.S. (2002) Identification and ranking of genetic and laboratory environment factors influencing a behavioral trait, thermal nociception, via computational analysis of a large data archive. *Neuroscience and Biobehavioral Reviews*, **26**, 907–923.

40 Wilson, S.G. and Mogil, J.S. (2001) Measuring pain in the (knockout) mouse: big challenges in a small mammal. *Behavioural Brain Research*, **125**, 65–73.

41 Lai, Y.Y. and Chan, S.H. (1982) Shortened pain response time following repeated algesiometric tests in rats. *Physiology & Behavior*, **28**, 1111–1113.

42 Le Bars, D., Gozariu, M., and Cadden, S.W. (2001b) Acute pain measurement in animals. Part 1. *Annales Francaises d'anesthesie et de Reanimation's*, **20**, 347–365.

43 Hole, K. and Tjølsen, A. (1993) The tail-flick and formalin tests in rodents: changes in skin temperature as a confounding factor. *Pain*, **53**, 247–254.

44 Benoist, J.-M., Pincedé, I., Ballantyne, K., Plaghki, L., and Le Bars, D. (2008) Peripheral and central determinants of a nociceptive reaction: an approach to psychophysics in the rat. *PLoS One*, **3**, e3125.

45 Pincedé, I., Pollin, B., Meert, T., Plaghki, L., and Le Bars, D. (2012) Psychophysics of a nociceptive test in the mouse: ambient temperature as a key factor for variation. *PLoS One*, **7**, e36699.

46 Mallet, C., Barriere, D.A., Ermund, A., Jonsson, B.A., Eschalier, A., Zygmunt, P.M. et al. (2010) TRPV1 in brain is involved in acetaminophen-induced antinociception. *PLoS One*, **5** (9), e12748.

47 Lariviere, W.R., Wilson, S.G., Laughlin, T.M., Kokayeff, A., West, E.E., Adhikari, S.M. et al. (2002) Heritability of nociception. III. Genetic relationships among commonly used assays of nociception and hypersensitivity. *Pain*, **97**, 75–86.

48 Backonja, M.-M. and Stacey, B. (2004) Neuropathic pain symptoms relative to overall pain rating. *Journal of Pain*, **5**, 491–497.

49 Maier, C., Baron, R., Tölle, T.R., Binder, A., Birbaumer, N., Birklein, F. et al. (2010) Quantitative sensory testing in the German Research Network on Neuropathic Pain (DFNS): somatosensory abnormalities in 1236 patients with different neuropathic pain syndromes. *Pain*, **150**, 439–450.

50 Scholz, J., Mannion, R.J., Hord, D.E., Griffin, R.S., Rawal, B., Zheng, H. et al. (2009) A novel tool for the assessment of pain: validation in low back pain. *PLoS Medicine*, **6**, e1000047.

51 Hendershot, L.C. and Forsaith, J. (1959) Antagonism of the frequency of phenylquinone-induced writhing in the mouse by weak analgesics and nonanalgesics. *The Journal of Pharmacology and Experimental Therapeutics*, **125**, 237–240.

52 Vissers, K., Hoffmann, V., Geenen, F., Biermans, R., and Meert, T. (2003) Is the second phase of the formalin test useful to predict activity in chronic constriction injury models? A pharmacological comparison in different species. *Pain Practice*, **3**, 298–309.

53 Vissers, K.C.P., Geenen, F., Biermans, R., and Meert, T.F. (2006) Pharmacological correlation between the formalin test and the neuropathic pain behavior in different species with chronic constriction injury. *Pharmacology, Biochemistry, and Behavior*, **84**, 479–486.

54 Grégoire, S., Etienne, M., Gaulmin, M., Caussade, F., Neuzeret, D., and Ardid, D. (2012) New method to discriminate sedative and analgesic effects of drugs in the automated formalin test in rats. *Journal of Neuroscience Research*, **72**, 194–198.

55 Yaksh, T.L., Ozaki, G., McCumber, D., Rathbun, M., Svensson, C., Malkmus, S. et al. (2001) An automated flinch detecting system for use in the formalin nociceptive bioassay. *Journal of Applied Physiology*, **90**, 2386–2402.

56 Ness, T.J. and Gebhart, G.F. (1988) Colorectal distension as a noxious visceral stimulus: physiologic and pharmacologic characterization of pseudoaffective reflexes in the rat. *Brain Research*, **450**, 153–169.

57 Rouzade, M.L., Fioramonti, J., and Bueno, L. (1998) A model for evaluation of gastric sensitivity in awake rats. *Neurogastroenterology and Motility*, **10** (2), 157–163.

58 Tammpere, A., Brusberg, M., Axenborg, J., Hirsch, I., Larsson, H., and Lindström, E. (2005) Evaluation of pseudo-affective responses to noxious colorectal distension in rats by manometric recordings. *Pain*, **116** (3), 220–226.

59 Bourdu, S., Dapoigny, M., Chapuy, E., Artigue, F., Vasson, M.P., Dechelotte, P., Bommelaer, G., Eschalier, A., and Ardid, D. (2005) Rectal instillation of butyrate provides a novel clinically relevant model of noninflammatory colonic hypersensitivity in rats. *Gastroenterology*, **128** (7), 1996–2008.

60 Al Chaer, E.D., Kawasaki, M., and Pasricha, P.J. (2000) A new model of chronic visceral hypersensitivity in adult rats induced by colon irritation during postnatal development. *Gastroenterology*, **119**, 1276–1285.

61 Giamberardino, M.A., Valente, R., de Bigontina, P., and Vecchiet, L. (1995) Artificial ureteral calculosis in rats: behavioural characterization of visceral pain episodes and their relationship with referred lumbar muscle hyperalgesia. *Pain*, **61** (3), 459–469.

62 Giamberardino, M.A., Rampin, O., Laplace, J.P., Vecchiet, L., and Albe-Fessard, D. (1988) Muscular hyperalgesia and hypoalgesia after stimulation of the ureter in rats. *Neuroscience Letters*, **87** (1–2), 29–34.

63 Giamberardino, M.A., Vecchiet, L., and Albe-Fessard, D. (1990) Comparison of the effects of ureteral calculosis and occlusion on muscular sensitivity to painful stimulation in rats. *Pain*, **43** (2), 227–234.

64 Matsumoto, G., Vizzard, M.A., Hisamitsu, T., and de Groat, W.C. (1996) Increased c-fos expression in spinal neurons induced by electrical stimulation of the ureter in the rat. *Brain Research*, **709** (2), 197–204.

65 Roza, C. and Laird, J.M. (1995) Pressor responses to distension of the ureter in anaesthetised rats: characterisation of a model of acute visceral pain. *Neuroscience Letters*, **198** (1), 9–12.

66 Roza, C., Laird, J.M., and Cervero, F. (1998) Spinal mechanisms underlying persistent pain and referred hyperalgesia in rats with an experimental ureteric stone. *Journal of Neurophysiology*, **79** (4), 1603–1612.

67 Guilbaud, G., Berkley, K.J., Benoist, J.M., and Gautron, M. (1993) Responses of neurons in thalamic ventrobasal complex of rats to graded distension of uterus and vagina and to uterine suprafusion with bradykinin and prostaglandin F2 alpha. *Brain Research*, **614** (1–2), 285–290.

68 Bradshaw, H.B., Temple, J.L., Wood, E., and Berkley, K.J. (1999) Estrous variations in behavioral responses to vaginal and uterine distention in the rat. *Pain*, **82** (2), 187–197.

69 Wesselmann, U. and Lai, J. (1997) Mechanisms of referred visceral pain: uterine inflammation in the adult virgin rat results in neurogenic plasma extravasation in the skin. *Pain*, **73** (3), 309–317.

70 Sandner-Kiesling, A., Pan, H.L., Chen, S.R., James, R.L., DeHaven-Hudkins, D.L., Dewan, D.M., and Eisenach, J.C. (2002) Effect of kappa opioid agonists on visceral nociception induced by uterine cervical distension in rats. *Pain*, **96** (1–2), 13–22.

71 Vizzard, M.A. (2000) Alterations in spinal cord Fos protein expression induced by bladder stimulation following cystitis. *American Journal of Physiology. Regulatory, Integrative and Comparative Physiology*, **278** (4), R1027–R1039.

72 Ness, T.J., Lewis-Sides, A., and Castroman, P. (2001) Characterization of pressor and visceromotor reflex responses to bladder distention in rats: sources of variability and

effect of analgesics. *The Journal of Urology*, **165** (3), 968–974.

73 Buffington, C.A. (2001) Visceral pain in humans: lessons from animals. *Current Pain and Headache Reports*, **5** (1), 44–51.

74 Brock, N., Stekar, J., Pohl, J., Niemeyer, U., and Scheffler, G. (1979) Acrolein, the causative factor of urotoxic side-effects of cyclophosphamide, ifosfamide, trofosfamide and sufosfamide. *Arzneimittel-Forschung*, **29** (4), 659–661.

75 Boucher, M., Meen, M., Codron, J.P., Coudore, F., Kemeny, J.L., and Eschalier, A. (2000) Cyclophosphamide-induced cystitis in freely-moving conscious rats: behavioral approach to a new model of visceral pain. *The Journal of Urology*, **164** (1), 203–208.

76 Olivar, T. and Laird, J.M. (1999) Cyclophosphamide cystitis in mice: behavioural characterisation and correlation with bladder inflammation. *European Journal of Pain*, **3** (2), 141–149.

77 Guerios, S.D., Wang, Z.Y., and Bjorling, D.E. (2006) Nerve growth factor mediates peripheral mechanical hypersensitivity that accompanies experimental cystitis in mice. *Neuroscience Letters*, **392** (3), 193–197.

78 Abelli, L., Conte, B., Somma, V., Maggi, C.A., Giuliani, S., Geppetti, P., Alessandri, M., Theodorsson, E., and Meli, A. (1988) The contribution of capsaicin-sensitive sensory nerves to xylene-induced visceral pain in conscious, freely moving rats. *Naunyn-Schmiedeberg's Archives of Pharmacology*, **337** (5), 545–551.

79 McMahon, S.B. and Abel, C. (1987) A model for the study of visceral pain states: chronic inflammation of the chronic decerebrate rat urinary bladder by irritant chemicals. *Pain*, **28** (1), 109–127.

80 Jaggar, S.I., Scott, H.C., and Rice, A.S. (1999) Inflammation of the rat urinary bladder is associated with a referred thermal hyperalgesia which is nerve growth factor dependent. *British Journal of Anaesthesia*, **83** (3), 442–448.

81 Farquhar-Smith, W.P., Jaggar, S.I., and Rice, A.S. (2002) Attenuation of nerve growth factor-induced visceral hyperalgesia via cannabinoid CB1 and CB2-like receptors. *Pain*, **97** (1–2), 11–21.

82 Ribeiro, R.A., Freitas, H.C., Campos, M.C., Santos, C.C., Figueiredo, F.C., Brito, G.A., and Cunha, F.Q. (2002) Tumor necrosis factor-alpha and interleukin-1beta mediate the production of nitric oxide involved in the pathogenesis of ifosfamide induced hemorrhagic cystitis in mice. *The Journal of Urology*, **167** (5), 2229–2234.

83 Cruz, Y. and Downie, J.W. (2006) Abdominal muscle activity during voiding in female rats with normal or irritated bladder. *American Journal of Physiology. Regulatory, Integrative and Comparative Physiology*, **290** (5), R1436–R1445.

84 Randich, A., Uzzell, T., Cannon, R., and Ness, T.J. (2006) Inflammation and enhanced nociceptive responses to bladder distension produced by intravesical zymosan in the rat. *BMC Urology*, **6**, 2.

85 Vykhovanets, E.V., Resnick, M.I., MacLennan, G.T., and Gupta, S. (2007) Experimental rodent models of prostatitis: limitations and potential. *Prostate Cancer and Prostatic Diseases*, **10** (1), 15–29.

86 Rudick, C.N., Schaeffer, A.J., and Thumbikat, P. (2008) Experimental autoimmune prostatitis induces chronic pelvic pain. *American Journal of Physiology. Regulatory, Integrative and Comparative Physiology*, **294** (4), R1268–R1275.

87 Mizoguchi, A. (2012) Animal models of inflammatory bowel disease. *Progress in Molecular Biology and Translational Science*, **105**, 263–320.

88 Morris, G.P., Beck, P.L., Herridge, M.S., Depew, W.T., Szewczuk, M.R., and Wallace, J.L. (1989) Hapten-induced model of chronic inflammation and ulceration in the rat colon. *Gastroenterology*, **96** (3), 795–803.

89 Coutinho, S.V., Meller, S.T., and Gebhart, G.F. (1996) Intracolonic zymosan produces visceral hyperalgesia in the rat that is mediated by spinal NMDA and non-NMDA receptors. *Brain Research*, **736** (1–2), 7–15.

90 Okayasu, I., Hatakeyama, S., Yamada, M., Ohkusa, T., Inagaki, Y., and Nakaya, R. (1990) A novel method in the induction of reliable experimental acute and chronic ulcerative colitis in mice. *Gastroenterology*, **98** (3), 694–702.

91 Larauche, M., Mulak, A., and Taché, Y. (2012) Stress and visceral pain: from

animal models to clinical therapies. *Experimental Neurology*, **233** (1), 49–67.

92 Qin, H.Y., Wu, J.C., Tong, X.D., Sung, J.J., Xu, H.X., and Bian, Z.X. (2011) Systematic review of animal models of post-infectious/post-inflammatory irritable bowel syndrome. *Journal of Gastroenterology*, **46** (2), 164–174.

93 Silberer, H., Küppers, B., Mickisch, O., Baniewicz, W., Drescher, M., Traber, L., Kempf, A., and Schmidt-Gayk, H. (2005) Fecal leukocyte proteins in inflammatory bowel disease and irritable bowel syndrome. *Clinical Laboratory*, **51** (3–4), 117–126.

94 Gecse, K., Róka, R., Ferrier, L., Leveque, M., Eutamene, H., Cartier, C., Ait-Belgnaoui, A., Rosztóczy, A., Izbéki, F., Fioramonti, J., Wittmann, T., and Bueno, L. (2008) Increased faecal serine protease activity in diarrhoeic IBS patients: a colonic lumenal factor impairing colonic permeability and sensitivity. *Gut*, **57** (5), 591–599.

95 Brigatte, P., Sampaio, S.C., Gutierrez, V.P., Guerra, J.L., Sinhorini, I.L., Curi, R., and Cury, Y. (2007) Walker 256 tumor-bearing rats as a model to study cancer pain. *Journal of Pain*, **8** (5), 412–421.

96 Mantyh, P.W. (2006) Cancer pain and its impact on diagnosis, survival and quality of life. *Nature Reviews. Neuroscience*, **7** (10), 797–809.

97 Sasamura, T., Nakamura, S., Iida, Y., Fujii, H., Murata, J., Saiki, I., Nojima, H., and Kuraishi, Y. (2002) Morphine analgesia suppresses tumor growth and metastasis in a mouse model of cancer pain produced by orthotopic tumor inoculation. *European Journal of Pharmacology*, **441** (3), 185–191.

98 Menéndez, L., Lastra, A., Fresno, M.F., Llames, S., Meana, A., Hidalgo, A., and Baamonde, A. (2003) Initial thermal heat hypoalgesia and delayed hyperalgesia in a murine model of bone cancer pain. *Brain Research*, **969** (1–2), 102–109.

99 Schwei, M.J., Honore, P., Rogers, S.D., Salak-Johnson, J.L., Finke, M.P., Ramnaraine, M.L., Clohisy, D.R., and Mantyh, P.W. (1999) Neurochemical and cellular reorganization of the spinal cord in a murine model of bone cancer pain. *The Journal of Neuroscience*, **19** (24), 10886–10897.

100 Sevcik, M.A., Jonas, B.M., Lindsay, T.H., Halvorson, K.G., Ghilardi, J.R., Kuskowski, M.A., Mukherjee, P., Maggio, J.E., and Mantyh, P.W. (2006) Endogenous opioids inhibit early-stage pancreatic pain in a mouse model of pancreatic cancer. *Gastroenterology*, **131** (3), 900–910.

101 Khasabova, I.A., Gielissen, J., Chandiramani, A., Harding-Rose, C., Odeh, D.A., Simone, D.A., and Seybold, V.S. (2011) CB1 and CB2 receptor agonists promote analgesia through synergy in a murine model of tumor pain. *Behavioural Pharmacology*, **22** (5–6), 607–616.

102 Kim, W.M., Jeong, C.W., Lee, S.H., Kim, Y.O., Cui, J.H., and Yoon, M.H. (2011) The intrathecally administered kappa-2 opioid agonist GR89696 and interleukin-10 attenuate bone cancer-induced pain through synergistic interaction. *Anesthesia and Analgesia*, **113** (4), 934–940.

103 Ono, K., Harano, N., Nagahata, S., Seta, Y., Tsujisawa, T., Inenaga, K., and Nakanishi, O. (2009) Behavioral characteristics and c-Fos expression in the medullary dorsal horn in a rat model for orofacial cancer pain. *European Journal of Pain*, **13** (4), 373–379.

104 Bloom, A.P., Jimenez-Andrade, J.M., Taylor, R.N., Castañeda-Corral, G., Kaczmarska, M.J., Freeman, K.T., Coughlin, K.A., Ghilardi, J.R., Kuskowski, M.A., and Mantyh, P.W. (2011) Breast cancer-induced bone remodeling, skeletal pain, and sprouting of sensory nerve fibers. *Journal of Pain*, **12** (6), 698–711.

105 Quang, P.N. and Schmidt, B.L. (2010) Endothelin-A receptor antagonism attenuates carcinoma-induced pain through opioids in mice. *Journal of Pain*, **11** (7), 663–671.

106 Beyreuther, B.K., Callizot, N., Brot, M.D., Feldman, R., Bain, S.C., and Stöhr, T. (2007) Antinociceptive efficacy of lacosamide in rat models for tumor- and chemotherapy-induced cancer pain. *European Journal of Pharmacology*, **565** (1–3), 98–104.

107 Shimoyama, M., Tanaka, K., Hasue, F., and Shimoyama, N. (2002) A mouse model of neuropathic cancer pain. *Pain*, **99** (1–2), 167–174.

108 Ono, K., Harano, N., Inenaga, K., and Nakanishi, O. (2012) A rat pain model of facial cancer. *Methods in Molecular Biology*, **851**, 149–157.

109 Nagamine, K., Ozaki, N., Shinoda, M., Asai, H., Nishiguchi, H., Mitsudo, K., Tohnai, I., Ueda, M., and Sugiura, Y. (2006) Mechanical allodynia and thermal hyperalgesia induced by experimental squamous cell carcinoma of the lower gingiva in rats. *Journal of Pain*, **7** (9), 659–670.

110 Asai, H., Ozaki, N., Shinoda, M., Nagamine, K., Tohnai, I., Ueda, M., and Sugiura, Y. (2005) Heat and mechanical hyperalgesia in mice model of cancer pain. *Pain*, **117** (1–2), 19–29.

111 Wacnik, P.W., Eikmeier, L.J., Ruggles, T.R., Ramnaraine, M.L., Walcheck, B.K., Beitz, A.J., and Wilcox, G.L. (2001) Functional interactions between tumor and peripheral nerve: morphology, algogen identification, and behavioral characterization of a new murine model of cancer pain. *The Journal of Neuroscience*, **21** (23), 9355–9366.

112 Siegel, R., Naishadham, D., and Jemal, A. (2013) Cancer statistics, 2013. *CA: A Cancer Journal for Clinicians*, **63** (1), 11–30.

113 Bubendorf, L., Schöpfer, A., Wagner, U., Sauter, G., Moch, H., Willi, N., Gasser, T.C., and Mihatsch, M.J. (2000) Metastatic patterns of prostate cancer: an autopsy study of 1,589 patients. *Human Pathology*, **31** (5), 578–583.

114 Roughan, J.V., Flecknell, P.A., and Davies, B.R. (2004) Behavioural assessment of the effects of tumour growth in rats and the influence of the analgesics carprofen and meloxicam. *Laboratory Animals*, **38** (3), 286–296.

115 Jimenez-Andrade, J.M., Mantyh, W.G., Bloom, A.P., Ferng, A.S., Geffre, C.P., and Mantyh, P.W. (2010) Bone cancer pain. *Annals of the New York Academy of Sciences*, **1198**, 173–181.

116 Halvorson, K.G., Sevcik, M.A., Ghilardi, J.R., Sullivan, L.J., Koewler, N.J., Bauss, F., and Mantyh, P.W. (2008) Intravenous ibandronate rapidly reduces pain, neurochemical indices of central sensitization, tumor burden, and skeletal destruction in a mouse model of bone cancer. *Journal of Pain and Symptom Management*, **36** (3), 289–303.

117 Sittig, H.B. (2012) Pathogenesis and bisphosphonate treatment of skeletal events and bone pain in metastatic cancer: focus on ibandronate. *Onkologie*, **35** (6), 380–387.

118 Hans, G., Schmidt, B.L., and Strichartz, G. (2009) Nociceptive sensitization by endothelin-1. *Brain Research Reviews*, **60** (1), 36–42.

119 Jimenez-Andrade, J.M., Ghilardi, J.R., Castañeda-Corral, G., Kuskowski, M.A., and Mantyh, P.W. (2011) Preventive or late administration of anti-NGF therapy attenuates tumor-induced nerve sprouting, neuroma formation, and cancer pain. *Pain*, **152** (11), 2564–2574.

120 Balayssac, D., Ferrier, J., Descoeur, J., Ling, B., Pezet, D., Eschalier, A., and Authier, N. (2011) Chemotherapy-induced peripheral neuropathies: from clinical relevance to preclinical evidence. *Expert Opinion on Drug Safety*, **10** (3), 407–417.

121 Levin, L.A. and Danesh-Meyer, H.V. (2010) Lost in translation: bumps in the road between bench and bedside. *The Journal of the American Medical Association*, **303**, 1533–1534.

13
Inflammatory, Musculoskeletal/Joint (OA and RA), and Postoperative Pain

Laurent Diop and Yassine Darbaky

13.1
Introduction: Evaluation of Pain in Animal Models

The sensory-discriminative dimension of pain has been widely studied in animal models, and almost all currently used analgesics were tested in classical preclinical models in rodents. Numerous animal models have been developed to simulate specific human painful conditions, mostly by producing diseases or traumatic injuries that have painful sequelae, providing useful systems to study various pain situations. Animals cannot self-report, but their behaviors in response to noxious stimuli can be reliably and objectively quantified. Indeed, because pain cannot be measured directly, evoked pain – hyperalgesia (enhanced response to a normally painful stimulus) and allodynia (pain resulting from a normally innocuous stimulus) – is often used as outcome measure [1,2]. The evaluation of pain sensitivity is thus essentially correlated with withdrawal responses from thermal or mechanical stimuli applied on the body surface (Table 13.1). In parallel, signs of paw guarding, lifting and limping, excessive grooming and biting, changes in exploratory behavior, posture, gait, and weight bearing can also be suggested as indications for the presence of spontaneous pain (Table 13.1) [3]. Pain can also impact emotional/affective and cognitive functions, limiting the capacity of chronic pain patients to react appropriately to pain and challenges of daily life. The emotional/affective component, which confers the unpleasant and intrusive sensation of pain, can induce anxious and depressive episodes. The cognitive processes can modulate pain perception, and conversely, pain can affect cognitive functions. These components of pain are difficult to explore in animals, but in recent years, a growing interest has been reported for these novel behavioral approaches to assess emotional/affective and cognitive impairments associated with pain in animals (Table 13.1) [4]. The choice of a particular animal model is multifactorial. It seems necessary to improve the preclinical evaluation of new analgesic drugs and enhance the predictability of their efficacy in subsequent clinical trials.

In Vivo Models for Drug Discovery, First Edition. Edited by José M. Vela, Rafael Maldonado, and Michel Hamon.
© 2014 Wiley-VCH Verlag GmbH & Co. KGaA. Published 2014 by Wiley-VCH Verlag GmbH & Co. KGaA.

Table 13.1 Methods of evaluation of the various components of pain in rodents.

Pain condition	Modality	Test name	Test method/stimulus	Species	Testing site	Outcome parameter
Evoked pain	Mechanical	von Frey test	Application of nonnoxious calibrated static hair on skin	Rat, mouse	Hind paw, face, back	Withdrawal threshold
		Brush test	Innocuous brushing of skin	Rat, mouse	Hind paw	Number of paw withdrawal responses
		Randall–Selitto	Application of linearly increasing mechanical force in noxious range	Rat	Hind paw	Withdrawal threshold
		Strain gauges	Application of linearly increasing mechanical force in noxious range	Rat, mouse	Hind paw/ knee	Withdrawal threshold
		Colorectal distension	Noxious mechanical stimulation to viscera	Rat, mouse	Colon	Behavioral response (abdominal cramp)
		Tail flick	Application of radiant heat on tail or tail immersion in hot water	Rat, mouse	Tail	Withdrawal latency
	Thermal (heat)	Hargreaves	Application of radiant heat on skin	Rat, mouse	Hind paw	Withdrawal latency
		Hot plate	Animal placed on heated metal plate	Mouse	Hind paw	Latency to elicit nociceptive or escape behavior
		Acetone	Application of acetone on skin	Rat, mouse	Hind paw	Duration/intensity of nociceptive behavior
	Thermal (cold)	Cold plate	Animal placed on cooled metal plate	Rat, mouse	Hind paw	Latency to elicit nociceptive or escape behavior

13.1 Introduction: Evaluation of Pain in Animal Models

	Cold water	Animal placed in a cold water bath	Rat, mouse	Hind paw, tail	Withdrawal latency
Chemical	Formalin test	Injection of a formalin solution	Rat, mouse	Hind paw/face	Paw licking time
	Writhing test	Injection of acetic acid/PBQ	Rat, mouse	Viscera	Number of writhing
Posture	Incapacitance test	Animal positioned on two separated sensor plates	Rat, mouse	Hind paw	Percentage of weight distribution
Gait	Gait score	Limping of the affected paw	Rat, mouse	Hind paw	Gait score
	Dynamic weight bearing	Freely moving rodents on an instrumented floor cage	Rat, mouse	Paws	Weight ratio measurements on freely moving rodents
	Catwalk	Locomotor ability of rodents placed in a corridor	Rat, mouse	Paws	Automated gait analysis in rodents measuring the intensity of the illumination caused by paw contact with a glass floor
Nocifensive signs	Behavioral observations	Paw licking	Rat, mouse	Hind paw	Number of licking
		Excessive grooming	Rat, mouse	—	Number of grooming
		Excessive exploratory behavior	Rat, mouse	—	Time spent to explore
		Guarding behavior	Rat, mouse	Hind paw	Guarding score
Autotomy	Behavioral observations	Self-mutilation and attack of the denervated areas	Rat, mouse	Hind paw	Behavioral observations
Choice	Condition place preference	Analgesic-induced place preference	Rat, mouse	—	Time spent in each compartment
	Condition place aversion	Formalin-induced place aversion	Rat, mouse	—	Time spent in each compartment
					Scoring and response threshold ($t°$)

(continued)

Table 13.1 (Continued)

Pain condition	Modality	Test name	Test method/stimulus	Species	Testing site	Outcome parameter
		Dynamic hot plate	Temperature ramp or two-temperature choice	Rat, mouse	Hind paw	
		Dynamic cold plate	Temperature ramp or two-temperature choice	Rat, mouse	Hind paw	Scoring and response threshold ($t°$)
		Saccharine preference test		Rat, mouse	—	Measurement of saccharine solution intake and water intake
	Facial expression	Rat grimace scale	Behavioral observations	Rat, mouse	Face	Scoring of facial expressions
Cognitive component of pain		Social interaction	Behavioral observations of a pair of rats	Rat, mouse	—	Time spent in active social interaction
		Social recognition	Introduction of a juvenile rat into the home cage of the adult rat	Rat	—	Time spent in active social interaction
		Y-maze	Behavioral observations	Rat, mouse	—	Total number of entries and the percentage of time spent in each arm
		Morris water maze	Animal capacity to learn platform location	Rat, mouse	—	Distance swam to reach the platform
		Five-choice serial reaction time task		Rat	—	Total number of rewarded responses
		Rodent gambling task		Rat, mouse	—	Ratio between advantageous and disadvantageous options

13.2
Inflammatory Pain

The injection of different inflammatory agents produces inflammation. Inflammation may be acute or chronic. Inflammatory response occurs in three distinct phases. The first phase is caused by an increase in vascular permeability resulting in exudation of fluids from the blood into the interstitial space, the second phase involves the infiltration of leukocytes from the blood into the tissue, and in the third phase granuloma formation and tissue repair take place. Mediators of inflammation originate either from plasma or from cells (i.e., histamine, prostaglandins (PGs), NGF, CGRP, cytokines, etc.). Generally, the mediators of inflammation are histamine, PGs, leukotrienes (LTB_4), nitric oxide (NO), platelet-activating factor (PAF), bradykinin, serotonin, cytokines, and growth factors. These inflammation responses are associated with pain syndromes (hyperalgesia and allodynia).

13.2.1
Formalin Test

Formalin test is the most common procedure to evaluate the potency of analgesic drugs. The injection of formalin in the dorsal part of plantar surface of the paw produces behavioral responses such as licking, shaking, grooming, rearing, guarding, or paw withdrawal. The behavioral responses – frequency, duration, and level – depend on the specific concentration and the site of injection. Indeed, injections into the proximal plantar region produce more pain than that in the distal plantar region. In rodents, the behavioral reactions produce a biphasic response: (a) early phase occurring in the first 10 min and (b) late phase lasting 10–40 min [5]. The early phase is related to local or direct stimulation of nociceptors. The initial phase of the response (early phase), likely caused by a burst of activity from C fibers, begins immediately after the formalin injection. The second phase involves inflammatory and central mechanisms. This phase involves a central sensitization during which inflammatory phenomena occur. The opiates or local anesthetics act on both phases. Nonsteroidal anti-inflammatory drugs (NSAIDs), *N*-methyl-D-aspartate (NMDA) receptor antagonists, gabapentin, and pregabalin act only in the late phase, indicating these drugs are antihyperalgesic.

13.2.2
Carrageenan-Induced Hyperalgesia

Carrageenan, a polysaccharide obtained from various seaweeds, when injected into the plantar paw or the knee joint results in a localized inflammation, and therefore decreases weight bearing and modifies guarding of the treated limb, and thermal and mechanical hyperalgesia.

Windup of Aδ and C fibers of flexor motor neurons has been observed after injection of carrageenan. The release of local inhibitory controls and direct excitatory controls participates in the mechanisms of the windup. In this model, primary hyperalgesia is observed after an intraplantar injection followed by thermal stimulation, whereas the intra-articular injection induces secondary hyperalgesia. Inflammation is induced by intraplantar injection of carrageenan (2% w/v) into the hind paw of the rat. After 3 h, reaction thresholds are measured using the paw pressure test. Pressure is gradually applied to the inflamed and noninflamed hind paws of the rat, and reaction thresholds are determined as the pressure (g) required to induce paw withdrawal or vocalization. This assay is widely and reliably used for revealing the efficacy of new analgesics in a model of inflammatory pain in conscious rats [6]. The electronic von Frey and thermal plantar stimulation can also be applied to this condition. Anti-inflammatory drugs (indomethacin, diclofenac, and meloxicam) have been used as reference compounds. Morphine and local application of bupivacaine (local anesthetic) are active in this model.

The carrageenan models have been extensively used to demonstrate the efficacy of many analgesic compounds in a model of inflammatory pain. This model is a useful screening test for new analgesic compounds.

13.2.3
Complete Freund's Adjuvant-Induced Hyperalgesia

The complete Freund's adjuvant (CFA) is a water-in-oil emulsion containing heat-killed mycobacteria or mycobacterial cell wall components. The chronic CFA-induced hyperalgesia is due to the prolonged presence of antigens at the site of injection. It is associated with the more effective transport of the antigens to the lymphatic system and to the lungs, where the adjuvant promotes the accumulation of cells concerned with the immune response. The exact mechanisms, in particular the activation of T and B lymphocytes, remain unidentified. Early events include rapid uptake of adjuvant components by dendritic cells, enhanced phagocytosis, production of cytokines by mononuclear phagocytes, and transient activation and proliferation of CD41 lymphocytes. The immune-mediated disease results from the overproduction of proinflammatory (e.g., IL-1, IL-6, IL-17, and TNF-α) and proerosive (i.e., receptor activator of NF-κB ligand) factors, hyperactivity of proinflammatory and proerosive signaling pathways, or a reduction in cytokines (i.e., IL-4, IL-10, and transforming growth factor-β) and soluble receptors (i.e., IL-1ra and soluble TNF receptor) that antagonize the proinflammatory response. The late-produced cytokines may play a role not only in bringing about the arrest of T-cell expansion and activation but also in the gradual buildup of myelopoiesis.

13.2.4
Capsaicin-Induced Hyperalgesia

Capsaicin is the pungent ingredient in hot peppers. Topically applied to the human skin, it gives rise to burning pain as well as mechanical and thermal hyperalgesia at the site of application (i.e., primary hyperalgesia) and mechanical hyperalgesia/allodynia within a large surrounding area (i.e., secondary hyperalgesia). Burning pain and hyperalgesia following capsaicin application are believed to occur, at least in part, by excitation and sensitization of C-fiber nociceptors. These sensory symptoms in humans resemble those of some neuropathic patients [7].

In animals, intraplantar injection of capsaicin produces primary and secondary hyperalgesia not only in rats but also in monkeys. The primary thermal and mechanical hyperalgesia is mediated by the stimulation of TRPV1 on peripheral Aδ and C fibers. The windup phenomenon occurs for a short term only during the primary hyperalgesia. In contrast, central sensitization and long-term potentiation can induce long-term changes. CGRP is an important neuropeptide involving central sensitization. The blockage of CGRP receptors by CGRP8–37 (CGRP antagonist) reduced and suppressed the hyperalgesia and allodynia induced by capsaicin. This assay is widely and reliably used for revealing the efficacy of new analgesics in a model of inflammatory pain in conscious rats [7].

13.3
Musculoskeletal/Joint Osteoarthritis (OA) and Rheumatoid Arthritis (RA) Pain

Musculoskeletal disorders represent the fourth most common cause of disability following neuropsychiatric disorders, neoplasms, and cardiovascular disease in both developed and developing countries [8]. These injuries include a variety of disorders that cause pain in bones, joints, muscles, and surrounding structures. Musculoskeletal pain is a known consequence of repetitive strain, overuse, and work-related musculoskeletal disorders. Pain can be acute or chronic, focal or diffuse, and associated with worse functional outcomes and poorer quality of life compared with a range of other chronic conditions [9]. The pathophysiology of musculoskeletal pain is not completely clear and the repertoire of analgesics available is limited. Osteoarthritis (OA) and, to a lesser extent, rheumatoid arthritis (RA) are considered as the most common articular disorders and are frequently cited as the leading cause of persistent musculoskeletal pain [10]. Inflammation, fibrosis, tissue degradation, neurotransmitters, and neurosensory disturbances have been implicated in the induction, sensation, and maintenance of chronic arthritic joint pain. Several preclinical models of musculoskeletal pain have been developed for the understanding of the mechanisms that drive different types of musculoskeletal pain and the development of new analgesics, which could have significant clinical, economic, and societal benefits. Among the variety of common conditions that cause musculoskeletal pain, this chapter will focus specifically on OA and RA.

13.3.1
Osteoarthritis Pain Models

Osteoarthritis is a degenerative process involving all the major joint tissues, characterized by damages to the articular cartilage, changes in subchondral and marginal bone, synovitis, and capsular thickening, resulting in structural and functional failure of synovial joints [11]. This progressive joint failure may cause pain, physical disability, and psychological distress [12]. The quality of life in the majority of patients with OA is significantly impaired by severe, often intractable, pain. Pain in OA is localized (asymmetrical) and use related, occurring during movement or weight bearing. Current analgesic agents such as paracetamol and NSAIDs show partial efficacy. NSAIDs have increased morbidity in the elderly population due to gastric ulceration and cardiovascular complications. Preclinically, a range of animal models are used for the study of OA progression and for evaluating the efficacy of drugs acting on this progression. Conversely, until recently, mechanisms of pain generation in OA have been difficult to study due to the lack of clinically relevant animal models, as well as sensitive methods for measuring pain behavior.

Commonly used animal models of OA are based on the histopathological similarities to human disease and thus focused on the study of the pathogenesis of cartilage degeneration. They have been used extensively for the testing of potential antiarthritic drugs. They are generally either naturally occurring or chemically or surgically induced [13]. Spontaneous OA (i.e., based on genetic predisposition) occurs in the knee joints of various strains of mice and transgenic or mutant mouse models of OA and also in guinea pigs, Syrian hamsters, and larger animal species such as rabbit, dog, nonhuman primate, sheep/goat, and horse [14]. Naturally occurring or transgenically induced, the pathology and pathogenesis are probably similar to those occurring in the most common forms of human disease. The slow progression of the disease is, however, not really appropriate for preclinical pain approaches. Surgically induced instability models of OA (partial/total meniscectomy combined with transection of collateral and/or cruciate ligaments) have been described in various animal species [14]. Traumatic OA does occur in humans (athletes, joint surgery), and even if the disease progression is much more rapid in these animal models, they may mimic aspects of the pathogenesis and pathology in a period of time compatible with preclinical pain studies. Chemical models involve intra-articular injections of compounds that cause joint pathology through inhibition of chondrocyte metabolism (papain, monosodium iodoacetate (MIA)) and damage of ligaments and tendons (collagenase). In the field of pain, there is no single gold standard animal model for knee osteoarthritis, taking notably into account that mechanical factors differ considerably between a small quadruped and humans. Each animal model has unique advantages and disadvantages (Table 13.2) and particular attention has to be given to the scientific question under investigation and the hypothesis being tested, in order to choose the appropriate animal model [3]. In this context, the MIA model has emerged as a particularly useful and well-characterized animal model for pharmaceutical testing in OA pain because it is reproducible and mimics pathological changes and OA pain in humans. A single intra-articular injection of MIA into the femorotibial joint produces progressive joint degeneration through inhibition of glycolysis and subsequent chondrocyte death that develops over several weeks. Similar to human osteoarthritis, joint pathology is characterized by chondrocyte necrosis resulting in decreased thickness of the articular cartilage and fibrillation of the cartilage surface, separation of the necrotic cartilage from the

Table 13.2 Rodent models commonly used for pain studies in osteoarthritis.

Categories	Induction method	Induction site	Model primary mechanism	Model name	Species	Mechanical sensitivity	Thermal sensitivity	Spontaneous pain	Key advantages	Disadvantages
Spontaneous	—	—	—	STR/ort mouse model	Mouse	—	—	—	Genetically predisposed to develop a pronounced instability in the knee joint	Duration of disease progression not adapted with preclinical pain studies. Generally used for basic experiments to explore proposed molecular mechanisms
Chemical	Monosodium iodoacetate	Knee	Progressive joint degeneration, inhibition of chondrocyte metabolism	MIA-induced osteoarthritis	Rat, mouse	X	—	X	Widely used for analgesic drug effects, reproducible, mimics human pathological changes and pain	Nonspecific for articular cells at high concentrations
	Papain			Papain-induced osteoarthritis		—	—	No	Weak/no spontaneous pain	No chronic alteration of the cartilage

(continued)

Table 13.2 (Continued)

Categories	Induction method	Induction site	Model primary mechanism	Model name	Species	Mechanical sensitivity	Thermal sensitivity	Spontaneous pain	Key advantages	Disadvantages
	Collagenase		Damages of ligaments and tendons	Collagenase-induced osteoarthritis	Rat	—	—	X	Mimics human pathological changes	Need of repeated injections
Surgical	Partial or total meniscectomy + transection of collateral and/or cruciate ligaments	Knee	Joint instability, progressive cartilage degenerative changes characterized by chondrocyte and proteoglycan loss, fibrillation, osteophyte formation, and chondrocyte cloning	Medial meniscus tear		X	No	X	Mimics predisposing factor: meniscal damage (athletes, patients undergoing articular surgical intervention). Rapid progression of the disease	Rapid progression of the disease
				Partial medial meniscectomy		X	—	No		
				ACL transection		X	No	X		
				ACL transection with partial medial meniscectomy		X	No	X		
				Destabilization of the medial meniscus (DMM) model	Mouse	X	X	X		

underlying bone and exposure of the subchondral bone, osteolysis and swelling, and reduction in bone mineral content and density [15]. Acetaminophen, NSAIDs, COX-2 inhibitors, and opiates are effective in reducing evoked and spontaneous pain in this model, depending on the dose of MIA used and the time point tested. Consistent results have also been obtained using gabapentin, indicating that the secondary mechanical allodynia, or referred pain, present in the MIA model can be reversed with drugs designed to target neuropathic pain, such as anticonvulsants that can be of interest for therapeutic intervention in OA [16]. Pain-related behavior obtained using the MIA model in rats was compared with that obtained after partial meniscectomy [17]. In the latter model, the patella is dislocated laterally to expose and incise the medial collateral ligament of the femorotibial joint. A 3 mm cut is made on the medial meniscus to free it from the medial tibial plateau before being grasped to simulate a meniscal tear. Histopathologically, the partial meniscectomy model presents similarities to human OA with cartilage damage with loss of proteoglycan, complete loss of the cartilage layer, exposure of the subchondral bone, and presence of osteophytes. Symptomatically, the partial meniscectomy model induces evoked pain (tactile allodynia but not mechanical hyperalgesia) and a weak alteration in hind paw weight distribution compared with the MIA model. Pharmacologically, it has been shown that in another model of surgically induced OA in rats (medial meniscal tear model), acetaminophen, NSAIDs, and COX-2 inhibitors are all efficacious against nociceptive pain, whereas gabapentin effectively reverses referred pain [16].

13.3.2
Rheumatoid Arthritis Pain Models

The classic immune-mediated joint disease in humans is rheumatoid arthritis. RA is a chronic systemic inflammatory autoimmune disorder that may affect many tissues and organs (skin, blood vessels, heart, lungs, and muscles), but principally attacks the joints (synovium). The exact etiology and pathogenesis of the disease remain uncertain. Current thinking is that the primary arthropathic immunological defects may include constitutive activation of immune surveillance cells resulting in persistent relative overproduction of proinflammatory and proerosive cytokines and abnormal recognition of self-antigens as nonself due to their similarity with a foreign protein [18]. RA is characterized by a palindromic presentation (symmetrical pattern of affected joints), joint swelling and tenderness, and morning stiffness generally resolved by movement. RA is often associated with severe pain, suffering, and diminished function, thereby detracting from an optimal quality of life. The usual drugs used for treating the inflammation of RA are NSAIDs, disease-modifying antirheumatic drugs (DMARDs) such as methotrexate or sulfasalazine, biologics including anti-TNF therapies, and corticosteroids. Paracetamol, opiates, or antidepressants can also be used to relieve pain.

Animal models of arthritis are used extensively in the pharmaceutical industry in the testing of potential antiarthritis agents and analgesics. They are generally spontaneous, genetically engineered, or chemically induced (Table 13.3) [18].

Table 13.3 Rodent models commonly used for pain studies in rheumatoid arthritis.

Categories	Induction method	Induction site	Model primary mechanism	Model name	Species	Mechanical sensitivity	Thermal sensitivity	Spontaneous pain	Key advantages	Disadvantages
Spontaneous	—	—	MRL/Mpj-lpr/lpr	MRL/lpr	Mouse	—	—	—	—	—
Chemical	CFA	Ankle, knee	Joint inflammation, cartilage destruction, and bone erosion	CFA-induced monoarthritis	Rat, mouse	X	X	X	Persist several weeks in rats after a single CFA injection	Murine CFA-induced monoarthritis needs repeated injections of a much higher concentration of CFA into the knee to produce long-lasting effects
	Kaolin/carrageenan	Ankle, knee	Inflammation of the synovia and synovial fluid exudate	K/C arthritis model	Rat, mouse	X	X	X	Rapid development and long-lasting effects (weeks)	
	Zymosan	Ankle, knee	Erosive synovitis	Zymosan-induced arthritis	Rat, mouse	X	X	X	Rapid development (acute phase) and long-lasting effects (chronic phase)	
	SCW (streptococcal cell wall)	Knee		SCW-induced monoarthritis	Rat, mouse	—	—	—	—	—

13.3 Musculoskeletal/Joint Osteoarthritis (OA) and Rheumatoid Arthritis (RA) Pain

	CFA	Systemic	Robust polyarticular inflammation, marked bone resorption, and periosteal bone proliferation	CFA-induced polyarthritis	Rat	X	X	X	Model of chronic immune-mediated joint inflammation	Systemic nature of this arthritis may affect the overall condition and well-being of the animals and may confound pain assessment. CFA polyarthritis model is well established and reproducible in rats but not in mice
	CIA, type II collagen (bovine, porcine, rodent)	Systemic	Severe erosive polyarthritis, marked cartilage destruction associated with immune complex deposition on articular surfaces, bone resorption and periosteal inflammation	CIA-induced polyarthritis	Rat, mouse	X	X	X	Model of chronic immune-mediated joint inflammation	Ethical issue
	Pristane	Systemic		AIA	Rat, mouse	X	X	X	Model of chronic immune-mediated joint inflammation	Ethical issue
	SCW	Systemic	Human leukocyte antigen (HLA) B27 and	SCW-induced polyarthritis	Rat, mouse	—	—	—		Ethical issue
Genetically engineered	Genetic alteration	—		HLA-B27 transgenic rat	Rat	—	—	—	—	—

(continued)

Table 13.3 (Continued)

Categories	Induction method	Induction site	Model primary mechanism	Model name	Species	Mechanical sensitivity	Thermal sensitivity	Spontaneous pain	Key advantages	Disadvantages
			human β$_2$-microglobulin							
		—	Expression of MHC class II allele HLA-DR	HLA-DR transgenic mouse	Mouse	—	—	—	—	—
		—	Overexpression of TNF-α	TNF-α transgenic mouse		—	—	—	—	—
		—	Human T-cell receptor (KRN) and a human MHC class II molecule	K/BxN mouse		—	—	—	—	—
		—	Interleukin-1 receptor antagonist	IL-1ra knockout mouse		—	—	—	—	—

Guinea pigs, cats, and nonhuman primates are employed occasionally in immune-mediated arthritis research, primarily to explore basic mechanisms. But rats and mice remain the most common species used for pain investigation in arthritis. Most models of chronic inflammatory pain mimicking RA rely on the administration of substances that induce an immune response or the administration of inflammatory mediators themselves. They can be categorized depending on the type of exogenous material used and the location of administration. Indeed, adjuvant-induced arthritis (AIA) results from administration of various oil-based chemicals. The traditional example is based on the intra-articular (knee and ankle) administration of CFA, a water-in-oil emulsion of heat-killed *Mycobacterium butyricum* or *Mycobacterium tuberculosum*. Adjuvant activity is the result of sustained release of antigen from the oily deposit and stimulation of a local innate immune response. An essential component of this response is an intense inflammatory reaction at the site of antigen deposition associated with pain. The CFA injection produced a strong and long-lasting inflammatory reaction on the site of injection and in the draining lymph nodes. This inflammation may be painful to the animal. This model produces a disorder of the spontaneous behavior between the second and the fourth week postinjection and mechanical and thermal hyperalgesia during 8 weeks following induction. The CFA model is reliable in rats, but more difficult in mice for which either repeated injections at high concentrations or the use of sensitive strains might be required [3]. Knee or ankle joint injections of carrageenan (a polysaccharide obtained from various seaweeds), kaolin/carrageenan mix, or zymosan (yeast cell wall component) are also used as painful inflammatory monoarthritis models and are known to induce both thermal and mechanical allodynia and hyperalgesia [3]. The time course of local inflammation and the alteration of the synovia, cartilage, and bone differ between these models of arthritis. More chronic autoinflammatory or autoimmune painful conditions can also be modeled in rodents. These animal models of polyarthritis may raise, however, ethical issues related to their duration (weeks to months) and their pain-related consequences even if they are important for preclinical translational research on rheumatoid arthritis and its treatment [1]. Pharmacologically, animal models show good track records for predictability. Anti-inflammatory drugs (indomethacin, diclofenac, and meloxicam) have been used as reference compounds. Opiates are active in these models. The injection of neurotensin antagonists or NMDA receptor antagonists blocks the facilitation of the thermal paw withdrawal response. However, the mechanisms of sensitization are different for thermal and mechanical hyperalgesia.

13.4
Postoperative Pain

For decades, the data from animal research with various pain models have been translated to the field of postoperative pain (POP), although they may not represent properly this clinical situation. Indeed, some models were too short and mild to induce lesions observed during surgery, some were too specific of a chemical pathway, and some were too representative of chronic situations. Models of POP have been developed since, providing a better knowledge on the mechanisms [19]. However, these new models do not reflect all types of surgeries performed in humans. Surgery aims either to repair a part of the body by reshaping or replacing it or to remove dysfunctional elements. For this, various procedures are needed, which may transiently but extremely strongly activate the nociceptive network, thus inducing central sensitization. For this reason, the anesthetists – when they do not block the nerves by locoregional anesthesia – give a high dose of opioids during surgery, which may induce opiate-induced hyperalgesia [20,21]. Furthermore, some procedures (such as incision of the skin and deeper tissues, dissection, and electrocoagulation) are lesions induced on tissues, which will need healing processes in the postoperative period; this can be considered as a subacute model of inflammation.

Data from animal research [19] and clinical observations (mostly made on and around the wounded cutaneous area) [22,23] have evidenced processes related to both peripheral (primary hyperalgesia) [24] and central sensitization (secondary hyperalgesia) [22], which are quite well understood [25]. Sensitization of the nociceptive pathways is here represented at both the peripheral (Aδ- and C-fiber nociceptors) and the central (spinal dorsal horn and above) level, moving from activation (transient) via modulation (subacute but still reversible functional changes) to modification (structural and architectural alterations, basis of chronicization of pain) [21]. Secondary hyperalgesia involves activation of the spontaneous activity in dorsal horn neurons corresponding to the central sensitization.

13.4.1
Incisional Pain

Mechanical hyperalgesia is observed by applying force directly on the surgical wounds of patients after inguinal herniorrhaphy, open cholecystectomy, and abdominal hysterectomy. Several models of POP [19,26] have been proposed to mimic surgical wounds. In animals, nociceptive behaviors can be measured after incisional procedure, using the electronic von Frey. The withdrawal threshold induced by the application of von Frey filaments is markedly decreased after the plantar incision and this mechanical allodynia lasts for several days. Mechanical withdrawal threshold (Randall–Selitto test) and weight bearing alterations are also observed. In this model, behavioral changes are observed such as guarding, indicating the spontaneous pain induced by the surgical act. The magnitude of spontaneous activity of nociceptors and dorsal horn neurons is increased after incision. The spontaneous activity of Aδ and C fibers is increased after incision, whereas no afferents are spontaneously active in the sham group. This indicates an aspect of sensitization occurring after surgery. A 1 cm longitudinal incision is made through skin, fascia, and muscle of the plantar aspect of the hind paw in anesthetized rats. Twenty-four hours after surgery, a mechanical allodynia produced by the incision is quantified using the von Frey test. In this test, an increasing pressure is applied on both ipsilateral and contralateral hind paws and the paw withdrawal threshold is measured. Locally applied bupivacaine is also potent on tactile allodynia. The gabapentinoid compounds, NMDA antagonists, κ-opioid receptor agonists, and partial μ-opioid receptor agonists are active in this model.

The incisional pain model allows assessment of the mechanisms of increased mechanical sensitivity following a surgical incision and is widely used for revealing the potency of new analgesics in a model of POP in conscious rats.

13.4.2
Laparotomy

The abdominal incision (laparotomy) represents a relevant model of POP for gastrointestinal surgery. The surgery produces spontaneous behaviors, locomotion changes, immune response, and postoperative ileus. Cramping visceral pain commonly occurs after abdominal, genitourinary, and gynecologic surgery. These abdominal wounds are particularly painful and result in postoperative ileus associated with food-seeking behavioral changes. The ability of abdominal incision to induce postoperative ileus has been extensively studied [27]. These models are able to distinguish different types of activities in assessing the behavioral effects of surgery and are useful in assessing beneficial and harmful effects of analgesic agents in the postoperative state.

13.4.3
Ovariohysterectomy

In rats and dogs, ovariohysterectomy is considered as a relevant model of POP [28,29]. Indeed, compared with the incisional pain model, this model closely reflects the major proportion of elective surgery that involves operative invasion of the body cavities, including abdominal and thoracic surgical procedures. In such cases, there is a significant activation and sensitization of visceral afferents, giving rise to inputs that are processed differently from those of somatic sensory neurons. The behavioral responses shown by female rats following ovariohysterectomy are represented by abdominal postures, referred hyperalgesia, and two distinct types of referred mechanical allodynia (static and dynamic) in the rat hind paws. Interestingly, in patients, following surgery, allodynia constitutes a great postoperative problem because relevant stimuli (i.e., clothes touching skin, breathing, coughing, and movement of joints) are almost unavoidable.

13.4.4
Other Models of Postoperative Pain

A postoperative model has been developed to mimic chronic postthoracotomy pain induced by thoracotomy and rib retraction [30]. Buvanendran *et al.* [31] described a new simple, reproducible rat model to assess function and discomfort after knee surgery, and one that responds to therapeutic interventions. In these models, the efficacies of some drugs such as morphine and gabapentin have shown beneficial effects in postoperative pain.

13.5
Translation to Clinics: Limitations and Difficulties

Translational animal research plays a critical role in understanding the mechanisms of diseases and identifying/investigating potential treatment targets. The aim of a translational animal model is to facilitate the translation of findings from basic science to practical applications that enhance human health and well-being. No (induced) animal model can reproduce accurately the full complexity of the human disease, but important criteria in selection of a model for drug testing can be defined as similarity with the human disease, capacity to predict efficacy in humans, reproducibility of the data, ease of use, reasonable duration of test period, and cost, as well as the study of various components of pain [3,14]. Animal models provide practical approaches to study both the natural history of the disease and the response to relevant treatments. The most important point remains the particular attention that has to be given to the scientific question under investigation in order to choose an appropriate animal model [3]. In this context, spontaneous models mimicking the natural occurrence and progression of the human disease would be preferred. In the field of OA, larger animal species offer this advantage with close similarities to human knee pathology. On the contrary, disadvantages include the slow progression of the disease not really appropriate for the assessment of analgesics, the cost, and the public perception. Smaller animals (i.e., rodents) are also widely used. They are easier to use and less costly, but the information gathered may be less applicable to human pathologies. Actually, most of them are chemically or surgically induced. Chemical stimulations involve several mechanisms of action that are difficult to transpose to pathophysiological mechanisms involved in human diseases. Indeed, the existing models using inflammatory mediators such as formalin, carrageenan, and CFA are too drastic in terms of inflammatory process to mimic arthritis, osteoarthritis, and postsurgical pain. For chronic situations, little similarity exists between the development of MIA-induced OA (rapidly progressive model) and the long-term progression and development of OA in humans, but this model (chemically induced) is currently used for discerning therapeutic approaches for OA pain intervention.

Another limitation in the translation of animal models to clinics is represented by the drug doses and paradigms of treatments used in pharmacological pain studies. In the past decades, many analgesic targets emerged from basic science studies, but the corresponding treatments that have shown efficacy in animal models produce disappointing results in humans. Range of doses used in rodents and humans differs significantly because of different drug metabolisms or differences in affinities. It limits the relevance of the study when doses are out of selectivity range or when they induce overall behavioral perturbations that interfere with the nociceptive measures [1]. Typically, nonopioid drugs are often insufficient in relieving pain to the normal level of sensitivity in patients suffering from severe pain. The treatment with the classical μ-opioid agonists is not optimal and pain relief is closely associated with side effects such as constipation, nausea, sedation, and euphoria. A benefit of treatment may also be greater in animals because the treatment is initiated at the time the injury is induced, before the development of the disease, whereas patients are treated much later in the disease process.

Attrition also raises the question of preclinical validity of basic pain tests used in animals compared with the complexity of chronic pain in humans [32]. The evaluation of pain is subjective depending on sex, social aspects, and psychology. In the last years, gender influences on pain and analgesia and data regarding gender differences in response to pharmacological pain treatments have become hot topics. In particular, females seem to be more sensitive to pain than males. Depression is a common mental disorder with various symptoms and often accompanied with unexplained painful physical symptoms. In experimental models, it is important to have robust and reproducible pain measures to evaluate the analgesic effects of drugs. These studies have thus to be controlled in terms of pain stimulation (i.e., modality, localization, intensity, frequency, and duration). The clinical aspects of sensitization are expressed as increased pain for a given stimulus. Such "hyperalgesia" may be detrimental in the early postoperative period, as it increases the amount of experienced POP and may induce stress with all the possible negative consequences of it [21], and it is strongly linked to movement-evoked POP, against which the patient may behave by avoiding any painful movement. This may relevantly affect rehabilitation; for example, interventions reducing movement-evoked POP are associated with fewer postoperative thrombo-embolic complications [33] and improve pulmonary outcomes [34]. The guarding behavior observed in the rat model of hind paw incision could be considered as a good surrogate of this avoidance behavior [19]. Moreover, the primary symptoms of chronic pain in patients are spontaneous pain. For musculoskeletal disorders, pain is usually localized in a precise area, increases with pressure on the area involved, can be caused/exacerbated by weight bearing, and is often felt at night. Mechanical pain thresholds, range of motion, weight bearing, and gait analysis are commonly used in the clinical setting to assess pain in patients with arthritis. In animal models of arthritis, behavioral tests that use indirect measures of knee joint pain include, as in humans, static and dynamic weight bearing, foot posture and gait analysis, and mechanical or heat sensitivity of the paw. A potential limitation of dynamic weight bearing measurements is that animals are required to move, which can be influenced by a number of factors such as motivation. In fact, pain should not be reduced to its sensory-discriminative component because it also involves motivational/affective and cognitive-evaluative dimensions. Dissecting out the factors that contribute to changes in patients' nociceptive capabilities and those that are related to the communication of their pain as a central/cognitive perception is a real challenge for future clinical research. In animals, assessing these behavioral modifications are of interest not only for the study of pathophysiological mechanisms involved in chronic inflammatory pain but also for the preclinical assessment of analgesic drug effects [35].

In conclusion, the animal models in inflammatory, musculoskeletal/joint, and postoperative pain are necessary to evaluate the potency of antihyperalgesic and/or antiallodynic drugs. The need for more predictive pain models with better understanding of their pathophysiology should be useful in developing the new analgesics. Progress in clinical pain research has been aided by the development of more sophisticated animal models based notably on the study of the various dimensions of pain in rodents with chronic pain.

References

1 Barrot, M. (2012) Tests and models of nociception and pain in rodents. *Neuroscience*, **211**, 39–50.

2 Sandkuhler, J. (2009) Models and mechanisms of hyperalgesia and allodynia. *Physiological Reviews*, **89**, 707–758.

3 Neugebauer, V., Han, J.S., Adwanikar, H., Fu, Y., and Ji, G. (2007) Techniques for assessing knee joint pain in arthritis. *Molecular Pain*, **3**, 8.

4 Gregoire, S., Michaud, V., Chapuy, E., Eschalier, A., and Ardid, D. (2012) Study of emotional and cognitive impairments in mononeuropathic rats: effect of duloxetine and gabapentin. *Pain*, **153**, 1657–1663.

5 Dubuisson, D. and Dennis, S.G. (1977) The formalin test: a quantitative study of the analgesic effects of morphine, meperidine, and brain stem stimulation in rats and cats. *Pain*, **4**, 161–174.

6 Morris, C.J. (2003) Carrageenan-induced paw edema in the rat and mouse. *Methods in Molecular Biology (Clifton, NJ)*, **225**, 115–121.

7 O'Neill, J., Brock, C., Olesen, A.E., Andresen, T., Nilsson, M., and Dickenson, A.H. (2012) Unravelling the mystery of capsaicin: a tool to understand and treat pain. *Pharmacological Reviews*, **64**, 939–971.

8 Schopper, D., Pereira, J., Torres, A., Cuende, N., Alonso, M., Baylin, A., Ammon, C., and Rougemont, A. (2000) Estimating the burden of disease in one Swiss canton: what do disability adjusted life years (DALY) tell us? *International Journal of Epidemiology*, **29**, 871–877.

9 Sprangers, M.A., de Regt, E.B., Andries, F., van Agt, H.M., Bijl, R.V., de Boer, J.B., Foets, M., Hoeymans, N., Jacobs, A.E., Kempen, G.I., Miedema, H.S., Tijhuis, M.A., and de Haes, H.C. (2000) Which chronic conditions are associated with better or poorer quality of life? *Journal of Clinical Epidemiology*, **53**, 895–907.

10 Brooks, P.M. (2002) Impact of osteoarthritis on individuals and society: how much disability? Social consequences and health economic implications. *Current Opinion in Rheumatology*, **14**, 573–577.

11 Kidd, B.L. (2006) Osteoarthritis and joint pain. *Pain*, **123**, 6–9.

12 Guccione, A.A., Felson, D.T., Anderson, J.J., Anthony, J.M., Zhang, Y., Wilson, P.W., Kelly-Hayes, M., Wolf, P.A., Kreger, B.E., and Kannel, W.B. (1994) The effects of specific medical conditions on the functional limitations of elders in the Framingham Study. *American Journal of Public Health*, **84**, 351–358.

13 Bendele, A. (2001) Animal models of rheumatoid arthritis. *Journal of Musculoskeletal & Neuronal Interactions*, **1**, 377–385.

14 Gregory, M.H., Capito, N., Kuroki, K., Stoker, A.M., Cook, J.L., and Sherman, S.L. (2012) A review of translational animal models for knee osteoarthritis. *Arthritis*, **2012**, 764621.

15 Guzman, R.E., Evans, M.G., Bove, S., Morenko, B., and Kilgore, K. (2003) Mono-iodoacetate-induced histologic changes in subchondral bone and articular cartilage of rat femorotibial joints: an animal model of osteoarthritis. *Toxicologic Pathology*, **31**, 619–624.

16 Bove, S.E., Flatters, S.J., Inglis, J.J., and Mantyh, P.W. (2009) New advances in

musculoskeletal pain. *Brain Research Reviews*, **60**, 187–201.
17 Fernihough, J., Gentry, C., Malcangio, M., Fox, A., Rediske, J., Pellas, T., Kidd, B., Bevan, S., and Winter, J. (2004) Pain related behaviour in two models of osteoarthritis in the rat knee. *Pain*, **112**, 83–93.
18 Bolon, B., Stolina, M., King, C., Middleton, S., Gasser, J., Zack, D., and Feige, U. (2011) Rodent preclinical models for developing novel antiarthritic molecules: comparative biology and preferred methods for evaluating efficacy. *Journal of Biomedicine & Biotechnology*, **2011**, 569068.
19 Brennan, T.J. (2011) Pathophysiology of postoperative pain. *Pain*, **152**, S33–S40.
20 Chu, L.F., Angst, M.S., and Clark, D. (2008) Opioid-induced hyperalgesia in humans: molecular mechanisms and clinical considerations. *The Clinical Journal of Pain*, **24**, 479–496.
21 Wilder-Smith, O.H. and Arendt-Nielsen, L. (2006) Postoperative hyperalgesia: its clinical importance and relevance. *Anesthesiology*, **104**, 601–607.
22 Groetzner, P. and Weidner, C. (2010) The human vasodilator axon reflex: an exclusively peripheral phenomenon? *Pain*, **149**, 71–75.
23 Martinez, V., Fletcher, D., Bouhassira, D., Sessler, D.I., and Chauvin, M. (2007) The evolution of primary hyperalgesia in orthopedic surgery: quantitative sensory testing and clinical evaluation before and after total knee arthroplasty. *Anesthesia and Analgesia*, **105**, 815–821.
24 Sumikura, H., Andersen, O.K., Drewes, A.M., and Arendt-Nielsen, L. (2003) Spatial and temporal profiles of flare and hyperalgesia after intradermal capsaicin. *Pain*, **105**, 285–291.
25 Basbaum, A.I., Bautista, D.M., Scherrer, G., and Julius, D. (2009) Cellular and molecular mechanisms of pain. *Cell*, **139**, 267–284.
26 Pogatzki, E.M., Niemeier, J.S., Sorkin, L.S., and Brennan, T.J. (2003) Spinal glutamate receptor antagonists differentiate primary and secondary mechanical hyperalgesia caused by incision. *Pain*, **105**, 97–107.
27 De Winter, B.Y. (2003) Study of the pathogenesis of paralytic ileus in animal models of experimentally induced postoperative and septic ileus. *Verhandelingen: Koninklijke Academie voor Geneeskunde van Belgie*, **65**, 293–324.
28 Gonzalez, M.I., Field, M.J., Bramwell, S., McCleary, S., and Singh, L. (2000) Ovariohysterectomy in the rat: a model of surgical pain for evaluation of pre-emptive analgesia? *Pain*, **88**, 79–88.
29 Lascelles, B.D., Waterman, A.E., Cripps, P.J., Livingston, A., and Henderson, G. (1995) Central sensitization as a result of surgical pain: investigation of the pre-emptive value of pethidine for ovariohysterectomy in the rat. *Pain*, **62**, 201–212.
30 Buvanendran, A., Kroin, J.S., Kerns, J.M., Nagalla, S.N., and Tuman, K.J. (2004) Characterization of a new animal model for evaluation of persistent postthoracotomy pain. *Anesthesia and Analgesia*, **99**, 1453–1460.
31 Buvanendran, A., Kroin, J.S., Kari, M.R., and Tuman, K.J. (2008) A new knee surgery model in rats to evaluate functional measures of postoperative pain. *Anesthesia and Analgesia*, **107**, 300–308.
32 Mogil, J.S. (2009) Animal models of pain: progress and challenges. *Nature Reviews. Neuroscience*, **10**, 283–294.
33 Paul, J.E., Arya, A., Hurlburt, L., Cheng, J., Thabane, L., Tidy, A., and Murthy, Y. (2010) Femoral nerve block improves analgesia outcomes after total knee arthroplasty: a meta-analysis of randomized controlled trials. *Anesthesiology*, **113**, 1144–1162.
34 Gilron, I., Orr, E., Tu, D., O'Neill, J.P., Zamora, J.E., and Bell, A.C. (2005) A placebo-controlled randomized clinical trial of perioperative administration of gabapentin, rofecoxib and their combination for spontaneous and movement-evoked pain after abdominal hysterectomy. *Pain*, **113**, 191–200.
35 Han, J.S. and Neugebauer, V. (2005) mGluR1 and mGluR5 antagonists in the amygdala inhibit different components of audible and ultrasonic vocalizations in a model of arthritic pain. *Pain*, **113**, 211–222.

14
Neuropathic Pain
Said M'Dahoma, Sylvie Bourgoin, and Michel Hamon

14.1
Introduction

Pain is considered chronic when it persists, with or without treatment, for more than 6 months [1]. Among the different types of chronic pain, neuropathic pain is caused by lesion or dysfunction of the central or peripheral nervous system. It can be the consequence of various insults, such as surgical intervention, trauma with nerve compression or section, spinal cord contusion, viral infection (HIV, herpes zoster and varicella zoster), neurotoxic chemicals (notably anticancer and antiretrovirus drugs), or metabolic pathologies such as diabetes mellitus. In addition, neuropathic pain constitutes one of the most deleterious symptoms of several neurological syndromes (multiple sclerosis, amyotrophic lateral sclerosis, Parkinson's disease, Guillain–Barré syndrome, stroke, etc.). Estimates of prevalence of neuropathic pain vary widely, ranging from 1 to 7% of the population, with a commonly adopted midrange estimate of 3%. This percentage means that nowadays, at the beginning of the twenty-first century, about 63 million people worldwide suffer from neuropathic pain. Actually, this number is currently increasing notably because of the progression of diabetes prevalence, with unavoidable downstream increase in diabetic neuropathy, especially in the United States and in Europe.

To date, neuropathic pain is a major public health problem not only because of its increasing prevalence but also because of the limited efficacy of available treatments. Classical analgesic drugs are usually poorly effective or even completely ineffective, and, mainly because of the limited understanding of the precise etiology of many neuropathic pain conditions, current pharmacological treatments are based on empirical data. Thus, treatments encompass an array of drug classes originally targeted on other pathological conditions, especially some (not all) antidepressants, anticonvulsants, and topical anesthetics. Accordingly, thorough investigations of pathophysiological mechanisms underlying neuropathic pain are mandatory for the potential development of rational, innovative, really effective, and well-tolerated treatments. To reach this goal, experimental pain models are an absolute requirement, and, indeed, a large panel of animal models of neuropathic

In Vivo Models for Drug Discovery, First Edition. Edited by José M. Vela, Rafael Maldonado, and Michel Hamon.
© 2014 Wiley-VCH Verlag GmbH & Co. KGaA. Published 2014 by Wiley-VCH Verlag GmbH & Co. KGaA.

pain has been set up during the last 40 years. Their main characteristics, usefulness, and also limitations are critically assessed in this chapter.

14.2
Main Types of Neuropathic Pain in Humans

Most of the time, neuropathic pain is described as persistent and diffuse burning-like sensation with no specific location in given organs or tissues. In addition, patients suffer from paroxystic pain, which is described as electric shock-like sensations of short duration alternating with remission periods.

Evoked painful sensations vary with the intensity of the stimulus (mechanical, thermal, or chemical). Two types of sensations are reported by patients: *hyperalgesia*, which corresponds to exacerbated pain from a stimulus that normally induces only moderate pain, and *allodynia*, which is pain caused by a stimulus that does not normally evoke pain in healthy subjects. Allodynia can be particularly debilitating because patients have to change their way of living and their social behavior, by avoiding every mechanical contact (with clothes, sheets, shower) that could eventually trigger pain in the body part concerned. In all cases, animal models will aim at reproducing hyperalgesia and allodynia in response to various mechanical, thermal, and/or chemical-driven sensory stimulations.

14.2.1
Neuropathic Pain Caused by Peripheral Nerve Lesions

14.2.1.1 Diabetes-Induced Neuropathic Pain
Diabetes-induced neuropathy concerns about 9–14% of patients with insulin-dependent diabetes mellitus and 7–9% of patients with noninsulin-dependent diabetes mellitus [2,3] and comes as a late complication of these metabolic pathologies.

Patients develop not only abnormal sensations such as paresthesia, allodynia, and hyperalgesia but also spontaneous pain that coexists with loss of normal sensory function. The pathological features of diabetic neuropathy include consequences of Schwann cell disruption such as nodal widening and segmental demyelination, axonal degeneration, and microvascular lesions [4].

14.2.1.2 Human Immunodeficiency Virus-Related Pain
AIDS patients suffer from neurological disorders, notably the neuropathic pain called distal sensory polyneuropathy, which affects one-third of the patients at advanced stages [5,6]. Distal sensory polyneuropathy is especially refractory to analgesic drugs. In particular, morphine, which relieves most pains from other origins, can even be pronociceptive in HIV neuropathic patients [7]. On the other hand, only few reports mention some improvement of the pain status with treatments aimed at HIV viral suppression [8]. Indeed, antiretroviral drugs have toxic effects on nerves. This is the case with didanosine, $2',3'$-dideoxycytidine, and

stavudine, which cause peripheral neuropathy [9,10] and even increase distal sensory neuropathy.

14.2.1.3 Postherpetic Neuralgia

Usually, the herpes zoster virus, whose first infection causes varicella, remains dormant in sensory ganglia. However, reactivation and transport of the virus from skin to sensory ganglia can cause herpes zoster (shingles) [11], particularly in old and/or immunodepressed patients. Acute herpes zoster induces a rash, which is accompanied by pain in the dermatome of the sensory ganglia infected by the virus. Postherpetic neuralgia, which is thought to be induced by nerve damage caused by the virus, can be severe, not responsive to classical analgesic treatments, and persistent for years [12].

14.2.1.4 Neuropathic Pain Caused by Anticancer Drugs

Chemotherapy is most frequently used for breast, lung, and gastrointestinal cancers. Because of their neurotoxic effects affecting essentially peripheral nerves, anticancer drugs do not reduce cancer-evoked pain but even cause additional neuropathic pain, which contributes to major deterioration of the quality of life of treated patients [13]. In particular, platinum salts such as cisplatin and oxaliplatin, as well as taxanes (paclitaxel), are well known to cause sensory dysfunctions (paresthesias and dysesthesias) and neuropathic-like pain, and these drugs are frequently used to generate neuropathic pain models in rodents (see below).

14.2.2 Neuropathic Pain Caused by Central Lesions

14.2.2.1 Spinal Cord Injury

In addition to motor and genitourinary deficits, pain resulting from spinal cord injury (SCI) is an especially debilitating issue. The prevalence of severe chronic pain in SCI patients ranges from 30 to 51% [14]. Their pain can be so severe that, when asked, SCI patients would rather renounce their sexual or bladder function than still feeling pain [15]. Indeed, it affects patient's quality of life much more than motor dysfunction and often leads to depression and even suicide [16].

Pain arising from SCI is multiple in terms of pathophysiology, symptoms, and body localization. SCI pain can be referred to as nociceptive (mainly musculoskeletal or visceral pain) or neuropathic (above, at, or below the level of the injury) pain. Musculoskeletal pain has the highest prevalence, with 58% of SCI patients suffering from it. Neuropathic pain is also frequent with 12–42% of patients reporting at-level pain and 23–34% reporting below-level pain [14,15].

A classification of the different cases of spinal cord injury has been proposed by the American Spinal Injury Association (ASIA) that distinguishes two main categories of patients with complete (ASIA A) or incomplete (ASIA B, C, or D) spinal cord injury [17]. ASIA A refers to a patient who does not have any sensory or motor function in the sacral segment S4–S5. Since a complete lesion is rarely seen, the definition of the zone of partial preservation (ZPP) has been proposed for a more appropriate classification of ASIA A patients. Indeed, ZPP is strictly applicable to ASIA A patients and refers to the most caudal zone with the dermatomes and/or myotomes still innervated, which preserve some sensory and/or motor functions.

14.2.2.2 The Various Types of Pain in SCI Patients

Musculoskeletal Pain Musculoskeletal pain arises from musculoskeletal structures (muscles, tendons, ligaments, joints, and bones) located above, at, or below the level of spinal cord injury. Typically, musculoskeletal pain arises when the patient moves and includes pain resulting from joint arthritis, spinal fractures, muscle injury, and/or muscle spasms [18]. Musculoskeletal structures show tenderness on palpation and imaging reveals the skeletal pathology, which fits with the pain representation. This pain, described as "dull" or "aching," can generally be alleviated by anti-inflammatory and opioid medications, at least better than neuropathic pain [14]. Pain located in musculoskeletal tissues without those characteristics is considered as neuropathic pain.

Visceral Pain Visceral pain is generated in visceral structures and located in the thorax, abdomen, or pelvis. Tenderness of visceral structures is evident on palpation of the abdomen and the pathology is further characterized by imaging, in consistence with the pain representation. It is temporally correlated with food intake or visceral functions/dysfunctions such as constipation. The pain is described as "cramping," "dull," or "tender," and is associated with nausea and sweating. Treatments with antispasmodic drugs, histamine H_2 receptor antagonists, and inhibitors of proton pump can produce significant alleviating effects, in addition to the use of "classical" analgetics (acetaminophen and opioids), which are effective against severe visceral pain. Pain located in the thorax, abdomen, or pelvis without these characteristics is considered as neuropathic pain.

Neuropathic Pain In SCI patients, neuropathic pain refers to a lesion or a disease of a nerve root or the spinal cord itself. Its onset can be almost immediately after the SCI or months later [15]. The faster the pain arises, the more likely the patient is to have ongoing pain for 3–5 years after the injury [19]. Neuropathic pain is mainly characterized by its severity, with typical symptoms such as allodynia (see above), which is an especially disabling feature because touch from clothes or taking a shower may cause intense pain, and even a gentle touch can be enough to trigger a burning sensation [15]. In SCI patients, induced neuropathic pain commonly occurs at level and below the lesion.

Pain develops first at level and then below injury level [19]. To be defined as at-level pain, it has to be perceived at least within the dermatome concerned with the lesion and/or in one dermatome above or three below [14]. Any pain experienced below three dermatomes should not be described as at-level neuropathic pain. Moreover, to be classified as at-level pain, neuropathic pain has to result from a lesion or disease affecting a nerve root and/or the spinal cord itself closely related to the location of injury-evoked somatosensory dysfunctions.

At-level SCI pain is characterized by sensory deficits along with allodynia and hyperalgesia. Words used to describe this pain are "hot burning," "tingling," "pricking," "pins and needles," "sharp," "shooting," "squeezing," "painful cold," and "electric shock-like" [14,16].

Below-level neuropathic pain is typically perceived beyond three dermatomes under the level of injury and may extend up to the at-level dermatome [14]. Like at-level pain, below-level neuropathic pain is characterized by sensory deficits along with allodynia and hyperalgesia within the affected dermatomes. In addition, the same words as those used to describe at-level pain are also used by the below-level suffering patients to depict their painful symptoms [14,16].

14.3
Modelization of Chronic Pain in Rodents

Extensive characterization of neuropathic pain in humans and identification of underlying causes allowed the development of numerous animal models, especially in rodents, aimed at filling the three main criteria, namely, *face validity*, *construct validity*, and *predictive validity*, for reliable studies of (i) pathophysiological mechanisms responsible for neuropathic pain at cellular and molecular levels, (ii) potential targets for setting up innovative alleviating treatments, and (iii) efficacy and tolerability of drugs, or combination of drugs, for improved therapeutic strategies in humans.

14.3.1
Models of Peripheral Nerve Injury

14.3.1.1 Nerve Section

Sciatic Nerve Section Unilateral transection of the sciatic nerve at mid-thigh level is the first nerve lesion model that has been developed [20]. In anesthetized rats, the sciatic nerve is exposed and two nylon sutures are tightly tied 1 cm apart, close to its bifurcation. The nerve is transected twice between the ligatures so as to remove a 5 mm fragment, thereby preventing any reconnection. Indeed, a neuroma develops at the proximal nerve stump as a result of regenerative nerve sprouting in all directions. With this procedure, the adjacent saphenous nerve is also lesioned, which leads to the complete denervation of the distal hind limb. This nerve lesion is considered as an approximate model of "anesthesia dolorosa" in humans [20], in which there is also an absence of any sensory input in the innervated area. Among the neuroplastic changes induced within the ipsilateral dorsal horn of the spinal cord in sciatic nerve-sectioned rats, a marked induction of CCK-B receptors of cholecystokinin (CCK) has been reported, especially within the superficial layers

[21]. Since CCK-B receptor signaling has clear-cut antiopioid effects, this adaptive change might explain, at least in part, why morphine is only poorly effective against neuropathic pain in such lesioned rats. Although this sciatic nerve section model undoubtedly contributed to a better knowledge of pathophysiological mechanisms underlying neuropathic pain, it has major limitations since it can lead to autotomy. Whether autotomy reflects pain or just an abnormal sensation or dysesthesia is a matter of debate [22,23], but, whatever the answer, this dramatic behavioral disorder caused by nerve section raised serious concerns for obvious ethical reasons [24].

Transection of Tibial and Sural Nerves In this model, tibial and sural nerves are tightly ligated with 5-0 silk thread and sectioned at the distal side of the ligation to remove 2 mm of the distal part of the nerves. In rats, this surgical operation produces mechanical allodynia, cold allodynia, and behavioral signs of spontaneous pain of greater amplitude than common peroneal nerve ligation [25].

14.3.1.2 Nerve Ligation, Compression, and Other Lesion Procedures

Complete Ligation of the Sciatic Nerve The model of chronic constriction injury (CCI), first developed by Bennett and Xie [26] in the rat, consists of the placement of four ligatures with silk (4-0) or chromic gut thread, approximately 1 mm apart, on one sciatic nerve (Figure 14.1). The ligatures are loosely tightened until a twitch is observed at the footpad. The purpose of this controlled procedure is to reduce the epineural blood flow without stopping it [26,27]. This results in sciatic nerve swelling, loss of axons distal to the ligatures, and neuroma formation at the level of the ligatures. The use of chromic gut tends to increase pain behavior because it promotes the inflammatory immune component of the neuropathy [28]. Unilateral CCI to the sciatic nerve induces mechanical allodynia and hyperalgesia as well as

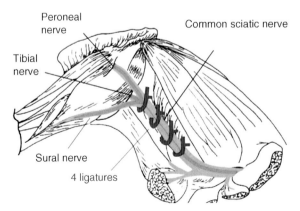

Figure 14.1 Model of chronic constriction injury to the sciatic nerve [26].

thermal (heat) hyperalgesia, which reach a plateau 2 weeks after the surgery and persists for at least 7 weeks thereafter [26,29]. Cold hyperalgesia has also been reported in sciatic nerve-ligated rats [30]. Even though initial reports indicated hyperalgesia and allodynia only on the lesioned side, more recent reports noted the occurrence of bilateral pain [31].

In addition to exacerbating provoked pain behavior, this model induces mild to moderate autotomy and altered posture. Although the pain relevance of such behavioral changes is still a matter of debate [32], the expected postural avoidance of placing body weight on the injury side (guarding) has been documented [33]. As a matter of fact, the sciatic nerve ligation model undoubtedly replicates most symptoms of the complex regional pain syndrome in patients [26]. However, because of difficulties inherent to the control of constriction tightness [34] and variations linked to the choice of ligation material [28], some variability in sciatic nerve ligation-evoked neuropathic pain-like symptoms is unavoidable from one operated rat to another. Indeed, usually only 60–70% of CCI rats developed hyperalgesia and/or allodynia, in spite of apparently identical nerve ligations.

Partial Ligation of the Sciatic Nerve In 1990, Seltzer *et al.* [35] developed a model that consists of unilateral tight ligation of one-third to one-half of the sciatic nerve with an 8-0 silk suture just distal to the point at which posterior biceps semitendinosus nerve branches off. Spontaneous pain, as suggested by guarding behavior of the ipsilateral hind paw and frequent licking, together with cold allodynia, chemical hyperreactivity, and mechanical hyperalgesia is induced from 1 to 6 weeks after surgery [36,37]. Because of the rapid onset and long-lasting continuation of touch-evoked allodynia and hyperalgesia, the partial sciatic nerve injury model is generally considered as mimicking causalgiform pain disorders in humans. In support of this assertion, mechanical hyperalgesia occurs bilaterally in rats with unilateral partial sciatic nerve ligation, like the "mirror image" pains reported by patients suffering from causalgia with excessive sympathetic activity.

Sciatic Nerve Cuffing Placement of a polyethylene cuff around the sciatic nerve has been developed as an alternative to nerve ligation, with the idea of reducing the interindividual variability already noted. Indeed, neuropathic pain similar to the one produced by the CCI model of Bennett and Xie [26] is induced by a polyethylene cuff (2 mm in length and 0.7 mm in inner diameter) placed around the common branch of the sciatic nerve in rats. Heat hyperalgesia and mechanical allodynia, which last for 3 weeks and 2 months, respectively, have been reported in rats and mice with sciatic nerve cuffing [38,39]. Comparison with the sciatic nerve ligation model seems to confirm that the cuffing model leads to less variability in the intensity of neuropathic pain-like symptoms from one operated rat to another [40,41].

Spared Nerve Injury Another variant of the Bennett and Xie's model consists of tight ligation of two of the three branches of the sciatic nerve, the tibial and the common peroneal nerves (see Figure 14.1), with 5-0 silk thread followed by axotomy of a 2 mm nerve segment between ligatures. The third branch, corresponding to the sural nerve, is spared [42]. This model induces mechanical allodynia as well as hot and cold allodynia at ipsilateral hind paw from 1 week to 6 months postinjury [42,43].

Laser-Induced Sciatic Nerve Injury In this model, rodents are first treated acutely with erythrosine B (32.5 mg/kg i.v.), a photosensitizing dye laser. The sciatic nerve is then exposed and irradiated with an argon ion laser to trigger a photochemical reaction that causes thrombosis and occlusion of small vessels supplying the nerve. This results in long-lasting bilateral mechanical allodynia and unilateral thermal hyperalgesia [44,45]. Ipsilateral pain is induced more rapidly and has a greater magnitude than that generated on the contralateral side. After such laser-induced ischemic nerve lesion, approximately 95% of the animals not only develop neuropathic pain but also show clear-cut behavioral signs of spontaneous pain [46].

Laser beam, on its own, can also induce neuropathic pain. Thus, without any photosensitizing dye, irradiation of the sciatic nerve by a 532 nm laser beam of 1 mm diameter at an output power of 100 mW for 30 s results in a marked reduction of the blood flow to the nerve, ending with neurodegeneration [47]. Under these conditions, rats develop thermal hyperalgesia and mechanical allodynia, which last for 4–9 weeks after the surgery.

Sciatic Nerve Cryoneurolysis Cold-induced lesion of the sciatic nerve has also been proposed as a model for generating neuropathic pain in rats. According to Willenbring *et al.* [48], the sciatic nerve is frozen proximal to its trifurcation with a cryoprobe cooled at $-60\,°C$ using a 2 mm diameter cryoprobe with nitrous oxide as the refrigerant (30 s/5 s/30 s, freeze–thaw–freeze cycle). This operation induces bilateral mechanical allodynia for up to 21 days [48], but no thermal hyperalgesia. Interestingly, sympathectomy does not reduce cryoneurolysis-induced mechanical allodynia, in contrast to that found in the case of mechanical allodynia in rats rendered neuropathic by spinal nerve ligation or partial ligation of the sciatic nerve [48], further indicating that freeze-induced lesion probably triggers structural and functional alterations of nociceptive signaling pathways different from those resulting from mechanical lesion of nerves. In line with such differences, autotomy seems to occur more frequently after sciatic nerve cryoneurolysis, which explains why this model did not give rise to extensive studies.

Common Peroneal Nerve Injury This lesion model has been elaborated in the mouse. It consists of a single ligature of the common peroneal nerve with chromic gut suture 5-0 [49]. The common peroneal nerve has been chosen because one of its branches, the superficial peroneal nerve, carries mainly sensory fibers from the dorsal part of the foot. The nerve is slowly tightened until contraction of the foot dorsiflexors. This model is characterized by allodynia and thermal hyperalgesia without apparent alterations in motor functions. It therefore contrasts with most other neuropathic pain models in which both sensory and motor nerve fibers are lesioned, thereby directly causing abnormal sensory and motor responses.

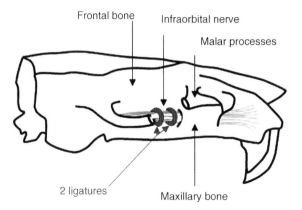

Figure 14.2 Chronic constriction injury to the infraorbital nerve [50].

Infraorbital Nerve Ligation The model of chronic constriction injury to the infraorbital nerve, first developed by Vos *et al.* [50] in the rat, consists of the placement of two ligatures with silk (4-0) or chromic gut thread, approximately 1 mm apart, on one infraorbital nerve (Figure 14.2). As expected of the specific lesion of a nerve (second branch of the trigeminal nerve) that comprises sensory fibers only, rats with CCI of the infraorbital nerve developed abnormal spontaneous pain-related behavior [51], thermal heat hyperalgesia [52], and mechanical allodynia located at the vibrissae pad 2 weeks after the surgery [29,50,53]. The purpose of this model is to reproduce and decipher the physiopathological mechanisms of typical cephalic pain such as "cluster headache" in humans. Interestingly, Kayser *et al.* [54] showed that, in rats, pain resulting from infraorbital nerve ligation can be reduced by antimigraine drugs such as triptans in contrast to neuropathic pain generated by sciatic nerve ligation. Therefore, this model seems to be especially appropriate to investigate specificities of neuropathic pain at the cephalic level and may be used to assess potential antimigraine effects of drugs. Indeed, not only triptans but also CGRP receptor antagonists have been found to alleviate mechanical allodynia induced by infraorbital nerve ligation, but not that due to sciatic nerve ligation.

Dorsal Rhizotomy This model has been extensively characterized by Lombard *et al.* [55]. It consists of unilateral sections of lumbar dorsal roots. Briefly, a dorsal hemilaminectomy is performed in deeply anesthetized rats and, through an opening of the dura mater, nine dorsal roots (T13–S2) are sectioned intradurally, proximal to the spinal cord, with great caution to avoid trauma to spinal tissues and ventral roots. This surgery results in mechanical allodynia and mechanical and cold hyperalgesia [55,56], which resemble the symptoms of nerve root avulsions in humans [57].

Spinal Nerve Ligation In this model, developed by Kim and Chung [58] in the rat, L5 and L6 spinal nerves are unilaterally ligated using 6-0 silk thread under deep anesthesia. This results in mechanical allodynia, cold allodynia, and thermal heat hyperalgesia. Spontaneous pain can also be observed in operated animals with ipsilateral hind limb in guarding position [58]. These behavioral manifestations start to develop within 48 h after spinal nerve ligation and last for 10–16 weeks [58–60]. Because of these well-established characteristics, the spinal nerve ligation model is frequently used in studies aimed at investigating pathophysiological features and potential therapeutic strategies relevant to causalgia resulting from peripheral nerves injury in patients.

Injury to Dorsal Root Ganglia Rather than nerves, dorsal root ganglia can also be injured to generate experimental neuropathic pain. Thus, Liu *et al.* [61] inserted a small stainless steel rod (4 mm in length and 0.5–0.8 mm in diameter) into the L5 and/or L4 intervertebral foramen to produce foramen stenosis. The resulting chronic steady compression of L5/L4 dorsal root ganglia induced heat hyperalgesia, as well as mechanical hyperalgesia and allodynia underlain by increased excitability of ganglion neurons with lowered threshold currents and action potential voltage thresholds and increased incidence of repetitive discharges [62,63]. Both hyperalgesia and allodynia on the one hand and associated electrophysiological changes on the other hand could be prevented/reversed by NMDA receptor antagonists, indicating their mediation through spinal glutamatergic neurotransmission [62].

14.3.1.3 Drug- and Virus-Induced Neuropathic Pain

Diabetes-Inducing Drugs The modelization of diabetes-induced neuropathy is generally made by injection of streptozotocin (STZ) [64,65] or alloxan [66] in rats and mice. These two agents that destroy β-cells in the pancreas produce an insulin-dependent diabetes mellitus with marked hyperglycemia.

A single injection of alloxan (40–120 mg/kg i.p.) induces thermal hyperalgesia associated with reduced analgesic efficacy of morphine compared with naïve rats [67,68]. Injection of STZ at the single dose of 70 mg/kg s.c. or 75 mg/kg i.p. induces not only mechanical and thermal hyperalgesia but also sensitization to chemical stimuli and hyperresponsiveness of C fibers, which persist for at least 4 weeks [65,69]. The major problem of this model is that rats also develop physical debility with weight loss, hypolocomotion, and major metabolic disorders, which complicate data interpretation in studies specifically dedicated to pain. However, much less secondary effects seem to occur when STZ is injected intravenously (50 mg/kg). This route of injection should therefore be preferred especially because hyperalgesia and allodynia are as pronounced but occur earlier than after i.p. or s.c. administration of STZ [70].

As a matter of fact, similarities of these rodent models with the human pathology extend beyond chronic peripheral pain since they also include increased vascular permeability and inflammation, vulnerability to nerve ischemia, decrease in nerve conduction velocity, loss of motor and sensory fibers, axonal shrinkage, and demyelination [65]. In addition, extensive pharmacological studies showed that alloxan- or STZ-induced neuropathic-like pain, as assessed by the measurement of hyperalgesia and allodynia with validated tests, responds to antidepressants, in particular tricyclics, dual inhibitors of norepinephrine and serotonin reuptake such as paroxetine, duloxetine, venlafaxine, and milnacipran [65,71], and anticonvulsants such as gabapentin and pregabalin [72], but is relatively resistant to opioidergic analgesics, like that observed in diabetic patients suffering from neuropathic pain.

Antiretroviral Drugs and HIV-Related Pain In animal models aimed at studying HIV-induced neuropathy, the glycoprotein gp120, which is a major component of the HIV envelope, is injected directly onto the sciatic nerve [73–75], intrathecally [76], or into the plantar paw [73]. In rodents, these administration modes induce neuropathic pain with mechanical allodynia and thermal hyperalgesia, which persist from hours (intrathecally) to weeks (onto the sciatic nerve).

On the other hand, the potency of antiretroviral drugs to induce neuropathic pain has been demonstrated through their administration using intravenous or intraperitoneal route [77,78]. In those cases, pain, which can last for at least 3 weeks, develops rapidly after a single administration of these drugs. Thus, van Steenwinckel et al. [79] showed that thermal allodynia as well as mechanical hyperalgesia and allodynia are already striking 4 days after a single i.v. injection of 2′,3′-dideoxycytidine in rats. Interestingly, similar neuropathic-like pain symptoms develop after systemic administration of this drug in wild-type mice but not in knockout mutants deficient in the 5-HT$_{2A}$ subtype of serotonin receptors, suggesting that this receptor, whose activation contributes to facilitate NMDA receptor-mediated glutamatergic neurotransmission, plays a permissive role in 2′,3′-dideoxycytidine-induced neuropathic pain [79]. Furthermore, there is evidence that this antiretroviral drug produces marked alterations in mitochondrial functions in DRG neurons, but not in spinal neurons, thereby supporting the inference that neuropathic pain really results from injury to the peripheral nervous system [79].

Rather than administering antiretroviral drugs alone in healthy rodents, a treatment more relevant to the clinics consists of the combined administration of gp120 (to mimic HIV-induced neuropathy), directly to the sciatic nerve, and 2′,3′-dideoxycytidine, via a systemic (intraperitoneal) route. A clear-cut exacerbated neuropathic pain that markedly exceeds those produced by each treatment alone has been evidenced in rats after such a combined treatment [80]. Marked alterations in DRG cell phenotypes and microglia activation contribute to neuropathic pain because treatment with the microglial inhibitor, minocycline, has clear-cut efficacy to reduce hypersensitivity to mechanical stimuli by combined gp120/2′,3′-dideoxycytidine treatment. Interestingly, gabapentin and morphine, but not the tricyclic antidepressant amitriptyline, also reduced gp120/2′,3′-dideoxycytidine-induced neuropathic pain [80], indicating a different sensitivity to drugs, compared with diabetes-induced neuropathic pain (see above).

Postherpetic Neuralgia Modelization of herpes-evoked pain in rodents is usually done using the varicella zoster virus itself [81]. Rats are injected subcutaneously with CV-1 cells infected (4×10^6 infected cells; 50 µl) with the varicella zoster virus.

They develop mechanical allodynia and thermal hyperalgesia within 5 days postinfection, and both neuropathic pain-like symptoms last for at least 2 months, together with the presence of active virus in DRG neurons [82].

Another virus of the same Herpesviridae family that has been used for the modelization of postherpetic pain in rodents is the herpes simplex virus type 1 (HSV-1). Injection of the HSV-1 complex (1×10^6 plaque forming units) into the hind paw skin of mice causes not only allodynia and hyperalgesia but also skin lesions as in humans [83]. The pain behaviors start 5 days postinjection and persist for at least 8 days. HSV-induced neuropathic pain has also been reported in rats injected with HSV-1 (10^7 plaque forming units) into glabrous skin [84].

Working on these viruses requires specially dedicated rooms and specific qualifications, which can make these models rather difficult to set up in common laboratories.

Interestingly, acute treatment with resiniferatoxin, an ultrapotent TRPV1 agonist, has been reported to reproduce at least some of the characteristics of postherpetic neuralgia in rats, thereby avoiding the special setups for the use of viruses. A single i.p. injection of resiniferatoxin at the dose of 200 µg/kg induces a reduction in thermal sensitivity but a marked increase in mechanical sensitivity, as shown by profound and persistent tactile allodynia [85]. These changes are associated with a marked loss of unmyelinated fibers and extensive ultrastructural damage of myelinated fibers in the sciatic nerve of resiniferatoxin-treated rats [85]. Furthermore, abnormal sprouting and connections of myelinated primary afferent fibers within the dorsal horn of the spinal cord (notably in lamina II) have been noted, which might also contribute to resiniferatoxin-induced mechanical allodynia. Because both a reduced thermal sensitivity and a profound tactile allodynia also occur in the dermatomes affected by postherpetic neuralgia in patients [86], systemic treatment of resiniferatoxin has been proposed as a model for understanding pathophysiological mechanisms underlying this chronic painful condition [85].

Neuropathic Pain Caused by Anticancer Drugs Several models using the different anticancer treatments have been developed in rodents with the dual aim of understanding underlying pathophysiological mechanisms and setting up appropriate antipain treatments.

Relevant studies have notably been performed with paclitaxel also known as Taxol. This drug induces impairment of myelinated fiber function at the origin of sensory neuropathy mostly characterized by tingling, numbness, mechanical allodynia, cold allodynia, and ongoing spontaneous burning pain [87–89]. Peripheral neuropathy can be induced in rodents by repeated i.p. injections of paclitaxel at the dose of 0.5–1 or 2 mg/kg, four times with 2-day intervals. This protocol induces cold allodynia and long-lasting mechanical allodynia, reproducing the same features as those seen with early usage of paclitaxel in humans [87,88]. When injected daily at the dose of 2 mg/kg for 5 days, rats also develop heat hyperalgesia [89] with the maximum on day 10 after the first injection. Mechanical allodynia usually disappears within 21 days, but cold allodynia still persists even after 4 weeks. Neither systemic toxicity nor motor impairments have been reported in rodents after such treatments.

Higher dosages of paclitaxel, such as those achieved with either 16 mg/kg i.p. of the drug once a week for 5 weeks, two intravenous injections at 18 mg/kg with a 3-day interval, or a single i.p. injection at 32 mg/kg, induce thermal hypoalgesia in addition to the other symptoms already noted in low-dosage models [90,91]. However, systemic toxicity of paclitaxel at high dosages interferes with behavioral tests to assess nociceptive functions, which explains why low dosage is usually preferred in animal studies.

Some studies have also been performed with docetaxel, another anticancer drug of the taxane family. Docetaxel injected i.v. once a week for 5 weeks increases thermal sensitivity and causes degeneration of skin nerves in the foot pad in rats [92].

To date, cisplatin and oxaliplatin are the most commonly used anticancer drugs of the platinum salt family. Repeated administration of low doses of cisplatin (1 mg/kg i.p. once weekly for 9 weeks or 2 mg/kg i.p. twice a week for 5 weeks) in rats induces behavioral, anatomical, and electrophysiological changes similar to those observed in humans treated with this drug. In particular, cisplatin-treated rats exhibit mechanical and cold allodynia as well as thermal heat hyperalgesia [93–95].

Oxaliplatin is less toxic than cisplatin on peripheral organs and functions, but is more toxic on sensory nerves. Neurotoxicity induced by oxaliplatin is reversible and characterized by dysesthesia and paresthesia. Injections of oxaliplatin at 1–4 mg/kg i.p. twice weekly for 4–5 weeks induce mechanical and cold allodynia and hyperalgesia, as well as thermal heat hyperalgesia with no signs of motor dysfunction [96]. To fit better with the clinics in humans, notably for the treatment of the metastatic colorectal cancer, a model that consists of a single administration of oxaliplatin has been developed with different doses: 3, 6, and 12 mg/kg i.p. This treatment induces both mechanical allodynia and hyperalgesia and cold allodynia and hyperalgesia, but no heat hyperalgesia or allodynia [97]. This model essentially replicates the clinical signs seen in humans after a single injection of oxaliplatin, namely, cold allodynia and hyperalgesia.

Another treatment that consists of three injections of oxaliplatin at 10 mg/kg i.p. with 3-day intervals between them was recently developed to induce mechanical and thermal allodynia at both extracephalic and cephalic levels in rats [98]. Data reported using this model further confirmed that neuropathic pain involving trigeminal versus spinal mechanisms has different pathophysiological features and responds differentially to alleviating drugs. In particular, morphine at a low dose (3 mg/kg s.c.) completely reversed oxaliplatin-induced increase in nocifensive responses due to subcutaneous injection of formalin into a hind paw (extracephalic) territory, but was only marginally active against oxaliplatin-induced neuropathic-like pain at cephalic (vibrissal pad) level [98]. No sign of microglial activation could be detected in the spinal cord of oxaliplatin-treated rats, indicating that this neuropathic pain model involves pathophysiological mechanisms distinct from those evoked by physical nerve lesion. Indeed, oxaliplatin does not induce direct axonal lesions, but causes a decrease of the size of somas and nucleus of DRG neurons and atrophy of intraepidermal fibers [99,100]. Thorough examinations of receptor channels of the TRP family also indicated a modest but significant overexpression of TRPA1 in DRG, which very probably contributes to supersensitivity to mechanical, cold, and chemical/inflammatory stimuli in rodents rendered neuropathic by subchronic administration of oxaliplatin [98,101].

In humans, vincristine is used notably to reduce breast cancer and primary brain tumors. It induces neuropathy symptoms, especially paresthesia and thermal hyperalgesia, in all patients [102].

Also in rats, vincristine injected daily at the dose of 75 μg/kg i.v for up to 9 days induces the development of mechanical hyperalgesia and allodynia with maxima on day 11 [103]. An alternative to this treatment consists of five administrations of vincristine at the dose of 150 μg/kg i.v. every other day. This treatment schedule produces mechanical and thermal hyperalgesia and allodynia correlated with electrophysiological alterations and histopathological changes in myelinated nerve fibers without altering motor performance and general physiological status [104]. Neuroanatomical studies clearly showed that vincristine-induced neuropathic pain is not associated with any loss of DRG cells or degeneration of proximal sensory axons. However, vincristine-treated rats show marked alterations in mitochondria, characterized by a swelling and disappearance of cristae in lumbar DRG, like those observed with other neuropathic pain-inducing anticancer drugs such as paclitaxel [105]. A causal relationship could be evidenced between mitochondria alterations and neuropathic pain, notably from data obtained with L-acetylcarnitine, which reverses, at least partially, mitochondrial dysfunction and can prevent and partly reverse chemotherapy-induced neuropathy [106].

14.3.2
Models of Spinal Cord Injury

14.3.2.1 Spinal Cord Contusion

It is the oldest and still the most widely used model of SCI. It consists of the contusion of the spinal cord with an impactor such as a weight drop impactor. Under deep anesthesia, spinal cord is exposed after laminectomy and injured by dropping a rod from a specified height. The resulting lesion induces severe paraplegia underlain by neuronal death and marked neuronal dysfunctions above, at, and below impact levels [107,108]. Because cervical contusion can be life threatening through dramatic consequences on heart or lung functions, contusion is usually made at the thoracic or lumbar level only. Thermal hyperalgesia [109] and mechanical hyperalgesia and allodynia [110] have been described after such spinal cord lesions in rats. However, a large interindividual variability exists in this regard because not all of the rats develop pain behavior. Indeed, unavoidable differences in the extent and location of the spinal cord damage induced by the rod in one rat to another very probably account for this high degree of variability [111].

14.3.2.2 Clip Compression Injury

Under deep anesthesia, rats undergo a laminectomy and a moderate to severe incomplete injury to the spinal cord is made by clip compression (of 35–50 g) of the cord for 1 min, usually at the thoracic level (T13). After such a procedure, rats develop mechanical allodynia and hyperalgesia at, below, and above the site of injury [112,113], as well as thermal heat and cold hyperalgesia below the level of injury [114], which can be reduced by amitriptyline, morphine, and gabapentin, all drugs used for alleviating neuropathic pain in patients with spinal cord injury. These pharmacological data support the idea that this spinal cord injury model in rats meets most of the *face*, *construct*, and *predictive* validities expected for reliable assessment of the potential therapeutic value of innovative drugs aimed at reducing SCI-evoked pain in patients.

14.3.2.3 Spinal Cord Transection

Under deep anesthesia, rats undergo a laminectomy, and the spinal cord is transected usually at the thoracic level (T8–T9). A gel foam is inserted between the two ends in order to reduce bleeding and to make sure that the transection is complete. This model has notably been used to study specifically the central pattern generator at the lumbar level (below the lesion), which controls extensor and flexor muscles involved in locomotor movements of hind limbs [115,116]. In addition, it has allowed thorough investigation of physiopathological mechanisms underlying spasticity and hyperreflexia, which are classical symptoms in paraplegic and tetraplegic patients [117,118]. Regarding pain, nociceptive messages generated below the lesion no longer reach the brain, and this model can be used only for studying above- and at-level neuropathic pain after the transection. Indeed, rats with complete transection of the spinal cord do not develop above-level neuropathic pain, but a strong at-level neuropathic pain is triggered for months with a maximum 4 weeks after the surgery [113,119,120]. Long-lasting mechanical allodynia is particularly pronounced in cutaneous territory around the transection, together with increased neuronal activity in the two to three spinal segments located just rostrally [120]. Although complete lesion of the spinal cord is rather rare after injury in humans, the model of complete transection in rats has some translational relevance because the resulting at-level mechanical allodynia is responsive to drugs (ketamine, baclofen, morphine, and tapentadol) used for alleviating pain in paraplegic and tetraplegic patients.

A variant of this model consists of spinal cord hemisection, which also produces mechanical hyperalgesia along with mechanical and cold allodynia [121,122]. However, it suffers from interindividual variability because of unavoidable variations in the location and extent of lesion from one rat to another.

14.3.2.4 Spinal Cord Ischemia

The technique used for lesioning spinal cord tissues by laser-mediated ischemia is very close to the one already described for the sciatic nerve. The first step also consists of i.v. injection of a photosensitizing dye such as erythrosin B. Then, an argon ion laser beam is directly focused at the vertebrae level. The resulting blood vessel occlusion generates ischemia-induced spinal cord injury [123]. This model has the great advantage of avoiding laminectomy, which allows studies of the effects of spinal cord injury *sensu stricto*, and its intrinsic role in the resulting pain. Mechanical and cold allodynia at level and below the lesion have been regularly reported after such laser-induced spinal cord lesions in rats. Furthermore, evoked mechanical and thermal allodynia are both responsive to drugs that are effective in alleviating neuropathic pain in spinally lesioned patients [123,124], as expected of a relevant model for assessing the potential value of innovative treatments targeting this type of central pain.

14.3.3
Neuropathic-Like Pain Evoked by Chemicals Administered at the Spinal Level

14.3.3.1 Intrathecal Administration of ATP

ATP is abundantly released after neural injury, not only by the damaged cells but also by astrocytes and microglia within the spinal cord. The role and the importance of purinergic signaling in neuropathic pain have been clearly demonstrated [125,126], emphasizing that activation of ATP receptors, especially the ionotropic P2X4 and P2X7 types on activated microglia, is critical for the induction and maintenance of pain through the release of numerous synapse-sensitizing factors and activation of downstream signaling pathways [127,128]. Accordingly, the direct intrathecal injection of ATP itself (30, 100, 300 nmol/10 µl) or of the P2X agonist α-β-Me-ATP (10, 30 nmol/10 µl) induces mechanical allodynia, which persists for 1–3 weeks after acute administration [129]. Thermal hyperalgesia has also been reported after intrathecal injection of α-β-Me-ATP (30 µg/5 µl) as well as 2-methylthio-ATP (3 and 30 µg/5 µl) [130]. Pathophysiological mechanisms downstream of P2X receptor activation involve notably the release of proinflammatory chemokines (CXCL2) and cytokines (IL-1β) like those triggered by neural lesion causing neuropathic pain, in support of the idea that acute intrathecal administration of ATP has some relevance to model neuropathic pain in animals.

14.3.3.2 Intrathecal Administration of BDNF

Whereas BDNF seems to have an analgesic role in midbrain [131], its contribution to neuropathic pain states at the spinal level has been clearly demonstrated in several convergent studies [132]. Accordingly, intrathecal injection of BDNF (50 ng/25 µl) induces long-lasting thermal hyperalgesia and mechanical allodynia in both rats and mice [133]. Recently, Constandil *et al.* [134,135] showed that a single injection of a very low dose of BDNF, 0.003 ng/10 µl, is sufficient to trigger long-lasting mechanical hyperalgesia in the rat. These data further underline that BDNF is a key factor in the induction and maintenance of neuropathic pain after neural lesions [136] and support the idea that direct intrathecal administration of this neurotrophic factor produced by various cell types, especially activated microglia and astrocytes, could be a relevant paradigm to study downstream cellular and molecular mechanisms responsible for nociceptive pathways sensitization underlying neural lesion-induced pain.

14.3.3.3 Excitotoxic Injury to the Spinal Cord

Spinal cord injury can be made by intraspinal injection of excitotoxic agonists of glutamate receptors such as the AMPA-R agonist quisqualic acid, NMDA-R agonists, ibotenic acid or kainic acid. Indeed, SCI produces dramatic increase in extracellular glutamate concentration, up to excitotoxic levels, and the direct intraspinal administration of these agonists in fact triggers pathophysiological mechanisms similar to those resulting from other types of lesion, especially mechanical lesion of the spinal cord [137]. Usually, the reproducibility of lesions induced by direct intraspinal injection of excitotoxic agonists of ionotropic glutamate receptors is higher than that after mechanical injury, which explains why 100% of treated animals (rats and mice) develop long-lasting spontaneous pain, mechanical allodynia, and thermal hyperalgesia [138,139].

Numerous other compounds injected intrathecally, namely, proinflammatory cytokines, substance P, and chemokines, have been reported to trigger neuropathic pain-like symptoms in rodents. Like that found with dynorphin A, which can trigger long-lasting allodynia after a single intrathecal administration in rats [140], underlying mechanisms generally involve sensitization of NMDA receptor-mediated glutamatergic neurotransmission, supporting the idea that glutamatergic synapses, especially within the dorsal horn of the spinal cord, should be considered as a privileged target for the development of effective antineuropathic pain treatments.

14.4
Translation to Clinics: Limitations and Difficulties

Table 14.1 summarizes the main consequences regarding pain of the various mechanical, chemical, or ischemic injuries that have been made at peripheral nerves or at the spinal cord with the aim of developing validated models of neuropathic pain in rodents.

Some of these models closely reproduce human pathologies, notably through the use of the same causal event as that at the origin of neuropathic pain in humans. Thus, neuropathic-like pain evoked by administration of anticancer drugs or diabetes-induced drugs such as alloxan and streptozotocin in rats is generally considered as really reflecting neuropathic pain in humans. Indeed, clear-cut mechanical allodynia and hyperalgesia and thermal hyperalgesia are regularly observed in rats injected with these drugs (Table 14.1), and these symptoms can be significantly reduced by the same therapeutic approaches as those used in humans. Nevertheless, like in humans, only a limited percentage of animals develop hyperalgesia and/or allodynia in spite of perfectly controlled biological parameters, demonstrating that all animals injected with these neuropathic pain-inducing drugs develop the very same pathological features (i.e., the same level of hyperglycemia in streptozotocin-injected rats that develop or do not develop neuropathic-like pain symptoms). To date, no convincing explanation of such interindividual differences has yet been provided, and the use of these models is

Table 14.1 Main hyperalgesia and allodynia symptoms in the various models of neuropathic pain that have been developed in rodents.

Peripheral nerve injury		Mechanical allodynia	Mechanical hyperalgesia	Heat hyperalgesia	Cold hyperalgesia
Sciatic nerve	Nerve section	●	●	●	●
	Chronic constriction injury	●	●	●	●
	Partial ligation of the nerve	●	●	●	●
	Nerve cuffing	●	○	●	●
	Spared nerve injury	●	●	⊗	●
	Nerve cryoneurolysis	●	○	⊗	●
	Laser-induced nerve injury	●	○	●	●
Other neural tissues	Tibial and sural nerve transection	●	○	○	●
	Common peroneal nerve injury	●	○	●	●
	Spinal nerve ligation	●	●	●	●
	Dorsal rhizotomy	●	○	○	●
	Injury to dorsal root ganglia	●	●	●	⊗
	Chronic constriction injury to the infraorbital nerve	●	○	●	●

Drug- and virus-induced neuropathic pain		Mechanical allodynia	Mechanical hyperalgesia	Heat hyperalgesia	Cold hyperalgesia
Diabetes-induced neuropathic pain	Streptozotocin	●	●	●	●
	Alloxan	●	●	●	●
Anticancer-induced neuropathic pain	Paclitaxel	●	●	●	●
	Docetaxel	●	●	●	●
	Cisplatin	●	●	●	●
	Oxaliplatin	●	●	●	●
	Vincristine	●	●	●	●
Antiretroviral and HIV-induced neuropathic pain	Antiretroviral drugs (see text)	●	●	●	○
	gp120	●	●	●	○
Postherpetic neuralgia	Varicella zoster virus	●	○	●	○
	HSV1	●	●	●	○
	Resiniferatoxin	●	○	⊗	○

Spinal cord injuries	Mechanical allodynia	Mechanical hyperalgesia	Heat hyperalgesia	Cold hyperalgesia
Spinal cord contusion	●	●	●	○
Clip compression injury	●	●	●	●
Spinal cord transection	●	○	○	○
Spinal cord hemisection	●	○	●	●
Spinal cord ischemia	●	○	●	●

Chemicals injected directly at the spinal level	Mechanical allodynia	Mechanical hyperalgesia	Heat hyperalgesia	Cold hyperalgesia
ATP	●	○	●	○
BDNF	●	●	●	○
Excitotoxic drugs	●	○	●	○

(●) Extensively characterized symptom; (○) limited data in the literature; (⊗) noninduced symptom.

complicated because it cannot be predicted which rats will effectively develop neuropathic pain among those injected with diabetes-inducing or anticancer drugs.

Another limitation of these drug-induced neuropathic pain models is the fact that pathophysiological mechanisms underlying neuropathic pain differ, at least partly, from those responsible for neuropathic pain generated by trauma-induced nerve injury. In particular, a dramatic microglia activation develops only in the latter models.

As a matter of fact, all these models have allowed considerable progress in the knowledge of molecular and cellular mechanisms underlying allodynia and hyperalgesia generated by peripheral nerve lesion or spinal cord injury. Indeed, intercellular and intracellular signaling pathways responsible for sensitization of neural circuits transmitting pain messages up to cortical areas have been elucidated for their most part, and potential targets for the development of innovative treatments have been identified. Thus, pharmacological inhibition of microglia activation, p38 kinase, and tetrahydrobiopterin synthesis, among many other factors/events, has been shown to effectively reduce neuropathic-like symptoms in validated animal models. To date, however, none of effective compounds issued from preclinical research has led yet to an innovative medical treatment of neuropathic pain in humans.

Clearly, this (hopefully, transient) failure may lead to the conclusion that animal models of neuropathic pain are globally inappropriate for the development of innovative alleviating therapies. Indeed, neuropathic pain is characterized not only by pathophysiological features but also by affective and cognitive dysfunctions (depression is frequently comorbid with neuropathic pain), which are most often not considered in animal studies. Accordingly, focusing only on pathophysiological mechanisms is probably not enough to really model all aspects of neuropathic pain. Recent attempts to set up experimental paradigms aimed at assessing both sensory and emotional/affective/cognitive dysfunctions associated with neuropathic pain [141] may allow major improvements toward the development of innovative treatments for rational, effective, and well-tolerated antineuropathic pain therapies.

References

1 Bonica, J.J. (1990) Evolution and current status of pain programs. *Journal of Pain and Symptom Management*, **5**, 368–374.

2 Daousi, C., MacFarlane, I.A., Woodward, A., Nurmikko, T.J., Bundred, P.E., and Benbow, S.J. (2004) Chronic painful peripheral neuropathy in an urban community: a controlled comparison of people with and without diabetes. *Diabetic Medicine*, **21**, 976–982.

3 Wu, E.Q., Borton, J., Said, G., Le, T.K., Monz, B., Rosilio, M., and Avoinet, S. (2007) Estimated prevalence of peripheral neuropathy and associated pain in adults with diabetes in France. *Current Medical Research and Opinion*, **23**, 2035–2042.

4 Calcutt, N.A. (2002) Potential mechanisms of neuropathic pain in diabetes. *International Review of Neurobiology*, **50**, 205–228.

5 Schifitto, G., McDermott, M.P., McArthur, J.C., Marder, K., Sacktor, N., Epstein, L., and Kieburtz, K. (2002) Incidence of and risk factors for HIV-associated distal sensory polyneuropathy. *Neurology*, **58**, 1764–1768.

6 Finnerup, N.B., Otto, M., McQuay, H.J., Jensen, T.S., and Sindrup, S.H. (2005) Algorithm for neuropathic pain treatment: an evidence based proposal. *Pain*, **118**, 289–305.

7 Smith, H. (2011) Treatment considerations in painful HIV-related neuropathy. *Pain Physician*, **14**, E505–E524.

8 Martin, C., Solders, G., Sonnerborg, A., and Hansson, P. (2000) Antiretroviral therapy may improve sensory function in HIV-infected patients: a pilot study. *Neurology*, **54**, 2120–2127.

9 Williams, D., Geraci, A., and Simpson, D.M. (2001) AIDS and AIDS-treatment neuropathies. *Current Neurology and Neuroscience Reports*, **1**, 533–538.

10 Cherry, C.L., McArthur, J.C., Hoy, J.F., and Wesselingh, S.L. (2003) Nucleoside analogues and neuropathy in the era of HAART. *Journal of Clinical Virology*, **26**, 195–207.

11 Hope-Simpson, R.E. (1965) The nature of herpes zoster: a long-term study and a new hypothesis. *Proceedings of the Royal Society of Medicine*, **58**, 9–20.

12 Dworkin, R.H. and Portenoy, R.K. (1996) Pain and its persistence in herpes zoster. *Pain*, **67**, 241–251.

13 Farquhar-Smith, P. (2011) Chemotherapy-induced neuropathic pain. *Current Opinion in Supportive and Palliative Care*, **5**, 1–7.

14 Bryce, T.N., Biering-Sørensen, F., Finnerup, N.B., Cardenas, D.D., Defrin, R., Lundeberg, T., Norrbrink, C., Richards, J.S., Siddall, P., Stripling, T., Treede, R., Waxman, S.G., Widerström-Noga, E., Yezierski, R.P., and Dijkers, M. (2012) International spinal cord injury pain classification: part I. Background and description. *Spinal Cord*, **50**, 413–417.

15 Baastrup, C. and Finnerup, N.B. (2008) Pharmacological management of neuropathic pain following spinal cord injury. *CNS Drugs*, **22**, 455–475.

16 Attal, N., Cruccu, G., Baron, R., Haanpaa, M., Hansson, P., Jensen, T.S., and Nurmikko, T. (2010) EFNS guidelines on the pharmacological treatment of neuropathic pain: 2010 revision. *European Journal of Neurology*, **17**, 1113–e1188.

17 Kirshblum, S.C., Burns, S.P., Biering-Sorensen, F., Donovan, W., Graves, D.E., Jha, A., Johansen, M., Jones, L., Krassioukov, A., Mulcahey, M.J., Schmidt-Read, M., and Waring, W. (2011) International standards for neurological classification of spinal cord injury (revised 2011). *Journal of Spinal Cord Medicine*, **34**, 535–546.

18 Cardenas, D.D., Turner, J.A., Warms, C.A., and Marshall, H.M. (2002) Classification of chronic pain associated with spinal cord injuries. *Archives of Physical Medicine and Rehabilitation*, **83**, 1708–1714.

19 Siddall, P.J., McClelland, J.M., Rutkowski, S.B., and Cousins, M.J. (2003) A longitudinal study of the prevalence and characteristics of pain in the first 5 years following spinal cord injury. *Pain*, **103**, 249–257.

20 Wall, P.D., Devor, M., Inbal, R., Scadding, J.W., Schonfeld, D., Seltzer, Z., and Tomkiewicz, M.M. (1979) Autotomy following peripheral nerve lesions:

experimental anaesthesia dolorosa. *Pain*, **7**, 103–111.

21 Antunes Bras, J.M., Laporte, A.M., Benoliel, J.J., Bourgoin, S., Mauborgne, A., Hamon, M., Cesselin, F., and Pohl, M. (1999) Effects of peripheral axotomy on cholecystokinin neurotransmission in the rat spinal cord. *Journal of Neurochemistry*, **72**, 858–867.

22 Blumenkopf, B. and Lipman, J.J. (1991) Studies in autotomy: its pathophysiology and usefulness as a model of chronic pain. *Pain*, **45**, 203–209.

23 Kauppila, T. (1998) Correlation between autotomy-behavior and current theories of neuropathic pain. *Neuroscience and Biobehavioral Reviews*, **23**, 111–129.

24 Riopelle, J.M. (1992) The ethics of using animal models to study treatment of phantom pain. *Anesthesiology*, **76**, 1069–1071.

25 Lee, B.H., Won, R., Baik, E.J., Lee, S.H., and Moon, C.H. (2000) An animal model of neuropathic pain employing injury to the sciatic nerve branches. *Neuroreport*, **11**, 657–661.

26 Bennett, G.J. and Xie, Y.K. (1988) A peripheral mononeuropathy in rat that produces disorders of pain sensation like those seen in man. *Pain*, **33**, 87–107.

27 Muthuraman, A., Jaggi, A.S., Singh, N., and Singh, D. (2008) Ameliorative effects of amiloride and pralidoxime in chronic constriction injury and vincristine induced painful neuropathy in rats. *European Journal of Pharmacology*, **587**, 104–111.

28 Maves, T.J., Pechman, P.S., Gebhart, G.F., and Meller, S.T. (1993) Possible chemical contribution from chromic gut sutures produces disorders of pain sensation like those seen in man. *Pain*, **54**, 57–69.

29 Latrémolière, A., Mauborgne, A., Masson, J., Bourgoin, S., Kayser, V., Hamon, M., and Pohl, M. (2008) Differential implication of proinflammatory cytokine interleukin-6 in the development of cephalic versus extracephalic neuropathic pain in rats. *The Journal of Neuroscience*, **28**, 8489–8501.

30 Vierck, C.J., Acosta-Rua, A.J., and Johnson, R.D. (2005) Bilateral chronic constriction of the sciatic nerve: a model of long-term cold hyperalgesia. *Journal of Pain*, **6**, 507–517.

31 Hutchinson, M.R., Zhang, Y., Brown, K., Coats, B.D., Shridhar, M., Sholar, P.W., Patel, S.J., Crysdale, N.Y., Harrison, J.A., Maier, S.F., Rice, K.C., and Watkins, L.R. (2008) Non-stereoselective reversal of neuropathic pain by naloxone and naltrexone: involvement of toll-like receptor 4 (TLR4). *The European Journal of Neuroscience*, **28**, 20–29.

32 Mogil, J.S., Graham, A.C., Ritchie, J., Hughes, S.F., Austin, J.S., Schorscher-Petcu, A., Langford, D.J., and Bennett, G.J. (2010) Hypolocomotion, asymmetrically directed behaviors (licking, lifting, flinching, and shaking) and dynamic weight bearing (gait) changes are not measures of neuropathic pain in mice. *Molecular Pain*, **6**, 34.

33 Imamura, Y. and Bennett, G.J. (1995) Felbamate relieves several abnormal pain sensations in rats with an experimental peripheral neuropathy. *The Journal of Pharmacology and Experimental Therapeutics*, **275**, 177–182.

34 Ro, L.S. and Jacobs, J.M. (1993) The role of the saphenous nerve in experimental sciatic nerve mononeuropathy produced by loose ligatures: a behavioural study. *Pain*, **52**, 359–369.

35 Seltzer, Z., Dubner, R., and Shir, Y. (1990) A novel behavioral model of neuropathic pain disorders produced in rats by partial sciatic nerve injury. *Pain*, **43**, 205–218.

36 Dowdall, T., Robinson, I., and Meert, T.F. (2005) Comparison of five different rat models of peripheral nerve injury. *Pharmacology, Biochemistry, and Behavior*, **80**, 93–108.

37 Yi, H., Kim, M.A., Back, S.K., Eun, J.S., and Na, H.S. (2011) A novel rat forelimb model of neuropathic pain produced by partial injury of the median and ulnar nerves. *European Journal of Pain*, **15**, 459–466.

38 Pitcher, G.M., Ritchie, J., and Henry, J.L. (1999) Nerve constriction in the rat: model of neuropathic, surgical and central pain. *Pain*, **83**, 37–46.

39 Benbouzid, M., Choucair-Jaafar, N., Yalcin, I., Waltisperger, E., Muller, A., Freund-Mercier, M.J., and Barrot, M. (2008)

Chronic, but not acute, tricyclic antidepressant treatment alleviates neuropathic allodynia after sciatic nerve cuffing in mice. *European Journal of Pain*, **12**, 1008–1017.

40 Benbouzid, M., Pallage, V., Rajalu, M., Waltisperger, E., Doridot, S., Poisbeau, P., Freund-Mercier, M.J., and Barrot, M. (2008) Sciatic nerve cuffing in mice: a model of sustained neuropathic pain. *European Journal of Pain*, **12**, 591–599.

41 Barrot, M. (2012) Tests and models of nociception and pain in rodents. *Neuroscience*, **211**, 39–50.

42 Decosterd, I. and Woolf, C.J. (2000) Spared nerve injury: an animal model of persistent peripheral neuropathic pain. *Pain*, **87**, 149–158.

43 Bourquin, A.F., Süveges, M., Pertin, M., Gilliard, N., Sardy, S., Davison, A.C., Spahn, D.R., and Decosterd, I. (2006) Assessment and analysis of mechanical allodynia-like behavior induced by spared nerve injury (SNI) in the mouse. *Pain*, **122** (14), e1–e14.

44 Gazelius, B., Cui, J.G., Svensson, M., Meyerson, B., and Linderoth, B. (1996) Photochemically induced ischaemic lesion of the rat sciatic nerve. A novel method providing high incidence of mononeuropathy. *Neuroreport*, **7**, 2619–2623.

45 Hao, J.X., Xu, I.S., Xu, X.J., and Wiesenfeld-Hallin, Z. (1999) Effects of intrathecal morphine, clonidine and baclofen on allodynia after partial sciatic nerve injury in the rat. *Acta Anaesthesiologica Scandinavica*, **43**, 1027–1034.

46 Kupers, R., Yu, W., Persson, J.K., Xu, X.J., and Wiesenfeld-Hallin, Z. (1998) Photochemically-induced ischemia of the rat sciatic nerve produces a dose-dependent and highly reproducible mechanical, heat and cold allodynia, and signs of spontaneous pain. *Pain*, **76**, 45–59.

47 Chiang, H.Y., Chen, C.T., Chien, H.F., and Hsieh, S.T. (2005) Skin denervation, neuropathology, and neuropathic pain in a laser-induced focal neuropathy. *Neurobiology of Disease*, **18**, 40–53.

48 Willenbring, S., Beauprie, I.G., and DeLeo, J.A. (1995) Sciatic cryoneurolysis in rats: a model of sympathetically independent pain. Part 1: effects of sympathectomy. *Anesthesia and Analgesia*, **81**, 544–548.

49 Vadakkan, K.I., Jia, Y.H., and Zhuo, M. (2005) A behavioral model of neuropathic pain induced by ligation of the common peroneal nerve in mice. *Journal of Pain*, **6**, 747–756.

50 Vos, B.P., Strassman, A.M., and Maciewicz, R.J. (1994) Behavioral evidence of trigeminal neuropathic pain following chronic constriction injury to the rat's infraorbital nerve. *The Journal of Neuroscience*, **14**, 2708–2723.

51 Kryzhanovskii, G.N., Dolgikh, V.G., Gorizontova, M.P., and Mironova, I.V. (1993) The formation of a pathological system in rats with neuropathic trigeminal neuralgia. *Bulletin of Experimental Biology and Medicine*, **115**, 567–569.

52 Imamura, Y., Kawamoto, H., and Nakanishi, O. (1997) Characterization of heat-hyperalgesia in an experimental trigeminal neuropathy in rats. *Experimental Brain Research*, **116**, 97–103.

53 Idanpaan-Heikkila, J.J. and Guilbaud, G. (1999) Pharmacological studies on a rat model of trigeminal neuropathic pain: baclofen, but not carbamazepine, morphine or tricyclic antidepressants, attenuates the allodynia-like behaviour. *Pain*, **79**, 281–290.

54 Kayser, V., Aubel, B., Hamon, M., and Bourgoin, S. (2002) The antimigraine 5-HT$_{1B/1D}$ receptor agonists, sumatriptan, zolmitriptan and dihydroergotamine, attenuate pain-related behaviour in a rat model of trigeminal neuropathic pain. *British Journal of Pharmacology*, **137**, 1287–1297.

55 Lombard, M.C., Nashold, B.S., Jr., Albe-Fessard, D., Salman, N., and Sakr, C. (1979) Deafferentation hypersensitivity in the rat after dorsal rhizotomy: a possible animal model of chronic pain. *Pain*, **6**, 163–174.

56 Ramer, L.M., Borisoff, J.F., and Ramer, M.S. (2004) Rho-kinase inhibition enhances axonal plasticity and attenuates cold hyperalgesia after dorsal rhizotomy. *The Journal of Neuroscience*, **24**, 10796–10805.

57 Bruxelle, J., Travers, V., and Thiebaut, J.B. (1988) Occurrence and treatment of pain

after brachial plexus injury. *Clinical Orthopaedics and Related Research*, **237**, 87–95.

58 Kim, S.H. and Chung, J.M. (1992) An experimental model for peripheral neuropathy produced by segmental spinal nerve ligation in the rat. *Pain*, **50**, 355–363.

59 Choi, Y., Yoon, Y.W., Na, H.S., Kim, S.H., and Chung, J.M. (1994) Behavioral signs of ongoing pain and cold allodynia in a rat model of neuropathic pain. *Pain*, **59**, 369–376.

60 LaBuda, C.J. and Little, P.J. (2005) Pharmacological evaluation of the selective spinal nerve ligation model of neuropathic pain in the rat. *Journal of Neuroscience Methods*, **144**, 175–181.

61 Liu, B., Li, H., Brull, S.J., and Zhang, J.M. (2002) Increased sensitivity of sensory neurons to tumor necrosis factor alpha in rats with chronic compression of the lumbar ganglia. *Journal of Neurophysiology*, **88**, 1393–1399.

62 Song, X.J., Vizcarra, C., Xu, D.S., Rupert, R.L., and Wong, Z.N. (2003) Hyperalgesia and neural excitability following injuries to central and peripheral branches of axons and somata of dorsal root ganglion neurons. *Journal of Neurophysiology*, **89**, 2185–2193.

63 Zhang, J.M., Song, X.J., and LaMotte, R.H. (1999) Enhanced excitability of sensory neurons in rats with cutaneous hyperalgesia produced by chronic compression of the dorsal root ganglion. *Journal of Neurophysiology*, **82**, 3359–3366.

64 Courteix, C., Eschalier, A., and Lavarenne, J. (1993) Streptozocin-induced diabetic rats: behavioural evidence for a model of chronic pain. *Pain*, **53**, 81–88.

65 Aubel, B., Kayser, V., Mauborgne, A., Farré, A., Hamon, M., and Bourgoin, S. (2004) Antihyperalgesic effects of cizolirtine in diabetic rats: behavioral and biochemical studies. *Pain*, **110**, 22–32.

66 Lee, J.H., Cox, D.J., Mook, D.G., and McCarty, R.C. (1990) Effect of hyperglycemia on pain threshold in alloxan-diabetic rats. *Pain*, **40**, 105–107.

67 Ibironke, G.F. and Saba, O.J. (2006) Effect of hyperglycemia on the efficacy of morphine analgesia in rats. *African Journal of Medicine and Medical Sciences*, **35**, 443–445.

68 Ahmadi, S., Ebrahimi, S.S., Oryan, S., and Rafieenia, F. (2012) Blockades of ATP-sensitive potassium channels and L-type calcium channels improve analgesic effect of morphine in alloxan-induced diabetic mice. *Pathophysiology*, **19**, 171–177.

69 Chen, X. and Levine, J.D. (2003) Altered temporal pattern of mechanically evoked C-fiber activity in a model of diabetic neuropathy in the rat. *Neuroscience*, **121**, 1007–1015.

70 Aley, K.O. and Levine, J.D. (2001) Rapid onset pain induced by intravenous streptozotocin in the rat. *Journal of Pain*, **2**, 146–150.

71 Wattiez, A.S., Libert, F., Privat, A.M., Loiodice, S., Fialip, J., Eschalier, A., and Courteix, C. (2011) Evidence for a differential opioidergic involvement in the analgesic effect of antidepressants: prediction for efficacy in animal models of neuropathic pain? *British Journal of Pharmacology*, **163**, 792–803.

72 Field, M.J., McCleary, S., Hughes, J., and Singh, L. (1999) Gabapentin and pregabalin, but not morphine and amitriptyline, block both static and dynamic components of mechanical allodynia induced by streptozocin in the rat. *Pain*, **80**, 391–398.

73 Jolivalt, C.G., Dacunha, J.M., Esch, F.S., and Calcutt, N.A. (2008) Central action of prosaptide TX14(A) against gp120-induced allodynia in rats. *European Journal of Pain*, **12**, 76–81.

74 Bhangoo, S.K., Ripsch, M.S., Buchanan, D.J., Miller, R.J., and White, F.A. (2009) Increased chemokine signaling in a model of HIV1-associated peripheral neuropathy. *Molecular Pain*, **5**, 48.

75 Maratou, K., Wallace, V.C., Hasnie, F.S., Okuse, K., Hosseini, R., Jina, N., Blackbeard, J., Pheby, T., Orengo, C., Dickenson, A.H., McMahon, S.B., and Rice, A.S. (2009) Comparison of dorsal root ganglion gene expression in rat models of traumatic and HIV-associated neuropathic pain. *European Journal of Pain*, **13**, 387–398.

76 Milligan, E.D., O'Connor, K.A., Nguyen, K.T., Armstrong, C.B., Twining, C.,

Gaykema, R.P., Holguin, A., Martin, D., Maier, S.F., and Watkins, L.R. (2001) Intrathecal HIV-1 envelope glycoprotein gp120 induces enhanced pain states mediated by spinal cord proinflammatory cytokines. *The Journal of Neuroscience*, **21**, 2808–2819.

77 Joseph, E.K., Chen, X., Khasar, S.G., and Levine, J.D. (2004) Novel mechanism of enhanced nociception in a model of AIDS therapy-induced painful peripheral neuropathy in the rat. *Pain*, **107**, 147–158.

78 Huang, W., Calvo, M., Karu, K., Olausen, H.R., Bathgate, G., Okuse, K., Bennett, D.L., and Rice, A.S. (2013) A clinically relevant rodent model of the HIV antiretroviral drug stavudine induced painful peripheral neuropathy. *Pain*, **154**, 560–575.

79 Van Steenwinckel, J., Brisorgueil, M.J., Fischer, J., Vergé, D., Gingrich, J.A., Bourgoin, S., Hamon, M., Bernard, R., and Conrath, M. (2008) Role of spinal serotonin 5-HT$_{2A}$ receptor in 2′,3′-dideoxycytidine-induced neuropathic pain in the rat and the mouse. *Pain*, **137**, 66–80.

80 Wallace, V.C., Blackbeard, J., Segerdahl, A.R., Hasnie, F., Pheby, T., McMahon, S.B., and Rice, A.S. (2007) Characterization of rodent models of HIV-gp120 and anti-retroviral-associated neuropathic pain. *Brain*, **130**, 2688–2702.

81 Fleetwood-Walker, S.M., Quinn, J.P., Wallace, C., Blackburn-Munro, G., Kelly, B.G., Fiskerstrand, C.E., Nash, A.A., and Dalziel, R.G. (1999) Behavioural changes in the rat following infection with varicella-zoster virus. *The Journal of General Virology*, **80**, 2433–2436.

82 Zhang, G.H., Lv, M.M., Wang, S., Chen, L., Qian, N.S., Tang, Y., Zhang, X.D., Ren, P.C., Gao, C.J., Sun, X.D., and Xu, L.X. (2011) Spinal astrocytic activation is involved in a virally-induced rat model of neuropathic pain. *PLoS One*, **6**, e23059.

83 Takasaki, I., Andoh, T., Shiraki, K., and Kuraishi, Y. (2000) Allodynia and hyperalgesia induced by herpes simplex virus type-1 infection in mice. *Pain*, **86**, 95–101.

84 Dalziel, R.G., Bingham, S., Sutton, D., Grant, D., Champion, J.M., Dennis, S.A., Quinn, J.P., Bountra, C., and Mark, M.A. (2004) Allodynia in rats infected with varicella zoster virus: a small animal model for post-herpetic neuralgia. *Brain Research. Brain Research Reviews*, **46**, 234–242.

85 Pan, H.L., Khan, G.M., Alloway, K.D., and Chen, S.R. (2003) Resiniferatoxin induces paradoxical changes in thermal and mechanical sensitivities in rats: mechanism of action. *The Journal of Neuroscience*, **23**, 2911–2919.

86 Baron, R. and Saguer, M. (1993) Postherpetic neuralgia. Are C-nociceptors involved in signalling and maintenance of tactile allodynia? *Brain*, **116**, 1477–1496.

87 Polomano, R.C., Mannes, A.J., Clark, U.S., and Bennett, G.J. (2001) A painful peripheral neuropathy in the rat produced by the chemotherapeutic drug, paclitaxel. *Pain*, **94**, 293–304.

88 Flatters, S.J. and Bennett, G.J. (2006) Studies of peripheral sensory nerves in paclitaxel-induced painful peripheral neuropathy: evidence for mitochondrial dysfunction. *Pain*, **122**, 245–257.

89 Nieto, F.R., Entrena, J.M., Cendan, C.M., Pozo, E.D., Vela, J.M., and Baeyens, J.M. (2008) Tetrodotoxin inhibits the development and expression of neuropathic pain induced by paclitaxel in mice. *Pain*, **137**, 520–531.

90 Authier, N., Gillet, J.P., Fialip, J., Eschalier, A., and Coudore, F. (2000) Description of a short-term Taxol-induced nociceptive neuropathy in rats. *Brain Research*, **887**, 239–249.

91 Kilpatrick, T.J., Phan, S., Reardon, K., Lopes, E.C., and Cheema, S.S. (2001) Leukaemia inhibitory factor abrogates Paclitaxel-induced axonal atrophy in the Wistar rat. *Brain Research*, **911**, 163–167.

92 Roglio, I., Bianchi, R., Camozzi, F., Carozzi, V., Cervellini, I., Crippa, D., Lauria, G., Cavaletti, G., and Melcangi, R.C. (2009) Docetaxel-induced peripheral neuropathy: protective effects of dihydroprogesterone and progesterone in an experimental model. *Journal of the Peripheral Nervous System*, **14**, 36–44.

93 Cavaletti, G., Tredici, G., Marmiroli, P., Petruccioli, M.G., Barajon, I., and Fabbrica, D. (1992) Morphometric study of the sensory neuron and peripheral nerve changes induced by chronic cisplatin

(DDP) administration in rats. *Acta Neuropathologica*, **84**, 364–371.

94 Authier, N., Gillet, J.P., Fialip, J., Eschalier, A., and Coudore, F. (2003) An animal model of nociceptive peripheral neuropathy following repeated cisplatin injections. *Experimental Neurology*, **182**, 12–20.

95 Vera, G., Chiarlone, A., Cabezos, P.A., Pascual, D., Martin, M.I., and Abalo, R. (2007) WIN 55,212-2 prevents mechanical allodynia but not alterations in feeding behaviour induced by chronic cisplatin in the rat. *Life Sciences*, **81**, 468–479.

96 Ling, B., Authier, N., Balayssac, D., Eschalier, A., and Coudore, F. (2007) Behavioral and pharmacological description of oxaliplatin-induced painful neuropathy in rat. *Pain*, **128**, 225–234.

97 Ling, B., Coudoré-Civiale, M.A., Balayssac, D., Eschalier, A., Coudoré, F., and Authier, N. (2007) Behavioral and immunohistological assessment of painful neuropathy induced by a single oxaliplatin injection in the rat. *Toxicology*, **234**, 176–184.

98 Michot, B., Bourgoin, S., Kayser, V., and Hamon, M. (2013) Effects of tapentadol on mechanical hypersensitivity in rats with ligatures of the infraorbital nerve versus the sciatic nerve. *European Journal of Pain*, **17**, 867–880.

99 Jamieson, S.M., Liu, J., Connor, B., and McKeage, M.J. (2005) Oxaliplatin causes selective atrophy of a subpopulation of dorsal root ganglion neurons without inducing cell loss. *Cancer Chemotherapy and Pharmacology*, **56**, 391–399.

100 Meyer, L., Patte-Mensah, C., Taleb, O., and Mensah-Nyagan, A.G. (2011) Allopregnanolone prevents and suppresses oxaliplatin-evoked painful neuropathy: multi-parametric assessment and direct evidence. *Pain*, **152**, 170–181.

101 Descoeur, J., Pereira, V., Pizzocarro, A., François, A., Ling, B., Maffre, V., Couette, B., Brusserolles, J., Courteix, C., Noël, J., Lazdunski, M., Eschalier, A., Authier, N., and Bourinet, E. (2011) Oxaliplatin-induced cold hypersensitivity is due to remodeling of ion channel expression in nociceptors. *EMBO Molecular Medicine*, **3**, 266–278.

102 Pal, P.K. (1999) Clinical and electrophysiological studies in vincristine induced neuropathy. *Electromyography and Clinical Neurophysiology*, **39**, 323–330.

103 Sweitzer, S.M., Pahl, J.L., and DeLeo, J.A. (2006) Propentofylline attenuates vincristine-induced peripheral neuropathy in the rat. *Neuroscience Letters*, **400**, 258–261.

104 Authier, N., Gillet, J.P., Fialip, J., Eschalier, A., and Coudore, F. (2003) A new animal model of vincristine-induced nociceptive peripheral neuropathy. *Neurotoxicology*, **24**, 797–805.

105 Thibault, K., Van Steenwinckel, J., Brisorgueil, M.J., Fischer, J., Hamon, M., Calvino, B., and Conrath, M. (2008) Serotonin 5-HT$_{2A}$ receptor involvement and Fos expression at the spinal level in vincristine-induced neuropathy in the rat. *Pain*, **140**, 305–322.

106 Xiao, W.H. and Bennett, G.J. (2008) Chemotherapy-evoked neuropathic pain: abnormal spontaneous discharge in A-fiber and C-fiber primary afferent neurons and its suppression by acetylcarnitine. *Pain*, **135**, 262–270.

107 Hulsebosch, C.E., Xu, G.Y., Perez-Polo, J.R., Westlund, K.N., Taylor, C.P., and McAdoo, D.J. (2000) Rodent model of chronic central pain after spinal cord contusion injury and effects of gabapentin. *Journal of Neurotrauma*, **17**, 1205–1217.

108 Nakae, A., Nakai, K., Yano, K., Hosokawa, K., Shibata, M., and Mashimo, T. (2011) The animal model of spinal cord injury as an experimental pain model. *Journal of Biomedicine & Biotechnology*, **2011**, 939023.

109 Hoschouer, E.L., Yin, F.Q., and Jakeman, L.B. (2009) L1 cell adhesion molecule is essential for the maintenance of hyperalgesia after spinal cord injury. *Experimental Neurology*, **216**, 22–34.

110 Kerr, B.J. and David, S. (2007) Pain behaviors after spinal cord contusion injury in two commonly used mouse strains. *Experimental Neurology*, **206**, 240–247.

111 Basso, D.M., Beattie, M.S., and Bresnahan, J.C. (1996) Graded histological and locomotor outcomes after spinal cord contusion using the NYU weight-drop device versus transection. *Experimental Neurology*, **139**, 244–256.

112 Bruce, J.C., Oatway, M.A., and Weaver, L.C. (2002) Chronic pain after clip-compression injury of the rat spinal cord. *Experimental Neurology*, **178**, 33–48.

113 Densmore, V.S., Kalous, A., Keast, J.R., and Osborne, P.B. (2010) Above-level mechanical hyperalgesia in rats develops after incomplete spinal cord injury but not after cord transection, and is reversed by amitriptyline, morphine and gabapentin. *Pain*, **151**, 184–193.

114 Hama, A. and Sagen, J. (2007) Behavioral characterization and effect of clinical drugs in a rat model of pain following spinal cord compression. *Brain Research*, **1185**, 117–128.

115 Antri, M., Mouffle, C., Orsal, D., and Barthe, J.Y. (2003) 5-HT$_{1A}$ receptors are involved in short- and long-term processes responsible for 5-HT-induced locomotor function recovery in chronic spinal rat. *The European Journal of Neuroscience*, **18**, 1963–1972.

116 Antri, M., Barthe, J.Y., Mouffle, C., and Orsal, D. (2005) Long-lasting recovery of locomotor function in chronic spinal rat following chronic combined pharmacological stimulation of serotonergic receptors with 8-OH-DPAT and quipazine. *Neuroscience Letters*, **384**, 162–167.

117 Boulenguez, P., Liabeuf, S., Bos, R., Bras, H., Jean-Xavier, C., Brocard, C., Stil, A., Darbon, P., Cattaert, D., Delpire, E., Marsala, M., and Vinay, L. (2010) Down-regulation of the potassium-chloride cotransporter KCC2 contributes to spasticity after spinal cord injury. *Nature Medicine*, **16**, 302–307.

118 Yates, C., Garrison, K., Reese, N.B., Charlesworth, A., and Garcia-Rill, E. (2011) Novel mechanism for hyperreflexia and spasticity. *Progress in Brain Research*, **188**, 167–180.

119 Scheifer, C., Hoheisel, U., Trudrung, P., Unger, T., and Mense, S. (2002) Rats with chronic spinal cord transection as a possible model for the at-level pain of paraplegic patients. *Neuroscience Letters*, **323**, 117–120.

120 Hoheisel, U., Scheifer, C., Trudrung, P., Unger, T., and Mense, S. (2003) Pathophysiological activity in rat dorsal horn neurones in segments rostral to a chronic spinal cord injury. *Brain Research*, **974**, 134–145.

121 Hains, B.C., Johnson, K.M., Eaton, M.J., Willis, W.D., and Hulsebosch, C.E. (2003) Serotonergic neural precursor cell grafts attenuate bilateral hyperexcitability of dorsal horn neurons after spinal hemisection in rat. *Neuroscience*, **116**, 1097–1110.

122 Kim, J., Kim, J.H., Kim, Y., Cho, H.Y., Hong, S.K., and Yoon, Y.W. (2009) Role of spinal cholecystokinin in neuropathic pain after spinal cord hemisection in rats. *Neuroscience Letters*, **462**, 303–307.

123 Watson, B.D., Prado, R., Dietrich, W.D., Ginsberg, M.D., and Green, B.A. (1986) Photochemically induced spinal cord injury in the rat. *Brain Research*, **367**, 296–300.

124 Hao, J.X., Stohr, T., Selve, N., Wiesenfeld-Hallin, Z., and Xu, X.J. (2006) Lacosamide, a new anti-epileptic, alleviates neuropathic pain-like behaviors in rat models of spinal cord or trigeminal nerve injury. *European Journal of Pharmacology*, **553**, 135–140.

125 Burnstock, G. (2009) Purinergic receptors and pain. *Current Pharmaceutical Design*, **15**, 1717–1735.

126 Inoue, K. and Tsuda, M. (2012) Purinergic systems, neuropathic pain and the role of microglia. *Experimental Neurology*, **234**, 293–301.

127 Tsuda, M., Shigemoto-Mogami, Y., Koizumi, S., Mizokoshi, A., Kohsaka, S., Salter, M.W., and Inoue, K. (2003) P2X4 receptors induced in spinal microglia gate tactile allodynia after nerve injury. *Nature*, **424**, 778–783.

128 Honore, P., Donnelly-Roberts, D., Namovic, M.T., Hsieh, G., Zhu, C.Z., Mikusa, J.P., Hernandez, G., Zhong, C., Gauvin, D.M., Chandran, P., Harris, R., Medrano, A.P., Carroll, W., Marsh, K., Sullivan, J.P., Faltynek, C.R., and Jarvis, M.F. (2006) A-740003 [*N*-(1-{[(cyanoimino)(5-quinolinylamino) methyl]amino}-2,2-dimethylpropyl)-2-(3,4-dimethoxyphenyl) acetamide], a novel and selective P2X7 receptor antagonist, dose-dependently reduces neuropathic pain in the rat. *The Journal of Pharmacology and Experimental Therapeutics*, **319**, 1376–1385.

129 Nakagawa, T., Wakamatsu, K., Zhang, N., Maeda, S., Minami, M., Satoh, M., and Kaneko, S. (2007) Intrathecal administration of ATP produces long-lasting allodynia in rats: differential mechanisms in the phase of the induction and maintenance. *Neuroscience*, **147**, 445–455.

130 Tsuda, M., Ueno, S., and Inoue, K. (1999) Evidence for the involvement of spinal endogenous ATP and P2X receptors in nociceptive responses caused by formalin and capsaicin in mice. *British Journal of Pharmacology*, **128**, 1497–1504.

131 Siuciak, J.A., Altar, C.A., Wiegand, S.J., and Lindsay, R.M. (1994) Antinociceptive effect of brain-derived neurotrophic factor and neurotrophin-3. *Brain Research*, **633**, 326–330.

132 Trang, T., Beggs, S., and Salter, M.W. (2011) Brain-derived neurotrophic factor from microglia: a molecular substrate for neuropathic pain. *Neuron Glia Biology*, **7**, 99–108.

133 Zhang, X., Xu, Y., Wang, J., Zhou, Q., Pu, S., Jiang, W., and Du, D. (2012) The effect of intrathecal administration of glial activation inhibitors on dorsal horn BDNF overexpression and hind paw mechanical allodynia in spinal nerve ligated rats. *Journal of Neural Transmission*, **119**, 329–336.

134 Constandil, L., Aguilera, R., Goich, M., Hernandez, A., Alvarez, P., Infante, C., and Pelissier, T. (2011) Involvement of spinal cord BDNF in the generation and maintenance of chronic neuropathic pain in rats. *Brain Research Bulletin*, **86**, 454–459.

135 Constandil, L., Goich, M., Hernàndez, A., Bourgeais, L., Cazorla, M., Hamon, M., Villanueva, L., and Pelissier, T. (2012) Cyclotraxin-B, a new TrkB antagonist, and glial blockade by propentofylline, equally prevent and reverse cold allodynia induced by BDNF or partial infraorbital nerve constriction in mice. *Journal of Pain*, **13**, 579–589.

136 Wang, X., Ratnam, J., Zou, B., England, P.M., and Basbaum, A.I. (2009) TrkB signaling is required for both the induction and maintenance of tissue and nerve injury-induced persistent pain. *The Journal of Neuroscience*, **29**, 5508–5515.

137 Liu, D., Thangnipon, W., and McAdoo, D.J. (1991) Excitatory amino acids rise to toxic levels upon impact injury to the rat spinal cord. *Brain Research*, **547**, 344–348.

138 Fairbanks, C.A., Schreiber, K.L., Brewer, K.L., Yu, C.G., Stone, L.S., Kitto, K.F., Nguyen, H.O., Grocholski, B.M., Shoeman, D.W., Kehl, L.J., Regunathan, S., Reis, D.J., Yezierski, R.P., and Wilcox, G.L. (2000) Agmatine reverses pain induced by inflammation, neuropathy, and spinal cord injury. *Proceedings of the National Academy of Sciences of the United States of America*, **97**, 10584–10589.

139 Yezierski, R.P., Liu, S., Ruenes, G.L., Kajander, K.J., and Brewer, K.L. (1998) Excitotoxic spinal cord injury: behavioral and morphological characteristics of a central pain model. *Pain*, **75**, 141–155.

140 Vanderah, T.W., Laughlin, T., Lashbrook, J.M., Nichols, M.L., Wilcox, G.L., Ossipov, M.H., Malan, T.P., and Porreca, F. (1996) Single intrathecal injections of dynorphin A or *des*-Tyr-dynorphins produce long-lasting allodynia in rats: blockade by MK-801 but not naloxone. *Pain*, **68**, 275–281.

141 Navratilova, E., Xie, J.Y., King, T., and Porreca, F. (2013) Evaluation of reward from pain relief. *Annals of the New York Academy of Sciences*, **1282**, 1–11.

15
Obesity and Metabolic Syndrome
Sunil K. Panchal, Maharshi Bhaswant, and Lindsay Brown

15.1
Introduction

Animals have contributed significantly to the understanding of human biochemistry, physiology, pathophysiology, and pharmacology. Different models have been developed, characterized, and then successfully used for the development of preventive measures or cures for human diseases. One of the important human conditions is metabolic syndrome, and this can be successfully mimicked in rodents. We have already described the major characteristics of the most common rodent models used in metabolic syndrome research [1]. Here, we will revisit the important animal models for metabolic syndrome research and then discuss the limited translatability of these models to human trials.

15.2
Why Metabolic Syndrome?

Metabolic syndrome is the cluster of metabolic complications such as obesity, dyslipidemia, impaired glucose tolerance, and insulin resistance together with hypertension [2,3] influenced by environmental factors, including lifestyle and diet [4–6]. Different organizations have specified different requirements for classifying patients under the definition of metabolic syndrome [7–11]. These requirements have been summarized in Table 15.1. Many complications are not included in the definition of metabolic syndrome, such as fatty liver, oxidative stress, inflammation, and endothelial dysfunction, but these are frequently found in patients with metabolic syndrome [2,4]. The prevalence of metabolic syndrome has reached a level where it is considered a worldwide health problem. Table 15.2 summarizes the prevalence of metabolic syndrome in different countries according to the different definitions.

The high prevalence of metabolic syndrome makes it extremely important to find effective treatments or prevention. Hence, we need to understand the mechanisms associated with the development of metabolic syndrome in rodents,

Table 15.1 Definitions of metabolic syndrome.

	WHO (1998) [7]	EGIR (1999) [8]	NCEP ATP III (2005 revision) [9]	IDF (2005) [10]	Harmonized definition (2009) [11]
Compulsory	Insulin resistance	Hyperinsulinemia	None	Central obesity	None
Requirements	Insulin resistance or diabetes, plus any two of the five criteria	Hyperinsulinemia, plus any two of the four criteria	Any three of the five criteria	Central obesity, plus any two of the four criteria	Any three of the five criteria
Central obesity	Waist:hip ratio (>0.90 in males, >0.85 in females) or BMI ≥30 kg/m²	Waist circumference (≥94 cm in males, ≥80 cm in females)	Waist circumference (>102 cm in males, >88 in females)	Waist circumference (≥94 cm in males, ≥80 cm in females)	Population- and country-specific definitions
Hyperglycemia	Impaired glucose regulation, type 2 diabetes or insulin resistance	Hyperinsulinemia; fasting plasma glucose ≥6.1 mmol/l	Fasting glucose ≥100 mg/dl	Fasting glucose ≥100 mg/dl or previously diagnosed type 2 diabetes	Fasting glucose ≥100 mg/dl
Dyslipidemia (triglycerides)	Triglycerides ≥150 mg/dl or HDL-cholesterol (<35 mg/dl in males, <39 mg/dl in females)	Triglycerides ≥180 mg/dl or HDL-cholesterol <40 mg/dl or treated for dyslipidemia	Triglycerides ≥150 mg/dl or treated for dyslipidemia	Triglycerides ≥150 mg/dl or treated for dyslipidemia	Triglycerides ≥150 mg/dl or treated for dyslipidemia
Dyslipidemia (cholesterol)			HDL-cholesterol (<40 mg/dl in males, <50 mg/dl in females)	HDL-cholesterol (<40 mg/dl in males, <50 mg/dl in females) or treated for dyslipidemia	HDL-cholesterol (<40 mg/dl in males, <50 mg/dl in females) or treated for reduced HDL-cholesterol
Hypertension	≥160/90 mmHg	≥140/90 mmHg	>130/85 mmHg or treated for hypertension	>130/85 mmHg or treated for hypertension	≥130/85 mmHg or treated for hypertension
Other criteria	Microalbuminuria (urinary albumin excretion ≥20 μg/min or albumin:creatinine ratio ≥20 mg/g)				

WHO: World Health Organization; EGIR: European Group for the Study of Insulin Resistance; NCEP ATP III: National Cholesterol Education Program Adult Treatment Panel III; IDF: International Diabetes Federation; BMI: body mass index; HDL: high-density lipoprotein.

Table 15.2 Prevalence of metabolic syndrome.

Country of survey	Definition used	Year of survey	Age group	Prevalence
Johannesburg metropolitan area, South Africa [12]	Harmonized definition [11]	Started in 1990		29% in African population; 46% in Asian Indian population
Australia [13]	NCEP ATP III	2004–2005	25–74 years	27.1% in men; 28.3% in women
	IDF			33.7% in men; 30.1% in women
Kuwait [14]	IDF	2006	20–65 years	36.2%
	NCEP			24.8%
Australia [15]	ATP III	1999–2000	≥25 years	22.1%
	WHO			21.7%
	IDF			30.7%
	EGIR			13.4%
India [16]	NCEP ATP III	2010–2011	≥30 years	29% in women; 23% in men; overall 25.6%
Taiwan [17]	WHO	—	19–95 years	18.5% in men; 14.7% in women
USA [18]	NCEP	1999–2002	≥20 years	33.7% in men; 35.4% in women; 34.5% overall
	IDF			39.9% in men; 38.1% in women; 39% overall
USA [19]	NCEP ATP III	2003–2006	≥20 years	35.1% in men; 32.6% in women; 34% overall
Spain [20]	Revised NCEP ATP III	2001–2003	≥20 years	28.2% in men; 26.3% in women; overall 27.2%
	IDF			36.9% in men; 28.1% in women; overall 32.2%
	Harmonized definition			38.9% in men; 28.4% in women; overall 33.2%

WHO: World Health Organization; EGIR: European Group for the Study of Insulin Resistance; NCEP ATP III: National Cholesterol Education Program Adult Treatment Panel III; IDF: International Diabetes Federation.

the pathophysiological similarities and differences between humans and rodent models, and finally the translatability of results from rodent models to humans.

15.3
Classical Animal Models of Obesity and Metabolic Syndrome

Many animal models have been used in metabolic syndrome research to mimic the human conditions. These animal models have been consistently used to identify both the roles of various regulators in the body that may be responsible for the development of metabolic syndrome in humans and some of the treatment strategies against metabolic syndrome [1,21,22]. Review articles have identified the usefulness of these animal models; however, few models reproduce the range of changes that metabolic syndrome produces throughout the human body [1,21,23–31]. The animal models currently used include the genetic models that develop metabolic syndrome spontaneously, genetically modified models to induce metabolic syndrome, and the models in which the metabolic syndrome is induced using specialized diets.

15.3.1
Genetic Models of Obesity and Diabetes

Genetic models of obesity and diabetes include *db/db* mice, *ob/ob* mice, Zucker diabetic fatty rats, Otsuka Long–Evans Tokushima Fatty rats, and Goto–Kakizaki rats. These models are primarily useful in identifying treatments for metabolic syndrome consequent to genetic defects. However, the models also induce other pathological conditions associated with metabolic syndrome in humans [1].

ob/ob mice have a mutation in the leptin gene, being important since leptin controls energy intake and expenditure. These leptin-deficient mice become obese at a very early age. Obesity accompanies hyperinsulinemia, hyperglycemia, impaired glucose tolerance, and nonalcoholic fatty liver disease [1,32]. However, they do not develop hypertension or dyslipidemia [1]. *db/db* mice and Zucker diabetic fatty rats have a mutation in the gene for leptin receptor, impairing leptin signaling [33,34]. Similar to *ob/ob* mice, *db/db* mice and Zucker diabetic fatty rats show signs of early-life obesity, hyperinsulinemia, hyperglycemia, and cardiovascular complications along with dyslipidemia [1,34]. However, they fail to develop hypertension [1]. These three models suggest the importance of leptin in the control of metabolism in the body and also the role of leptin or leptin-signaling defects in the development of metabolic syndrome.

Otsuka Long–Evans Tokushima Fatty rats have decreased cholecystokinin-1 receptor density. Cholecystokinin is a peptide hormone secreted from L-cells of the intestine that regulates digestion and food intake. These rats show progression of obesity with increasing age, correlated with higher food intake due to deficiency of cholecystokinin-1 receptor. These rats also show dyslipidemia, hyperglycemia, impaired glucose tolerance, and insulin resistance along with hypertension and cardiovascular complications [1]. Goto–Kakizaki rats are nonobese and spontaneously diabetic. These rats develop hyperglycemia at a very early age; they also show cardiac hypertrophy and systolic dysfunction along with signs of kidney damage at later stages of life. The other symptoms of metabolic syndrome observed in this model are impaired glucose tolerance, dyslipidemia, insulin resistance, and hyperinsulinemia, but hypertension is not observed [1,35]. A relatively new inbred model for obesity has been identified at the National Institute of Nutrition, Hyderabad, India [36]. Both males and females from this strain show similar responses. This strain (WNIN/Ob) develops obesity, probably through hyperphagia, at a very early stage of life and hyperglycemia and hyperinsulinemia by 28 days of age. They have lower lean mass and much higher fat mass compared with their lean littermates along with dyslipidemia. These rats show hyperleptinemia probably with no change in leptin and leptin receptor locus. A defect on chromosome 5 near leptin receptor locus has been suggested as the cause of obesity [36,37,38].

Although these rodent models provide a reasonably reproducible pathological condition, they do not mimic the actual pathophysiology in humans as the occurrence of genetic defects in either leptin or cholecystokinin receptors leading to metabolic syndrome, obesity, and diabetes is quite rare [1,39].

15.3.2
Artificially Induced Metabolic Syndrome in Animals

Metabolic syndrome can be artificially induced in experimental animals, usually mice, through genetic engineering where a particular gene of interest is knocked out or made nonfunctional. These genetic models define the role of a particular protein or receptor in the pathophysiology of metabolic syndrome. For example, GLUT-4, IRS-1, IRS-2, and insulin receptor knockout mice have been studied [40–44]. These genetically engineered models do not mimic the human condition of metabolic syndrome, but they can provide useful information about a particular protein, its receptor, and the intracellular pathways involved in the regulation of metabolism [1].

A commonly used strategy to induce metabolic syndrome in animals, especially rodents, is the use of hypercaloric diets. We argued that the diet-induced models best mimic the human conditions as they share similar mechanisms in the development of metabolic syndrome [1]. The diets used to induce metabolic syndrome include fructose, sucrose, and animal and plant fats. Different research groups have characterized different combinations of these components in different species and strains of rodents. Some examples of the combinations of diets include high-carbohydrate diets (either fructose or sucrose as carbohydrate), high-fat diets (either animal or plant fats), and a combination of high-carbohydrate and high-fat diets [1]. These diets differ in the contribution of carbohydrate and fat to available calories and the sources of fat. Basically, the aim of these studies is to provide excess energy from diet, which is the major cause of human metabolic syndrome and obesity [27]. Most of the diet-induced models show symptoms of metabolic syndrome, including central obesity, dyslipidemia, impaired glucose tolerance, insulin resistance, and hypertension along with cardiovascular complications as well as nonalcoholic fatty liver disease [1].

We argued that a combination of simple sugars and animal fat serves as the best model to mimic metabolic syndrome in rodents [1]. This type of diet mimics the Western/cafeteria diet that is rich in fructose, sucrose, and animal fat. Also, the prevalence of metabolic syndrome is very high in developed countries (Table 15.2). This may directly reflect the role of high-carbohydrate, high-fat diets in the development of metabolic syndrome. Based on this assumption, we have characterized an animal model with complex diet composition, including fructose, condensed milk, and beef tallow, which induced a range of complications that are generally found in metabolic syndrome patients [45]. These complications include hyperinsulinemia, impaired glucose tolerance, central obesity, nonalcoholic fatty liver disease, cardiac remodeling, hypertension, and endothelial dysfunction along with mild renal damage and increased pancreatic islet mass [45]. The high-carbohydrate, high-fat diet mimics the full range of metabolic syndrome changes occurring in either vegetarian or nonvegetarian populations, depending on the source of the increased fats. However, the complexity and variability of the human diet cannot be mimicked by a fixed rodent diet on a day-to-day basis. An advantage of the rat model is the shortened time period to develop the syndrome of months rather than years or decades as in humans. We have also used this model to test natural products for the attenuation of metabolic syndrome [46–48]. The different responses shown by these interventions clearly suggest that this model is capable of responding to the pharmacological interventions.

15.3.2.1 Monosodium Glutamate-Induced Obesity

Monosodium glutamate given by subcutaneous injection induces obesity in mice and rats [49–51] together with impaired glucose tolerance, dyslipidemia, liver dysfunction, and hyperinsulinemia [50]. Monosodium glutamate in rats and mice did not affect body weight when it was given in diet (up to 20% of diet) or in drinking water (2%) [52]. It has been argued that monosodium glutamate does not reflect human obesity in rats and mice [52,53] since in humans monosodium glutamate is taken in foods and not as an injection. Thus, results with injected monosodium glutamate in mice and rats cannot be extrapolated to oral ingestion in humans.

15.3.2.2 Intrauterine Growth-Restricted Rats

This is also a very recently developed model based on Barker *et al.* hypothesis [54]. The rat model was developed through bilateral ligation of uterine artery to reduce the blood flow to the fetus [55]. At birth, rats showed lower insulin concentrations and body weight compared with control rats. After 7 weeks of age, fasting blood glucose and insulin concentrations were higher in these rats than controls. After 15 weeks of age, the growth-restricted rats showed lower insulin with higher fasting blood glucose concentrations than their normal controls. By 26 weeks of age, rats showed obesity and very high fasting blood glucose concentrations, a characteristic of type 2 diabetes [55,56]. A similar model has been developed by restricting the diet of the pregnant mothers [57].

Although there are differences between the physiology of humans, rats, and mice, appropriate animal models can provide an excellent initial point to study either the causes or the treatment strategies for metabolic syndrome. This provides the basic understanding of the intervention strategy before going into human trials. At this point, *in vitro* assays may help provide more information on the possible effects of the proposed intervention.

Table 15.3 Treatments used in humans against metabolic syndrome.

Subject	Study type and model	Study duration	Treatment and dose	Exclusion criteria	Effects
19 females; 11 males (18–75 years of age) [58]	Randomized, double-blind, two-arm, parallel group, placebo-controlled; in type 2 diabetes patients	2 weeks	5 µg exenatide (first week); 10 µg exenatide (second week)	Clinically important medical conditions or had used sulfonylureas, meglitinides, α-glucosidase inhibitors, pramlintide, exogenous insulin, or weight loss drugs within the prior 2 months; fasting triglycerides >4.5 mmol/l, >1 episode of severe hypoglycemia within 6 months, treatment with corticosteroids within 2 months, treatment with an investigational drug within 30 days, or current treatment with drugs known to affect gastrointestinal motility	Lowered postprandial increases in plasma glucose and triglycerides no change in free fatty acids
24 females; 5 males (18–30 years age) [59]	Randomized crossover; obese subjects (BMI ≥30)	Two study visits; at least 7 days apart	Cereal prepared with 6 g ground cassia cinnamon during study visit	Allergy to wheat, cinnamon, and sucralose; pregnancy; type 1 or type 2 diabetes	Lowered postprandial glucose
875 patients (55–80 years age); normal (n = 282); overweight (n = 405); obese (n = 150); severely obese (n = 38) [60]	Essential hypertension: double-blind treatment with losartan compared with atenolol	LIFE trial: cardiovascular death/fatal or nonfatal myocardial infection/stroke as endpoint	Losartan and atenolol	Underweight (BMI < 18.5 kg/m^2)	Shift from concentric to eccentric hypertrophy in both the treatment groups; higher cardiovascular mortality despite antihypertensive treatment in obese subjects

(continued)

Table 15.3 (Continued)

Subject	Study type and model	Study duration	Treatment and dose	Exclusion criteria	Effects
7447 subjects (57% females); (55–80 years age) [61]	PREDIMED trial; parallel group, multicenter, randomized; type 2 diabetes or any three of following: smoking, hypertension, higher LDL-c, lower HDL-c, obesity, family history of coronary heart disease	Primary endpoints: myocardial infarction, stroke and death from cardiovascular causes; secondary endpoints: stroke, myocardial infarction, death from cardiovascular causes, and death from any cause	Mediterranean diet with extravirgin olive oil (1 l/week) or Mediterranean diet with nuts (30 g/day)	—	Mediterranean diet without energy restriction reduces the risk of major cardiovascular events among high-risk persons
35 males (mean age: 53.8 ± 5.8 years) [62]	Mild hypercholesterolemia	18 weeks (6 weeks treatment followed by 6 weeks gap followed by 6 week treatment)	Chokeberry juice, 250 ml/day	No earlier pharmacological treatment	Decreased serum triglycerides, serum total/LDL-c, improved endothelial function,
42 males; 54 females (25–65 years age); BMI 25–35 kg/m² [63]	Double-blind, randomized, placebo controlled crossover trial; central obesity and high serum triglycerides	6 weeks treatment followed by 5 weeks washout	Quercetin, 150 mg/day	Smoking; insulin-dependent diabetes mellitus; liver, gastrointestinal, or inflammatory diseases; a history of cardiovascular events; abnormal thyroid function; use of antiobesity medications, dietary supplements, or anti-inflammatory drugs; cancer; recent major surgery or illness; pregnancy or breastfeeding; alcohol abuse; participation in a current weight loss program; necessity for a medically supervised diet; >5 kg weight loss within the 3 months prior to the study	apoE3 genotype- decreased blood pressure, serum TNFα, no change in serum total cholesterol, triglyceride, glucose; apoE4 genotype- reduction in HDL, serum TNFα, no change in serum total cholesterol, triglyceride, glucose, no change in blood pressure

30 males; 12 females (18–75 years age) [64]	Randomized, double-blind crossover trial; blood pressure: systolic 140–170 mmHg and diastolic 90–105 mmHg	4 weeks	Potassium bicarbonate or potassium chloride (potassium, 6.4 mmol/day)	Impaired renal function, secondary cause of hypertension, chronic diarrhea, history of ulcer disease, previous stroke, ischemic heart disease, heart failure, diabetes mellitus, malignancy, liver disease, pregnancy or breastfeeding, oral contraceptive pills	Improved endothelial function, reduced cardiovascular risk factors; potassium bicarbonate – improved calcium and bone metabolism
338 males; 352 females (25–64 years age) [66]	Randomized control trial	6 months	Increase in consumption of fruits and vegetables	Cardiovascular disease other than hypertension, gastrointestinal disease, cancer, serious psychiatric disorders, hypercholesterolemia, and recent traumatic events	Reduction in systolic and diastolic blood pressure by 4 and 1.5 mmHg, respectively
4 males; 44 females (mean age: 50 ± 3 years) [66]	Randomized controlled study	8 weeks	Freeze-dried blueberries, 50 g/day	<21 years age; taking medications for hypoglycemic, hypolipidemic, anti-inflammatory, or steroidal medications; liver, renal, or thyroid disorders; anemia; consuming antioxidants or fish oil supplements regularly; smokers; consuming alcohol regularly; pregnant or lactating females	Decrease in blood pressure; decreased LDL and lipid peroxidation; trend toward decrease in body weight

(continued)

Table 15.3 (Continued)

Subject	Study type and model	Study duration	Treatment and dose	Exclusion criteria	Effects
289 subjects; males (45–74 years age); females (55–74 years age) [67]	Randomized, double-blind, parallel trial; carotid intima–media thickness (0.7–2.0 mm on at least one side)	18 months	Pomegranate juice, 240 ml/day	Coronary heart disease, diabetes, BMI >40 kg/m², hepatic disease, cancer in previous 2 years, HIV, hepatitis B or C, uncontrolled hypertension, untreated or unstable hypothyroidism	Rate of carotid intima-media thickness progression was slowed
45 subjects (69–80 years age) [68]	Randomized, placebo-controlled, double-blinded study	3 months	Pomegranate juice, 240 ml/day	History of stroke or transient ischemic attack; myocardial infarction during the preceding 6 weeks; surgically untreated left main coronary artery lesion with >50% diameter narrowing; coronary revascularization procedure during the preceding 6 months; current unstable angina pectoris; abnormal lung uptake on previous scintigram or positron emission tomogram; class IV congestive heart failure; or ejection fraction <30% at time of study entry; significant comorbidity; current use of tobacco products; or alcohol or drug abuse	Decreased myocardial ischemia and improved myocardial perfusion; no negative effects on lipids, blood glucose, hemoglobin A1c, body weight or blood pressure

| 28 males; 28 females (30–60 years age) [69] | Randomized double-blind, placebo-controlled parallel trial; BMI ≥30 kg/m²; stable hypertension with systolic <160 mmHg and diastolic <100 mmHg for 6 months | 3 months | 379 mg green tea extract (including 208 mg of epigallocatechin-3-gallate) | Secondary hypertension and/or secondary obesity; diabetes; history of coronary artery disease; stroke congestive heart failure; malignancy; history of use of any dietary supplements within 3 months before the study; current need for modification of antihypertensive therapy; abnormal liver, kidney, or thyroid gland function; clinically significant inflammatory process within respiratory, digestive or genitourinary tract, or in the oral cavity, pharynx or paranasal sinuses; history of infection in the month before the study; nicotine or alcohol abuse | Decreased blood pressure, total plasma cholesterol, triglycerides and LDL-c with increase in HDL-c; decreased inflammatory markers like TNFα and C-reactive protein; improved insulin resistance |

15.4
Human Experimental Models

Human trials are essential in the development of drug therapies. New compounds are first identified in animal studies as potential human treatments. Experimental parameters such as dosage, dietary composition, and exercise can be controlled in animal studies, but are much more difficult to control in outpatient studies in humans. Table 15.3 describes some of the human trials for interventions against the symptoms of metabolic syndrome.

15.5
Translation to Clinics: Difficulties and Limitations

Translation of results from rodent studies to human trials remains a problem. For example, quercetin attenuated the symptoms of metabolic syndrome in rodent models [70,71]. It is one of the most commonly found flavonoids in the human diet, although prevalence of metabolic syndrome is increasing in the community. Two well-studied compounds against metabolic syndrome are curcumin and resveratrol, with an immense literature available for these compounds *in vitro* and *in vivo* [72–74]. However, the successful translation of these interventions to humans has not yet been reported.

Relevant human doses have been estimated from rodent doses [75,76], but these doses assume high oral bioavailability for compounds given in the food while drug metabolism may vary between rats and humans. Furthermore, the food matrix is a well-known variable affecting absorption of food components. The length of dosing is important, with the average life span of laboratory rats of ∼2 years being much less than the average human life span of 75–80 years in many countries. Thus, 8-week interventions in rats are ∼6-year interventions in humans, based on life span. Longer interventional studies in humans, at higher doses, may be necessary to show therapeutic benefits. This may impose safety issues in the use of new interventions in humans.

References

1 Panchal, S.K. and Brown, L. (2011) Rodent models for metabolic syndrome research. *Journal of Biomedicine & Biotechnology*, **2011**, 351982.

2 Kassi, E., Pervanidou, P., Kaltsas, G., and Chrousos, G. (2011) Metabolic syndrome: definitions and controversies. *BMC Medicine*, **9**, 48.

3 Kahn, R., Buse, J., Ferrannini, E., and Stern, M. (2005) The metabolic syndrome: time for a critical appraisal: joint statement from the American Diabetes Association and the European Association for the Study of Diabetes. *Diabetes Care*, **28**, 2289–2304.

4 Johnson, R.J., Stenvinkel, P., Martin, S.L., Jani, A., Sánchez-Lozada, L.G., Hill, J.O., and Lanaspa, M.A. (2012) Redefining metabolic syndrome as a fat storage condition based on studies of comparative physiology. *Obesity (Silver Spring)*, **21**, 659–664.

5 Cordain, L., Eaton, S.B., Sebastian, A., Mann, N., Lindeberg, S., Watkins, B.A., O'Keefe, J.H., and Brand-Miller, J. (2005)

Origins and evolution of the Western diet: health implications for the 21st century. *The American Journal of Clinical Nutrition*, **81**, 341–354.

6 Esmaillzadeh, A., Kimiagar, M., Mehrabi, Y., Azadbakht, L., Hu, F.B., and Willett, W.C. (2007) Dietary patterns, insulin resistance, and prevalence of the metabolic syndrome in women. *The American Journal of Clinical Nutrition*, **85**, 910–918.

7 Alberti, K.G. and Zimmet, P.Z. (1998) Definition, diagnosis and classification of diabetes mellitus and its complications. Part 1: diagnosis and classification of diabetes mellitus provisional report of a WHO consultation. *Diabetic Medicine*, **15**, 539–553.

8 Balkau, B. and Charles, M.A. (1999) Comment on the provisional report from the WHO consultation. European Group for the Study of Insulin Resistance (EGIR). *Diabetic Medicine*, **16**, 442–443.

9 Grundy, S.M., Cleeman, J.I., Daniels, S.R., Donato, K.A., Eckel, R.H., Franklin, B.A., Gordon, D.J., Krauss, R.M., Savage, P.J. et al. (2005) Diagnosis and management of the metabolic syndrome: an American Heart Association/National Heart, Lung, and Blood Institute Scientific Statement. *Circulation*, **112**, 2735–2752.

10 Reaven, G.M. (2006) The metabolic syndrome: is this diagnosis necessary? *The American Journal of Clinical Nutrition*, **83**, 1237–1247.

11 Alberti, K.G., Eckel, R.H., Grundy, S.M., Zimmet, P.Z., Cleeman, J.I., Donato, K.A., Fruchart, J.C., James, W.P., Loria, C.M. et al. (2009) Harmonizing the metabolic syndrome: a joint interim statement of the International Diabetes Federation Task Force on Epidemiology and Prevention; National Heart, Lung, and Blood Institute; American Heart Association; World Heart Federation; International Atherosclerosis Society; and International Association for the Study of Obesity. *Circulation*, **120**, 1640–1645.

12 George, J.A., Norris, S.A., van Deventer, H.E., and Crowther, N.J. (2013) The association of 25 hydroxyvitamin D and parathyroid hormone with metabolic syndrome in two ethnic groups in South Africa. *PLoS One*, **8**, e61282.

13 Janus, E.D., Laatikainen, T., Dunbar, J.A., Kilkkinen, A., Bunker, S.J., Philpot, B., Tideman, P.A., Tirimacco, R., and Heistaro, S. (2007) Overweight, obesity and metabolic syndrome in rural southeastern Australia. *The Medical Journal of Australia*, **187**, 147–152.

14 Al Rashdan, I. and Al Nesef, Y. (2010) Prevalence of overweight, obesity, and metabolic syndrome among adult Kuwaitis: results from community-based national survey. *Angiology*, **61**, 42–48.

15 Cameron, A.J., Magliano, D.J., Zimmet, P.Z., Welborn, T., and Shaw, J.E. (2007) The metabolic syndrome in Australia: prevalence using four definitions. *Diabetes Research and Clinical Practice*, **77**, 471–478.

16 Beigh, S.H. and Jain, S. (2012) Prevalence of metabolic syndrome and gender differences. *Bioinformation*, **8**, 613–616.

17 Lin, J.D., Chiou, W.K., Weng, H.F., Fang, J.T., and Liu, T.H. (2004) Application of three-dimensional body scanner: observation of prevalence of metabolic syndrome. *Clinical Nutrition*, **23**, 1313–1323.

18 Ford, E.S. (2005) Prevalence of the metabolic syndrome defined by the International Diabetes Federation among adults in the U.S. *Diabetes Care*, **28**, 2745–2749.

19 Irwin, R.B. (2009) Prevalence of metabolic syndrome among adults 20 years of age and over, by sex, age, race and ethnicity, and body mass index: United States, 2003–2006. *National Health Statistics Reports*, **13**, 1–7.

20 Gavrila, D., Salmerón, D., Egea-Caparrós, J.M., Huerta, J.M., Pérez-Martínez, A., Navarro, C., and Tormo, M.J. (2011) Prevalence of metabolic syndrome in Murcia Region, a southern European Mediterranean area with low cardiovascular risk and high obesity. *BMC Public Health*, **11**, 562.

21 Fellmann, L., Nascimento, A.R., Tibirica, E., and Bousquet, P. (2013) Murine models for pharmacological studies of the metabolic syndrome. *Pharmacology & Therapeutics*, **137**, 331–340.

22 Karimi, I. (2012) Animal models as tools for translational research: focus on atherosclerosis, metabolic syndrome and

22. type-II diabetes mellitus, in *Lipoproteins: Role in Health and Diseases* (eds S. Frank and G. Kostner), InTech.
23. Speakman, J., Hambly, C., Mitchell, S., and Król, E. (2008) The contribution of animal models to the study of obesity. *Laboratory Animals*, **42**, 413–432.
24. Kanasaki, K. and Koya, D. (2011) Biology of obesity: lessons from animal models of obesity. *Journal of Biomedicine & Biotechnology*, **2011**, 197636.
25. Lutz, T.A. and Woods, S.C. (2012) Overview of animal models of obesity. *Current Protocols in Pharmacology*, 58:5.61.1–5.61.18.
26. Bagnol, D., Al-Shamma, H.A., Behan, D., Whelan, K., and Grottick, A.J. (2012) Diet-induced models of obesity (DIO) in rodents. *Current Protocols in Neuroscience*, 59:9.38.1–9.38.13.
27. Nilsson, C., Raun, K., Yan, F.F., Larsen, M.O., and Tang-Christensen, M. (2012) Laboratory animals as surrogate models of human obesity. *Acta Pharmacologica Sinica*, **33**, 173–181.
28. Wang, C.Y. and Liao, J.K. (2012) A mouse model of diet-induced obesity and insulin resistance. *Methods in Molecular Biology*, **821**, 421–433.
29. Angelova, P. and Boyadjie, N. (2013) A review of the models of obesity and metabolic syndrome in rat. *Trakia Journal of Sciences*, **11**, 5–12.
30. Guerre-Millo, M. (2013) Animal models of obesity, in *Physiology and Physiopathology of Adipose Tissue* (eds J.P. Bastard and B. Fève), Springer, Paris, pp. 255–266.
31. Segal-Lieberman, G. and Rosenthal, T. (2013) Animal models in obesity and hypertension. *Current Hypertension Reports*, **15**, 190–195.
32. Perfield, J.W. II, Ortinau, L.C., Pickering, R.T., Ruebel, M.L., Meers, G.M., and Rector, R.S. (2013) Altered hepatic lipid metabolism contributes to nonalcoholic fatty liver disease in leptin-deficient *ob/ob* mice. *Journal of Obesity*, **2013**, 296537.
33. Belke, D.D. and Severson, D.L. (2012) Diabetes in mice with monogenic obesity: the *db/db* mouse and its use in the study of cardiac consequences. *Methods in Molecular Biology*, **933**, 47–57.
34. Shiota, M. and Printz, R.L. (2012) Diabetes in Zucker diabetic fatty rat. *Methods in Molecular Biology*, **933**, 103–123.
35. Portha, B., Giroix, M.H., Tourrel-Cuzin, C., Le-Stunff, H., and Movassat, J. (2012) The GK rat: a prototype for the study of non-overweight type 2 diabetes. *Methods in Molecular Biology*, **933**, 125–159.
36. Harishankar, N., Vajreswari, A., and Giridharan, N.V. (2011) WNIN/GR-Ob: an insulin-resistant obese rat model from inbred WNIN strain. *The Indian Journal of Medical Research*, **134**, 320–329.
37. Prasad Sakamuri, S.S.V., Sukapaka, M., Prathipati, V.K., Nemani, H., Putcha, U.K., Pothana, S., Koppala, S.R., Ponday, L.R.K., Acharya, V. *et al.* (2012) Carbenoxolone treatment ameliorated metabolic syndrome in WNIN/Ob obese rats, but induced severe fat loss and glucose intolerance in lean rats. *PLoS One*, **7**, e50216.
38. Kalashikam, R.R., Battula, K.K., Kirlampalli, V., Friedman, J.M., and Nappanveettil, G. (2013) Obese locus in WNIN/obese rat maps on chromosome 5 upstream of leptin receptor. *PLoS ONE*, **8**, e77679.
39. Dubern, B. and Clement, K. (2012) Leptin and leptin receptor-related monogenic obesity. *Biochimie*, **94**, 2111–2115.
40. Brüning, J.C., Michael, M.D., Winnay, J.N., Hayashi, T., Hörsch, D., Accili, D., Goodyear, L.J., and Kahn, C.R. (1998) A muscle-specific insulin receptor knockout exhibits features of the metabolic syndrome of NIDDM without altering glucose tolerance. *Molecular Cell*, **2**, 559–569.
41. Jackerott, M., Baudry, A., Lamothe, B., Bucchini, D., Jami, J., and Joshi, R.L. (2001) Endocrine pancreas in insulin receptor-deficient mouse pups. *Diabetes*, **50** (Suppl. 1), S146–S149.
42. Kitamura, T., Kahn, C.R., and Accili, D. (2003) Insulin receptor knockout mice. *Annual Review of Physiology*, **65**, 313–332.
43. Shirakami, A., Toyonaga, T., Tsuruzoe, K., Shirotani, T., Matsumoto, K., Yoshizato, K., Kawashima, J., Hirashima, Y., Miyamura, N. *et al.* (2002) Heterozygous knockout of the IRS-1 gene in mice enhances obesity-linked insulin resistance: a possible model for the development of type 2 diabetes. *The Journal of Endocrinology*, **174**, 309–319.

44 Stenbit, A.E., Tsao, T.S., Li, J., Burcelin, R., Geenen, D.L., Factor, S.M., Houseknecht, K., Katz, E.B., and Charron, M.J. (1997) GLUT4 heterozygous knockout mice develop muscle insulin resistance and diabetes. *Nature Medicine*, **3**, 1096–1101.

45 Panchal, S.K., Poudyal, H., Iyer, A., Nazer, R., Alam, M.A., Diwan, V., Kauter, K., Sernia, C., Campbell, F. *et al.* (2011) High-carbohydrate, high-fat diet-induced metabolic syndrome and cardiovascular remodeling in rats. *Journal of Cardiovascular Pharmacology*, **57**, 611–624.

46 Panchal, S.K., Poudyal, H., Waanders, J., and Brown, L. (2012) Coffee extract attenuates changes in cardiovascular and hepatic structure and function without decreasing obesity in high-carbohydrate, high-fat diet-fed male rats. *The Journal of Nutrition*, **142**, 690–697.

47 Panchal, S.K., Wong, W.-Y., Kauter, K., Ward, L.C., and Brown, L. (2012) Caffeine attenuates metabolic syndrome in diet-induced obese rats. *Nutrition*, **28**, 1055–1062.

48 Poudyal, H., Panchal, S.K., Waanders, J., Ward, L., and Brown, L. (2012) Lipid redistribution by α-linolenic acid-rich chia seed inhibits stearoyl-CoA desaturase-1 and induces cardiac and hepatic protection in diet-induced obese rats. *The Journal of Nutritional Biochemistry*, **23**, 153–162.

49 Nascimento, O.V., Boleti, A.P., Yuyama, L.K., and Lima, E.S. (2013) Effects of diet supplementation with Camu-camu (*Myrciaria dubia* HBK McVaugh) fruit in a rat model of diet-induced obesity. *Anais da Academia Brasileira de Ciencias*, **85**, 355–363.

50 Seiva, F.R., Chuffa, L.G., Braga, C.P., Amorim, J.P., and Fernandes, A.A. (2012) Quercetin ameliorates glucose and lipid metabolism and improves antioxidant status in postnatally monosodium glutamate-induced metabolic alterations. *Food and Chemical Toxicology*, **50**, 3556–3561.

51 Bunyan, J., Murrell, E.A., and Shah, P.P. (1976) The induction of obesity in rodents by means of monosodium glutamate. *The British Journal of Nutrition*, **35**, 25–39.

52 Tordoff, M.G., Aleman, T.R., and Murphy, M.C. (2012) No effects of monosodium glutamate consumption on the body weight or composition of adult rats and mice. *Physiology & Behavior*, **107**, 338–345.

53 Wu, X., Xie, C.Y., Yin, Y., and Deng, Z.Y. (2013) The results of some studies involving animal models of obesity induced by monosodium glutamate are not conclusive. *European Journal of Clinical Nutrition*, **67**, 228.

54 Barker, D.J., Hales, C.N., Fall, C.H., Osmond, C., Phipps, K., and Clark, P.M. (1993) Type 2 (non-insulin-dependent) diabetes mellitus, hypertension and hyperlipidaemia (syndrome X): relation to reduced fetal growth. *Diabetologia*, **36**, 62–67.

55 Simmons, R.A., Templeton, L.J., and Gertz, S.J. (2001) Intrauterine growth retardation leads to the development of type 2 diabetes in the rat. *Diabetes*, **50**, 2279–2286.

56 Islam, M.S. and Wilson, R.D. (2012) Experimentally induced rodent models of type 2 diabetes. *Methods in Molecular Biology*, **933**, 161–174.

57 Somm, E., Vauthay, D.M., Guérardel, A., Toulotte, A., Cettour-Rose, P., Klee, P., Meda, P., Aubert, M.L., Hüppi, P.S., and Schwitzgebel, V.M. (2012) Early metabolic defects in dexamethasone-exposed and undernourished intrauterine growth restricted rats. *PLoS One*, **7**, e50131.

58 Schwartz, S.L., Ratner, R.E., Kim, D.D., Qu, Y., Fechner, L.L., Lenox, S.M., and Holcombe, J.H. (2008) Effect of exenatide on 24-hour blood glucose profile compared with placebo in patients with type 2 diabetes: a randomized, double-blind, two-arm, parallel-group, placebo-controlled, 2-week study. *Clinical Therapeutics*, **30**, 858–867.

59 Magistrelli, A. and Chezem, J.C. (2012) Effect of ground cinnamon on postprandial blood glucose concentration in normal-weight and obese adults. *Journal of the Academy of Nutrition and Dietetics*, **112**, 1806–1809.

60 Gerdts, E., de Simone, G., Lund, B.P., Okin, P.M., Wachtell, K., Boman, K., Nieminen, M.S., Dahlöf, B., and Devereux, R.B. (2013) Impact of overweight and obesity on cardiac benefit of antihypertensive treatment. *Nutrition, Metabolism, and Cardiovascular Diseases*, **23**, 122–129.

61 Estruch, R., Ros, E., Salas-Salvadó, J., Covas, M.I., Corella, D., Arós, F., Gómez-Gracia, E., Ruiz-Gutiérrez, V., Fiol, M. et al. (2013) Primary prevention of cardiovascular disease with a Mediterranean diet. *The New England Journal of Medicine*, **368**, 1279–1290.

62 Poreba, R., Skoczynska, A., Gac, P., Poreba, M., Jedrychowska, I., Affelska-Jercha, A., Turczyn, B., Wojakowska, A., Oszmianski, J., and Andrzejak, R. (2009) Drinking of chokeberry juice from the ecological farm Dzieciolowo and distensibility of brachial artery in men with mild hypercholesterolemia. *Annals of Agricultural and Environmental Medicine*, **16**, 305–308.

63 Egert, S., Boesch-Saadatmandi, C., Wolffram, S., Rimbach, G., and Müller, M.J. (2010) Serum lipid and blood pressure responses to quercetin vary in overweight patients by apolipoprotein E genotype. *The Journal of Nutrition*, **140**, 278–284.

64 He, F.J., Marciniak, M., Carney, C., Markandu, N.D., Anand, V., Fraser, W.D., Dalton, R.N., Kaski, J.C., and MacGregor, G.A. (2010) Effects of potassium chloride and potassium bicarbonate on endothelial function, cardiovascular risk factors, and bone turnover in mild hypertensives. *Hypertension*, **55**, 681–688.

65 John, J.H., Ziebland, S., Yudkin, P., Roe, L.S., Neil, H.A., and Oxford Fruit and Vegetable Study Group (2002) Effects of fruit and vegetable consumption on plasma antioxidant concentrations and blood pressure: a randomised controlled trial. *Lancet*, **359**, 1969–1974.

66 Basu, A., Du, M., Leyva, M.J., Sanchez, K., Betts, N.M., Wu, M., Aston, C.E., and Lyons, T.J. (2010) Blueberries decrease cardiovascular risk factors in obese men and women with metabolic syndrome. *The Journal of Nutrition*, **140**, 1582–1587.

67 Davidson, M.H., Maki, K.C., Dicklin, M.R., Feinstein, S.B., Witchger, M., Bell, M., McGuire, D.K., Provost, J.C., Liker, H., and Aviram, M. (2009) Effects of consumption of pomegranate juice on carotid intima-media thickness in men and women at moderate risk for coronary heart disease. *The American Journal of Cardiology*, **104**, 936–942.

68 Sumner, M.D., Elliott-Eller, M., Weidner, G., Daubenmier, J.J., Chew, M.H., Marlin, R., Raisin, C.J., and Ornish, D. (2005) Effects of pomegranate juice consumption on myocardial perfusion in patients with coronary heart disease. *The American Journal of Cardiology*, **96**, 810–814.

69 Bogdanski, P., Suliburska, J., Szulinska, M., Stepien, M., Pupek-Musialik, D., and Jablecka, A. (2012) Green tea extract reduces blood pressure, inflammatory biomarkers, and oxidative stress and improves parameters associated with insulin resistance in obese, hypertensive patients. *Nutrition Research*, **32**, 421–427.

70 Perez-Vizcaino, F., Duarte, J., Jimenez, R., Santos-Buelga, C., and Osuna, A. (2009) Antihypertensive effects of the flavonoid quercetin. *Pharmacological Reports*, **61**, 67–75.

71 Egert, S., Bosy-Westphal, A., Seiberl, J., Kürbitz, C., Settler, U., Plachta-Danielzik, S., Wagner, A.E., Frank, J., Schrezenmeir, J. et al. (2009) Quercetin reduces systolic blood pressure and plasma oxidised low-density lipoprotein concentrations in overweight subjects with a high-cardiovascular disease risk phenotype: a double-blinded, placebo-controlled cross-over study. *The British Journal of Nutrition*, **102**, 1065–1074.

72 Aggarwal, B.B., Sundaram, C., Malani, N., and Ichikawa, H. (2007) Curcumin: the Indian solid gold. *Advances in Experimental Medicine and Biology*, **595**, 1–75.

73 Brown, L., Kroon, P.A., Das, D.K., Das, S., Tosaki, A., Chan, V., Singer, M.V., and Feick, P. (2009) The biological responses to resveratrol and other polyphenols from alcoholic beverages. *Alcoholism, Clinical and Experimental Research*, **33**, 1513–1523.

74 Kroon, P.A., Iyer, A., Chunduri, P., Chan, V., and Brown, L. (2010) The cardiovascular nutrapharmacology of resveratrol: pharmacokinetics, molecular mechanisms and therapeutic potential. *Current Medicinal Chemistry*, **17**, 2442–2455.

75 Bachmann, K., Pardoe, D., and White, D. (1996) Scaling basic toxicokinetic parameters from rat to man. *Environmental Health Perspectives*, **104**, 400–407.

76 Reagan-Shaw, S., Nihal, M., and Ahmad, N. (2008) Dose translation from animal to human studies revisited. *The FASEB Journal*, **22**, 659–661.

16
Cognitive Disorders: Impairment, Aging, and Dementia

Nick P. van Goethem, Roy Lardenoije, Konstantinos Kompotis, Bart P.F. Rutten, Jos Prickaerts, and Harry W.M. Steinbusch

16.1
Introduction

Cognitive dysfunction is a feature often encountered in a broad spectrum of neurological and psychiatric conditions. The property of animal models to study the development of a disease, and not just late-stage pathology, is crucial for disease models involving cognitive deficits, as such deficits are often the result of neurodegeneration. Considering the limited regenerative capacity of the brain, it is thus pivotal to treat neurodegenerative diseases as early as possible [1]. Since ameliorating these dysfunctions can dramatically improve the quality of life of patients, developing treatments, or "cognition enhancers," is a major area of interest for the pharmaceutical industry. Accordingly, over the past few decades certain drugs have been approved for the treatment of cognitive impairments related to specific neurological and psychiatric conditions (for a recent review, see Ref. [2]). A diverse range of animal models are being used to identify potential cognition-enhancing drugs and such models can be based on pharmacological deficits, the naturally occurring aging process, and/or introduction of transgenic constructs in rodents. The first part of this chapter describes the most commonly used rodent pharmacological deficit models. Hereafter, animal models of aging and transgenic animal models will be discussed.

16.2
Pharmacological Models

In pharmacological deficit models, specific drugs are administered to animals in order to induce cognitive deficits. The targets of these cognition-impairing drugs are hypothesis based and are often directed to alter distinct neurotransmitter systems, with different disorders showing specific dysregulation or impairments.

In Vivo Models for Drug Discovery, First Edition. Edited by José M. Vela, Rafael Maldonado, and Michel Hamon.
© 2014 Wiley-VCH Verlag GmbH & Co. KGaA. Published 2014 by Wiley-VCH Verlag GmbH & Co. KGaA.

16.2.1
Inhibition of Energy/Glucose Metabolism

A variety of studies in both rodents and humans have shown that slight increases in circulating glucose concentrations exhibit beneficial effects in brain functions relating to learning and memory [3]. Administrating glucose has been shown to facilitate rodent performance and furthermore reverses both drug- and age-related cognitive deficits. The putative mechanism of action underlying these procognitive effects probably relates to altered neuronal metabolism, neuronal activity, or neurotransmitter synthesis [4].

The most straightforward way of inhibiting energy/glucose metabolism is glucose deprivation. *In vitro* studies often use oxygen–glucose deprivation to mimic ischemic injury and subsequently study acute stroke pathology [5]. *In vivo* studies, which use oxygen–glucose deprivation, mostly do this via middle cerebral artery occlusion [6]. *N*-methyl-D-aspartate (NMDA) receptor antagonists have been shown to be neuroprotective against excitotoxicity in both *in vitro* and *in vivo* models of ischemia or neurodegeneration [7,8]. Another way of inhibiting energy/glucose metabolism is by treatment with the glycolytic inhibitor, 2-deoxyglucose. Although mostly used for glucose uptake measurement, 2-deoxyglucose has been shown to dose-dependently affect cognitive performance of rodents [9].

Another possible animal model for metabolic dysfunction (and/or generation of oxidative stress) is intracerebral ventricular (i.c.v.) administration of streptozotocin [10,11]. Streptozotocin is a naturally occurring chemical that was discovered in the late 1950s and a little later identified as an antibacterial antibiotic [12]. Subsequently, it was discovered that i.c.v. administration of streptozotocin decreases the central metabolism of glucose and hence offers a useful animal/rodent model of neurodegeneration (e.g., Alzheimer's disease) [13]. Furthermore, i.c.v. streptozotocin administration also reduces the concentrations of different neurotransmitters, including acetylcholine (ACh) [14,15]. As will be described in the next section, this cholinergic reduction further contributes to the use of this animal model of neurodegeneration. Accordingly, middle-aged and old rats that have been treated with streptozotocin (i.c.v.) show cognitive deficits in tasks assessing learning and memory. These deficits can be reversed with specific cognition-enhancing drugs [13,16].

16.2.2
Cholinergic Interventions

Cholinergic Toxins The use of pharmacological deficit models targeting the cholinergic system became popular after the cholinergic hypothesis of geriatric memory dysfunction was postulated. This hypothesis states that the age-related decline in cognition is predominately caused by a decrement of cholinergic neurotransmission [17]. Nowadays, with the exception of one NMDA receptor antagonist (see also above), all approved drugs for the treatment of cognitive dysfunction in Alzheimer's disease aim at increasing cholinergic neurotransmission. Different approaches have been used to induce cholinergic hypofunction in order to mimic Alzheimer's disease-, and age-related cognitive decline. To achieve chronic dysregulation of the cholinergic system, cholinergic toxins have been used. The exact role of ACh in cognition is not fully understood, but ACh regulation has been associated with attention, learning, and memory processes [18].

Many of the early rat studies made use of excitotoxic lesions by means of central administrations of ibotenic acid or quisqualic acid. The excitotoxic lesions (especially with ibotenic acid) of cholinergic neurons revealed a vast range of cognitive impairments [19,20]. However, a fundamental problem with this approach was the lack of a specific cholinergic toxin, introducing the possibility that such impairments may be due to damage to noncholinergic neurons. A more selective way to destruct cholinergic cells can be accomplished by locally injecting 192 IgG-saporin. 192 IgG-saporin is an antineuronal immunotoxin that consists of a monoclonal antibody (192 IgG) to the nerve growth factor (NGF) receptor that has been armed with saporin, a ribosome-inactivating protein [21,22]. Injection of this 192 IgG-saporin complex produces long-lasting depletions in cholinergic markers throughout the forebrain of rats [23]. 192 IgG-saporin administration has been used to induce cognitive impairments in rodents to investigate the role of the cholinergic system in particular brain structures [24,25].

Cholinergic Antagonists Induction of more transient or acute disruption of the cholinergic system can be induced with cholinergic antagonists. ACh has two types of receptors: the metabotropic muscarinic receptors (five subtypes in CNS) and the ionotropic nicotinic receptors (two major subtypes in CNS). There are specific antagonists for each ACh receptor type. A further division can be made between selective and nonselective cholinergic antagonists. This applies to the selectivity/affinity of an antagonist to the isoforms of ACh receptor (sub)types.

The most widely used nonselective competitive cholinergic antagonists are the tropane alkaloids scopolamine hydrobromide and atropine. The nonselective muscarinic antagonist scopolamine is probably the most often used cognition-deficit-inducing drug in (preclinical) rodent research. Since scopolamine induces amnesia that is caused by a blockade of cholinergic signaling, this drug is used to model cognitive deficits associated with aging and dementia [26]. In preclinical testing, scopolamine is often coadministered with putative cognition-enhancing drugs in order to test whether a new drug is effective in reversing a scopolamine-induced cognitive deficit [27]. The rationale is that if a new experimental drug can reverse such a deficit, it might also improve cognitive function in healthy participants or people diagnosed with a neuropsychiatric disorder [26].

Since scopolamine is a nonselective muscarinic antagonist, efforts have been made to promote the use of more selective muscarinic antagonists. Since muscarinic receptors are both centrally and peripherally present, it would be more "clean" to use a more centrally selective muscarinic antagonist. Of the five known muscarinic receptors (M1–M5), M1 might be a promising target since this receptor is predominantly located in the cortex and the hippocampus, brain regions known to be important for attention, learning, and memory. Peripheral presence of the M1 receptor is relatively limited [28]. The selective muscarinic M1 receptor antagonist biperiden is, therefore, an interesting drug candidate to more selectively induce cognitive, in particular memory, deficits in rodent models [29].

The other class of cholinergic receptors is the class of ionotropic nicotinic receptors (nAChRs). These receptors belong to a family of ligand-gated ion channel receptors that include type 3 serotonin (5HT3), $GABA_A$ and strychnine-sensitive glycine receptors. nAChRs in the brain are composed of five subunits, which can be either α-subunits (nine identified subunits: α2–α10) or β-subunits (three identified subunits: β2–β4). These subunits can combine to result in different isoforms. In the CNS, the heteropentameric α4β2 and the homopentameric α7 nAChRs comprise >90% of the nAChR subtypes [30]. Since nAChRs have been shown to be involved in learning and memory [27] and postmortem research shows that nAChR densities are markedly decreased in the brains of both patients with Alzheimer's disease and schizophrenia, the pharmaceutical industry has been developing different nAChR agonists in order to try to ameliorate the cognitive deficits that accompany these disorders [30]. Accordingly, antagonists of these nAChRs cause cognitive impairments in rodents, and hence certain drugs are used to mimic cognitive deficits seen in both Alzheimer's disease and schizophrenia.

Mecamylamine is such a nonselective nAChR antagonist shown to induce learning and memory deficits (at high enough doses) in rodents [31]. In order to more specifically investigate the role of the different nAChR subtypes, selective nAChR antagonists are used. Methyllycaconitine (MLA) is a selective α7 nAChR competitive antagonist, and dihydro-beta-erythroidine (DHβE) is a selective α4β2 nAChR competitive antagonist. Both of these drugs have been shown to induce memory deficits in rodents [32], when administered at a high enough dose [33]. Besides inducing cognitive deficits on their own, these drugs are also used to counteract the procognitive effect of agonists at their corresponding nAChR subtype. This approach is used in order to confirm that the procognitive effects of a selective nAChR agonist are indeed mediated via a specific nAChR [27,33].

16.2.3
Glutamatergic Antagonists

Another important neurotransmitter directly involved in cognitive processes is glutamate. Glutamate is an abundantly present excitatory neurotransmitter, which acts through the ionotropic NMDA receptor (besides the AMPA receptor). NMDA receptors have been implicated in cognitive processes, in particular memory formation [34].

Following this rationale, NMDA antagonists have been used to function as cognition-deficit models in rodents and of these the most widely used cognition impairers are noncompetitive NMDA receptor-channel blockers. The most frequently used NMDA receptor-channel blockers in rodent models are MK-801 (dizocilpine), phencyclidine (PCP), and ketamine. These receptor-channel blockers bind to specific sites within the NMDA receptor channel pore and subsequently block the channel, thereby inducing cognitive impairments.

MK-801 has been assessed in a broad range of rodent test paradigms and is considered a valid model to induce acute cognitive dysfunction provided the right dose is used (without inducing noncognitive side effects) [34]. PCP in rodents is mainly used in a (sub)chronic manner to mimic the impairments seen in schizophrenia patients. In contrast to MK-801, PCP was also tested in humans; hence, more direct comparisons between rodent and human behavior can be made [35]. PCP is believed to bind to a site within the NMDA receptor-channel pore (the PCP binding site) that is only accessible when the channel is open. Therefore, the antagonism is "use dependent." PCP thus acts at the same site as other "open-channel" blockers such as MK-801 or ketamine [36]. Besides acting on the NMDA receptor channel, PCP also binds to the dopamine uptake site. MK-801 is considerably more potent than PCP in producing a noncompetitive blockade at the NMDA receptor. However, MK-801 lacks the direct action on dopamine uptake, which accounts for the argument that PCP might be a more suitable deficit model for schizophrenia specifically, since PCP intoxication is associated with more psychotic features. Ketamine also acts as a type 2 dopamine partial agonist, but is a weaker blocker of the NMDA ion channel. Therefore, for mimicking psychosis, PCP might represent a more (and ketamine a less) complete model. Although MK-801 is much less complex in its pharmacological profile, it has proved to be valuable in animal studies because of its high selectivity for the NMDA receptor [35]. After scopolamine, MK-801 is probably the most widely used drug for the induction of cognitive impairments in rodents [34].

16.2.4
Serotonergic Intervention

The serotonergic system has been implicated in cognitive processes as well. This system may have only minor effects on cognitive function on its own, but is assumed to interact with the cholinergic system. This serotonergic–cholinergic interaction probably plays an important role in the mediation of behavioral, including cognitive, performance [37].

A model used to decrease serotonin (5HT) entails the lowering of 5HT levels. Decreasing 5HT levels can be accomplished by manipulating the availability of the essential amino acid tryptophan via the food. Tryptophan has multiple functions, one of which is that it functions as a biochemical precursor for 5HT. Acute tryptophan depletion is used as a pharmacological deficit model to lower central 5HT levels. The acute tryptophan depletion method is widely used both preclinically and clinically as a model to investigate the implication of the 5HT system in affective disorders [38,39]. This serotonergic-deficit model has been frequently used to study putative cognition enhancers in rats [39,40].

16.3
Aging and Transgenic Models

Over the past few decades, ample transgenic rodent models modeling specific diseases and exhibiting cognitive deficits have been generated. It should, however, be noted that most of the diseases discussed below are not of simple genetic origin. Indeed, the exact etiology of most remains to be elucidated. This means that the specific mutations used to create a model may only have a small hand in the actual pathology. Single mutations might not even result in any detectable pathology and multiple mutations, or specific environmental interactions may be required to instigate disease pathology [41]. Described in this section is a selection of transgenic rodent models of some of the most common neurodegenerative diseases involving cognitive impairments, which are most widely used or have provided critical insights.

16.3.1
Normal Aging

Of most cognitive disorders, aging is the top risk factor, while at the same time aging itself is also associated with cognitive decline [42]. Although aging is a natural process, it can result in quite severe functional limitations at the end of the life span, resulting inevitably in death. Rats and mice are useful laboratory species for studying the aging process, as they have relatively short life spans (up to 4 years for mice and up to 5 years for rats), are small and thus easy to keep, and reproduce fast [43]. For instance, nontransgenic mice can be used to study epigenetic, physiological, morphological, and behavioral changes as they occur during the aging process [44–46]. Importantly, interventions that may have a positive effect on age-related decline, such as caloric restriction, can be tested in these animals in a relatively short amount of time [46]. An even faster rodent model of aging is the senescence-accelerated mouse (SAM). This model consists of a collection of series created through the selective breeding of AKR/J mice, which already showed signs of accelerated aging, including multiple senescence-prone (P series) and senescence-resistant (R series) series [47,48]. Of particular interest are the SAMP8 mice, which show ample age-related changes early in life, leading to a median survival time of only around 10 months. SAMP8 mice naturally present with neuropathological and neurochemical changes, including Aβ deposition, hyperphosphorylation of tau, and hampered dendritic spine development, as well as NMDA-, acetylcholine-, and noradrenaline-associated abnormalities [49]. This makes the SAMP8 model attractive for the study of, for example, age-related Parkinson's and Alzheimer's diseases (AD). SAMP8 mice develop learning and memory impairments at a young age. Such deficits start at 2 months of age, as assessed with such tests as the water maze, T-maze, passive avoidance, and one-way active avoidance paradigms [49,50].

The greatest advantage of mice and rats may, however, also be one of their greatest limitations as models of human aging: The large gap between the life spans of humans, and that of mice and rats, may be indicative of the latter being unable to fully elucidate the mechanisms influencing human aging [43]. For this reason, some investigators have chosen to use animal models that live longer, among which are also other rodent models. Some of these model organisms, including the naked mole rat, porcupines, and beavers, reach life span of over 20 years. Comparing species of the same order of Rodentia with such diverging life spans may offer insights into the general mechanisms that increase a species age.

16.3.2
Alzheimer's Disease

APP Despite its relative rarity, familial AD (fAD) has garnered the most attention due to its large genetic component. It is thus not surprising that the first transgenic mouse model for AD, the PDAPP model made in 1995, is based on a mutation in the fAD-associated amyloid precursor protein (APP) gene [51,52]. PDAPP mice express human APP cDNA with the Indiana mutation (V717F). In this model, plaque pathology arises between 6 and 9 months, paired with synapse, but no severe cell loss, or neurofibrillary tangle (NFT) deposition. Aged mice of this model display an impaired learning ability in the Morris water maze, the radial arm water maze, the cue task, and serial spatial reversal task [53].

Although some neuropathology occurs in this first model, it is the second transgenic model, Tg2576, implementing a double APP mutation (K670N and M671L), that successfully models an age-dependent buildup of amyloid plaques and related cognitive decline, as associated with AD [54]. The mutant APP expressed by Tg2576 mice is also referred to as APPSWE, and is under control of the hamster prion promoter. Cognitive decline in these widely used mice occurs progressively from 6 to 9 months of age. By the age of 12 months, this model shows an impaired performance on spatial and working memory tasks, including the Y-maze spontaneous alternation and visible platform recognition tasks, as well as amygdala-dependent fear conditioning tasks.

A more aggressive AD model, the TgCRND8 transgenic mouse model, combines the Swedish and Indiana mutations, expressing the human βAPP695 transgene under control of the Syrian hamster prion promoter, on a C3H/B6 background [55]. This combination results in rapid extracellular plaque formation in the hippocampus and frontal cortex, similar to human AD, paired with defunct spatial learning in the Morris water maze task at 3 months of age, and impaired nonspatial episodic memory, as determined with the object recognition task at 8 weeks of age.

PS1, PS2, and PS1 × APP Apart from mutations in the APP gene, mutations in presenilin (PS) genes have also been used to generate transgenic mouse models. For instance, the PS1M146L, PS1M146V, and PS2N141I models were used to demonstrate *in vivo* that mutant PS1 and PS2 are able to selectively enhance Aβ42 levels [56]. This increased Aβ42 presence is, however, without significant plaque pathology and cognitive deficits. It seems that the interaction between the presenilin and APP genes is of vital importance in the pathophysiology of AD and, therefore, presenilin mutations are usually combined with a mutated APP transgene. The biogenic PSAPP model, a crossing between APP and PS1 transgenic models (e.g., Tg2576 × PS1M146L, PS1-A246 + APPSWE, and APP$_{swe}$/PS1dE9), shows a grave acceleration in pathology, compared with mutant APP-only models [57]. This includes an earlier onset of cognitive impairments, as measured with the Morris water maze and radial arm water maze tests for working memory.

One of the most early-onset and aggressive amyloid models is the 5XFAD transgenic mouse model, sporting five fAD-associated mutations [58]. 5XFAD mice carry two transgenes under the mouse Thy-1 promoter: APPswe/Ind/fl and PS1M146L/L286V (on a B6/SJL background), resulting in a grossly exaggerated Aβ42 production. Consequently, amyloid deposits in the hippocampus start to form at the young age of 2 months. By the age of 6 months, massive amyloid pathology can be observed throughout the hippocampus and cortex of these mice, paired with impaired spatial working memory, as tested with the spontaneous alternation Y-maze. At this age 5XFAD mice also show impaired hippocampal-dependent contextual fear memory [59].

MAPT APP, PS1, and PS2 transgenic models are able to capture some of the Aβ-associated pathology seen in AD. Most of these models, however, fail to recapitulate the widespread neurodegeneration and tangle pathology, which is critical for a suitable phenocopy of AD. A model that achieves just that is the TauP301S transgenic mouse model, based on the shortest isoform of 4R microtubule-associated protein tau (MAPT) with the P301S mutation, controlled by the mouse Thy-1 promoter on a C57BL/J background [60]. Around 5–6 months of age, widespread NFT pathology can be observed in the brain and spinal cord, as well as neuronal loss in the latter area, paired with severe paraparesis in mice of this model. Cognitive deficits at 5–6 months of age include decreased spontaneous alternation in the Y-maze test, impaired sociability and object recognition memory in Crawley's social interaction test, hampered spatial memory in the Morris water maze test, and slightly impaired contextual memory in the contextual and cued fear conditioning tests.

The peculiar TauV337M model, which expresses 4R MAPT with the V337M mutation controlled by the platelet-derived growth factor promoter (also exists with the mouse Thy-1 promoter) on a B6SJL background, is characterized by a low-level synthesis of 4R MAPT, which is only 1/10 of endogenous mouse MAPT production [61]. The observation of neurofibrillary pathology in this model indicates that it may not be the absolute MAPT levels, but the nature of MAPT that instigates tangle pathology. At the age of 12 months, TauV337M mice seem to have defunct olfactory memory, as tested with the social transmission of food preferences task, and deficits in impulse control, as determined with the five-choice serial reaction time task, at 24 months of age and at 12 months of age when the intertrial intervals were increased. Note that in contrast to most other tau-based models, this model does not exhibit motor abnormalities until at least 24 months of age.

To investigate the reversibility of tangle pathology, the rTg4510 model was created [62]. These transgenic mice express MAPT with the P301L mutation under control of the TET-off system, making the transgene inducible. When the mutant MAPT is expressed, these mice show progressive NFT development and cell loss from 1 month of age, including severe hippocampal CA1 neuron death at the age of 5 months. From the age of 2.5 months, this model starts to display impaired spatial reference memory, as examined with the Morris water maze. Interestingly, turning off production of the mutant MAPT after 4 months of age leads to a recovery of cognitive performance, but a worsening of the tangle pathology, indicating that at this age tau pathology becomes independent of transgenic MAPT expression.

When considering the MAPT-based models discussed earlier as models for AD, it is important to realize that NFT pathology in AD arises in the absence of mutations in the MAPT gene; indeed, most of the mutations these models are based on are from other tauopathies such as frontotemporal dementia (FTD) [56]. Furthermore, most of the other transgenic models do not take into account endogenous gene expression of the model organism. For instance, all of the above-mentioned transgenic mouse models that express a mutant form of MAPT also express mouse MAPT. The htau transgenic mouse model was created keeping the following point in mind: expressing nonmutant human genomic MAPT in a mouse MAPT knockout background (maintained on a Swiss Webster/129/SvJae/C57BL/6 background) [63]. This model presents with AD-like tau pathology, starting with pretangle-like hyperphosphorylated MAPT accumulation after 3 months, spreading at an age of 9 months through hippocampal and neocortical regions. At the age of 12 months, these htau mice start displaying cognitive impairments in the object recognition task and the Morris water maze, paired with disrupted long-term potentiation in the hippocampal CA1 region [64].

PS1 × APP × MAPT One of the most used transgenic models for AD is the triple transgenic mouse model, which combines mutated PS1, APP, and MAPT genes into one model. This 3xTgAD model expresses mutant APPSWE and MAPTP301L, under control of the mouse Thy-1 promoter, on a PSEN1M146V knock-in background (PSEN1-KI) [65]. Plaques develop from an age of 6 months in 3xTgAD mice, and tangle pathology arises by the age of 12 months. Although not completely mimicking AD, this is one of the best models available – developing progressive synaptic dysfunction, amyloid plaques, and neurofibrillary tangles in a temporal and spatial pattern that is similar to human AD. Around 4 months of age, 3xTgAD mice start to present with impaired spatial memory and long-term retention, as tested with the Morris water maze task, and at 6 months their short- and long-term retention for contextual fear also becomes significantly reduced [66]. Aged 3xTgAD mice show deficits in object discrimination memory in the object discrimination task, together with derailed long-term potentiation and paired-pulse facilitation.

APOE4 When looking at the genes used in the triple transgenic AD model, it can be argued that it is primarily a model of fAD and not of the far more common sporadic AD (sAD). Models employing the highest genetic risk factor for sAD, allele APOE4, have been constructed – expressing human APOE4 under control of the neuron-specific enolase (NSE) promoter in transgenic mice devoid of endogenous mouse APOE [67]. This NSE-APOE4 model exhibits a less severe phenotype than most other transgenic models of AD, failing to recapitulate most of the pathological hallmarks associated with the disease. Nevertheless, the NSE-APOE4 model displays impaired excitatory synaptic transmission, a decline in dendritic density and complexity, and cognitive impairments in a water maze task at the age of 6 months.

16.3.3
Parkinson's Disease

α-Syn α-Synuclein transgenic mice overexpress human wild-type or mutant alpha-synuclein usually under the regulatory control of the human PDGF-ß promoter. α-Synuclein is expressed in high levels, resulting in an age-dependent increase of brain inclusions consisting of α-Synuclein (α-Syn), ubiquitin, and other proteins. Severity of the brain pathology correlates with increasing age. By 6 months of age, these transgenic mice exhibit deficits in cognition shown by an increased time to find the platform in the water maze task [68]. Mice overexpressing wild-type α-Syn under regulation of the human PDGF-β promoter also display a progressive increase in α-Syn aggregation in multiple brain regions, a loss of dopaminergic terminals in the striatum, and mild changes in motor activity as shown by a decreased latency to fall on a rotarod. Another variation of these mice uses the human Thy1 as a promoter for overexpressing α-Syn. Cognitive changes (Y-maze, novel object recognition, and operant reversal learning) are also evident in the Thy1-α-Syn mice beginning ∼4–6 months of age [69,70].

Nuber *et al.* in 2008 [71] created a conditional mouse model for the overexpression of WT α-Syn under the calcium/calmodulin-dependent protein kinase IIα (CaM) promoter, using a tetracycline-regulated TET-off system (tTA). These mice displayed a progressive motor decline after 7 months (rotarod) of age, modest impairment in reference memory after 12 months (water maze), and α-Syn accumulation in the substantia nigra, hippocampus, and olfactory bulb.

DJ1(PARK7)KO DJ1KO mice have a deficiency in expressing the Park7 protein, due to a knockout of the respective gene, namely, DJ1. $DJ1^{-/-}$ mice between 13 and 14 months of age show cognitive deficits, as characterized by reduced performance in an object recognition task [72].

Parkin(PARK2)KO This PD mouse model is produced by a knockout in the PARK2 gene, responsible for the expression of a protein called parkin. $Parkin^{-/-}$ mice display increased anxiety, as shown in the open-field and light/dark preference tests, and cognitive impairment exhibited as spatial memory deficits in the Morris water maze [73]. Mice that lack exon 3 in the parkin gene do not demonstrate loss of dopaminergic neurons; nevertheless, they show signs of altered synaptic transmission in the nigrostriatal circuit [74].

16.3.4
Huntington's Disease

Various transgenic rodent models of HD have been found to exhibit affective and cognitive abnormalities reflecting clinical data in HD patients. For example, R6/1 and R6/2 transgenic lines of HD mice have behavioral deficits that include impaired hippocampal-dependent spatial cognition [75,76]. However, depression-like behavior also manifests in R6/1 HD mice prior to cognitive and motor symptoms [77].

R6/2 Of the transgenic chimeric models that express truncated forms of the human mutant HD allele, the R6/2 line is the most widely used. This line expresses an exon 1 fragment of htt with a range of 148–153 repeats, expressed from an unknown location in the mouse genome. R6/2 mice exhibit learning and memory tasks abnormalities as early as 3.5 weeks of age (water Morris maze), which follow them throughout their life span, as evaluated by various cognitive tests (T-maze, two-choice swim tank, and visual discriminate learning) [78–80]. Moreover, they show behavioral deficits by 5 weeks, neuroanatomic abnormalities including progressive reduction in brain and striatal volume, substantially reduced striatal neuron number by 12 weeks, and death by 12–15 weeks [80–82]. As the R6/2 model exhibits severe, early-onset and diffuse pathology, it is potentially a good model of juvenile-onset HD, displaying an aggressive phenotype and provides clear experimental endpoints.

YAC128 The YAC128 is a widely used yeast-artificial-chromosome full-length human mutant HD transgenic model generated and characterized by the Hayden laboratory [83,84]. Van Raamsdonk *et al.* in 2005 evaluated YAC128 mice with a variety of more cognitively oriented tests, demonstrating progressive cognitive deficits at 8 weeks (accelerated rotarod) and 32 weeks (water Morris maze, open-field habituation, and T-maze). Unlike the R6/2 mice, where there is probably a diffuse loss of brain volume, some regions of the YAC128 brain, such as the cerebellum and hippocampus, exhibit normal volume [85]. YAC128 mice also exhibit motor abnormalities as early as 3 months with increased open field activity, followed by rotarod performance abnormalities at 6 months.

tgHD Rats This transgenic rat model of HD, with a mutated huntingtin gene containing 51 CAG repeats, expresses adult-onset neurological phenotypes, cognitive impairments, progressive motor dysfunction, and neuronal nuclear inclusions in the brain [86]. The transgenic rat model exhibits a late-onset neurological phenotype, cognitive decline in spatial learning at 10 months (radial arm maze), and significantly impaired object recognition performance at 16 months [87], develops gradually progressive motor abnormalities, and dies between 15 and 24 months. However, according to a recent report by Fielding *et al.* in 2012 [88], the tgHD rat model does not show consistent, reliable, and progressive impairment in a range of cognitive tests. The consistent failure to reveal impairments at any age on a range of tests of cognition and learning suggest that the tgHD rat is not a reliable model of the cognitive and behavioral impairments of human HD.

16.3.5
Frontotemporal Dementia

TDP43 Transgenic murine models used in FTLD-TDP research overexpress either wild-type or mutant human TDP43KI via a human TDP promoter. TDP43 is a multifunctional, nuclear protein that binds both DNA and RNA, as well as a member of the heterogeneous nuclear ribonuclear protein (hnRNP) family, and regulates several aspects of RNA processing, including alternative splicing, miRNA production, and mRNA trafficking and stabilization. Missense changes in the glycine-rich domain of TDP-43 lead to a shift in its localization from the nucleus to the cytoplasm, resulting in FTLD-TDP pathology [89]. This mouse model exhibits cognitive deficits at the age of 7 or 9 months, depending on the use of a mutated or a wild-type TDP43KI, respectively, as shown by passive avoidance test and Barns maze. Cognitive impairments for this murine model reach a peak at the age of 11–13 months [89,90].

16.3.6
Down Syndrome

TgDyrk1A Apart from the trisomic mice used in Down syndrome research, transgenic models have also been constructed carrying human genes mapped in the repeated fragment of chromosome 21. One such model, namely, TgDyrk1a, overexpresses DYRK1A, a gene encoding a serine–threonine kinase, which is probably involved in neuroblast proliferation [91]. In the Morris water maze, TgDyrk1A mice show significant deficits in spatial learning and cognitive flexibility, due to hippocampal and prefrontal cortical dysfunction, a defect that was related specifically to reference memory. TgDyrk1A mice also exhibit delayed craniocaudal maturation, altered motor skill acquisition, and hyperactivity [92].

16.4
Translation to Clinics: Limitations and Difficulties

To date, pharmacological, transgenic, and naturally aging rodent models have provided new insights into behavioral function. Although these models have given invaluable information, it is important to remember that they only provide approximations of the molecular and cellular mechanisms and cognitive impairments as seen in humans. In addition, whereas motor phenotypes can be readily assessed in rodent models, it is more challenging to characterize cognitive phenotypes. The frontal cortex of rodents is anatomically different from that of humans [93], and it is therefore difficult to model executive dysfunction, not to mention the existence of significant limitations in modeling complex behaviors in rats and mice, since they already differ in their own cognitive and social functions. Due to these obstacles, face validity gets compromised (see Table 16.1). It has thus been suggested that the research community should take an "agnostic" approach as new models emerge and characterize their behavior as fully as possible. At present, face validity of the behavioral tests used is, in general, the same for pharmacological, aging, and transgenic rodent models (see Tables 16.2 and 16.3). This results from the fact that, independent of the manipulation used (pharmacological, age, or genetic), the same symptoms are being screened for. In addition, it is important to recognize that not all animal models currently in use or under development will be appropriate for mechanistic research, whereas other certain models exhibit

Table 16.1 Descriptions of construct, face, and, predictive validity.

Validity	Description
Validity	The extent to which a test measures what it purports to measure. It is vital for a test to be valid so that the results are accurately applied and interpreted
Construct validity	This is generally considered the most fundamental and all-inclusive validity concept, insofar as it specifies what the test measures. Construct validity holds that the model has a correct theoretical background compared with the human pathology. Therefore, it addresses the qualities contributing to the relation between X and Y. Overall, construct validity deals with the question – Does the measure or observation in a test or model show behavior that corresponds to how the theory says a measure or observation of that construct should behave?
Face validity	The extent to which a test seems on its surface to be measuring what it purports to measure. Face validity refers not to what the test measures but only to how it looks. The concept of face validity is that the animal shows the same kind of behavior and has the same symptoms as humans have. In short, do the measures in a test or model *appear* to be relevant?
Predictive validity	The extent to which a test or model can predict future outcomes. Predictive validity implies that the manipulations and treatments that are beneficial in the appropriate animal model should also have the same effect in humans/patients, and vice versa

phenotypes that are practical for therapy development. Compared with pharmacological models, transgenic models comprise more construct validity, and hence are more suited for mechanistic and fundamental research. On the other hand, pharmacological models comprise more predictive validity, and therefore contribute to more reliable testing of new (pharmacological) therapies (see Tables 16.2 and 16.3). Subjecting rodents to a comprehensive battery of tests provides a better framework not only for understanding the overall behavioral phenotype of the animal but also for more fully recognizing the limitations of the specific model. Nevertheless, it should be emphasized that the goal of animal research is to mimic

Table 16.2 Validity of pharmacological models.

Pharmacological models	Validity		
	Construct validity	Face validity	Predictive validity
Inhibition of energy/glucose metabolism	+++	++	+
Cholinergic toxins	+++	++	+
Cholinergic antagonists	++	++	++
Glutamatergic antagonists	++	++	++
Serotonergic intervention	+	++	+

++++: meets validity perfectly, +++: meets validity good, ++: meets validity somewhat, +: meets validity poorly.

Table 16.3 Validity of aging and transgenic models in general.

Aging and transgenic models	Validity		
	Construct validity	Face validity	Predictive validity
Normal aging	++++	++	++
Alzheimer's disease models	+++	++	+
Parkinson's disease models	+++	++	+
Huntington's disease models	+++	++	+
Frontotemporal dementia TDP43 model	+++	++	+
Down syndrome TgDyrk model	+++	++	+

++++: meets validity perfectly, +++: meets validity good, ++: meets validity somewhat, +: meets validity poorly.

as much as possible the human disease pathophysiology, and thus improving construct and face validity will provide greater insights into basic genetic and molecular mechanisms involved in expression of the behavior [94]. At the same time, once these mechanisms are better understood, predictive validity will improve and better efficacious therapeutic strategies can be explored and developed for treating cognitive deficits in human patients.

References

1 Faigle, R. and Song, H. (2013) Signaling mechanisms regulating adult neural stem cells and neurogenesis. *Biochimica et Biophysica Acta*, **1830** (2), 2435–2448.

2 Froestl, W., Muhs, A., and Pfeifer, A. (2012) Cognitive enhancers (nootropics). Part 1: drugs interacting with receptors. *Journal of Alzheimer's Disease*, **32**, 793–887.

3 Gold, P.E. (1995) Role of glucose in regulating the brain and cognition. *The American Journal of Clinical Nutrition*, **61** (4), 987S–995S.

4 Korol, D.L. and Gold, P.E. (1998) Glucose, memory, and aging. *The American Journal of Clinical Nutrition*, **67** (4), 764S–771S.

5 Cho, S., Wood, A., and Bowlby, M.R. (2007) Brain slices as models for neurodegenerative disease and screening platforms to identify novel therapeutics. *Current Neuropharmacology*, **5** (1), 19–33.

6 Bederson, J.B. et al. (1986) Rat middle cerebral artery occlusion: evaluation of the model and development of a neurologic examination. *Stroke*, **17** (3), 472–476.

7 Arias, R.L., Tasse, J.R.P., and Bowlby, M.R. (1999) Neuroprotective interaction effects of NMDA and AMPA receptor antagonists in an *in vitro* model of cerebral ischemia. *Brain Research*, **816** (2), 299–308.

8 Danysz, W. and Parsons, C.G. (2003) The NMDA receptor antagonist memantine as a symptomatological and neuroprotective treatment for Alzheimer's disease: preclinical evidence. *International Journal of Geriatric Psychiatry*, **18** (S1), S23–S32.

9 Ockuly, J.C. et al. (2012) Behavioral, cognitive, and safety profile of 2-deoxy-2-glucose (2DG) in adult rats. *Epilepsy Research*, **101**, 246–252.

10 Mayer, G., Nitsch, R., and Hoyer, S. (1990) Effects of changes in peripheral and cerebral glucose metabolism on locomotor activity, learning and memory in adult male rats. *Brain Research*, **532** (1), 95–100.

11 Nitsch, R., Mayer, G., and Hoyer, S. (1989) The intracerebroventriculary streptozotocin-treated rat: impairment of cerebral glucose metabolism resembles the alterations of carbohydrate metabolism of the brain in Alzheimer's disease. *Journal of Neural Transmission: Parkinson's Disease and Dementia Section*, **1** (1), 109–110.

12 Vavra, J. *et al.* (1959) Streptozotocin, a new antibacterial antibiotic. *Antibiotics Annual*, **7**, 230–235.

13 Prickaerts, J. *et al.* (1995) Spatial discrimination learning and choline acetyltransferase activity in streptozotocin-treated rats: effects of chronic treatment with acetyl-L-carnitine. *Brain Research*, **674** (1), 142–146.

14 Ding, A., Nitsch, R., and Hoyer, S. (1992) Changes in brain monoaminergic neurotransmitter concentrations in rat after intracerebroventricular injection of streptozotocin. *Journal of Cerebral Blood Flow and Metabolism*, **12**, 103–109.

15 Hellweg, R. *et al.* (1992) Nerve growth factor and choline acetyltransferase activity levels in the rat brain following experimental impairment of cerebral glucose and energy metabolism. *Journal of Neuroscience Research*, **31** (3), 479–486.

16 Blokland, A. and Jolles, J. (1993) Spatial learning deficit and reduced hippocampal ChAT activity in rats after an ICV injection of streptozotocin. *Pharmacology, Biochemistry, and Behavior*, **44** (2), 491–494.

17 Bartus, R.T. *et al.* (1982) The cholinergic hypothesis of geriatric memory dysfunction. *Science*, **217**, 408–417.

18 Blokland, A. (1995) Acetylcholine: a neurotransmitter for learning and memory? *Brain Research. Brain Research Reviews*. **21** (3), 285–300.

19 Steckler, T. *et al.* (1993) Effects of NBM lesions with two neurotoxins on spatial memory and autoshaping. *Pharmacology, Biochemistry, and Behavior*, **44** (4), 877–889.

20 Peternel, A. *et al.* (1988) Basal forebrain and memory: neurotoxic lesions impair serial reversals of a spatial discrimination. *Psychobiology*, **16**, 54–58.

21 Wiley, R.G., Oeltmann, T.N., and Lappi, D.A. (1991) Immunolesioning: selective destruction of neurons using immunotoxin to rat NGF receptor. *Brain Research*, **562** (1), 149–153.

22 Wenk, G.L. *et al.* (1994) Behavioral, biochemical, histological, and electrophysiological effects of 192 IgG-saporin injections into the basal forebrain of rats. *The Journal of Neuroscience*, **14** (10), 5986–5995.

23 Book, A.A., Wiley, R.G., and Schweitzer, J.B. (1992) Specificity of 192 IgG-saporin for NGF receptor-positive cholinergic basal forebrain neurons in the rat. *Brain Research*, **590** (1), 350–355.

24 Walsh, T. *et al.* (1996) Injection of IgG 192-saporin into the medial septum produces cholinergic hypofunction and dose-dependent working memory deficits. *Brain Research*, **726** (1), 69–79.

25 Lehmann, O. *et al.* (2003) A double dissociation between serial reaction time and radial maze performance in rats subjected to 192 IgG-saporin lesions of the nucleus basalis and/or the septal region. *European Journal of Neuroscience*, **18** (3), 651–666.

26 Klinkenberg, I. and Blokland, A. (2010) The validity of scopolamine as a pharmacological model for cognitive impairment: a review of animal behavioral studies. *Neuroscience and Biobehavioral Reviews*, **34** (8), 1307–1350.

27 Prickaerts, J. *et al.* (2012) EVP-6124, a novel and selective α7 nicotinic acetylcholine receptor partial agonist, improves memory performance by potentiating the acetylcholine response of α7 nicotinic acetylcholine receptors. *Neuropharmacology*, **62**, 1099–1110.

28 Caulfield, M.P. (1993) Muscarinic receptors: characterization, coupling and function. *Pharmacology & Therapeutics*, **58** (3), 319–379.

29 Klinkenberg, I. and Blokland, A. (2011) A comparison of scopolamine and biperiden as a rodent model for cholinergic cognitive impairment. *Psychopharmacology*, **215** (3), 549–566.

30 Toyohara, J. and Hashimoto, K. (2010) α7 Nicotinic receptor agonists: potential therapeutic drugs for treatment of cognitive impairments in schizophrenia and Alzheimer's disease. *The Open Medicinal Chemistry Journal*, **4**, 37–56.

31 Levin, E.D. (1992) Nicotinic systems and cognitive function. *Psychopharmacology*, **108** (4), 417–431.

32 Addy, N.A., Nakijama, A., and Levin, E.D. (2003) Nicotinic mechanisms of memory: effects of acute local DHβE and MLA infusions in the basolateral amygdala. *Brain Research. Cognitive Brain Research*, **16** (1), 51–57.

33 Hahn, B., Shoaib, M., and Stolerman, I.P. (2011) Selective nicotinic receptor antagonists: effects on attention and nicotine-induced attentional enhancement. *Psychopharmacology*, **217** (1), 75–82.

34 van der Staay, F.J. *et al.* (2011) Effects of the cognition impairer MK-801 on learning and memory in mice and rats. *Behavioural Brain Research*, **220** (1), 215–229.

35 Ellison, G. (1995) The *N*-methyl-D-aspartate antagonists phencyclidine, ketamine and dizocilpine as both behavioral and anatomical models of the dementias. *Brain Research Reviews*, **20** (2), 250–267.

36 Morris, B.J., Cochran, S.M., and Pratt, J.A. (2005) PCP: from pharmacology to modelling schizophrenia. *Current Opinion in Pharmacology*, **5** (1), 101–106.

37 Steckler, T. and Sahgal, A. (1995) The role of serotonergic–cholinergic interactions in the mediation of cognitive behaviour. *Behavioural Brain Research*, **67** (2), 165–199.

38 Booij, L., Van der Does, A., and Riedel, W. (2003) Monoamine depletion in psychiatric and healthy populations: review. *Molecular Psychiatry*, **8** (12), 951–973.

39 van Donkelaar, E.L. *et al.* (2008) Phosphodiesterase 2 and 5 inhibition attenuates the object memory deficit induced by acute tryptophan depletion. *European Journal of Pharmacology*, **600** (1), 98–104.

40 Rutten, K. *et al.* (2007) The PDE4 inhibitor rolipram reverses object memory impairment induced by acute tryptophan depletion in the rat. *Psychopharmacology*, **192** (2), 275–282.

41 Chouliaras, L. *et al.* (2010) Gene–environment interaction research and transgenic mouse models of Alzheimer's disease. *International Journal of Alzheimer's Disease*, **2010**, 859101.

42 Gu, Y. *et al.* (2010) Drinking hydrogen water ameliorated cognitive impairment in senescence-accelerated mice. *Journal of Clinical Biochemistry and Nutrition*, **46** (3), 269–276.

43 Gorbunova, V., Bozzella, M.J., and Seluanov, A. (2008) Rodents for comparative aging studies: from mice to beavers. *Age*, **30** (2–3), 111–119.

44 Chouliaras, L. *et al.* (2011) Caloric restriction attenuates age-related changes of DNA methyltransferase 3a in mouse hippocampus. *Brain, Behavior, and Immunity*, **25** (4), 616–623.

45 Chouliaras, L. *et al.* (2011) Prevention of age-related changes in hippocampal levels of 5-methylcytidine by caloric restriction. *Neurobiology of Aging*, **33** (8), 1672–1681.

46 Rutten, B.P. *et al.* (2010) Caloric restriction and aging but not overexpression of SOD1 affect hippocampal volumes in mice. *Mechanisms of Ageing and Development*, **131** (9), 574–579.

47 Takeda, T., Hosokawa, M., and Higuchi, K. (1991) Senescence-accelerated mouse (SAM): a novel murine model of accelerated senescence. *Journal of the American Geriatrics Society*, **39** (9), 911–919.

48 Takeda, T. *et al.* (1981) A new murine model of accelerated senescence. *Mechanisms of Ageing and Development*, **17** (2), 183–194.

49 Tomobe, K. and Nomura, Y. (2009) Neurochemistry, neuropathology, and heredity in SAMP8: a mouse model of senescence. *Neurochemical Research*, **34** (4), 660–669.

50 Miyamoto, M. *et al.* (1986) Age-related changes in learning and memory in the senescence-accelerated mouse (SAM). *Physiology & Behavior*, **38** (3), 399–406.

51 Giuliani, F. *et al.* (2009) Decreased behavioral impairments in an Alzheimer mice model by interfering with TNF-alpha metabolism. *Brain Research Bulletin*, **80** (4–5), 302–308.

52 Nilsson, L.N. *et al.* (2004) Cognitive impairment in PDAPP mice depends on ApoE and ACT-catalyzed amyloid formation. *Neurobiology of Aging*, **25** (9), 1153–1167.

53 Chen, G. *et al.* (2007) Active β-amyloid immunization restores spatial learning in PDAPP mice displaying very low levels of β-amyloid. *The Journal of Neuroscience*, **27** (10), 2654–2662.

54 King, D.L. and Arendash, G.W. (2002) Behavioral characterization of the Tg2576

transgenic model of Alzheimer's disease through 19 months. *Physiology & Behavior*, **75** (5), 627–642.

55 Francis, B.M. *et al.* (2012) Object recognition memory and BDNF expression are reduced in young TgCRND8 mice. *Neurobiology of Aging*, **33** (3), 555–563.

56 McGowan, E., Eriksen, J., and Hutton, M. (2006) A decade of modeling Alzheimer's disease in transgenic mice. *Trends in Genetics*, **22** (5), 281–289.

57 Arendash, G.W. *et al.* (2001) Progressive, age-related behavioral impairments in transgenic mice carrying both mutant amyloid precursor protein and presenilin-1 transgenes. *Brain Research*, **891** (1–2), 42–53.

58 Ohno, M. *et al.* (2007) BACE1 gene deletion prevents neuron loss and memory deficits in 5XFAD APP/PS1 transgenic mice. *Neurobiology of Disease*, **26** (1), 134–145.

59 Kimura, R. and Ohno, M. (2009) Impairments in remote memory stabilization precede hippocampal synaptic and cognitive failures in 5XFAD Alzheimer mouse model. *Neurobiology of Disease*, **33** (2), 229–235.

60 Takeuchi, H. *et al.* (2011) P301S mutant human tau transgenic mice manifest early symptoms of human tauopathies with dementia and altered sensorimotor gating. *PloS One*, **6** (6), e21050.

61 Lambourne, S.L. *et al.* (2005) Increased tau phosphorylation on mitogen-activated protein kinase consensus sites and cognitive decline in transgenic models for Alzheimer's disease and FTDP-17: evidence for distinct molecular processes underlying tau abnormalities. *Molecular and Cellular Biology*, **25** (1), 278–293.

62 Santacruz, K. *et al.* (2005) Tau suppression in a neurodegenerative mouse model improves memory function. *Science*, **309** (5733), 476–481.

63 Andorfer, C. *et al.* (2003) Hyperphosphorylation and aggregation of tau in mice expressing normal human tau isoforms. *Journal of Neurochemistry*, **86** (3), 582–590.

64 Polydoro, M. *et al.* (2009) Age-dependent impairment of cognitive and synaptic function in the htau mouse model of tau pathology. *The Journal of Neuroscience*, **29** (34), 10741–10749.

65 Oddo, S. *et al.* (2003) Amyloid deposition precedes tangle formation in a triple transgenic model of Alzheimer's disease. *Neurobiology of Aging*, **24** (8), 1063–1070.

66 Billings, L.M. *et al.* (2005) Intraneuronal Abeta causes the onset of early Alzheimer's disease-related cognitive deficits in transgenic mice. *Neuron*, **45** (5), 675–688.

67 Raber, J. *et al.* (1998) Isoform-specific effects of human apolipoprotein E on brain function revealed in ApoE knockout mice: increased susceptibility of females. *Proceedings of the National Academy of Sciences of the United States of America*, **95** (18), 10914–10919.

68 Masliah, E. *et al.* (2011) Passive immunization reduces behavioral and neuropathological deficits in an alpha-synuclein transgenic model of Lewy body disease. *PloS One*, **6** (4), e19338.

69 Fleming, S.M. *et al.* (2008) Impaired reversal learning in transgenic mice overexpressing human wildtype alpha synuclein. *Neuroscience Abstracts*, **341**, 1.

70 Magen, I. and Chesselet, M.F. (2010) Genetic mouse models of Parkinson's disease: the state of the art. *Progress in Brain Research*, **184**, 53–87.

71 Nuber, S. *et al.* (2008) Neurodegeneration and motor dysfunction in a conditional model of Parkinson's disease. *The Journal of Neuroscience*, **28** (10), 2471–2484.

72 Pham, T. *et al.* (2010) DJ-1-deficient mice show less TH-positive neurons in the ventral tegmental area and exhibit non-motoric behavioural impairments. *Genes, Brain, and Behavior*, **9** (3), 305–317.

73 Zhu, X.R. *et al.* (2007) Non-motor behavioural impairments in parkin-deficient mice. *European Journal of Neuroscience*, **26** (7), 1902–1911.

74 Goldberg, M.S. *et al.* (2003) Parkin-deficient mice exhibit nigrostriatal deficits but not loss of dopaminergic neurons. *Journal of Biological Chemistry*, **278** (44), 43628–43635.

75 Nithianantharajah, J. *et al.* (2008) Gene–environment interactions modulating cognitive function and molecular correlates of synaptic plasticity in Huntington's disease transgenic mice. *Neurobiology of Disease*, **29** (3), 490–504.

76 Pang, T. et al. (2006) Differential effects of voluntary physical exercise on behavioral and brain-derived neurotrophic factor expression deficits in Huntington's disease transgenic mice. *Neuroscience*, **141** (2), 569.

77 Pang, T.Y. et al. (2009) Altered serotonin receptor expression is associated with depression-related behavior in the R6/1 transgenic mouse model of Huntington's disease. *Human Molecular Genetics*, **18** (4), 753–766.

78 Carter, R.J. et al. (1999) Characterization of progressive motor deficits in mice transgenic for the human Huntington's disease mutation. *The Journal of Neuroscience*, **19** (8), 3248–3257.

79 Lione, L.A. et al. (1999) Selective discrimination learning impairments in mice expressing the human Huntington's disease mutation. *The Journal of Neuroscience*, **19** (23), 10428–10437.

80 Stack, E.C. et al. (2005) Chronology of behavioral symptoms and neuropathological sequela in R6/2 Huntington's disease transgenic mice. *The Journal of Comparative Neurology*, **490** (4), 354–370.

81 Hickey, M. et al. (2005) Early behavioral deficits in R6/2 mice suitable for use in preclinical drug testing. *Neurobiology of Disease*, **20** (1), 1–11.

82 Morton, A.J. et al. (2005) A combination drug therapy improves cognition and reverses gene expression changes in a mouse model of Huntington's disease. *The European Journal of Neuroscience*, **21** (4), 855–870.

83 Slow, E.J. et al. (2003) Selective striatal neuronal loss in a YAC128 mouse model of Huntington disease. *Human Molecular Genetics*, **12** (13), 1555–1567.

84 Van Raamsdonk, J.M. et al. (2005) Cystamine treatment is neuroprotective in the YAC128 mouse model of Huntington disease. *Journal of Neurochemistry*, **95** (1), 210–220.

85 Van Raamsdonk, J.M. et al. (2005) Cognitive dysfunction precedes neuropathology and motor abnormalities in the YAC128 mouse model of Huntington's disease. *The Journal of Neuroscience*, **25** (16), 4169–4180.

86 von Horsten, S. et al. (2003) Transgenic rat model of Huntington's disease. *Human Molecular Genetics*, **12** (6), 617–624.

87 Zeef, D.H. et al. (2012) Memory deficits in the transgenic rat model of Huntington's disease. *Behavioural Brain Research*, **227** (1), 194–198.

88 Fielding, S.A. et al. (2012) Profiles of motor and cognitive impairment in the transgenic rat model of Huntington's disease. *Brain Research Bulletin*, **88** (2–3), 223–236.

89 Swarup, V. et al. (2011) Pathological hallmarks of amyotrophic lateral sclerosis/frontotemporal lobar degeneration in transgenic mice produced with TDP-43 genomic fragments. *Brain*, **134** (Part 9), 2610–2626.

90 Tsai, K.-J. et al. (2010) Elevated expression of TDP-43 in the forebrain of mice is sufficient to cause neurological and pathological phenotypes mimicking FTLD-U. *The Journal of Experimental Medicine*, **207** (8), 1661–1673.

91 Altafaj, X. et al. (2001) Neurodevelopmental delay, motor abnormalities and cognitive deficits in transgenic mice overexpressing Dyrk1A (minibrain), a murine model of Down's syndrome. *Human Molecular Genetics*, **10** (18), 1915–1923.

92 Ahn, K.-J. et al. (2006) DYRK1A BAC transgenic mice show altered synaptic plasticity with learning and memory defects. *Neurobiology of Disease*, **22** (3), 463–472.

93 Uylings, H., Groenewegen, H.J., and Kolb, B. (2003) Do rats have a prefrontal cortex? *Behavioural Brain Research*, **146** (1), 3–17.

94 D'Mello, G.D. and Steckler, T. (1996) Animal models in cognitive behavioural pharmacology: an overview. *Brain Research. Cognitive Brain Research*, **3** (3–4), 345–352.

17
Stroke and Traumatic Brain Injury

Dominique Lerouet, Valérie C. Besson, and Michel Plotkine

17.1
Introduction

Stroke and traumatic brain injury (TBI) constitute two major health problems worldwide. Both of these pathologies are leading causes of death and disability, in the elderly for stroke and in young individuals for TBI, contributing to devastating socioeconomic consequences. Despite considerable efforts, no therapeutic progress has emerged. Fourteen years after the original STAIR recommendations [1], the only stroke treatment, first approved by the Food and Drug Administration in 1996, is the reperfusion of the ischemic area by thrombolysis with recombinant tissue plasminogen activator (rt-PA) [2]. Nevertheless, its use remains limited to less than 5% of patients, partly due to its short therapeutic window. Until now, despite the thousands of chemical products reported as neuroprotective in preclinical studies, the translation into clinical trials has failed, albeit the great diversity of therapeutic targets [3]. This has led pharmaceutical industry to give up research on these acute neurological pathologies and to focus on chronic neurodegenerative diseases such as Alzheimer's and Parkinson's. In 2013, there is still an urgent need for efficient pharmacological intervention. The international academic community continues with preclinical studies and highlights more and more mechanisms contributing to the injury, particularly by introducing new experimental models that mimic the clinical situation much better than previous models.

Similarities between Stroke and Traumatic Brain Injury Despite a different initial insult between stroke and TBI, numerous similar molecular and cellular mechanisms contribute to the injury [4]. Notably, TBI commonly induces marked reduction in local cerebral blood flow (CBF) that may reach ischemic levels and contribute to secondary injury. Both stroke and TBI also lead to vascular disturbances. Endothelial alterations may increase vascular permeability, thus contributing to brain edema. In addition, platelet activation may alter local cerebral perfusion. Last but not least, stroke and TBI also induce a marked inflammation that plays a key role in the development of injury. All these similarities strongly suggest that therapeutic strategy may likely protect from both pathologies.

In Vivo Models for Drug Discovery, First Edition. Edited by José M. Vela, Rafael Maldonado, and Michel Hamon.
© 2014 Wiley-VCH Verlag GmbH & Co. KGaA. Published 2014 by Wiley-VCH Verlag GmbH & Co. KGaA.

In this chapter, we will describe the commonest models of stroke and TBI. The term model is defined as a "simplified representation of a phenomenon." The models are designed to reliably reproduce the clinical sequels. The large variety of animal models reflects the heterogeneity of stroke and TBI in humans, but the difficulty is to select the appropriate one, as no model can reproduce the entire spectrum of these pathologies [5,6]. The model to choose is then determined by a number of compromises and questions that each researcher has to consider with respect to the aims of his experiments. Advantages and disadvantages of these models have been detailed by others [6–13]. In addition, several variables such as regulation of CBF, temperature, blood gases concentration, blood pressure, and pH should also be taken into consideration as they have the potential to affect outcomes [6,8]. Moreover, the use of different anesthesia paradigms may alter the extent of injury *via* neuroprotective or vascular effects, thereby complicating the result interpretation across different laboratories [14–18].

For ethical, economical, and practical reasons, the most widely used animals are rodents, mainly rats and mice, but experiments in larger animals, such as nonhuman primates, also exist. The latter offer the great advantage of large gyrencephalic brains with gray/white matter proportions closer to the human one. However, mice are increasingly being used due to the availability of transgenic lines.

17.2
Stroke Models

Stroke models can be divided into global and focal cerebral ischemia. Global ischemia is defined by a blood flow reduction in the entire brain or forebrain, whereas in focal ischemia the reduction of blood flow affects only a specific region of the brain.

After a brief description of global stroke models, we will focus mainly on focal stroke models.

17.2.1
Global Stroke Models

Global models of cerebral ischemia reproduce the brain damage occurring after severe reduction in blood flow supply, such as after cardiac arrest, severe hypotension, or strangulation.

Among the different approaches (see extensive reviews, [19–21]), the most widely used models in rats are the so-called "four-vessel occlusion model" (4VO), involving permanent electrocoagulation of the vertebral arteries and temporary ligation of both common carotid arteries (CCA) [22] and the 2VO model combining occlusion of both CCA with hypotension [23]. In Mongolian gerbils, hypotension induction is not required to produce the 2VO model because of an incomplete circle of Willis in this species (absence of posterior communicating arteries). The mouse model of global stroke is similar to the rat 2VO model, using bilateral occlusion of CCA combined with hypotension or basilar artery occlusion (3VO).

17.2.2
Focal Stroke Models

Because the occlusion of the middle cerebral artery (MCA) is the most commonly identified type of ischemic stroke in human, many animal models of permanent or transient (vessels are occluded for periods of up to 3 h) and proximal or distal MCA occlusion have been developed over the years (see Refs [8,10,11,19–21] for reviews). Technical and procedural features of models are available in Ref. [21] and also on JoVE web site (*The Journal of Visualized Experiments*; http://www.jove.com; accessed March 29, 2013).

Permanent ischemia induces severe brain damage (core) surrounded by a zone of less damaged tissue (penumbra), and transient ischemia results in various degrees of ischemic damage (depending on the occlusion duration), due to both the MCA occlusion and the effect of reperfusion [24]. Although permanent models only mimic a minority of human strokes, both models are necessary prior to clinical drug development studies.

In proximal occlusion, MCA is occluded close to its origin, before the origin of the lenticulostriate arteries, and results in infarct involving only striatum or both striatum and cortex (depending on the duration of ischemia), whereas distal MCA occlusion affects only the cortex.

Briefly, there are two surgical approaches to access cerebral vasculature. The first one consists of opening the skull *via* a craniotomy to allow direct access to cerebral arteries, and the second one uses an intra-arterial access to avoid opening the skull. As the craniotomy prevents the increase of intracranial pressure, these models are associated with low or the absence of mortality.

17.2.2.1 **Extravascular Models**
The initial model of Tamura [25] consists, after craniotomy and opening of the dura mater, of electrocoagulation of the MCA and then of sectioning the artery portion occluded. Although this model results in a rather reproducible damage, the main disadvantage is the permanency of the ischemia. Reperfusion was achieved later in alternative models by using surgical clip [26], snare ligature [27], or hook [28]. In these models, the greater variability of brain lesion compared with electrocoagulation was improved by combining MCA occlusion with the occlusion of one or both CCA [29,30].

In the early 1990s, endothelin-1, a potent vasoconstrictor agent, was topically applied to the surface of exposed MCA, after craniotomy, to induce ischemia [31]. This model was later modified for a stereotaxic intracerebral injection method [32]. The main disadvantage is that ischemia duration cannot be easily controlled unless the dose is carefully standardized.

17.2.2.2 Photothrombosis Model

Chemically induced thromboembolism can be achieved by systemic injection of a photosensitive dye, Rose Bengal, in combination with irradiation by a light beam positioned onto the skull. Initially developed in rats [33], this model was later modified for mice [34]. Local activation of Rose Bengal results in free radical formation, disturbance of endothelial function, and thrombus formation. A disadvantage of this model is early vasogenic edema and blood-brain barrier (BBB) breakdown, resulting in a rapid evolving ischemic damage without salvageable penumbra; the infarct size is then hardly responsive to neuroprotective therapies, which limits the use of this model. However, photochemically induced infarcts cause long-term sensorimotor deficits, allow long-term survival, and are particularly suitable to assess the effectiveness of neuroregenerative therapies in chronic stroke studies [35].

More recently, new models, developed after several modifications of the "Watson's model," demonstrated evidence of a penumbra region and ischemia reversal after rt-PA treatment [11].

17.2.2.3 Intraluminal Occlusion Model

This model, originally described in Ref. [36] in rats, was later modified by others [37] and adapted for mice [38]. This method, which requires no craniotomy, has many variants depending on the thread used and the additional occluded vessels, but basically it consists of inserting a thread into the internal carotid artery (ICA) and advancing it until its tip occludes the origin of the MCA. The great advantage is that the thread can be either left into place for permanent occlusion or withdrawn at any time to allow reperfusion. A laser Doppler flowmetry probe, placed directly onto the skull downstream the occlusion site, is commonly used to verify the correct placement of the thread. Among the technical factors that may influence the severity of brain damage [10,39], the thread employed appears to play a key role (discussed in Ref. [6]). Moreover, one important complication is the onset of subarachnoid hemorrhages secondary to arterial rupture after thread insertion, which can be reduced by coating the thread tip. Although this model is currently the most widely used model of focal cerebral ischemia, it does not mimic the mechanism of occlusion in humans, as human strokes are most often caused by thromboembolism.

17.2.2.4 Thromboembolic Models

Thromboembolic ischemia can be induced by various approaches and the most common one consists of injecting *blood clots* (auto- or heterologous) directly into the circulation, without craniotomy. First described in dogs [40], this model was subsequently adapted for rats almost 30 years later [41]. As these early models had several disadvantages, such as variable and inhomogeneous infarction caused by multiple small clots, spontaneous recanalization, or controlateral strokes, they were later improved: the injection of a suspension of small clot fragments into the ICA was then replaced by introducing a single larger and standardized blood clot close to the MCA origin *via* a catheter, using an approach similar to the intraluminal occlusion model [42]. Another important point to take into consideration is the choice of the blood clot [6], as fibrin-rich clots appear more sensitive to thrombolysis with rt-PA.

Besides blood clots, microspheres have also been used to produce *artificial embolization* [43]. However, the resulting infarcts were multifocal and the reproducibility was quite low, which led to replace microspheres with macrospheres to surmount these issues [44]. In any case, the major disadvantage of these approaches is the permanency of ischemia.

An alternative approach is the *in situ induction of thrombus formation*. To this end, thrombin can be injected either at the origin of the MCA *via* an intraluminal catheter introduced into the ICA [45] or directly into the distal MCA after craniotomy [46]. In this latter model, we have demonstrated that rt-PA infusion at an early or delayed stage after MCA occlusion closely mimics both beneficial and deleterious effects of thrombolysis observed in clinical situation [47]. Moreover, a magnetic resonance imaging (MRI) study confirmed the invaluable value of this model, although with a slight note of caution [48]. Indeed, the authors reported a significant rate of spontaneous reperfusion in the first hours of clot formation, suggesting differential evolution of the clot like in human stroke, and consequently they call for extended MRI follow-up at the acute stage in studies. More recently, Karatas *et al.* [49] introduced a novel model produced by topical application of a $FeCl_3$-soaked filter paper strip on the dura mater over the trunk of the distal MCA, but contrary to other thromboembolic models, reperfusion with rt-PA was obtained in only half of the mice. Clot composition may certainly explain the lower efficiency of thrombolysis in this model. Indeed, thrombin cleaves fibrinogen and activates factor XIII to generate a fibrin-rich clot containing a low number of cells and platelets, whereas $FeCl_3$ induces free radical formation and endothelial damage resulting in the production of a mixed thrombus containing fibrin, platelets, and red blood cells.

The great advantage of all these thromboembolic models (except micro- or macrospheres) is their close similarity to human ischemic stroke and, most importantly, they are suitable for studying thrombolysis with rt-PA. Indeed, transient mechanical occlusion of the MCA, by intraluminal thread insertion for example, induces prompt recirculation, whereas, after thrombolysis with rt-PA, recirculation is gradually restored and then reflects the hemodynamic aspect of thrombolysis that commonly occurs in clinical situation [24].

17.3
Traumatic Brain Injury Models

A critical point to take into account about TBI concerns the type of damage: focal or diffuse injury. However, it is largely demonstrated that a defined focal brain injury model also induces diffuse injury throughout the brain. Thus, this distinction has been progressively replaced by another classification of TBI models based on the presence or absence of craniotomy before brain trauma.

17.3.1
TBI Models with Craniotomy

In these models, the dura mater is surgically exposed in order to deliver the calibrated cortical impact. Different severity can be achieved by the modulation of pressure, velocity, diameter, and localization of the impact.

17.3.1.1 Weight-Drop Model
This model developed by Feeney induces a direct cortical contusion through the intact dura mater [50].

17.3.1.2 Lateral Fluid Percussion Model
Initially developed in cats and rabbits [51,52], this model was then adapted for rodents [53,54]. Injury is produced by a rapid impact of a fluid bolus against the intact dural surface. This model reproduces aspects of mechanical, physiological, neurological, and histological responses of the human TBI. Two types of fluid percussion (FP) can be found in the literature: midline or central FP (CFP) model, which involves central (vertex) positioning of the craniotomy site at the midline between bregma and lambda; and the lateral model of FP (LFP), which positions the craniotomy site over the temporoparietal region [55]. CFP injury is limited to mild and moderate severity as higher severity is associated with brain stem compression and respiratory arrest. With the LFP, mild severity injury occurs at 1.8–2.2 atm, moderate injury at 2.4–2.8 atm, and severe injury at pressures higher than 2.8 atm. This model is associated with sensorimotor and cognitive deficits from days to months after TBI [56–58]. However, despite its widespread use during the 1990s, this model is variable as the generation of a pressure wave is highly sensitive to external factors.

17.3.1.3 Controlled Cortical Impact Model
The controlled cortical impact (CCI) was adapted from similar methods employed in experimental spinal cord injury studies. Even if CCI model has numerous similarities with the FP model, it employs pressurized air to drive a rigid impactor delivering mechanical energy onto the exposed and intact dura mater. A number of advantages include the ability to control deformation parameters such as time, velocity, and depth impact. In addition, the risk for a rebound injury is absent, which makes this model superior to devices that are guided by gravity of a free-falling guided weight. This injury was first characterized in the ferret [59] and was later adapted for rodents. Different variants of CCI have been proposed such as central and lateral impact with dura mater, and direct cortical impact without dura mater [60]. It is the most often used TBI model.

17.3.2
TBI Models without Craniotomy

These models reproduce a direct impact of the skull (impact/acceleration) or an acceleration/deceleration. The impact initiates the propagation of a wave through the skull and the brain and mimics the results of a fall. In contrast, acceleration/deceleration brain injury results from unrestricted head movement at the moment of injury such as seen in motor vehicle accidents.

The severity of head trauma can be achieved by using different weights and/or heights of the weight-drop model. The high mortality rate can be reduced by early respiratory support and the use of animals with a certain age and weight. In general, mild injury is associated with a diffuse injury pattern, whereas more severe injury produces a focal contusion. A major advantage of these models is that they can be performed quickly.

17.3.2.1 Weight-Drop Model
The skull is exposed to a free-falling guided weight [61–64]. Later, Shohami and coworkers introduced a new rodent model using a more standardized weight-drop device [65].

17.3.2.2 Impact/Acceleration Model
This model, also called "Marmarou's model," is induced by a free-falling guided weight to produce focal brain injury that is distributed widely over the skull through a protection helmet to avoid skull fracture. The impact from a large blunt weight causes acceleration of the head and minor contact phenomena leading predominantly to diffuse shear forces [66,67]. Since the mass and height of the weight can be varied, the post-traumatic response to this model has been characterized over a broad range of severities. The impact/acceleration remains a useful model for the production of diffuse brain injury.

17.3.2.3 Acceleration/Deceleration Model
Because a high percentage of patients are subjected to rotational forces leading to diffuse brain injury, a model of inertial acceleration injury was originally developed in the 1970s using the nonhuman primate [68]. This model, more recently characterized using the minipig, is the only available model inducing an axonal injury widely and deeply distributed in the white matter and at the junction between the white and the gray matter. However, due to high cost, and lack of availability to multiple laboratories and of neurobehavioral characterization, this model remains rarely used.

17.3.3
Blast Injury Models

Recently, new experimental models of TBI have appeared as exposure to blast has become frequent in military populations. Blast-related neurological lesion research began in 1915 during World War I, when many soldiers were exposed to a detonation with no external head injury but suffered from neurological disorders. This form of trauma is often described as combat stress or post-traumatic stress disorder (PTSD). Blast wave has a significant role in promoting brain injury. In addition, localized pulmonary blast injury provokes indirect brain injury as it has been reported that the primary effects of the blast on the lungs can result in air emboli [69]. The latter obstruct the blood vessels and subsequently reduce the blood supply to different organs including the brain. The blast injury can be classified into four types:

- *Primary blast injury:* This results from the infiltration of the blast wave through tissues and is determined by factors such as peak pressure, duration, and shape of the wave.
- *Secondary blast injury:* This is due to the impact of flying objects such as fragments and generates penetrating injuries.
- *Tertiary blast injury:* This occurs when the victim's body or head strikes surrounding objects or the ground and subsequently causes head injury and skull fracture.
- *Quaternary blast injury:* This results from heat, smoke, toxic gases, dust, or emission of electromagnetic pulses.

Models of blast injury include *open-field exposure to blast* in desert areas of different animal species and sizes [70,71]. *Blast tubes for explosives* can also be used. Anesthetized rat is mounted in the blast tube at a distance of 1 m from 5 g pentaerythritol tetranitrate, creating a peak pressure exceeding 10 bar during detonation [72]. Alternatively, *shock tubes with compressed air or gas* are used [73]. Compressed gas is loaded into one of the two chambers separated by a diaphragm. The rupture of the latter causes the entry of compressed gas and simulates a propagating blast wave [74–76]. An experimental *model of fragment penetration* has recently been published [77]. Anesthetized rat is placed in a stereotaxic frame and a craniotomy is performed. A lead bullet is accelerated by air pressure in a designed rifle and impacts a secondary projectile. The pin of the secondary guided projectile penetrates the surface of the brain with a speed of 100 m/s. The base of the projectile is surrounded by a compressible ring that provides control of the penetration depth into the brain, usually set to 5 mm. Finally, *penetrating ballistic brain injury model* has been designed to mimic both the permanent injury tract created by the path of the bullet itself and the large temporary cavity generated by energy dissipation from a penetrating object [78].

17.3.4
Repetitive TBI Models

In the United States, 1 000 000 people sustained a TBI every year. A significant proportion is sports-related TBI with an annual estimated incidence of 300 000 cases [79]. In order to fix this problem, researchers performed repeated TBI experiments. It is defined as an initial mechanical injury on the head followed by another mechanical insult on the head of the same or different degree. Until the previous century, only few studies were published showing selflessness in this field [80–82]. Thereafter, repetitive TBI models have been developed in the mouse using the weight-drop model [83,84] and in the rat using the FP model [85]. Unlike more severe levels of brain injury, mild TBI do not induce preconditioning or tolerance to repeated mild insult. These studies are particularly interesting as there is a correlation between the occurrence of TBI and further development of neurodegenerative disease later in life. TBI is considered to be one of the major risk factors for developing Alzheimer's disease [86].

17.4
Outcome Assessment

As suggested in STAIR and other recommendations [1,7,87], preclinical studies must follow more than one outcome measure. The two most common are infarct sizes and neurobehavioral deficits (generally, sensorimotor deficit).

The first concern with *infarct assessment* is "what to count, what to measure, and when?" [88]. Traditional methods include staining with triphenyltetrazolium chloride, hematoxylin/eosin, Nissl, or cresyl violet (Figure 17.1). A correction factor is usually applied based on the swelling of the ipsilateral hemisphere to avoid overestimation of infarct volume [11]. One has to consider the day of assessment as brain infiltration of blood cells and astrogliosis may be a source of an underestimation of the lesion. Although these techniques are generally simple and reproducible, they lack the ability to specify which cell type is degenerating. Some methods are considered more specific for a cell type, such as Fluoro-Jade, which labels degenerative neuron [89]. Noninvasive MRI methods, which are increasingly used to assess treatment efficiency in animal models, play a pivotal role in stroke and TBI management and also present the advantage to allow monitoring the progression of brain damage [20,48,90].

Behavioral assessment represents an essential component of the preclinical testing of drugs targeting the acute and chronic stages of stroke and TBI, but is also more challenging to accurately assess in animal models as neurological deficit can rapidly resolve in rodents. Over the years, several behavioral tests were developed for quantifying the injury severity and the efficiency of a treatment (see Refs [10,91–93] for reviews). The choice of functional tests strongly depends on the animal model used. As each test is sensitive to measuring deficits associated with a

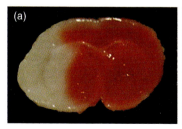
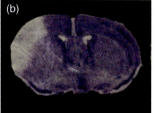

Figure 17.1 Representative photographs of coronal brain sections after (a) triphenyltetrazolium chloride and (b) cresyl violet staining. Mouse brain sections were obtained 24 h after permanent MCA occlusion induced by (a) thread insertion and (b) thrombin *in situ* injection. Infarcts appear as pale areas.

particular area of damage, it is useful to employ a battery of tests. Some complications of stroke and TBI models may have direct impact on behavioral outcomes. Indeed, body weight loss, muscle atrophy, stress, hyperthermia, immunodepression, or infections may impair performance in certain behavioral tasks and bias the treatment effect. For reasons such as smaller size and lesser intelligence, behavioral testing can be more challenging in mice than in rats. Strain differences in the response of stroke and TBI have also been reported. One has to be aware of the fact that testing functional outcome needs to be performed in a blinded fashion, and is extremely time-consuming and labor intensive.

Among deficits, some reflexes are transiently lost [94,95]. Individual reflexes reflect reasonably well motor components of the clinical scales that are commonly used in the acute phase in ischemic and traumatized patients. Currently, the authors use composite scores such as Bederson scale, neurological severity score (NSS), and a modified version (mNSS) (Table 17.1) [91]. In addition, vestibulomotor

Table 17.1 Detailed description of the mNSS.

Motor tests	
Raising rat by tail (normal = 0, maximum = 3)	3
Flexion of forelimb	1
Flexion of hind limb	1
Head moved >10° to vertical axis within 30 s	1
Placing rat on floor (normal = 0, maximum = 3)	3
Normal walk	0
Inability to walk straight	1
Circling toward the paretic side	2
Falls down to paretic side	3
Sensory tests (normal = 0, maximum = 2)	2
Placing test (visual and tactile tests)	1
Proprioceptive test (deep sensation, pushing paw against table edge to stimulate limb muscles)	1
Beam balance tests (normal = 0, maximum = 6)	6
Balance with steady posture	0
Grasps side of beam	1
Hugs beam and one limb falls down from beam	2
Hugs beam and two limbs fall down from beam, or spins on beam (>60 s)	3
Attempts to balance on but falls off (>40 s)	4
Attempts to balance on but falls off (>20 s)	5
Falls off; no attempt to balance or hang on the beam (<20 s)	6
Reflex absence and abnormal movements (normal = 0, maximum = 4)	4
Pinna reflex (head shake when auditory meatus is touched)	1
Corneal reflex (eye blink when cornea is lightly touched with cotton)	1
Startle reflex (motor response to a brief noise from clapping hands)	1
Seizures, myoclonus, myodystonia	1
Total maximum points	18

One point is given for an absent reflex tested or for the animal's inability to perform a task.
Final score: 1–6 = mild injury, 7–12 = moderate injury, 13–18 = severe injury.

tests determine the degree of motor coordination using rotating pole [96,97], beam balance [98,99], beam walk [100], rotarod [99,101], and rope grip [102]. Sensorimotor deficits could be assessed using adhesive removal test [103,104]. The most common and persistent deficits are cognitive functions. These dysfunctions may directly contribute to poor outcomes causing personal, social, and educational consequences. Unfortunately, most cognitive tests, including neuropsychological tests, are not designed to reflect the complexity of the "real life." However, laboratory tests typically rely on performance in a variety of hippocampal-dependent spatial mazes such as the commonly used Morris water maze evaluating the learning memory [91,99,105] and the 8-arm radial maze evaluating the working memory [91,96].

Similar to clinical trials, long-term outcome measures should be performed to evaluate a new pharmacological agent and ascertain that experimental results bear sufficient clinical relevance [104,106,107].

17.5
Translation to Clinics: Limitations and Difficulties

17.5.1
The Actual Target: From the Neuron to the Neurogliovascular Unit

Although stroke and TBI affect all brain cells in both gray and white matters, researchers mainly focused on neuronal death for many years. Today it is well established that protective strategies have to target not only neurons, the noble but the more vulnerable of CNS cells, but also other cell types such as glial (astrocytes, microglia, and oligodendrocytes) and vascular cells (endothelial cells, smooth muscle cells, and pericytes).

Besides its beneficial fibrinolytic activity leading to reperfusion, rt-PA also induces neuronal [108] and vascular toxicity [109]. Indeed, rt-PA-induced reperfusion alters microcirculation notably by oxidative and nitrosative stresses leading to BBB permeability, hemorrhagic transformation, and vasogenic edema [47,110,111]. This emphasizes the need to identify adjunct therapy in order to improve its safety. Moreover, microvascular protection is necessary for successful neuroprotection, indicating the critical importance of the "neurovascular unit" [112].

The implication of these multiple cell types can be illustrated by the various effects of oligodendrocyte precursor cells that migrate toward the lesion and participate in matrix metalloproteinase-9 release, early BBB leakage, polymorphonuclear neutrophil infiltration, demyelination, and cognitive deficits in a mouse model of prolonged cerebral hypoperfusion [113].

Considering the interrelationship between all the different cells, a future therapeutic strategy should target the "neurogliovascular unit." As numerous molecular mechanisms contribute to the complexity of stroke and TBI, drugs targeting only one mechanism failed to protect the whole unit. Consequently, pleiotropic drugs controlling multiple deleterious biochemical pathways demonstrated considerable beneficial effects in experimental studies and show maximum promise for success in clinical trials [100,114–119].

17.5.2
From Bench to Bedside to Bench: Recommendations for Improving the Translational Research

Animal models of stroke and TBI are an essential step toward a better understanding of the pathophysiology of these pathologies and the development of novel therapies. The failure of bench to bedside translation might be overcome by modifying several preclinical practices [7,120]. In particular, to increase translation potential of preclinical studies, an important consideration should be to incorporate more testing in females, as the susceptibility to injury differs between genders [121,122]. Indeed, it is recognized that women carry a higher stroke burden than the male population [123,124]. Moreover, preclinical studies have clearly shown that the death pathways activated by ischemia differ between males and females [125]. For example, PARP-1 activation and NAD depletion play an important role in ischemic cell death in males but not in females. Indeed, PARP-1 deletion reduces infarct volume in males, whereas it increases brain lesion in females. Among other mechanisms implicated in gender vulnerability to ischemic brain damage, a greater increase in NADPH oxidase 2-dependent superoxide production by T lymphocytes has been shown in male mice after reperfusion [126]. This sexual dimorphism may be related to the marked anti-inflammatory effect of estrogen and shows the urge to include females in preclinical studies.

In addition, preclinical studies should also take into account comorbidities such as age, hypertension, a major cause of stroke, and diabetes mellitus that increases cerebrovascular inflammation and constitutes a major limitation to thrombolysis [127]. Most studies are mainly performed in young animals and too rarely in aged subjects [128]. However, advanced age results in a reduced capacity of tissue regeneration and impairs neovascularization and endothelial precursor cells recruitment to the injury site [129]. To date, several animal models of stroke-related risk factors have been developed [130,131].

Finally, experimental studies should also enlarge the scope to white matter as it plays an important role in some of the neurobehavioral consequences of stroke and TBI [132]. In light of the growing interest in the understanding of white matter events [133], it is essential to develop appropriate animal models. Some have been well detailed in recently published reviews [133–135].

In conclusion, the ground for a robust and relevant preclinical evaluation of drugs requires testing on different experimental models to mimic at best the heterogeneity of clinical situations [136,137]. The decades of failure from bench to bedside translation clearly demonstrates that research in this field is especially difficult, but we should not give up as the potential therapeutic applications are so great!

References

1 STAIR (1999) Recommendations for standards regarding preclinical neuroprotective and restorative drug development. *Stroke*, **30** (12), 2752–2758.

2 Wechsler, L.R. (2011) Intravenous thrombolytic therapy for acute ischemic stroke. *The New England Journal of Medicine*, **364** (22), 2138–2146.

3 Ginsberg, M.D. (2008) Neuroprotection for ischemic stroke: past, present and future. *Neuropharmacology*, **55** (3), 363–389.

4 Bramlett, H.M. and Dietrich, W.D. (2004) Pathophysiology of cerebral ischemia and brain trauma: similarities and differences. *Journal of Cerebral Blood Flow and Metabolism*, **24** (2), 133–150.

5 Laplaca, M.C., Simon, C.R., Prado, G.R., and Cullen, D.K. (2007) CNS injury biomechanics and experimental models. *Progress in Brain Research*, **161**, 13–26.

6 Howells, D.W., Porritt, M.J., Rewell, S.S., O'Collins, V., Sena, E.S., van der Worp, H.B., Traystman, R.J., and Macleod, M.R. (2010) Different strokes for different folks: the rich diversity of animal models of focal cerebral ischemia. *Journal of Cerebral Blood Flow and Metabolism*, **30** (8), 1412–1431.

7 Marklund, N. and Hillered, L. (2011) Animal modelling of traumatic brain injury in preclinical drug development: where do we go from here? *British Journal of Pharmacology*, **164**, 1207–1229.

8 Braeuninger, S. and Kleinschnitz, C. (2009) Rodent models of focal cerebral ischemia: procedural pitfalls and translational problems. *Experimental & Translational Stroke Medicine*, **1**, 8.

9 Albert-Weissenberger, C. and Sirén, A.L. (2010) Experimental traumatic brain injury. *Experimental & Translational Stroke Medicine*, **2** (1), 16.

10 Lipsanen, A. and Jolkkonen, J. (2011) Experimental approaches to study functional recovery following cerebral ischemia. *Cellular and Molecular Life Sciences*, **68** (18), 3007–3017.

11 Macrae, I.M. (2011) Preclinical stroke research: advantages and disadvantages of the most common rodent models of focal ischaemia. *British Journal of Pharmacology*, **164** (4), 1062–1078.

12 Mergenthaler, P. and Meisel, A. (2012) Do stroke models model stroke? *Disease Models & Mechanisms*, **5** (6), 718–725.

13 Xiong, Y., Mahmood, A., and Chopp, M. (2013) Animal models of traumatic brain injury. *Nature Reviews. Neuroscience*, **14** (2), 128–142.

14 Statler, K.D., Kochanek, P.M., Dixon, C.E., Alexander, H.L., Warner, D.S., Clark, R.S., Wisniewski, S.R., Graham, S.H., Jenkins, L.W., Marion, D.W., and Safar, P.J. (2000) Isoflurane improves long-term neurological outcome versus fentanyl after traumatic brain injury in rats. *Journal of Neurotrauma*, **17**, 1179–1189.

15 Tecoult, E., Mésenge, C., Stutzmann, A.M., Plotkine, M., and Wahl, F. (2000) Influence of anesthesia protocol in experimental traumatic brain injury. *Journal of Neurosurgical Anesthesiology*, **12** (3), 255–261.

16 O'Connor, C.A., Cernak, I., and Vink, R. (2003) Interaction between anesthesia, gender, and functional outcome task following diffuse traumatic brain injury in rats. *Journal of Neurotrauma*, **20** (6), 533–541.

17 Luh, C., Gierth, K., Timaru-Kast, R., Engelhard, K., Werner, C., and Thal, S.C. (2011) Influence of a brief episode of anesthesia during the induction of experimental brain trauma on secondary brain damage and inflammation. *PLoS One*, **6** (5), e19948.

18 Thal, S.C., Luh, C., Schaible, E.V., Timaru-Kast, R., Hedrich, J., Luhmann, H.J., Engelhard, K., and Zehendner, C.M. (2012) Volatile anesthetics influence blood–brain barrier integrity by modulation of tight junction protein expression in traumatic brain injury. *PLoS One*, **7** (12), e50752.

19 Traystman, R.J. (2003) Animal models of focal and global cerebral ischemia. *The ILAR Journal*, **44** (2), 85–95.

20 Hossmann, K.A. (2008) Cerebral ischemia: models, methods and outcomes. *Neuropharmacology*, **55** (3), 257–270.

21 Woodruff, T.M., Thundyil, J., Tang, S.C., Sobey, C.G., Taylor, S.M., and Arumugam, T.V. (2011) Pathophysiology, treatment, and animal and cellular models of human

22 Pulsinelli, W.A. and Brierley, J.B. (1979) A new model of bilateral hemispheric ischemia in the unanesthetized rat. *Stroke*, **10** (3), 267–272.

23 Smith, M.L., Auer, R.N., and Siesjö, B.K. (1984) The density and distribution of ischemic brain injury in the rat following 2–10 min of forebrain ischemia. *Acta Neuropathologica*, **64** (4), 319–332.

24 Hossmann, K.A. (2012) The two pathophysiologies of focal brain ischemia: implications for translational stroke rescarch. *Journal of Cerebral Blood Flow and Metabolism*, **32** (7), 1310–1316.

25 Tamura, A., Graham, D.I., McCulloch, J., and Teasdale, G.M. (1981) Focal cerebral ischaemia in the rat: 1. Description of technique and early neuropathological consequences following middle cerebral artery occlusion. *Journal of Cerebral Blood Flow and Metabolism*, **1** (1), 53–60.

26 Dietrich, W.D., Nakayama, H., Watson, B.D., and Kanemitsu, H. (1989) Morphological consequences of early reperfusion following thrombotic or mechanical occlusion of the rat middle cerebral artery. *Acta Neuropathologica*, **78** (6), 605–614.

27 Shigeno, T., Teasdale, G.M., McCulloch, J., and Graham, DI. (1985) Recirculation model following MCA occlusion in rats. Cerebral blood flow, cerebrovascular permeability, and brain edema. *Journal of Neurosurgery*, **63** (2), 272–277.

28 Kaplan, B., Brint, S., Tanabe, J., Jacewicz, M., Wang, X.J., and Pulsinelli, W. (1991) Temporal thresholds for neocortical infarction in rats subjected to reversible focal cerebral ischemia. *Stroke*, **22** (8), 1032–1039.

29 Chen, S.T., Hsu, C.Y., Hogan, E.L., Maricq, H., and Balentine, J.D. (1986) A model of focal ischemic stroke in the rat: reproducible extensive cortical infarction. *Stroke*, **17** (4), 738–743.

30 Brint, S., Jacewicz, M., Kiessling, M., Tanabe, J., and Pulsinelli, W. (1988) Focal brain ischemia in the rat: methods for reproducible neocortical infarction using tandem occlusion of the distal middle cerebral and ipsilateral common carotid arteries. *Journal of Cerebral Blood Flow and Metabolism*, **8** (4), 474–485.

31 Robinson, M.J., Macrae, I.M., Todd, M., Reid, J.L., and McCulloch, J. (1990) Reduction of local cerebral blood flow to pathological levels by endothelin-1 applied to the middle cerebral artery in the rat. *Neuroscience Letters*, **118** (2), 269–272.

32 Sharkey, J., Ritchie, I.M., and Kelly, P.A. (1993) Perivascular microapplication of endothelin-1: a new model of focal cerebral ischaemia in the rat. *Journal of Cerebral Blood Flow and Metabolism*, **13** (5), 865–871.

33 Watson, B.D., Dietrich, W.D., Busto, R., Wachtel, M.S., and Ginsberg, M.D. (1985) Induction of reproducible brain infarction by photochemically initiated thrombosis. *Annals of Neurology*, **17** (5), 497–504.

34 Schroeter, M., Jander, S., and Stoll, G. (2002) Non-invasive induction of focal cerebral ischemia in mice by photothrombosis of cortical microvessels: characterization of inflammatory responses. *Journal of Neuroscience Methods*, **117** (1), 43–49.

35 Schmidt, A., Hoppen, M., Strecker, J.K., Diederich, K., Schäbitz, W.R., Schilling, M., and Minnerup, J. (2012) Photochemically induced ischemic stroke in rats. *Experimental & Translational Stroke Medicine*, **4** (1), 13.

36 Koizumi, J., Yoshida, Y., Nakazawa, T., and Ooneda, G. (1986) Experimental studies of ischemic brain edema. 1. A new experimental model of experimental embolism in rats in which recirculation can be reintroduced in the ischemic area. *Japanese Journal of Stroke*, **8**, 1–8.

37 Longa, E.Z., Weinstein, P.R., Carlson, S., and Cummins, R. (1989) Reversible middle cerebral artery occlusion without craniectomy in rats. *Stroke*, **20** (1), 84–91.

38 Clark, W.M., Lessov, N.S., Dixon, M.P., and Eckenstein, F. (1997) Monofilament intraluminal middle cerebral artery occlusion in the mouse. *Neurological Research*, **19** (6), 641–648.

39 Sicard, K.M. and Fisher, M. (2009) Animal models of focal brain ischemia. *Experimental & Translational Stroke Medicine*, **1**, 7.

40. Hill, N.C., Millikan, C.H., Wakim, K.G., and Sayre, G.P. (1955) Studies in cerebrovascular disease. VII. Experimental production of cerebral infarction by intracarotid injection of homologous blood clot; preliminary report. *Proceedings of the Staff Meetings of the Mayo Clinic*, **30** (26), 625–633.

41. Kudo, M., Aoyama, A., Ichimori, S., and Fukunaga, N. (1982) An animal model of cerebral infarction. Homologous blood clot emboli in rats. *Stroke*, **13** (4), 505–508.

42. Dinapoli, V.A., Rosen, C.L., Nagamine, T., and Crocco, T. (2006) Selective MCA occlusion: a precise embolic stroke model. *Journal of Neuroscience Methods*, **154** (1–2), 233–238.

43. Zivin, J.A., DeGirolami, U., Kochhar, A., Lyden, P.D., Mazzarella, V., Hemenway, C.C., and Henry, M.E. (1987) A model for quantitative evaluation of embolic stroke therapy. *Brain Research*, **435** (1–2), 305–309.

44. Gerriets, T., Li, F., Silva, M.D., Meng, X., Brevard, M., Sotak, C.H., and Fisher, M. (2003) The macrosphere model: evaluation of a new stroke model for permanent middle cerebral artery occlusion in rats. *Journal of Neuroscience Methods*, **122** (2), 201–211.

45. Zhang, Z., Zhang, R.L., Jiang, Q., Raman, S.B., Cantwell, L., and Chopp, M. (1997) A new rat model of thrombotic focal cerebral ischemia. *Journal of Cerebral Blood Flow and Metabolism*, **17** (2), 123–135.

46. Orset, C., Macrez, R., Young, A.R., Panthou, D., Angles-Cano, E., Maubert, E., Agin, V., and Vivien, D. (2007) Mouse model of *in situ* thromboembolic stroke and reperfusion. *Stroke*, **38** (10), 2771–2778.

47. El Amki, M., Lerouet, D., Coqueran, B., Curis, E., Orset, C., Vivien, D., Plotkine, M., Marchand-Leroux, C., and Margaill, I. (2012) Experimental modeling of recombinant tissue plasminogen activator effects after ischemic stroke. *Experimental Neurology*, **238** (2), 138–144.

48. Durand, A., Chauveau, F., Cho, T.H., Bolbos, R., Langlois, J.B., Hermitte, L., Wiart, M., Berthezène, Y., and Nighoghossian, N. (2012) Spontaneous reperfusion after *in situ* thromboembolic stroke in mice. *PLoS One*, **7** (11), e50083.

49. Karatas, H., Erdener, S.E., Gursoy-Ozdemir, Y., Gurer, G., Soylemezoglu, F., Dunn, A.K., and Dalkara, T. (2011) Thrombotic distal middle cerebral artery occlusion produced by topical $FeCl_3$ application: a novel model suitable for intravital microscopy and thrombolysis studies. *Journal of Cerebral Blood Flow and Metabolism*, **31** (6), 1452–1460.

50. Feeney, D.M., Boyeson, M.G., Linn, R.T., Murray, H.M., and Dail, W.G. (1981) Responses to cortical injury: I. Methodology and local effects of contusions in the rat. *Brain Research*, **211**, 67–77.

51. Hayes, R.L., Stalhammar, D., Povlishock, J.T., Allen, A.M., Galinat, B.J., Becker, D.P., and Stonnington, H.H. (1987) A new model of concussive brain injury in the cat produced by extradural fluid volume loading: II. Physiological and neuropathological observations. *Brain Injury*, **1**, 93–112.

52. Stalhammar, D., Galinat, B.J., Allen, A.M., Becker, D.P., Stonnington, H., and Hayes, R.L. (1987) A new model of concussive brain injury in the cat produced by extradural fluid volume loading: I. Biomechanical properties. *Brain Injury*, **1**, 73–91.

53. Dixon, C.E., Lyeth, B.G., Povlishock, J.T., Findling, R.L., Hamm, R.J., Marmarou, A., Young, H.F., and Hayes, R.L. (1987) A fluid percussion model of experimental brain injury in the rat. *Journal of Neurosurgery*, **67** (1), 110–119.

54. McIntosh, T.K., Vink, R., Noble, L., Yamakami, I., Fernyak, S., Soares, H., and Faden, A.L. (1989) Traumatic brain injury in the rat: characterization of a lateral fluid-percussion model. *Neuroscience*, **28** (1), 233–244.

55. Besson, V.C., Croci, N., Boulu, R.G., Plotkine, M., and Marchand-Verrecchia, C. (2003) Deleterious poly(ADP-ribose) polymerase-1 pathway activation in traumatic brain injury in rat. *Brain Research*, **989** (1), 58–66.

56. Thompson, H.J., Lifshitz, J., Marklund, N., Sean Grady, M., Graham, D.I., Hovda, D.A., and McIntosh, T.K. (2005) Lateral fluid

percussion brain injury: a 15-year review and evaluation. *Journal of Neurotrauma*, **22** (1), 42–75.

57 Kabadi, S.V., Hilton, G.D., Stoica, B.A., Zapple, D.N., and Faden, A.I. (2010) Fluid percussion-induced traumatic brain injury model in rat. *Nature Protocols*, **5** (8), 1–12.

58 Alder, J., Fujioka, W., Lifshitz, J., Crockett, D.P., and Thakker-Varia, S. (2011) Lateral fluid percussion: model of traumatic brain injury in mice. *Journal of Visualized Experiments*, **54**, 3063. doi: 10.3791/3063.

59 Lighthall, J.W., Dixon, C.E., and Anderson, T.E. (1988) Experimental models of brain injury. *Journal of Neurotrauma*, **6** (2), 83–97.

60 Cernak, I. (2005) Animal models of head trauma. *NeuroRx*, **2** (3), 410–422.

61 Hall, E.D. (1985) High-dose glucocorticoid treatment improves neurological recovery in head-injured mice. *Journal of Neurosurgery*, **62** (6), 882–887.

62 Mésenge, C., Verrecchia, C., Allix, M., Boulu, R.R., and Plotkine, M. (1996) Reduction of the neurological deficit in mice with traumatic brain injury by nitric oxide synthase inhibitors. *Journal of Neurotrauma*, **13** (4), 209–214.

63 Kupina, N.C., Nath, R., Bernath, E.E., Inoue, J., Mitsuyoshi, A., Yuen, P.W., Wang, K.K.W., and Hall, E.D. (2001) The novel calpain inhibitor SJA6017 improves functional outcome after delayed administration in a mouse model of diffuse brain injury. *Journal of Neurotrauma*, **18** (11), 1229–1240.

64 Hellal, F., Pruneau, D., Palmier, B., Faye, P., Croci, N., Plotkine, M., and Marchand-Verrecchia, C. (2003) Detrimental role of bradykinin B2 receptor in a murine model of diffuse brain injury. *Journal of Neurotrauma*, **20** (9), 841–851.

65 Flierl, M.A., Stahel, P.F., Beauchamp, K.M., Morgan, S.J., Smith, W.R., and Shohami, E. (2009) Mouse closed head injury model induced by a weight-drop device. *Nature Protocols*, **4** (9), 1328–1337.

66 Marmarou, A., Foda, M.A., van den Brink, W., Campbell, J., Kita, H., and Demetriadou, K. (1994) A new model of diffuse brain injury in rats. Part I: pathophysiology and biomechanics. *Journal of Neurosurgery*, **80**, 291–300.

67 Foda, M.A. and Marmarou, A. (1994) A new model of diffuse brain injury in rats. Part II: morphological characterization. *Journal of Neurosurgery*, **80**, 301–313.

68 Gennarelli, T.A., Thibault, L.E., Adams, J.H., Graham, D.I., Thompson, C., and Marcincin, R.P. (1982) Diffuse axonal injury and traumatic coma in the primate. *Annals of Neurology*, **12**, 564–574.

69 Bass, C.R., Panzer, M.B., Rafaels, K.A., Wood, G., Shridharani, J., and Capehart, B. (2012) Brain injuries from blast. *Annals of Biomedical Engineering*, **40** (1), 185–202.

70 Rubovitch, V., Ten-Bosch, M., Zohar, O., Harrison, C.R., Tempel-Brami, C., Stein, E., Hoffer, B.J., Balaban, C.D., Schreiber, S., Chiu, W.T., and Pick, C.G. (2011) A mouse model of blast-induced mild traumatic brain injury. *Experimental Neurology*, **232**, 280–289.

71 Lu, J., Ng, K.C., Ling, G., Wu, J., Poon, D.J., Kan, E.M., Tan, M.H., Wu, Y.J., Li, P., Moochhala, S., Yap, E., Lee, L.K., Teo, M., Yeh, I.B., Sergio, D.M., Chua, F., Kumar, S.D., and Ling, E. (2011) Effect of blast exposure on the brain structure and cognition in *Macaca fascicularis*. *Journal of Neurotrauma*, **29** (7), 1434–1454.

72 Risling, M. and Davidsson, J. (2012) Experimental animal models for studies on the mechanisms of blast-induced neurotrauma. *Frontiers in Neurology*, **3**, 1–9.

73 Cernak, I., Merkle, A.C., Koliatsos, V.E., Bilik, J.M., Luong, Q.T., Mahota, T.M., Xu, L., Slack, N., Windle, D., and Ahmed, F.A. (2011) The pathobiology of blast injuries and blast-induced neurotrauma as identified using a new experimental model of injury in mice. *Neurobiology of Disease*, **41**, 538–551.

74 Alhers, S.T., Vasserman-Stokes, E., Saughness, M.C., Hall, A.A., Shera, D.A., Chavko, M., McCarron, R.M., and Stone, J.D. (2012) Assessment of the effects of acute repeated exposure to blast overpressure in rodents: toward a greater understanding of blast and the potential ramifications for injury in humans exposed to blast. *Frontiers in Neurology*, **3**, 1–12.

75 Arun, P., Oguntayo, S., Alamneh, Y., Honnold, C., Wang, Y., Valiyaveetil, M., Long, J.B., and Nambiar, M.P. (2012) Rapid release of tissue enzymes into blood after blast exposure: potential use as biological dosimeters. *PLoS One*, **7** (4), e33798.

76 Panzer, M.B., Matthews, K.A., Yu, A.W., Morrisson, B., 3rd, Meaney, D.F., and Bass, C.R. (2012) A multiscale approach to blast neurotrauma modelling: Part I. Development of novel test devices for *in vivo* and *in vitro* blast injury models. *Frontiers in Neurology*, **3**, 1–11.

77 Risling, M., Plantman, S., Ageria, M., Rostami, E., Bellander, B.M., Kirkegaard, M., Arborelius, U., and Davidsson, J. (2011) Mechanisms of blast induced brain injuries, experimental studies in rats. *NeuroImage*, **54** (1), S89–S97.

78 Williams, A.J., Hartings, J.A., Lu, X.C., Rolli, M.L., Dave, J.R., and Tortella, F.C. (2005) Characterization of a new rat model of penetrating ballistic brain injury. *Journal of Neurotrauma*, **22**, 313–331.

79 Sosin, D., Sniezek, J., and Thurman, D. (1999) Incidence of mild and moderate brain injury in the United States: a public health perspective. *The Journal of Head Trauma Rehabilitation*, **14**, 602–615.

80 Olsson, Y., Rinder, L., Lindgren, S., and Stalhammar, D. (1971) Studies on vascular permeability changes in experimental brain concussion: 3. A comparison between the effects of single and repeated sudden mechanical loading of the brain. *Acta Neuropathologica*, **19** (3), 225–233.

81 Weitbrecht, W.U. and Noetzel, H. (1976) Autoradiographic investigations in repeated experimental brain concussion. *Archiv für Psychiatrie und Nervenkrankheiten*, **223** (1), 59–68.

82 Kanayama, G., Takeda, M., Niigawa, H., Ikura, Y., Tamii, H., Taniguchi, N., Kudo, T., Miyamae, Y., Morihara, T., and Nishimura, T. (1996) The effects of repetitive mild brain injury on cytoskeletal protein and behavior. *Methods and Findings in Experimental and Clinical Pharmacology*, **18** (2), 105–115.

83 DeFord, S.M., Wilson, M.S., Rice, A.C., Clausen, T., Rice, L.K., Barabnova, A., Bullock, R., and Hamm, R.J. (2002) Repeated mild traumatic brain injuries result in cognitive impairment in B6C3F1. *Journal of Neurotrauma*, **19**, 427–438.

84 Creeley, C.E., Wozniak, D.F., Bayly, P.V., Olney, J.W., and Lewis, L.M. (2004) Multiple episodes of mild traumatic brain injury result in impaired cognitive performance in mice. *Academic Emergency Medicine*, **11**, 809–819.

85 DeRoss, A.L., Adams, J.E., Vane, D.W., Russell, S.J., Terella, A.M., and Wald, S.L. (2002) Multiple head injuries in rats: effects on behaviour. *Journal of Trauma*, **52**, 708–714.

86 Weber, J.T. (2007) Experimental models of repetitive brain injuries. *Progress in Brain Research*, **161**, 253–261.

87 Fisher, M., Feuerstein, G., Howells, D.W., Hurn, P.D., Kent, T.A., Savitz, S.I., and Lo, E.H. (2009) Update of the Stroke Therapy Academic Industry Roundtable Preclinical Recommendations. *Stroke*, **40** (6), 2244–2250.

88 Kazanis, I. (2005) CNS injury research; reviewing the last decade: methodological errors and a proposal for a new strategy. *Brain Research. Brain Research Reviews*, **50** (2), 377–386.

89 Gu, Q., Schmued, L.C., Sarkar, S., Paule, M.G., and Raymick, B. (2012) One-step labeling of degenerative neurons in unfixed brain tissue samples using Fluoro-Jade C. *Journal of Neuroscience Methods*, **208** (1), 40–43.

90 Kim, J.J. and Gean, A.D. (2011) Imaging for the diagnosis and management of traumatic brain injury. *Neurotherapeutics*, **8** (1), 39–53.

91 Schaar, K.L., Brenneman, M.M., and Savitz, S.I. (2010) Functional assessments in the rodent stroke model. *Experimental & Translational Stroke Medicine*, **2** (1), 13.

92 Balkaya, M., Kröber, J.M., Rex, A., and Endres, M. (2013) Assessing post-stroke behavior in mouse models of focal ischemia. *Journal of Cerebral Blood Flow and Metabolism*, **33** (3), 330–338.

93 Livingston-Thomas, J.M. and Tasker, R.A. (2013) Animal models of post-ischemic forced use rehabilitation: methods, considerations, and limitations. *Experimental & Translational Stroke Medicine*, **5** (1), 2.

94 Floyd, C.L., Golden, K.M., Black, R.T., Hamm, R.J., and Lyeth, B.G. (2002) Craniectomy position affects Morris water maze performance and hippocampal cell loss after parasagittal fluid percussion. *Journal of Neurotrauma*, **19**, 303–316.

95 Hallam, T.M., Floyd, C.L., Folkerts, M.M., Lee, L.L., Gong, Q.Z., Lyeth, B.G., Muizelaar, J.P., and Berman, R.F. (2004) Comparison of behavioural deficits and acute neuronal degeneration in rat lateral fluid percussion and weight-drop brain injury models. *Journal of Neurotrauma*, **21**, 521–539.

96 Piot-Grosjean, O., Wahl, F., Gobbo, O., and Stutzmann, J.M. (2001) Assessment of sensorimotor and cognitive deficits induced by a moderate traumatic brain injury in the right parietal cortex of the rat. *Neurobiology of Disease*, **8**, 1082–1093.

97 Hoover, R.C., Motta, M., Davis, J., Saatman, K.E., Fujimoto, S.T., Thompson, H.J., Stover, J.F., Ditcher, M.A., Twyman, R., White, H.S., and McIntosh, T.K. (2004) Differential effects of the anticonvulsant topiramate on neurobehavioral and histological outcomes following traumatic brain injury in rats. *Journal of Neurotrauma*, **21** (5), 501–512.

98 Alessandri, B., Rice, A.C., Levasseur, J., Deford, M., Hamm, R.J., and Bullock, M.R. (2002) Cyclosporin A improves brain tissue oxygen consumption and learning/memory performance after lateral fluid percussion injury in rats. *Journal of Neurotrauma*, **19**, 829–841.

99 Shear, D.A., Lu, X.C., Bombard, M.C., Pederson, R., Chen, Z., Davis, A., and Tortella, F.C. (2010) Longitudinal characterization of motor and cognitive deficits in a model of penetrating ballistic-like brain injury. *Journal of Neurotrauma*, **27** (10), 1911–1923.

100 Chen, X.R., Besson, V.C., Béziaud, T., Plotkine, M., and Marchand-Leroux, C. (2008) Fenofibrate and simvastatin synergistically exert neuroprotective effects in traumatic brain injury. *The Journal of Pharmacology and Experimental Therapeutics*, **326** (3), 966–974.

101 Hamm, R.J. (2001) Neurobehavioral assessment of outcome following traumatic brain injury in rats: an evaluation of selected measures. *Journal of Neurotrauma*, **18**, 1207–1216.

102 Long, J.B., Gordon, J., Bettencourt, J.A., and Bolt, S.L. (1996) Laser-Doppler flowmetry measurements of subcortical blood flow changes after fluid percussion brain injury in rats. *Journal of Neurotrauma*, **13** (3), 149–162.

103 Hoane, M.R., Tan, A.A., Pierce, J.L., Anderson, G.D., and Smith, D.C. (2006) Nicotinamide treatment reduces behavioural impairments and provides cortical protection after fluid percussion injury in the rat. *Journal of Neurotrauma*, **23** (10), 1535–1548.

104 Bouët, V., Freret, T., Toutain, J., Divoux, D., Boulouard, M., and Schumann-Bard, P. (2007) Sensorimotor and cognitive deficits after transient middle cerebral artery occlusion in the mouse. *Experimental Neurology*, **203** (2), 555–567.

105 Dixon, C.E., Ma, X., Kline, A.E., Yan, H.Q., Ferimer, H., Kochanek, P.M., Wisniewski, S.R., Jenkins, L.W., and Marion, D.W. (2003) Acute etomidate treatment reduces cognitive deficits and histopathology in rats with traumatic brain injury. *Critical Care Medicine*, **31** (8), 2222–2227.

106 Washington, P.M., Forcelli, P.A., Wilkins, T., Zapple, D.N., Parsadanian, M., and Burns, M.P. (2012) The effect of injury severity on behavior: a phenotypic study of cognitive and emotional deficits after mild, moderate and severe controlled cortical impact injury in mice. *Journal of Neurotrauma*, **29**, 2283–2296.

107 Balkaya, M., Kröber, J., Gertz, K., Peruzzaro, S., and Endres, M. (2013) Characterization of long-term functional outcome in a murine model of mild brain ischemia. *Journal of Neuroscience Methods*, **213** (2), 179–187.

108 Montagne, A., Hébert, M., Jullienne, A., Lesept, F., Le Béhot, A., Louessard, M., Gauberti, M., Orset, C., Ali, C., Agin, V., Maubert, E., and Vivien, D. (2012) Memantine improves safety of thrombolysis for stroke. *Stroke*, **43** (10), 2774–2781.

109 Lemarchant, S., Docagne, F., Emery, E., Vivien, D., Ali, C., and Rubio, M. (2012) tPA in the injured central nervous system:

different scenarios starring the same actor? *Neuropharmacology*, **62** (2), 749–756.

110 Machado, L.S., Sazonova, I.Y., Kozak, A., Wiley, D.C., El-Remessy, A.B., Ergul, A., Hess, D.C., Waller, J.L., and Fagan, S.C. (2009) Minocycline and tissue-type plasminogen activator for stroke: assessment of interaction potential. *Stroke*, **40** (9), 3028–3033.

111 Haddad, M., Beray-Berthat, V., Coqueran, B., Plotkine, M., Marchand-Leroux, C., and Margaill, I. (2012) Combined therapy with PJ34, a poly(ADP-ribose)polymerase inhibitor, reduces tissue plasminogen activator-induced hemorrhagic transformations in cerebral ischemia in mice. *Fundamental & Clinical Pharmacology*, **27** (4), 393–401.

112 Gursoy-Ozdemir, Y., Yemisci, M., and Dalkara, T. (2012) Microvascular protection is essential for successful neuroprotection in stroke. *Journal of Neurochemistry*, **123** (Suppl. 2), 2–11.

113 Seo, J.H., Miyamoto, N., Hayakawa, K., Pham, L.D., Maki, T., Ayata, C., Kim, K.W., Lo, E.H., and Arai, K. (2013) Oligodendrocyte precursors induce early blood–brain barrier opening after white matter injury. *The Journal of Clinical Investigation*, **123** (2), 782–786.

114 Besson, V.C., Zsengeller, Z., Plotkine, M., Szabó, C., and Marchand-Verrecchia, C. (2005) Beneficial effects of PJ34 and INO-1001, two novel water-soluble poly(ADP-ribose) polymerase inhibitors, on the consequences of traumatic brain injury in rat. *Brain Research*, **1041** (2), 150–157.

115 Chen, X.R., Besson, V.C., Palmier, B., Garcia, Y., Plotkine, M., and Marchand, C. (2007) Neurological recovery promoting, anti-inflammatory and anti-oxidative effects afforded by fenofibrate, a PPAR alpha agonist, after traumatic brain injury. *Journal of Neurotrauma*, **24** (7), 1119–1131.

116 Vink, R. and Nimmo, A.J. (2009) Multifunctional drugs for head injury. *Neurotherapeutics*, **6**, 28–42.

117 Béziaud, T., Chen, X.R., El Shafey, N., Frechou, M., Teng, F., Palmier, B., Beray-Berthat, V., Soustrat, M., Margaill, I., Plotkine, M., Marchand-Leroux, C., and Besson, V.C. (2011) Simvastatin, an HMG-CoA reductase inhibitor, in traumatic brain injury: effect on brain edema mechanisms. *Critical Care Medicine*, **39** (10), 2300–2307.

118 O'Collins, V.E., Macleod, M.R., Donnan, G.A., and Howells, D.W. (2012) Evaluation of combination therapy in animal models of cerebral ischemia. *Journal of Cerebral Blood Flow and Metabolism*, **32** (4), 585–597.

119 Zhang, L., Zhang, Z.G., and Chopp, M. (2012) The neurovascular unit and combination treatment strategies for stroke. *Trends in Pharmacological Sciences*, **33** (8), 415–422.

120 Kahle, M.P. and Bix, G.J. (2012) Successfully climbing the "STAIRs": surmounting failed translation of experimental ischemic stroke treatments. *Stroke Research and Treatment*, **2012**, 374098.

121 Stein, D.G. (2007) Sex differences in brain damage and recovery of function: experimental and clinical findings. *Progress in Brain Research*, **161**, 339–351.

122 Wilson, M.E. (2013) Stroke: understanding the differences between males and females. *Pflügers Archiv: European Journal of Physiology*, **465** (5), 595–600.

123 Bushnell, C.D. (2008) Stroke and the female brain. *Nature Clinical Practice Neurology*, **4** (1), 22–33.

124 Haast, R.A., Gustafson, D.R., and Kiliaan, A.J. (2012) Sex differences in stroke. *Journal of Cerebral Blood Flow and Metabolism*, **32** (12), 2100–2107.

125 Siegel, C.S. and McCullough, L.D. (2013) NAD^+ and nicotinamide: sex differences in cerebral ischemia. *Neuroscience*, **237**, 223–231.

126 Brait, V.H., Jackman, K.A., Walduck, A.K., Selemidis, S., Diep, H., Mast, A.E., Guida, E., Broughton, B.R., Drummond, G.R., and Sobey, C.G. (2010) Mechanisms contributing to cerebral infarct size after stroke: gender, reperfusion, T lymphocytes, and Nox2-derived superoxide. *Journal of Cerebral Blood Flow and Metabolism*, **30** (7), 1306–1317.

127 Fan, X., Lo, E.H., and Wang, X. (2013) Effects of minocycline plus tissue plasminogen activator combination therapy after focal embolic stroke in type 1 diabetic rats. *Stroke*, **44** (3), 745–752.

128 Li, Z., Wang, B., Kan, Z., Zhang, B., Yang, Z., Chen, J., Wang, D., Wei, H., Zhang, J.N., and Jiang, R. (2012) Progesterone increases circulating endothelial progenitor cells and induces neural regeneration after traumatic brain injury in aged rats. *Journal of Neurotrauma*, **29** (2), 343–353.

129 Chang, E.I., Loh, S.A., Ceradini, D.J., Chang, E.I., Lin, S.E., Bastidas, N., Aarabi, S., Chan, D.A., Freedman, M.L., Giaccia, A.J., and Gurtner, G.C. (2007) Age decreases endothelial progenitor cell recruitment through decreases in hypoxia-inducible factor 1alpha stabilization during ischemia. *Circulation*, **116** (24), 2818–2829.

130 Bacigaluppi, M., Comi, G., and Hermann, D.M. (2010) Animal models of ischemic stroke. Part one: modeling risk factors. *The Open Neurology Journal*, **4**, 26–33.

131 Ankolekar, S., Rewell, S., Howells, D.W., and Bath, P.M. (2012) The influence of stroke risk factors and comorbidities on assessment of stroke therapies in humans and animals. *International Journal of Stroke*, **7** (5), 386–397.

132 Levine, B., Fujiwara, E., O'Connor, C., Richard, N., Kovacevic, N., Mandic, M., Restagno, A., Easdon, C., Robertson, I.H., Graham, S.J., Cheung, G., Gao, F., Schwartz, M.L., and Black, S.E. (2006) *In vivo* characterization of traumatic brain injury neuropathology with structural and functional neuroimaging. *Journal of Neurotrauma*, **23** (10), 1396–1411.

133 Smith, D.H., Hicks, R., and Povlishock, J.T. (2013) Therapy development for diffuse axonal injury. *Journal of Neurotrauma*, **30** (5), 307–323.

134 Morales, D.M., Marklund, N., Lebold, D., Thompson, H.J., Pitkanen, A., Maxwell, W.L., Longhi, L., Laurer, H., Maegele, M., Neugebauer, E., Graham, D.I., Stocchetti, N., and McIntosh, T.K. (2005) Experimental models of traumatic brain injury: do we really need to build a better mousetrap? *Neuroscience*, **136** (4), 971–989.

135 Sozmen, E.G., Hinman, J.D., and Carmichael, S.T. (2012) Models that matter: white matter stroke models. *Neurotherapeutics*, **9** (2), 349–358.

136 Hall, E.D. and Traystman, R.J. (2009) Role of animal studies in the design of clinical trials. *Frontiers of Neurology and Neuroscience*, **25**, 10–33.

137 Landis, S.C., Amara, S.G., Asadullah, K., Austin, C.P., Blumenstein, R., Bradley, E.W., Crystal, R.G., Darnell, R.B., Ferrante, R.J., Fillit, H., Finkelstein, R., Fisher, M., Gendelman, H.E., Golub, R.M., Goudreau, J.L., Gross, R.A., Gubitz, A.K., Hesterlee, S.E., Howells, D.W., Huguenard, J., Kelner, K., Koroshetz, W., Krainc, D., Lazic, S.E., Levine, M.S., Macleod, M.R., McCall, J.M., Moxley, R.T., 3rd, Narasimhan, K., Noble, L.J., Perrin, S., Porter, J.D., Steward, O., Unger, E., Utz, U., and Silberberg, S.D. (2012) A call for transparent reporting to optimize the predictive value of preclinical research. *Nature*, **490** (7419), 187–191.

18
Movement Disorders: Parkinson's Disease

Houman Homayoun and Christopher G. Goetz

18.1
Introduction

Movement disorders is the area of neurology that deals with diseases involving aberrant timing and coordination of movement. Hypokinetic disorders are characterized by bradykinesia or slowness of movement, and hyperkinetic disorders are characterized by involuntary and excessive movements. The prototypic movement disorder is Parkinson's disease (PD), and because animal models have been so pivotal to drug development for this disease, the chapter focuses on this disorder. Other movement disorders such as Huntington's disease, various choreic disorders, dystonia, tics, and myoclonus have made less rapid advances in terms of drug development because accurate animal models have not been well established.

18.1.1
Parkinson's Disease

Parkinson's disease is the most common and best-studied hypokinetic movement disorder. It is characterized by the cardinal features of rest tremor, rigidity, bradykinesia, and postural instability. Animal models involving both rodents and primates have played a critical role in the process of drug discovery in PD and continue to be pivotal to the further characterization of the neurochemical, neurophysiological, and pathophysiological bases of this condition. In addition, a number of conditions known as atypical parkinsonism, which include multiple system atrophy (MSA), progressive supranuclear palsy (PSP), corticobasal degeneration (CBG), and dementia with Lewy body (DLB), share some of the clinical features of PD, and despite their distinct underlying pathophysiology, have benefited from drug discoveries based on PD animal models.

The classical animal models for PD have been based on the use of neurotoxins. The two most commonly used models include unilateral stereotaxic lesioning of basal ganglia structures in rodents by 6-hydroxydopamine (6-OHDA or 2,4,5-trihydroxyphenylethylamine) and systemic injection of 1-methyl-4-phenyl-1,2,3,6-

In Vivo Models for Drug Discovery, First Edition. Edited by José M. Vela, Rafael Maldonado, and Michel Hamon.
© 2014 Wiley-VCH Verlag GmbH & Co. KGaA. Published 2014 by Wiley-VCH Verlag GmbH & Co. KGaA.

tetrahydropyridine (MPTP) to primates (or less commonly rodents) [1–3]. Earlier or less utilized models are those based on the depletion of monoamine transmitters, including the key neurotransmitter dopamine (e.g., reserpine), blockade of dopamine D_2 receptors (e.g., haloperidol), and selective disruption of the mitochondrial respiratory chain (e.g., rotenone) [4–6]. Another group of animal models is based on the genetic changes that are either associated with the inherited forms of PD or predispose to pathological processes relevant to PD (e.g., accumulation of the presynaptic phosphoprotein α-synuclein and focal activation of microglia) [7]. Here, we will briefly review drug/toxin and genetic models and examples of each approach, focusing on their significance in the drug discovery process and their face, construct, and predictive validity.

Face validity refers to clinical or pathological similarity between the animal models and PD in humans. Although some of the earlier animal models were developed based on their face validity in reproducing PD-like motor symptoms, the emphasis has shifted to reproducing the key pathological findings involved in PD. Thus, there has been an interest in models that reproduce aggregation of α-synuclein protein and formation of intracellular Lewy body inclusions, degeneration of substantia nigra pars compacta (SNc) dopaminergic neurons, and loss of their terminals in striatum. In general, the toxin-based models remain superior in terms of their phenomenological face validity, but none of the current models demonstrate the full range of pathological changes seen in PD. Importantly, none of the models adequately exhibit the progressive and chronic degeneration of nigral dopamine neurons and the involvement of selective extranigral areas relevant to PD.

Construct validity refers to the extent of similarity between mechanisms involved in the animal model and those understood to be pathophysiologically important to PD. Different models have variable, and at times complementary, degrees of construct validity relative to the evolving multifaceted pathophysiology of PD. Current evidence suggests that mitochondrial dysfunction, oxidative stress, malfunctioning of protein breakdown machinery, and intracellular neuroprotective mechanisms are among the key mechanisms involved in PD, leading to development of models that focus on one or more of these underlying mechanisms. As such, although each model provides only partial construct validity, some of the newer models, specifically the genetic and function-based ones, may prove to be more comprehensive than others.

Finally, predictive validity refers to the extent to which the animal model allows scientists to predict the efficacy and the side effect profile of a therapeutic intervention for PD. The classical models have also shown strong predictive validity in the area of symptomatic therapy for motor deficits in PD. On the other hand, all of the current models have so far been limited in their predictive validity for development of disease-modifying interventions. This current limitation remains an area in which further progress is likely to be driven by refinements in current models as well as development of novel mechanistic models. Each model is discussed herein in terms of face, construct, and predictive validity (see Table 18.1).

Table 18.1 A comparison of the face, construct and predictive validity of main animal models of Parkinson's disease.

	Face validity – clinical	Face validity – pathological	Construct validity	Predictive validity – symptomatic[a]
Reserpine	Fair	Poor	Poor	Good
Haloperidol	Fair	Poor	Poor	Fair
6-OHDA	Fair	Good but no LB	Fair	Good
MPTP	Good	Good but no LB	Good	Good
Rotenone	Fair	Good	Good	Fair
Paraquat	Poor	Fair	Good	Poor
Transgenic dominant genes	Poor	Poor	Fair	Poor
A53 α-synuclein	Fair	Fair	Fair	Poor
Transgenic recessive genes (parkin, DJ1, etc.)	Poor	Fair	Fair	Poor
Adult-onset conditional genetic models	Fair	Fair	Good	Fair
MitoPark	Fair	Good	Good	Fair
Function-based models	Poor	Fair	Fair	Poor
Nonrodent genetic models	Poor	Poor (some fair)	Fair (some good)	Poor

a) Predictive validity for neuroprotective strategies remains uncertain since so far no such strategy has been successfully translated clinically.

18.2
Drug- and Toxin-Based Models of PD

18.2.1
Reserpine

Reserpine is an agent that blocks vesicular storage of monoamines, including dopamine, and thereby depletes their reserves. In the 1950s, the use of reserpine in rabbits, rats, and mice led to an akinetic motor phenomenology similar to clinical parkinsonism [4]. The partial face validity provided by this finding opened the door to the discovery of the key role of basal ganglia dopamine in the pathophysiology of PD [4]. In addition, the reserpine model was the key in the discovery of the therapeutic effects of levodopa against parkinsonian motor deficits, a finding that was successfully translated into clinical practice in the early 1960s (predictive validity). It has been argued that the reserpine model has poor construct validity for the neurochemical profile of PD in that its main mechanism of action is based on the blockade of vesicular monoamine transporter 2 (VMAT2), and therefore nonselective depletion of serotonin and noradrenaline occurs along with dopamine [8]. Furthermore, reserpine acts diffusely and depletes other dopaminergic systems than the nigrostriatal system that is the hallmark of PD. Finally, the model is reversible, and dopaminergic cells do not degenerate. Nevertheless, reserpine can lead to a prominent and rapid depletion of dopamine in the striatum (95% depletion within 2 h) and this seems to be the predominant mechanism mediating its akinetic effect [9]. For this reason, it is an easy and inexpensive screening tool for behavioral assessments. Reserpine remains a useful model with good predictive validity for the drug screening aimed at symptomatic therapies of parkinsonian akinetic rigid state, and all of the clinically available dopaminergic medications have shown efficacy in this model [8]. In addition, amantadine and anticholinergic agents also show efficacy in this model, whereas inhibitors of monoamine oxidase-B (MAO-B) and catechol-O-methyltransferase (COMT) potentiate the effect of levodopa. Limitations include the acute and reversible paradigm, systemic injection (although unilateral intracerebral and intraventricular injections have also been used), and the confounding effects of blocking nondopaminergic pathways.

Another monoamine-depleting toxin that is used as a model for akinetic symptoms of PD involves α-methyl-paratyrosine, an inhibitor of tyrosine hydroxylase that is the rate-limiting enzyme in the dopamine synthesis pathway. Like reserpine, construct validity of this model remains limited.

18.2.2
Haloperidol

Haloperidol is another agent used to model some motor aspects of parkinsonism. This agent is a dopamine D_2 receptor antagonist and its systemic administration to rodents can cause acute and reversible rigidity and cataplexy [5,10]. The latter can be quantified by the bar test, which measures the latency of removing the forepaws from an elevated bar. This test has been used to screen agents with dopaminergic efficacy, which can reverse the effect of haloperidol, or nondopaminergic agents such as anticholinergics and amantadine, which can potentiate the effects of levodopa in this model. In addition, this model continues to be used in the discovery of the potential antiparkinsonian properties of novel therapeutic strategies, including more recently the adenosine receptor antagonists and the allosteric modulators of metabotropic glutamate receptor [8]. It remains to be seen if the predictive validity of this model for efficacy against motor deficits of PD would extend to these novel agents. Absence of construct validity for the pathophysiological process underlying PD is a major limitation of this model. Instead, chronic use of haloperidol provides a better model to study the phenomenon of parkinsonism secondary to chronic use of antipsychotic agents (drug-induced parkinsonism).

18.2.3
6-OHDA

6-OHDA is a neurotoxin that selectively targets catecholaminergic neurons. This model was introduced in 1968 by Ungerstedt and since then has become one of the most widely studied animal models to characterize the dopaminergic dysfunction in PD [2]. Given low penetrance through the blood–brain barrier, 6-OHDA is delivered through stereotaxic intracerebral administration. Because bilateral delivery leads to high mortality, unilateral delivery has become the standard model, enabling comparison with the nonlesioned side as a within-subject control. Three main targets for delivery of toxin include substantia nigra pars compacta, medial forebrain bundle (MFB), and striatum [1,8,11,12]. The intrastriatal injection method does not specifically induce the behavioral hallmarks of PD, but it is associated with a slow and progressive rate of dopaminergic cell death that provides pathological face validity [13]. Two other injection sites (SNc and MFB) are associated with faster demise of dopaminergic neurons. When injected unilaterally, the toxin leads to ipsilateral nigral dopamine loss and striatal dopamine depletion, causing a host of downstream effects that reflect both pathological and compensatory mechanisms associated with dopaminergic denervation. The model has allowed extensive studies of mechanisms involved in neurotoxicity and neuroplasticity of dopaminergic pathways of basal ganglia and their modulation by other nondopaminergic mechanisms such as glutamatergic, cholinergic, serotoninergic, and other pathways. The cellular mechanisms of neurotoxicity caused by 6-OHDA include primarily oxidative stress caused by the production of reactive oxygen species and the reduction of natural antioxidants such as glutathione [8,14,15]. Additional mechanisms involve the interruption of mitochondrial respiratory chain and the activation of inflammatory processes mediated by microglia, although the role of these latter mechanisms is likely indirect or secondary to primary oxidative stress [1,8,11,14]. Given that all of these mechanisms are believed to play key roles in the pathogenesis of PD, the 6-OHDA model has good construct validity. There are also similarities in downstream molecular change, for example, both PD patients and 6-OHDA-treated subjects demonstrate glutamatergic upregulation and changes in the expression of protective transcription factors in output nuclei of basal ganglia [14,15]. In addition, neurophysiological data suggest a good degree of concordance between the effects of this toxin on the rate and pattern of neuronal firing in subthalamic nucleus (STN) and globus pallidus interna (GPi) and intraoperative recordings from same regions in PD patients [16,17]. Despite these similarities, this model is limited in that it is not associated with the formation of Lewy bodies, the key pathological hallmark in PD. This limitation, however, is shared by many of the available animal models of PD.

Behaviorally, unilateral 6-OHDA lesioning in rodents is associated with ipsilateral turning, given the extent of dopaminergic damage is sufficiently extensive (typically loss of more than 80% of SNc dopaminergic neurons) [18,19]. Apart from this spontaneous ipsilateral rotation, amphetamine, a blocker of dopamine reuptake, can induce or potentiate ipsilateral rotation through increased synaptic availability of dopamine on the nonlesioned side. A different behavioral outcome, namely, contralateral rotation, can be induced by apomorphine, a nonselective dopamine agonist, mediated by supersensitivity of dopamine receptors in the dopamine-denervated lesioned side. This latter effect also requires a high degree of dopaminergic degeneration (more than 90% of dopamine neurons) [8,18]. Apart from rotational behavior, a number of other behavioral parameters can be assessed, including the preferential use of nonaffected limb in exploratory vertical rearing behavior or in forward stepping the paw over a rocking platform. These motor outcomes, as well as associated pathological changes, are dependent on the regimen of 6-OHDA administration (including the site of administration, dose, and duration) as well as on the strain of mice used [18]. A key factor is the degree of damage to dopaminergic pathways. Higher doses of 6-OHDA directly targeting SNc or MFB can cause rapid degeneration of a high fraction of dopaminergic neurons, leading to a robust and reproducible behavioral profile that can be used in drug discovery efforts aimed at symptomatic treatment of PD motor deficits. In fact, this paradigm has been helpful in identifying agents that can potentially reverse the parkinsonian akinesia, and has shown good predictive validity for levodopa and dopamine agonists [20,21]. In contrast, slow introduction of lower doses of 6-OHDA, specially into striatum, can produce a partial and slower progressive degeneration of dopaminergic system, characterized by initial destruction at striatal terminals and followed by retrograde degeneration of nigral dopamine neurons few weeks later. This model provides a better tool to assess pathological and neurochemical changes relevant to the earlier stages of PD, in which the degree of dopaminergic damage is similarly incomplete, and notably would allow a window of opportunity to study potential neuroprotective strategies [8,15,18]. A limitation for this partial lesioning paradigm is the higher degree of variability at the behavioral level because rodents with partial dopaminergic lesions exhibit a wide range of behaviors ranging from normal movement without akinesia to typical deficits already described. Therefore, the latter paradigm would be less suitable to study potential symptomatic motor benefits of a certain drug, given the inherent variability in motor manifestations, but rather is appropriate to study agents aimed at halting neurotoxicity or promoting neuroplasticity [1].

In terms of predictive validity, the 6-OHDA model has been instrumental in studying the mechanisms underlying the beneficial motor effects of levodopa and dopamine agonists in PD. Except for anticholinergics, other current medications used in the treatment of PD show efficacy in this model. Dopaminergic agents, including levodopa, can replicate the effect of apomorphine and induce contralateral rotations [22,23]. Adjunctive therapies such as inhibitors of MAO-B and COMT can potentiate the effects of dopaminergic agents in this model [21]. Thus, this model is often used in the pharmacological assessment of new agents for symptomatic treatment of motor deficits in PD. There has also been interest in the potential predictive validity of this model in the assessment of nondopaminergic symptomatic therapies in PD. Among current therapies, amantadine, a weak glutamate NMDA receptor antagonist, shows efficacy in this model [22]. Among other candidate anti-PD drugs, adenosine receptor antagonists, including istradefylline, have been promising in this model [24]. Other novel therapeutic strategies showing promise in this model and subsequently assessed through clinical trials include dopamine D_2 partial agonists, serotonin $5HT_{1A}$ agonists, serotonin 5HT2A inverse agonists, glutamate AMPA (2-amino-3-(3-hydroxy-5-methyl-isoxazol-4-yl)-propanoic acid) receptor antagonists, and glutamate release inhibitors [8,25]. As already indicated, variations of this model have been used in the studies of potential neuroprotective strategies, in some cases in parallel to MPTP primate model. Since the neuroprotective drug candidates have not shown clinical efficacy in Parkinson's disease so far, this aspect of predictive validity of 6-OHDA and other models does not appear promising, with the current clinical methodologies being used to chart disease progression.

This model has also made major contributions to the study of the motor complications of current dopaminergic therapies, a major clinical issue that can impact the quality of life of PD patients receiving long-term treatment. These complications include wearing-off of the beneficial motor effects of levodopa, and levodopa-induced dyskinesia, which consists of involuntary movements seen in a portion of chronically treated PD patients. Although dyskinesia has been more consistently studied in primate models, its equivalent has been described in 6-OHDA rats treated with repeated doses of levodopa [3,26]. In these rats, a series of abnormal involuntary movements, including stereotyped orolingual dyskinesia, repetitive head turning, and appendicular dystonia, emerge as a result of prolonged exposure to repeated doses of levodopa [26]. Therapies that are effective against drug-induced dyskinesia in clinical setting or in primates are usually effective in this model as well. Therefore, this rat model is part of the test array used to detect antidyskinetic properties of novel drugs [1,11,26]. A recent example includes antagonists of metabotropic glutamate receptor 5 that have shown efficacy against levodopa-induced dyskinesia in 6-OHDA-treated rats, MPTP-treated primates, and, more recently, in a couple of small clinical trials in humans [27]. Similarly, medications that modulate serotonin receptors, for example, piclozotan, a serotonin 5HT1A receptor partial agonist, show efficacy against levodopa-induced dyskinesia in this model. Other novel strategies against levodopa-induced dyskinesia that have been tested in this model and await clinical validation include antiepileptic agent topiramate, adenosine receptor antagonists, and sodium channel inhibitor and glutamate release inhibitor safinamide [25,26].

18.2.4
MPTP

MPTP was initially discovered as a human toxin causing permanent parkinsonism in intravenous heroin abusers [28]. Since then, it has been extensively used as a research tool in both primates and rodents. MPTP is converted *in vivo* to the active component 1-methyl-4-pyridinium (MPP^+), which in turn would inhibit the mitochondrial complex I and lead to cell death. MPP^+ is dependent on the selective uptake by dopamine transporter (DAT) in order to enter the neuron and activate the cell death process; therefore, its effects are selective and most prominent in dopaminergic neurons that express a high level of DAT on their surface [11,12,29]. Although MPTP predominantly targets dopaminergic neurons in SNc, it can also cause less extensive degeneration in other nuclei including dopaminergic neurons in ventral tegmental area, noradrenergic neurons in locus coeruleus (LC), and a fraction of hypothalamic cells. This pattern is similar to PD that is also associated with major damage to SNc dopaminergic neurons and a lower degree of damage to these other nuclei (pathological face validity).

Like 6-OHDA model, the schedule and dose of administration of MPTP and species used can lead to a spectrum of experimental outcomes [29,30]. In general, the MPTP administration leads to a rapid development of parkinsonism. The motor deficits reverse quickly in case of acute treatment, but more slowly when subacute and chronic administration regimens are used. The intensity of residual motor deficits is dependent on the dose and duration of initial toxin exposure. One of the methods of delivery of MPTP involves unilateral intracarotid injection of MPTP in primates, leading to selective unilateral lesioning of nigral dopaminergic neurons [31]. Another treatment regimen is based on repeated administration of small doses of MPTP, leading to progressive accumulation of neurological deficits, thus providing a model with improved face validity for the progressive course of PD. In most instances, systemic administration of MPTP is used, leading to rapid development of pathological deficits and motor phenotype, followed by at least partial reversal. Part of the rapid recovery from early MPTP-induced motor deficits has been attributed to a transient reserpine-like depletion of dopamine reserves, but it is clear that compensatory and neuroprotective mechanisms are also important in the long-term recovery from these deficits [8,29].

In primates, MPTP causes a selective destruction of dopaminergic neurons and provides an excellent degree of clinical face validity with a wide range of parkinsonian symptoms similar to those in MPTP-exposed humans and PD [28,29]. These include bradykinesia, rigidity, and even postural instability, but may not commonly involve the classical parkinsonian rest tremor, although postural tremor can be present. Notably, a number of nonmotor symptoms may also be seen in the MPTP model in primates (including constipation, sialorrhea, sleep abnormalities, and cognitive deficits), although it remains unclear if their genesis is mediated by pathological processes similar to those in PD or alternatively is a result of less specific toxic effects of MPTP on other tissues.

Whereas rats generally do not show a robust response to MPTP, some strains of mice, for example, C57BL mice, are sensitive and have been developed as a PD animal model [30]. Some other strains either are not sensitive or do not show similar selective sensitivity of SNc dopaminergic pathways as seen in primates. In this setting, mice undergoing systemic injection of MPTP provide a relatively inexpensive screening tool. However, because mice are not as sensitive to MPTP as primates, this rodent model has relatively limited utility in behavioral assessments and drug screening for potential symptomatic therapies. This model is also complicated by high mortality rates caused by higher doses of toxin necessary to induce reliable parkinsonism in mice. The behavioral deficits assessed in this model include spontaneous locomotor hypoactivity and diminished exploratory rearing behavior. Given systemic administration of the toxin, this mice model does not have the advantage of within-subject control that is present in 6-OHDA-treated rodents. A more recent mice model has also been developed based on the intranasal delivery of MPTP [32]. This mode of delivery aims at modeling a potentially more realistic pattern of human exposure to environmental toxins. Another recent mice model has used the chronic administration of low doses of MPTP through osmotic pumps and will be discussed later [33].

The mechanisms underlying MPTP neurotoxicity have been closely studied to establish construct validity. A number of these mechanisms are also believed to play key roles in the pathogenesis of PD and include toxic effects on mitochondria, impairment of ATP production, production of reactive oxygen species, and activation of intracellular cell death signaling pathways [1,6,11,29]. The detrimental impact of MPTP on mitochondrial complex I is of particular interest, given this pathway has been strongly implicated in both MPTP-induced toxicity and PD pathogenesis. An example is the identification of key molecules such as glycogen synthase kinase-3$_\beta$, which mediate the toxic depolarization of mitochondrial membrane and lead to the activation of cell death cascade, providing a suitable target for drug development efforts. The MPTP model is also associated with widespread effects downstream from dopaminergic degeneration that include reduction in striatal dopamine content and tyrosine hydroxylase level (rate-limiting enzyme in the dopamine synthesis pathway), imbalance in the expression of various dopamine receptor subtypes, increased basal ganglia inflammatory markers and subsequent reactive gliosis, elevated glutamate levels in the output nuclei of basal ganglia, and increased firing rates as well as abnormal oscillatory activity in these nuclei [1,6,8,11,12,29,30]. This model has been instrumental in our understanding of the neurophysiological changes within basal ganglia circuitry associated with parkinsonian motor deficits and is specially considered a good model for understanding nigral degeneration in advanced PD. Despite these advantages, a major limitation is the absence of Lewy bodies, although at least one report had indicated the presence of Lewy body-like inclusions in MPTP-treated baboons.

In addition, although MPTP impacts some extranigral structures (e.g., LC), it spares other structures known to be affected by pathological changes in PD (e.g., raphe nucleus and dorsal motor nucleus of vagus). However, it is noteworthy that a recent study in mice MPTP model reported evidence of extranigral dopaminergic degeneration in the enteric nervous system, indicating the potential of this paradigm to be used as a potential preclinical model for PD. Also, as indicated, MPTP model is an acute rather than progressive model. To address this problem, various modifications in the delivery protocol of MPTP have been attempted. For example, recently a model of chronic delivery of low-dose MPTP through osmotic pumps was developed in mice, and was associated with a slower and progressive accumulation of pathological changes and motor deficits, notably nigral inclusions with immunoreactivity for α-synuclein and ubiquitin [33]. These methodological advances need to be replicated and refined. Overall, MPTP is not a perfect model for the pathophysiological processes involved in the development and progression of PD, but rather provides a good model to understand the neurotoxic mechanisms involved in degeneration of dopaminergic cells and the neuroprotective mechanisms that may oppose this process.

The MPTP model offers a high degree of predictive validity for efficacy against parkinsonian motor deficits such that all the currently available antiparkinsonian agents have shown effectiveness in this model in primates [1,8,30]. The predictive validity is less consistent in mice, partly because of the limitations noted earlier. The MPTP primate model has also proved helpful in studying motor complications including levodopa-induced dyskinesia [3]. The model is also commonly used in studies aimed at the development of neuroprotective agents, but so far these efforts have not been successfully translated clinically [1,11]. Several agents have shown promising neuroprotective results in MPTP and other toxin-based models, but have failed clinically, including monoamine oxidase-B inhibitors, antiapoptotic agents inhibiting JNK kinase, L-type calcium channel antagonists isradipine, riluzole, creatine, and coenzyme Q10, among others [8,25,29]. Some other candidate agents, for example, the neurotrophic factor inducer PYM-50028 (Cogane), are being evaluated in clinical trials after showing neuroprotective efficacy in these models.

In addition to medical therapies, the MPTP model has been instrumental in the advancement of surgical therapies for PD, including targeted lesioning and deep brain stimulation implantation of basal ganglia output nuclei [34]. These surgical therapies are beyond the scope of this chapter, but it should be noted that a better understanding of the neurophysiological basis of deep brain stimulation may lead to future drug discovery efforts that can target the same mechanisms. For example, recent human data have revealed the presence of abnormal oscillatory activity, especially in the beta-frequency band, in the subthalamic nuclei of PD patients [35]. These aberrant oscillations can be disrupted with both deep brain stimulation and levodopa and apomorphine, predicting that other drugs capable of disrupting these oscillatory activities may provide symptomatic benefit in PD. Comparable oscillatory activities, though at different frequency bands, have been suggested in MPTP primates and, if confirmed, may allow preclinical assessment of such candidate drugs in future [36].

Another important aspect of the predictive validity of the MPTP model is its application in predicting potential neuroprotective strategies against PD. In fact, this model has been at the forefront of research aimed at neuroprotection and neurorestoration in PD. Efforts aimed at transplantation of neuroprotective grafts, including autologous grafts, have been pioneered in this model [37]. In addition, some of the main complications of these initial efforts, including excessive dyskinesia caused by dopamine-producing grafts, have been studied in the MPTP model [38]. Ongoing research on the more sophisticated methods to cultivate and transplant neurorestorative tissues, including stem cells and growth factors, are also heavily based on the primate MPTP models. Some of the rodent MPTP models, however, have been used as an initial and less expensive tool to screen the efficacy and technical feasibility of some of these neurorestorative methods before their implementation in the more expensive and labor-intensive primate models. So far, these efforts have not been successfully translated to clinical use and there is certainly a concern that some of the neuroprotective strategies with proven efficacy in the MPTP model have failed in PD patients, highlighting the limitations in this aspect of the predictive validity of the MPTP model and underscoring the need to develop more innovative models.

18.2.5
Rotenone

Epidemiological studies suggesting that exposure to pesticides and herbicides increases the risk for PD have led to the development of animal models based on exposure to these toxins [39]. The best-known model from this group is the rotenone model. Like MPTP, rotenone has toxic effects on mitochondrial complex I. The subsequent cascade of toxicity involves the production of reactive oxygen species and the activation of cell death pathways. The exact mechanism mediating cell death in this model has been extensively researched and likely involves a combination of bioenergetics crisis caused by reduced ATP, mitochondrial calcium overload, and glutamate-mediated excitotoxicity converging on mitochondrial membrane depolarization, leading to cellular demise [1,6,40]. These mechanisms echo processes involved in the current understanding of pivotal processes in PD and therefore allow the conclusion that this model has strong construct validity. The profile of nigrostriatal damage caused by this model is notable for loss of nigral dopamine neurons, loss of striatal dopamine terminals, pathological nigral microglial activation, and most remarkably nigral Lewy body-like cytoplasmic inclusions that contain α-synuclein and ubiquitin (pathological face validity) [40,41]. The latter finding has been of special interest, since classical models involving 6-OHDA and MPTP are not typically associated with inclusions. Thus, this model has shown promise for assessment of potential neuroprotective agents, especially those aimed at disruption of α-synuclein aggregation and Lewy body formation. Another feature of this model is that the process of dopaminergic degeneration starts in striatal terminals and progresses in a retrograde manner. The face validity of this model is fair with a behavioral profile that includes akinesia, rigidity, and flexed posture, but also non-parkinsonian features.

In spite of these strengths, use of this model has been challenging because of the dose-dependent high mortality rates caused by systemic rotenone delivery and difficulties with reproducibility of the findings that seems to be related to route- and dose-specific variations. The initial successful reports used an osmotic micropump for prolonged delivery of low doses of toxin, thus making this a labor-intensive model, although subcutaneous and intraperitoneal modes of delivery have also been reported [1,6,12]. There is also a high rate of mortality related to the systemic side effects of rotenone as well as a high rate of resistance to its toxic effects. This means that only a fraction of treated animals would develop the motor deficits that include decreased locomotion, akinesia, catalepsy, and postural instability. Further refinement of chronic intraperitoneal regimens has led to a more consistent behavioral and pathological profile. A more recent application of intragastric rotenone in mice has been reported to cause sequential emergence of α-synuclein containing inclusions in enteric neurons, dorsal motor nucleus of vagus, and later SNc, a pattern resembling recent influential models of progression of Lewy body pathology in PD [42].

The predictive validity of rotenone model for screening symptomatic treatments for motor deficits in PD is limited and only levodopa and apomorphine have shown efficacy in reversing motor outcomes in this model, whereas other currently used PD medications, including dopamine agonists, MAO-B inhibitors, and COMT inhibitors, have failed [8,40]. On the other hand and as already stated, this model may have the potential to offer better predictive validity for assessment of neuroprotective strategies, a promise that remains to be fulfilled. In addition, rotenone can exert synergistic toxic effects in some of the genetic models of PD (discussed later), providing a useful experimental setting to assess the role of neuroprotective agents that may specifically disrupt the interaction between genetic and environmental factors involved in the pathogenesis of PD.

18.2.6
Paraquat and Other Environmental Toxins

In addition to rotenone, some other environmental toxins capable of disrupting mitochondrial respiratory chain have been used to develop animal models of PD. One of these agents is the herbicide paraquat (N,N'-dimethyl-4,4'-bipyridinium dichloride), either alone or potentiated by concomitant addition of fungicide maneb. Like rotenone, cases of paraquat-induced PD have been reported based on epidemiological studies, usually with a history of simultaneous exposure to fungicides [39]. Paraquat is toxic for mitochondrial complex I, but its main mode of toxicity seems to be through generation of reactive oxygen species, and its toxicity can be blocked by increasing intracellular expression of antioxidant mechanisms such as superoxide dismutase. Maneb is an inhibitor for mitochondrial complex III. These models can increase immunoreactivity for α-synuclein in nigral dopamine cells, but in contrast to rotenone model, do not lead to Lewy body-like inclusions or marked nigral cell death [1,12]. As such, they have more limited pathological face validity. The spectrum of motor deficit caused by these models is also limited and not consistent, although certain akinetic behaviors that are reversible by levodopa have been reported [1,40]. These models also have limited predictive validity, as it is not clear if other PD medications, apart from levodopa, can ameliorate the behavioral deficits. Despite these limitations, they remain appropriate models to assess potential neuroprotective agents that may preserve mitochondrial function and inhibit the effectors of cell death.

Another recent model has been developed based on trichloroethylene, an industrial solvent and an environmental contaminant. Trichloroethylene has been linked to few cases of Parkinson's disease in industrial workers having long-term and excessive exposure to this agent. This agent is capable of inhibiting mitochondrial complex I *in vitro* and its *in vivo* application in rats has led to motor deficits as well as selective nigral dopaminergic degeneration, and notably α-synuclein aggregations in SNc and dorsal motor nucleus of vagus [43]. The latter finding, if replicated, may provide a model to study the involvement of extranigral strutures in the middle stages of PD pathology.

18.3
Genetic and Functional Models of PD

The discovery of genetic mutations underlying inherited forms of PD has led to the development of a number of genetic models that aim to replicate single gene defects associated with PD and to study their functional significance, their potential contribution to pathophysiology of PD, and their role in susceptibility to environmental toxins [1,7,12,44,45]. This effort is based on the assumption that sporadic PD, which constitutes the great majority of clinical population, shares some of the pathways and mechanisms responsible for disease progression in inherited cases. In this regard, main PD-associated genes include dominant genes (α-synuclein and LRRK2) and recessive genes (PINK1/parkin and DJ1). It is now clear that these genes are involved in key processes including the regulation of mitochondrial respiratory chain, protein folding, and protein breakdown. Although replicating the genetic defects directly implicated in clinical setting provides a good level of construct validity, the goal of simulating PD pathology in these models has remained mostly unmet to this date.

18.3.1
Rodent Genetic Models

In the case of autosomal dominant genes, transgenic and overexpressor mice have been created for α-synuclein (disease-associated mutations A30P and A53T) and LRRK2 (leucine-rich repeat kinase 2) [1,7,46]. In the transgenic models, the disease-associated mutation is induced in mice, whereas in overexpressor models, extra copies of human wild-type genes are overexpressed. The phenotype caused by α-synuclein overexpression is dependent on the type of promoter used in the development of the model [7]. The genetic models of α-synuclein mutation have been associated with major extranigral pathology, but not with reliable loss of dopaminergic neurons or formation of classical Lewy bodies in SNc [12,45]. However, one type of α-synuclein transgenic mice, the A53T mutation model under the control of mouse prion promoter, exhibits nigral aggregation of α-synuclein and progressive neurodegeneration [47]. This subtype also causes severe motor deficits, thus possessing good clinical and pathological face validity as well as construct validity. The α-synuclein models are important as a tool to study the early stages of α-synuclein accumulation and the significance of conversion from benign monomeric state to the more troublesome oligomeric and fibrillary states of α-synuclein, and could be used to determine the efficacy of drug development efforts aimed at stabilizing α-synuclein in its simpler monomeric state and preventing its intracellular aggregation [7]. The LRRK2 models have not shown any impact on dopaminergic cell death, α-synuclein aggregation, or motor behavior, but remain relevant in clarifying the possible role of LRRK2 in the pathophysiology of PD [1,12,45]. Overall, the autosomal dominant transgenic models, with the exception already indicated, do not possess convincing clinical or pathological face validity, or symptomatic face validity. Their usefulness in the assessment of neuroprotective strategies remains to be established, although it is likely that more sophisticated models based on the expression of these genes in adult rather than in young animals (discussed later) provide a superior model to assess neuroprotective predictive validity.

Among autosomal recessive genes, knockout models have been developed based on parkin, DJ1, and PINK1 (phosphatase and tensin homolog (PTEN)-induced novel kinase 1) [1,7,12,46]. Among these, parkin gene, which encodes a ligase in the ubiquitin proteasome system, is the most common cause of familial PD and responsible for around 20% of sporadic young-onset cases of PD [44]. Parkin knockout mice do not exhibit any consistent parkinsonian behavioral phenotype or dopaminergic degeneration. In general, recessive mice models have not reliably produced nigral dopaminergic cell loss, α-synuclein aggregation, or behavioral parkinsonian phenotype [1,7,46]. These models provide some degree of construct validity in that they impair mitochondrial function and modify striatal dopamine release, but the extent of these effects is limited and does not replicate the full spectrum of the pathology of PD. Thus, these mice models are not suitable for assessment of neuroprotective strategies and are primarily helpful in mechanistic studies. In addition, most PD medications are ineffective in this model or have not been tested [45,46]. Transgenic models of PD-related genes have also been developed in nonrodent organisms (discussed later), and efforts are underway to engineer corresponding knockout models in rats as well.

In addition to disease-causing genes, a number of other genetic targets have been used to model the pathophysiology of PD. For example, based on the findings that certain transcription factors such as Pitx3 and Nurr-1 are important for nigral neuronal maintenance and are depleted in the brain of PD patients, corresponding genetic models have been developed [1,48,49]. In the spontaneously occurring aphakia mice model, which lack the transcription factor Pitx3 in their midbrain dopamine progenitor cells, adult mice exhibit degeneration of SNc dopamine neurons, depletion of striatal dopamine levels, and hypokinetic motor manifestations that are reversible with levodopa [48]. A unique feature of this model is the development of levodopa-induced dyskinesia after prolonged exposure [1]. Likewise, Nurr-1 transgenic model has also helped to better understand the development and maintenance of nigral dopaminergic neurons. This model is also associated with marked dopaminergic degeneration and reduced locomotion, though not levodopa-induced dyskinesia [49].

Genetic models have also been used to study the interaction between genes and environmental factors, a concept that is particularly of interest in PD. Some of the toxins indicated earlier, including MPTP and rotenone, can exert increased toxicity in genetically modified models [7,8,12]. For example, the toxic effects of MPTP are potentiated in α-synuclein transgenic and DJ-1 knockout mice. Likewise, Nurr-1 knockout mice demonstrate enhanced susceptibility to toxins such as MPTP. An important concept is that current transgenic models, with evidence of minor alterations in their dopaminergic turnover and mild motor deficits, but lacking profound dopamine cell loss, may provide a model for prodromal phase of the disease, and their increased sensitivity to toxins can be used to assess the impact of potential neuroprotective strategies in this phase [45]. Furthermore, as potential environmental risk factors for PD are identified, the genetic models can allow us to study their specific neurotoxic pathways and, along the way, to identify potential therapeutic targets. An example of the latter approach is a recently developed invertebrate transgenic model expressing α-synuclein under the influence of manganese that can be used to study the clinical phenomenon of manganese-associated parkinsonism (manganism) [50].

18.3.1.1 Adult-Onset Rodent Gene-Based Models

It has been argued that genetic modifications at an early age, as is typical in most of the above-mentioned genetic models, can activate compensatory mechanisms that may not be typically involved in the late-onset PD. This compensatory plasticity may account for the failure of these genetic models in reproducing a reliable PD-like pathology and behavior. This notion is also supported by other lines of evidence including toxin-based models, for example, exposure to 6-OHDA at an early age causes only minimal dopaminergic changes without significant degeneration, whereas exposure at adult age leads to full behavioral and pathological profile, highlighting the potential for compensatory neuroplasticity to obstruct the detrimental effect of neurotoxins. To overcome this problem, some researchers have employed conditional knockout or overexpressor gene strategies that would enable targeted expression or deletion of a gene at adult age, and in certain settings in a selected tissue [7,12,45,51]. This novel approach provides a new level of control over the timing and region of the expression of target transgene that may prove invaluable in creating a window of opportunity to separate the signal from deficient gene from the noisy background of *in vivo* and developmental compensatory mechanisms. Using such methods, it was recently reported that knocking out parkin at adult age could cause nigral degeneration. Such a model may also prove more suitable for studying potential strategies for halting PD because the pathophysiological process likely begins a long time before clinical symptoms first appear.

Another example of this adult-onset conditional approach is the expression of wild-type α-synuclein gene under the control of a regulated tetracycline system. This state-of-the-art system combines the ability to express the transgene in a target tissue (such as SNc) using a tissue-specific promoter, with the ability to reversibly switch on and off the expression of the transgene based on the regulation of the promoter by an inhibitory mechanism sensitive to tetracycline analogs such as doxycycline [45]. The end result is the ability to control the expression of the target gene in a time- and region-specific manner, thus bypassing the developmental compensatory mechanisms. This α-synuclein model led to a progressive loss of SNc dopamine neurons and motor decline, which were halted when the conditional expression of α-synuclein was terminated, thus providing evidence that continued expression of α-synuclein is necessary for disease progression [45,52]. A similar conditional model based on LRRK2 gene instead of α-synuclein has yielded less promising results, failing to induce dopaminergic neuronal degeneration and parkinsonian motor deficits [53].

Perhaps one of the most promising of these adult-onset conditional expression models is the MitoPark mice, a model based on region-specific disruption of mitochondrial function in dopaminergic cells [12,51]. The production of this model is complex, labor intensive, and based on the principle of conditional knockout. These mice express a special recombinase enzyme under the control of a dopamine transporter. This would allow their recombinase to become selectively activated in the adult dopaminergic neurons, which express DAT, leading to deletion of the target gene TFAM-A (transcription factor A, mitochondrial) in this selective population. This model can produce nigral dopaminergic degeneration mediated by mitochondrial dysfunction as well as motor deficits and is considered a potentially useful tool in assessing the potential new therapies aimed at mitochondrial protection in PD. The MitoPark model exhibits a number of features that provide it with good construct validity. In addition to its deliberate targeting of mitochondrial respiratory chain in nigral cells, this model leads to adult-onset and slowly progressive motor impairment, nigral dopaminergic degeneration, and striatal dopamine depletion [12]. The MitoPark model can also lead to dopaminergic cytoplasmic inclusion bodies, but their significance is unclear since these do not contain α-synuclein, and can even be detected in MitoPark mice with null α-synuclein mutation. Notably, the motor impairment in this model, which includes akinesia and locomotor deficiency, is reversible by levodopa, but the degree of levodopa benefit varies based on the age of the mice and is less prominent in the aged mice, suggesting that this model may be helpful for assessment of the role of age and disease progression in symptomatic therapies in PD. This model has been used to assess the therapeutic potential of some novel symptomatic treatment strategies including positive allosteric modulators of group 4 metabotropic glutamate receptors and the antagonists of adenosine A2A receptors [12,54]. Both strategies have shown efficacy in the MitoPark model as well as in classical models such as the 6-OHDA model, indicating that MitoPark model may also provide a fair degree of symptomatic predictive validity. It is expected that conditional knockout strategy be applied to other molecules of interest in PD and, similar to the case already mentioned, be combined with additional genetic modifications, as well as toxicological exposures of interest.

Another novel method for improved control of transgene expression involves using large genomic inserts in the form of a bacterial artificial chromosome (BAC). These giant structures carry finely controllable gene promoters and endogenous gene regulatory elements, allowing a high level of control over the pattern of expression of delivered transgene [55,56]. For example, a parkin model has been developed using BAC-mediated delivery and under the control of a DAT promoter [55]. This model has been reported to cause progressive motor deficits and age-dependent nigral dopaminergic degeneration. One caveat is that the C-terminal-truncated parkin used in this model is a dominant gain-of-function mutation different from disease-related autosomal recessive mutation seen in the clinical setting. A LRRK2 BAC model has also been developed. This model also produces levodopa-responsive motor deficits and a reduction in dopamine levels, but no evidence of dopaminergic degeneration [56]. Overall, the adult-onset genetic models discussed herein provide a good degree of both construct and pathological face validity, with a variable degree of clinical face validity, and seem promising for assessment of neuroprotective therapies.

Given the limitations of genetic models so far, an alternative method for gene-related studies has included direct stereotaxic delivery of transgenes into the tissue of interest using viral vectors. These viral-based methods have been successfully implemented in rodents and primates, as well as in human clinical trials. A number of viral vectors are available, including herpes simplex virus (HSV), lentivirus, and recombinant adeno-associated virus (rAAV), that each offer distinct characteristics including the size of transduced tissue, the size of genes delivered, and, in the case of HSV, the ability for retrograde transport, for example, allowing delivery of the transgene to striatum with delayed transduction in SNc [45,57]. This method has facilitated the development of adult rat models of nigrostriatal α-synuclein and LRRK2 expression [57]. A more recent model has involved HSV-mediated delivery of LRRK2 (G2919s) to mice striatum, leading to significant nigral dopaminergic degeneration [45]. The fact that nigral degeneration could be achieved with this method suggests that prior failures with transgenic mice must have been related to subthreshold level of gene expression, or that the coactivation of glia, occurring in the case of viral-mediated model but not in the transgenic model, may be required. This model is likely to prove helpful in screening for potential neuroprotective strategies.

18.3.2
Rodent Function-Based Models

Some of the recent models of PD have been developed based on the replication of certain known aspects of PD pathophysiology in humans. For example, given the presence of inflammatory microglial activation as a pathological marker of ongoing damage within the SNc, methods have been developed to replicate focal nigral microglial activation using targeted injection of lipopolysaccharide [8,58,59]. This compound has shown the ability to destroy dopaminergic neurons both *in vitro* and *in vivo*. This is a process mediated by inflammatory cytokines and peroxynitrite, and when injected unilaterally into SNc, it can lead to nigrostriatal degeneration and unilateral motor deficit similar to the 6-OHDA model. Therefore, this model can be used particularly to assess the efficacy of novel anti-inflammatory treatments in slowing down nigral degeneration in PD [8]. Another model based on the known functional deficits in PD involves targeted disruption of proteasomal activity [59,60]. The rationale for this model is that in PD the catalytic activity of proteasome is decreased and this process is likely to play a key role in the inability of neurons to degrade mutated and misfolded proteins such as α-synuclein [60]. Several agents, including lactacystin, epoxomicin, and PSI, have been used to induce inhibition of the proteasome activity [59]. These models so far have been a mixed success; specifically their reproducibility has been debated and has not been completely established [59,61]. In certain mice strains, it has been reported that this strategy can lead to nigral dopaminergic degeneration and Lewy body-like inclusions [8]. However, other groups have been unable to reproduce similar results [61]. These function-based models provide poor clinical face validity and are unlikely to have symptomatic predictive validity, but their potential strength lies in providing at least a fair degree of construct validity with respect to specific mechanisms involved in the pathophysiology of PD.

Another function-based model comes from recent findings involving lysosomal glucocerebrosidase (GBA1), the gene responsible for Gaucher's disease. In humans, mutation in this gene is associated with a fivefold increase in PD risk in heterozygous carriers, making this the most common genetic risk factor for PD. From these findings, researchers have developed a mouse model of Gaucher-related synucleinopathy (Gba1$^{D409V/D409V}$), which behaviorally exhibits a range of cognitive and motor deficits. A recent study using this mice model reported that adeno-associated virus-mediated expression of human glucocerebrosidase in the brain of symptomatic Gba1$^{D409V/D409V}$ mice reverses the accumulation of α-synuclein aggregates [62]. Interestingly, the same strategy of overexpressing glucocerebrosidase, when applied to A53T α-synuclein mice, lowered the level of soluble α-synuclein [62]. Thus, the animal model based on Gaucher-related synucleinopathy may prove useful in the discovery of novel methods to disrupt α-synuclein aggregation that may be applicable to non-Gaucher-gene-related PD subjects. This model may also be relevant to studying aspects of cognitive impairment in PD as clinical studies have suggested that GBA1-carrier PD patients show lower cognitive performance than age-matched noncarrier PD patients.

18.3.3
Nonrodent Genetic Models of PD

Nonrodent genetic models of PD provide certain advantages over rodent models including lower expenses, faster reproduction time, and genomic simplicity that facilitates genetic modification [63–65]. The limitation clearly involves decreased face validity and lower complexity of their equivalent nervous system. The main nonrodent models include *Drosophila melanogaster* (fruit fly), *Caenorhabditis elegans* (nematode), and *Danio rerio* (zebrafish). *Drosophila* contains homologs of many of the PD-related genes including parkin, PINK-1, DJ-1, and LRRK2, but an exception is α-synuclein [63]. Transgenic *Drosophila* overexpressing wild-type human α-synuclein display behavioral deficits that are reminiscent of akinesia in higher organisms, for example, their ability to climb out of an open jar diminishes [64]. Similar behavioral deficits have been noted in a number of other *Drosophila* models, including parkin and LRRK2. These behavioral changes are associated with the loss of dopaminergic-type neurons and notably can be reversed by levodopa. In the case of α-synuclein overexpressor *Drosophila*, Lewy body-like filamentous inclusions containing α-synuclein and a progressive course of dopaminergic neuronal loss have been reported [63]. This is the only α-synuclein model that exhibits a progressive loss of dopaminergic neurons [7]. Similarly, parkin knockout *Drosophila* exhibit motor deficits, including locomotion deficits and wasting of their flight muscles, as well as dopaminergic degeneration, whereas parkin mice model does not demonstrate similar changes [7,63]. Studies in this model have also shown a shared pathogenic pathway between PINK-1 and parkin, but both models are limited by the presence of significant abnormalities outside the nervous system [7,63]. Thus, in contrast to mice, the *Drosophila* models exhibit a more reliable parkinsonian phenotype, although these results should be interpreted with caution given interspecies differences and the fact that *Drosophila* do not express wild-type α-synuclein [65]. A recent *Drosophila* model based on duplication of α-synuclein can lead to age-dependent dopaminergic neurodegeneration and is likely to be helpful in studying α-synuclein neurotoxicity [45].

Models based on the genetic manipulation of PD-associated genes in zebrafish include DJ-1, parkin, and LRRK2 [63,66]. In this species, knocking down LRRK2 can lead to a decrease in the density of tyrosine hydroxylase positive cells in association with impaired swimming ability. In addition, this model is also sensitive to the toxic effects of MPTP and may be suitable for future drug screening efforts for agents aimed at altering the interaction between susceptible genes and environmental toxins in PD.

The models based on *C. elegans* take advantage of a simple well-studied genome [67]. Although this simple organism does not contain equivalent, or orthologs, of PD genes such as α-synuclein, parkin, or DJ-1, these genes have been overexpressed in this model, either as wild type or in mutated form [63,67]. Moreover, *C. elegans* has equivalent of dopamine neurons and shows reliable feeding-related motor behavior that is dependent on dopamine. Overexpression of PD genes can lead to the degeneration of dopaminergic neurons and cause behavioral impairment that is reversible by dopamine agonists [67]. However, these results need to be interpreted with caution. For example, LRRK2 models in *C. elegans*, as well as in *Drosophila*, cause neurodegeneration, but in higher organisms this process involves α-synuclein, which is absent in these simpler organisms [7,63]. Therefore, despite the similarity, the involved mechanisms in these species are likely to be unrelated. Nevertheless, these simpler organisms provide an opportunity to identify potential pharmacological modulators of specific neurodegenerative pathways, in this case LRRK2-mediated neurodegeneration. It is also likely that *C. elegans* models based on the overexpression of α-synuclein may be helpful in drug screening efforts to identify modulators of α-synuclein aggregation and toxicity, leading to novel targets for drug development. Notably, *C. elegans* is also sensitive to toxic effects of rotenone, MPTP, and 6-OHDA, providing another potential platform for assessment of gene–environment interactions relevant to PD [68]. Overall, nonrodent genetic models provide limited clinical and pathological face validity, but they offer a fair degree of construct validity for some of the mechanisms involved in PD.

18.4
Translation to Clinics: Limitations and Difficulties

As noted earlier, the classical toxin-based models of PD have been instrumental in the development of symptomatic therapies for motor symptoms of PD and have illuminated important findings related to the complications of these therapies when they are used to treat the disease. These models remain essential in ongoing efforts to develop additional symptomatic therapies, especially with regard to novel nondopaminergic treatments and management of motor complications of current dopaminergic therapies [1,8,25]. On the other hand, these models have been limited by the acute, rather than progressive, nature of neuronal degeneration and by a paucity of extranigral pathology. In the recent years, modifications in the dosing and delivery protocols of these toxin-based methods have been developed with the goal of reproducing a more accurate pathological replica of PD. In models based on environmental toxins, for example, certain protocols have led to production of Lewy body-like inclusions and a gradual accumulation of nigral degeneration, whereas others have failed [40]. Therefore, the interpretation of new therapies in toxin-based models must take into consideration the specifics of dosing schedule and route of administration, both at the stage of choosing the appropriate protocol for a given research question and at the stage of interpreting the results.

The genetic models of PD were developed with the goal of a more accurate recapitulation of progressive pathology, but initial efforts were unsuccessful in reproducing a reliable and significant degree of dopaminergic neuronal degeneration [7]. As mentioned earlier, developmental neuroplasticity and *in vivo* compensatory mechanisms may be partly responsible for this failure, especially in young animals. Other factors such as interactions between genetic susceptibility and environmental toxic exposure, polygenic causation, and regulatory gene–gene interactions, may also be relevant to the question of why these transgenic rodent models do not express consistent dopaminergic degeneration. Success of transgenic models in reproducing more reliable PD-related degenerative features in simpler nonrodent animals clearly supports the significance of these genetic pathways in the pathophysiology of PD. This notion is further supported by more recent successful genetic efforts involving delivery of transgenes to adult rodents through vectors or conditional knockouts, leading to a more impressive pattern of neurodegeneration in targeted regions. These methods show great promise owing to their potential to express the PD-related genes in a time- and region-specific manner, and this may facilitate preclinical drug testing aimed at intervening at a certain stage of the disease based on the expected mechanism of action [51,52]. It would also be interesting to develop future genetic models carrying a combination of mutations, since polygenic causation is very likely in sporadic PD [7]. Overall, much is left to be achieved in this field, as we still lack a convincing model of progressive degeneration associated with corresponding Lewy body formation.

Nevertheless, current PD research focuses on the development of effective neuroprotective and neurorestorative therapies to modify the clinical course of the disease. There has been a clear translational gap between mechanisms that have shown efficacy in various animal models and their total failure in the clinical trials. A few factors seem to have contributed to this gap [25,69,70]. First, we should consider the limitations related to the models themselves. The issues that can cause significant variation within a model, including dosing and route of administration in toxin-based studies, genetic mutations and age and condition of expression in genetic models, and measured outcomes in all models, deserve special attention for future modifications. The results of preclinical studies need to be interpreted carefully considering these issues before moving into clinical trials [25]. For example, measurement of dopamine striatal levels as a surrogate for nigral dopaminergic degeneration may not be optimal if neuroprotection is the ultimate goal [8]. Likewise, an agent that shows neuroprotective efficacy in the α-synuclein overexpression model in *Drosophila* cannot be immediately considered as a potential neuroprotective strategy for PD before confirmation in models involving higher organisms.

Clearly, the construct validity of many of the available PD models is based on our currently limited, though expanding, understanding of the pathophysiology of PD. The understanding of exact causative mechanisms will open the field to the replication of these mechanisms in animal models, allowing targeted experiments to identify agents that deactivate and inhibit these processes and thereby suppress progressive neuronal death. Such advances will also allow the identification of upstream targets that can potentially be promoted and potentiated to effectively overwrite the pathophysiological processes involved in PD. It is likely that information gained from current models would provide pieces of the puzzle, but it is also likely that future and more comprehensive models with a higher degree of face and construct validity may need to be developed before we can expect a reliable degree of predictive validity for disease-modifying therapies. It is also possible that our changing understanding of the pathophysiology of PD may open up the doors to new therapeutic strategies. For example, a recent study has suggested that once α-synuclein is introduced into normal brain, it may use a prion-like template recruitment and transmission mechanism to spread to adjacent areas [71]. If confirmed, such a discovery would enrich our current understanding of the process underlying PD and suggest a number of potential immune-based therapies that can be tested with appropriate animal models before human trials.

A key limitation to all currently available models is their lack of focus on the progressive and treatment-refractory nonmotor symptoms that are a major cause of disability and diminished quality of life in advanced PD [69,70]. The inability of current animal models to recapitulate these aspects of PD remains a major limitation, especially in the assessment of potential neuroprotective processes. Some of the advances already reviewed hint at extranigral pathology that may be relevant to PD, but they are not definitive. For example, models exhibiting pathology in enteric nervous system and dorsal motor nucleus of vagus may be appropriate for evaluation of early neuroprotective intervention that may prove helpful to halt PD in a prodromal state, but clear outcome measures need to be defined and their relevance to PD needs to be established before such studies can be translated clinically. The issue of cognitive decline in advanced PD is another important aspect that deserves further attention. In fact, cognitive tasks capable of detecting subtle cognitive deficits have been developed and used in both rodent and primate models. Transgenic mice and simpler organisms are less appropriate for this purpose and primates are expensive and labor intensive. Development of transgenic rats would facilitate progress as rats are more cognitively complex and some sophisticated cognitive paradigms for rats have already been developed. In this case, the more realistic animal models should also be ideally based on the progressive accumulation of Lewy body pathology with both nigral and selective extranigral involvement.

Furthermore, modeling the interactions between genetic and environmental factors deserves further attention [6]. Although such interactions have been highlighted in the clinical epidemiological studies and modeled successfully in some of the genetic models exposed to subthreshold doses of toxins, they are not a focus of many neuroprotective drug screening efforts. One argument is that the current models perhaps do not replicate the exact type of toxins, or even gene defects, that may be clinically relevant in the majority of sporadic PD patients. Nonetheless, the pathways downstream to these interactions are likely to be shared with those involved in other potentially distinct gene–toxin interactions in sporadic PD. Thus, the application of established toxins in genetic models of PD provides a unique opportunity for studying the interactions between genes and environmental toxins specific to PD, and remains an area of interest in future drug development efforts.

Another factor limiting the translation of animal models to human PD is the clinical heterogeneity of PD itself [25,69,70]. Some patients are tremor dominant, whereas others lack tremor and have dominant akinesia and gait problems. Some patients have cognitive and psychiatric problems as part of their disease and others do not. Some patients deteriorate relatively rapidly over 10 years and others are much more indolent in their progression. This issue of heterogeneity is problematic for animal models that rely on a consistent population-based set of behaviors, pathological changes, and treatment responses. Findings of treatment efficacy in a homogenous model may prove unsuccessful when it is tested in the wider heterogeneity of human PD. This problem is evident in translating animal model data into clinical trials testing either symptomatic therapies or neuroprotective strategies, since a treatment identified in the laboratory may be effective for a certain subset of PD patients but not the whole group, leading to false negative results. A current limitation is the unavailability of translatable clinical biomarkers that can identify subsets of PD patients suitable for specific treatment interventions [25]. If such biomarkers become available, they can be also applied in experimental animal models, both to help delineate subset-specific pathophysiology and to allow drug discovery efforts aimed at subsets expressing certain biomarkers. This area has great potential for bidirectional translational research between bench and bedside.

Another limitation is that the impact of aging, which remains a major risk factor for the development of PD, is not taken into account in many animal studies [72]. This problem is, to some extent, related to the short half-life of simpler organisms and rodents, the high expense of long-term housing of aged animals, and the long duration and increasing ethical and public policy issues related to primate colonies. Despite these hurdles, the role of aging deserves more attention in neuroprotective drug development efforts and overlooking this factor would play a role in the translational disconnect already mentioned. Both primate models, with a closer face validity to human aging process, and simpler organisms, with their rapid reproduction cycles and multiple offspring, provide opportunities to study the interaction between aging and PD-related neurotoxicity and neuroplasticity processes.

Current animal models of PD have made significant contributions to our understanding of its pathophysiology as well as to the development of symptomatic therapies for PD motor deficits. Given the rapid expansion of recent genetic models of PD and the prospect for studying their interactions with well-characterized neurotoxins and neuroinflammatory triggers, animal model research remains a highly dynamic and continually evolving research field. Furthermore, focusing on modeling the key aspects of PD, including progressive course, Lewy body depositions, extranigral pathology, and gene–toxin interactions, is warranted to facilitate future neuroprotective drug development efforts.

References

1 Blesa, J., Phani, S., Kackson-Lewis, V., and Przedborski, S. (2012) Classic and new animal models of Parkinson's disease. *Journal of Biomedicine and Biotechnology*, **2012**, 845618.

2 Ungerstedt, U. (1968) 6-Hydroxy-dopamine induced degeneration of central monoamine neurons. *European Journal of Pharmacology*, **5**, 107–110.

3 Langston, J.W., Quik, M., Petzinger, G., Jakowec, M., and Di Monte, D.A. (2000) Investigating levodopa-induced dyskinesias in the parkinsonian primate. *Annals of Neurology*, **47** (4 Suppl. 1), S79–S89.

4 Carlsson, A., Linqvist, M., and Magnusson, T. (1957) 3,4-Dihydroxyphenylalanine and 5-hydroxytryptophan as reserpine antagonists. *Nature*, **180** (4596), 1200.

5 Sanberg, P.R. (1980) Haloperidol-induced catalepsy is mediated by postsynaptic dopamine receptors. *Nature*, **284**, 472–473.

6 Greenamyre, J.T., Cannon, J.R., Drolet, R., and Mastroberardino, P.G. (2010) Lessons from the rotenone model of Parkinson's disease. *Trends in Pharmacological Sciences*, **31** (4), 141–142.

7 Dawson, T.M., Ko, H.S., and Dawson, V.L. (2010) Genetic animal models of Parkinson's disease. *Neuron*, **66** (5), 646–661.

8 Duty, S. and Jenner, P. (2011) Animal models of Parkinson's disease: a source of novel treatments and clues to the cause of the disease. *British Journal of Pharmacology*, **164**, 1357–1391.

9 Heeringa, M.J. and Abercrombie, E.D. (1995) Biochemistry of somatodendritic dopamine release in substantia nigra: an *in vivo* comparison with striatal dopamine release. *Journal of Neurochemistry*, **65** (1), 192–200.

10 Foutz, A.S., Delashaw, J.B., Jr., Guilleminault, C., and Dement, W.C. (1981) Monoaminergic mechanisms and experimental cataplexy. *Annals of Neurology*, **10** (4), 369–376.

11 Schober, A. (2004) Classic toxin-induced animal models of Parkinson's disease: 6-OHDA and MPTP. *Cell Tissues Research*, **318**, 215–224.

12 Terzioglu, M. and Galter, D. (2008) Parkinson's disease: genetic versus toxin-induced rodent models. *FEBS Journal*, **275**, 1384–1391.

13 Przedborski, S., Levivier, M., Jiang, H., Ferreira, M., Jackson-Lewis, V., Donaldson, D., and Togasaki, D.M. (1995) Dose-dependent lesions of the dopaminergic nigrostriatal pathway induced by intrastriatal injection of 6-hydroxydopamine. *Neuroscience*, **67** (3), 631–647.

14 Bove, J. and Perier, C. (2012) Neurotoxin-based models of Parkinson's disease. *Neuroscience*, **211**, 51–76.

15 Sachs, C. and Jonsson, G. (1975) Mechanisms of action of 6-hydroxydopamine. *Biochemistry and Pharmacology*, **24** (1), 1–8.

16 Breit, S., Martin, A., Lessmann, L., Cerkez, D., Gasser, T., and Schulz, J.B. (2008) Bilateral changes in neuronal activity of the basal ganglia in the unilateral 6-hydroxydopamine rat model. *Journal of Neuroscience Research*, **86** (6), 1388–1396.

17 Wichmann, T. and Dostrovsky, J.O. (2011) Pathological basal ganglia activity in movement disorders. *Neuroscience*, **198**, 232–244.

18 Emborg, M.E. (2004) Evaluation of animal models of Parkinson's disease for neuroprotective strategies. *Journal of Neuroscience Methods*, **139**, 121–143.

19 Pienaar, I.S., Lu, B., and Schallert, T. (2012) Closing the gap between clinic and cage: sensori-motor and cognitive behavioural

testing regimens in neurotoxin-induced animal models of Parkinson's disease. *Neuroscience Biobehavior Review*, **36** (10), 2305–2324.

20 Schmidt, W.J., Lebsanft, H., Heindl, M., Gerlach, M., Gruenblatt, E., Riederer, P., Mayerhofer, A., and Scheller, D.K. (2008) Continuous versus pulsatile administration of rotigotine in 6-OHDA-lesioned rats: contralateral rotations and abnormal involuntary movements. *Journal of Neural Transmission*, **115** (10), 1385–1392.

21 Moses, D., Gross, A., and Finberg, J.P. (2004) Rasagiline enhances l-DOPA-induced contralateral turning in the unilateral 6-hydroxydopamine-lesioned guinea-pig. *Neuropharmacology*, **47** (1), 72–80.

22 Reavill, C., Jenner, P., and Marsden, C.D. (1983) Differentiation of dopamine agonists using drug-induced rotation in rats with unilateral or bilateral 6-hydroxydopamine destruction of ascending dopamine pathways. *Biochemistry and Pharmacology*, **32** (5), 865–870.

23 Robertson, H.A. (1992) Dopamine receptor interactions: some implications for the treatment of Parkinson's disease. *Trends in Neuroscience*, **15** (6), 201–206.

24 Koga, K., Kurokawa, M., Ochi, M., Nakamura, J., and Kuwana, Y. (2000) Adenosine A_{2A} receptor antagonists KF17837 and KW-6002 potentiate rotation induced by dopaminergic drugs in hemi-Parkinsonian rats. *European Journal of Pharmacology*, **408** (3), 249–255.

25 Meissner, W.G., Frasier, M., Gasser, T., Goetz, C.G., Lozano, A., Piccini, P., Obeso, J., Rascal, O., Schapira, A., Voon, V., Weiner, D.M., Tison, F., and Bezard, E. (2011) Priorities in Parkinson's disease research. *Nature Reviews. Drug Discovery*, **10**, 377–393.

26 Iderberg, H., Francardo, V., and Pioli, E.Y. (2012) Animal models of l-DOPA-induced dyskinesia: an update on the current options. *Neuroscience*, **211**, 13–27.

27 Johnson, K.A., Conn, P.J., and Niswender, C.M. (2009) Glutamate receptors as therapeutic targets for Parkinson's disease. *CNS Neurological Disorders Drug Targets*, **8** (6), 475–491.

28 Langston, J.W. and Ballard, P. (1984) Parkinsonism induced by 1-methyl-4-phenyl-1,2,3,6-tetrahydropyridine (MPTP): implications for treatment and the pathogenesis of Parkinson's disease. *Canadian Journal of Neurological Sciences*, **11** (1 Suppl.), 160–165.

29 Fox, S.H. and Brotchie, J.M. (2010) The MPTP-lesioned non-human primate models of Parkinson's disease. Past, present, and future. *Progress in Brain Research*, **184**, 133–157.

30 Luchtman, D.W., Shao, D., and Song, C. (2009) Behavior, neurotransmitters and inflammation in three regimens of the MPTP mouse model of Parkinson's disease. *Physiology & Behavior*, **98** (1–2), 130–138.

31 Bankiewicz, K.S., Oldfield, E.H., Chiueh, C.C., Doppman, J.L., Jacobowitz, D.M., and Kopin, I.J. (1986) Hemiparkinsonism in monkeys after unilateral internal carotid artery infusion of 1-methyl-4-phenyl-1,2,3,6-tetrahydropyridine (MPTP). *Life Sciences*, **39** (1), 7–16.

32 Prediger, R.D., Aguiar, A.S., Jr., Moreira, E.L., Matheus, F.C., Castro, A.A., Walz, R., De Bem, A.F., Latini, A., Tasca, C.I., Farina, M., and Raisman-Vozari, R. (2011) The intranasal administration of 1-methyl-4-phenyl-1,2,3,6-tetrahydropyridine (MPTP): a new rodent model to test palliative and neuroprotective agents for Parkinson's disease. *Current Pharmacological Design*, **17** (5), 489–507.

33 Alvarez-Fischer, D., Guerreiro, S., Hunot, S., Saurini, F., Marien, M., Sokoloff, P., Hirsch, E.C., Hartmann, A., and Michel, P.P. (2008) Modelling Parkinson-like neurodegeneration via osmotic minipump delivery of MPTP and probenecid. *Journal of Neurochemistry*, **107** (3), 701–711.

34 Wichmann, T., Bergman, H., and DeLong, M.R. (1994) The primate subthalamic nucleus. III. Changes in motor behavior and neuronal activity in the internal pallidum induced by subthalamic inactivation in the MPTP model of parkinsonism. *Journal of Neurophysiology*, **72** (2), 521–530.

35 Brown, P. and Williams, D. (2005) Basal ganglia local field potential activity: character and functional significance in the human. *Clinical Neurophysiology*, **116** (11), 2510–2519.

36 Meissner, W., Leblois, A., Hansel, D., Bioulac, B., Gross, C.E., Benazzouz, A., and

Boraud, T. (2005) Subthalamic high frequency stimulation resets subthalamic firing and reduces abnormal oscillations. *Brain*, **128** (10), 2372–2382.

37. Bankiewicz, K.S., Bringas, J.R., McLaughlin, W., Pivirotto, P., Hundal, R., Yang, B., Emborg, M.E., and Nagy, D. (1998) Application of gene therapy for Parkinson's disease: nonhuman primate experience. *Advances in Pharmacology*, **42**, 801–806.

38. Lane, E.L., Bjorklund, A., Dunnett, S.B., and Winkler, C. (2010) Neural grafting in Parkinson's disease unraveling the mechanisms underlying graft-induced dyskinesia. *Progress in Brain Research*, **184**, 295–309.

39. Tanner, C.M., Kamel, F., Ross, G.W., Hoppin, J.A., Goldman, S.M., Korell, M., Marras, C., Bhudhikanok, G.S., Kasten, M., Chade, A.R., Comyns, K., Richards, M.B., Meng, C., Priestley, B., Fernandez, H.H., Cambi, F., Umbach, D.M., Blair, A., Sandler, D.P., and Langston, J.W. (2011) Rotenone, paraquat, and Parkinson's disease. *Environmental Health Perspective*, **119** (6), 866–872.

40. Martinez, T.N. and Greenamyre, J.T. (2012) Toxin models of mitochondrial dysfunction in Parkinson's disease. *Antioxidants and Redox Signaling*, **16** (9), 920–934.

41. Betarbet, R. and Greenamyre, J.T. (2002) Animal models of Parkinson's disease. *BioEssays*, **24**, 308–318.

42. Pan-Montojo, F., Anichtchik, O., Dening, Y., Knels, L., Pursche, S., Jung, R., Jackson, S., Gille, G., Spillantini, MG., Reichmann, H., and Funk, RH. (2010) Progression of Parkinson's disease pathology is reproduced by intragastric administration of rotenone in mice. *PLoS One*, **5** (1), e8762.

43. Liu, M., Choi, D.Y., Hunter, R.L., Pandya, J.D., Cass, W.A., Sullivan, P.G., Kim, H.C., Gash, D.M., and Bing, G. (2010) Trichloroethylene induces dopaminergic neurodegeneration in Fisher 344 rats. *Journal of Neurochemistry*, **112** (3), 773–783.

44. Gasser, T. (2009) Molecular pathogenesis of Parkinson disease: insights from genetic studies. *Expert Reviews in Molecular Medicine*, **11**, e22.

45. Lee, Y., Dawson, V.L., and Dawson, T.M. (2012) Animal models of Parkinson's disease: vertebrate genetics. *Cold Spring Harbor Perspectives in Medicine*, **2**, a009324.

46. Lim, K.L. and Ng, C.H. (2009) Genetic models of Parkinson disease. *Biochimica et Biophysica Acta*, **1792** (7), 604–615.

47. Giasson, B.I., Duda, J.E., Quinn, S.M., Zhang, B., Trojanowski, J.Q., and Lee, V.M. (2002) Neuronal alpha-synucleinopathy with severe movement disorder in mice expressing A53T human alpha-synuclein. *Neuron*, **34** (4), 521–533.

48. Nunes, I., Tovmasian, L.T., Silva, R.M., Burke, R.E., and Goff, S.P. (2003) Pitx3 is required for development of substantia nigra dopaminergic neurons. *Proceedings of the National Academy of Sciences of the United States of America*, **100** (7), 4245–4250.

49. Wallen, A. and Perlmann, T. (2003) Transcriptional control of dopamine neuron development. *Annals of New York Academy of Sciences*, **991**, 48–60.

50. Settivari, R., Levora, J., and Nass, R. (2009) The divalent metal transporter homologues SMF-1/2 mediate dopamine neuron sensitivity in *Caenorhabditis elegans* models of manganism and Parkinson disease. *Journal of Biological Chemistry*, **284** (51), 35758–35768.

51. Ekstrand, M.I., Terzioglu, M., Galter, D., Zhu, S., Hofstetter, C., Lindqvist, E., Thams, S., Bergstrand, A., Hansson, F.S., Trifunovic, A., Hoffer, B., Cullheim, S., Mohammed, A.H., Olson, L., and Larsson, N.G. (2007) Progressive parkinsonism in mice with respiratory-chain-deficient dopamine neurons. *Proceedings of the National Academy of Sciences of the United States of America*, **104** (4), 1325–1330.

52. Lin, X., Parisiadou, L., Sgobio, C., Liu, G., Yu, J., Sun, L., Shim, H., Gu, X.L., Luo, J., Long, C.X., Ding, J., Mateo, Y., Sullivan, P.H., Wu, L.G., Goldstein, D.S., Lovinger, D., and Cai, H. (2012) Conditional expression of Parkinson's disease-related mutant α-synuclein in the midbrain dopaminergic neurons causes progressive neurodegeneration and degradation of transcription factor nuclear receptor related 1. *Journal of Neuroscience*, **32** (27), 9248–9264.

53. Sloan, M., Alegre-Abarrategui, J., and Wade-Martins, R. (2012) Insights into LRRK2 function and dysfunction from transgenic

54 Le Poul, E., Boléa, C., Girard, F., Poli, S., Charvin, D., Campo, B., Bortoli, J., Bessif, A., Luo, B., Koser, A.J., Hodge, L.M., Smith, K.M., DiLella, A.G., Liverton, N., Hess, F., Browne, S.E., and Reynolds, I.J. (2012) A potent and selective metabotropic glutamate receptor 4 positive allosteric modulator improves movement in rodent models of Parkinson's disease. *Journal of Pharmacology and Experimental Therapeutics*, **343** (1), 167–177.

55 Lu, X.H., Fleming, S.M., Meurers, B., Ackerson, L.C., Mortazavi, F., Lo, V., Hernandez, D., Sulzer, D., Jackson, G.R., Maidment, N.T., Chesselet, M.F., and Yang, X.W. (2009) Bacterial artificial chromosome transgenic mice expressing a truncated mutant parkin exhibit age-dependent hypokinetic motor deficits, dopaminergic neuron degeneration, and accumulation of proteinase K-resistant alpha-synuclein. *Journal of Neuroscience*, **29** (7), 1962–1976.

56 Johnson, S.J. and Wade-Martins, R. (2011) A BACwards glance at neurodegeneration: molecular insights into disease from LRRK2, SNCA and MAPT BAC-transgenic mice. *Biochemical Society Transactions*, **39** (4), 862–867.

57 Löw, K. and Aebischer, P. (2012) Use of viral vectors to create animal models for Parkinson's disease. *Neurobiology of Disease*, **48** (2), 189–201.

58 Iravani, M.M., Leung, C.C., Sadeghian, M., Haddon, C.O., Rose, S., and Jenner, P. (2005) The acute and the long-term effects of nigral lipopolysaccharide administration on dopaminergic dysfunction and glial cell activation. *European Journal of Neuroscience*, **22** (2), 317–330.

59 Jenner, P. (2008) Functional models of Parkinson's disease: a valuable tool in the development of novel therapies. *Annals of Neurology*, **64** (Suppl.), S16–S29.

60 McNaught, K.S., Perl, D.P., Brownell, A.L., and Olanow, C.W. (2004) Systemic exposure to proteasome inhibitors causes a progressive model of Parkinson's disease. *Annals of Neurology*, **56** (1), 149–162.

61 Kordower, J.H., Kanaan, N.M., Chu, Y., Suresh Babu, R., Stansell, J., Terpstra, B.T., Sortwell, C.E., Steece-Collier, K., and Collier, T.J. (2006) Failure of proteasome inhibitor administration to provide a model of Parkinson's disease in rats and monkeys. *Annals of Neurology*, **60** (2), 264–268.

62 Sardi, S.P., Clarke, J., Viel, C., Chan, M., Tamsett, T.J., Treleaven, C.M., Bu, J., Sweet, L., Passini, M.A., Dodge, J.C., Haung Yu, W., Sidman, R.L., Cheng, S.H., and Shihabuddin, L.S. (2012) Augmenting CNS glucocerebrosidase activity as a therapeutic strategy for parkinsonism and other Gaucher-related synucleinopathies. *Proceedings of the National Academy of Sciences of the United States of America*, **110** (9), 3537–3542.

63 Pienaar, I.S., Götz, J., and Feany, M.B. (2010) Parkinson's disease: insights from non-traditional model organisms. *Progress in Neurobiology*, **92** (4), 558–571.

64 Pendleton, R.G., Parvez, F., Sayed, M., and Hillman, R. (2002) Effects of pharmacological agents upon a transgenic model of Parkinson's disease in *Drosophila melanogaster*. *Journal of Pharmacology and Experimental Therapeutics*, **300** (1), 91–96.

65 Mizuno, H., Fujikake, N., Wada, K., and Nagai, Y. (2010) α-Synuclein transgenic *Drosophila* as a model of Parkinson's disease and related synucleinopathies. *Parkinson's Disease*, **2011**, 212706.

66 Xi, Y., Noble, S., and Ekker, M. (2011) Modeling neurodegeneration in zebrafish. *Current Neurology and Neuroscience Reports*, **11** (3), 274–282.

67 Harrington, A.J., Hamamichi, S., Caldwell, G.A., and Caldwell, K.A. (2010) *C. elegans* as a model organism to investigate molecular pathways involved with Parkinson's disease. *Developmental Dynamics*, **239** (5), 282–295.

68 Braungart, E., Gerlach, M., Riederer, P., Baumeister, R., and Hoener, M.C. (2004) *Caenorhabditis elegans* MPP$^+$ model of Parkinson's disease for high-throughput drug screenings. *Neurodegenerative Disorders*, **1** (4–5), 175–183.

69 Bezard, E., Yue, Z., Kirik, D., and Spillantini, M.G. (2013) Animal models of Parkinson's disease: limits and relevance to neuroprotection studies. *Movement Disorders*, **28** (1), 61–70.

70 Potashkin, J.A., Blume, S.R., and Runkle, N.K. (2010) Limitations of animal models of Parkinson's disease. *Parkinson's Disease*, **2011**, 658083.

71 Masuda-Suzukake, M., Nonaka, T., Hosokawa, M., Oikawa, T., Arai, T., Akiyama, H., Mann, D.M., and Hasegawa, M. (2013) Prion-like spreading of pathological α-synuclein in brain. *Brain*, **136**, 1128–1138.

72 Collier, T.J., Kanaan, N.M., and Kordower, J.H. (2011) Ageing as a primary risk factor for Parkinson's disease: evidence from studies of non-human primates. *Nature Reviews. Neuroscience*, **12** (6), 359–366.

19
Epilepsy: Animal Models to Reproduce Human Etiopathology

Isabelle Guillemain, Christophe Heinrich, and Antoine Depaulis

19.1
Introduction

Epilepsy is a family of brain disorders that are characterized by regular occurrences of epileptic seizures that can have different electroclinical expressions, but that are due to an abnormal and hypersynchronous neuronal activity in the brain. An epileptic seizure can be as subtle as a momentary lapse of attention in some patients, but can also be associated with brutal and involuntary contractions of muscles (convulsions), depending on the involved regions of the brain. Worldwide, the age-adjusted prevalence of epilepsy is ∼4–10 per 1000 people [1,2]. It is one of the most common neurological disorders and affects ∼50 million people worldwide. The different forms of epilepsies greatly impact the life of both the patients and their families, and the society at large. Indeed, this pathology can negatively affect cognitive functions and cause increased mortality. It is a source of social disturbances and is associated with an increased risk of psychiatric disorders. It is, therefore, a major burden on our society and there is a crucial need for new effective treatments to control epileptic seizures and cure epileptic patients. Since the discovery of the potent antiepileptic effects of barbiturates about a century ago, up to 30 different antiepileptic drugs (AEDs) have been developed and ∼20 of them are currently available for the treatment of epileptic seizures [3]. However, these AEDs remain ineffective in suppressing seizures in ∼30% of epileptic patients and new mechanisms/targets are required to help them control their disease. Furthermore, all of the available AEDs have multiple secondary effects, which may seriously affect the patients' quality of life. Finally, no treatments are yet available to prevent epileptogenesis, that is, the process by which a brain develops epilepsy following an initial insult or during brain maturation.

In the last 30 years, animal models have led to the discovery of most commonly prescribed AEDs. The diversity of these models has proven to be of inestimable value for investigating basic mechanisms underlying epileptogenicity. They range from *Drosophila* to nonhuman primates, rats and mice being the most used. However, most of these preparations are considered as models of *seizures* (i.e., in which acute seizures are artificially evoked) rather than *epilepsy*, which is defined by the recurrence of spontaneous seizures. Indeed, the understanding of epilepsy and the development of AED require the use of models where spontaneous seizures occur chronically. Even after several years of research on the mechanisms underlying epilepsies and the possibility of controlling seizures with better designed compounds, we have failed to provide innovative targets to treat drug-resistant focal epilepsies. One of the reasons appears to be a lack of relevant animal models corresponding to these forms of epilepsy that are especially diverse not only regarding their causes (malformative, vascular, posttraumatic, infectious, genetic, etc.) but also the brain regions that are involved (temporal, frontal, occipital, etc.). Currently used animal models are often very different from the clinical conditions. Although it is quite understandable that a biological model is a simplified representation of a disease [4], there are essential electroclinical and histological features that need to be modeled in order to provide data that can be transposed to the clinic. Several sophisticated animal models have been developed during the past 10–20 years either by classical (i.e., lesions, stimulations, and genetic selection) or by more modern methods (i.e., transgenesis, transfection, and RNA interference) that display several electroencephalography (EEG), behavioral, or histopathological features reminiscent of a given form of epilepsy. Several of these models display a complex variety of features and the question remains to select those that are the most relevant for the clinical situation.

With the development of sophisticated genomic tools to generate new animal models with chronic occurrence of seizures, there is an urgent need to reconsider the most critical features for a given form of epilepsy to provide transposable data. Recently, a survey was performed by European neurologists with a strong expertise in the treatment of epilepsies, in order to determine which features could be essential to model four different prototypic forms of epilepsy: idiopathic epilepsy with generalized convulsive seizures, absence epilepsy, and focal epilepsies associated with either focal cortical dysplasia or hippocampal sclerosis, the latter two forms being especially frequent in epileptic patients (Guillemain *et al.*, in preparation; [5]). In this chapter, we discuss different animal models for these corresponding forms of epilepsy in the light of the clinician's requirements.

19.2
What Animal Species to Use to Model Epilepsy?

When asked a panel of European clinicians about the type of animal model of epilepsy to obtain the most reliable data for the clinic, rodents and monkeys obtained the largest score (Guillemain *et al.*, in preparation; [5]). This is in agreement with what is generally done in laboratories, although nonhuman primates are less and less used for technical, economical, and ethical reasons. In the 1980s, animal models of epilepsy were studied using dogs [6,7]. Epileptic dogs are the only genetic animal model of epilepsy that allows selection of animals with both pharmaco-resistant and pharmaco-sensitive seizures. However, there are several drawbacks to this model. Almost all studies were conducted on dogs from private owners who do not allow invasive experiments or give away their animals for breeding purposes. Moreover, no attempts to select drug-resistant animals from subgroups of dog colonies have been reported. In this respect, the high prime and maintenance costs of dogs necessary for selection and breeding of epileptic sublines limit the usefulness of this species for drug evaluation or studies on mechanisms of drug resistance [4]. More recently, in order to dissect in more detail the epileptic mechanisms, new and atypical models appear, especially the *Drosophila* and the zebrafish [8,9]. Seizure-like neuronal activities and behaviors in the fruit fly are described, as well as a set of mutations that exhibit features resembling some human epilepsies and render the fly sensitive to seizures [10–12]. A zebrafish model of seizures where larvae are exposed to various concentrations of a well-known convulsant (pentylenetetrazole) was developed [13]. Zebrafish have now been used to study effects of AED (valproic acid) on seizure-induced learning deficits [14] to identify pathway mechanisms involved in epilepsy [15] and to determine the genetic aspects of epilepsy [16]. These models are currently used for their capacity to generate more easily than rodent genetic mutations and are envisaged to be used for AED testing. However, they are still considered as emerging models and not commonly used in the field of epilepsy.

19.3 Which Type of Models Provide the Most Reliable Information on the Pathophysiology of Epilepsies?

In epilepsy, the panel of models ranges from *in silico* models to nonhuman primates, including *ex vivo* preparations like slices from either normal or epileptic animals, but also from human patients. When asked about the relevance of the different models available, clinicians showed only limited interest for data collected in acute preparations like *ex vivo* slices from normal animals or models where acute seizures are artificially induced (Guillemain *et al.*, in preparation; [5]). This is likely due to the lack of recurrence of seizures in these models as well as the difficulty to transfer these kinds of laboratory data to the clinic. However, *ex vivo* models using brain slices (e.g., from hippocampus) maintained alive for several hours and the seizures induced here by several kinds of manipulations (e.g., low concentration of magnesium) have increased our understanding of ictiogenesis (i.e., the transition from normal bioelectrical activity to epileptiform activity) [17,18]. More recently, the possibility to maintain in *ex vivo* conditions both hippocampi of the same animal and to control individually the perfusion media of each one, keeping intact their connectivity, has greatly enhanced the possibility to address issues like the propagation of seizures and the formation of a mirror focus [19,20]. It is noteworthy that clinicians show a marked interest for data collected in slice preparations obtained from human patients after resective surgery (Guillemain *et al.*, in preparation; [5]). Although such approach is unique for studying the cellular mechanisms of a human brain disease, very few groups in the world have developed the expertise [21,22].

The clear tendencies in both academic and private laboratories are to prefer animal models (usually mice and rats) where seizures occur spontaneously with sufficient recurrence. These models, whether they are induced by an initial insult, genetic selection, or after transgenesis (see below), are strongly preferred by clinicians. By contrast, preparations using normal animals where one or a few seizures are induced by a convulsant (e.g., pentylenetetrazole, bicuculline, and strychnine) or an electroshock are considered less and less relevant or are limited to the study of epilepsies with generalized tonic–clonic seizures. Finally, it is interesting to note that clinicians show more interest in mathematical models than in acute animal models. Indeed, several recent studies have proposed different approaches that model either the behavior of a population of neurons able to produce discharges that can be compared with EEG recordings [23] or the behavior of a neuron able to generate a paroxysmal depolarization shift, often encountered in epileptic discharges [24].

Epilepsy is not a single disorder, but rather consists of multiple heterogeneous syndromes with many etiologies. Here, we propose to address the most available models in four characteristic forms of epilepsy with a preference for emerging ones.

19.4
Modeling Four Prototypic Forms of Epilepsy

19.4.1
Idiopathic Generalized Epilepsies with Convulsive Seizures

Idiopathic generalized epilepsies (IGEs) constitute about 20% (15–32% according to different studies) [25] of all epilepsies, but are often the form to which people refer to. Indeed, IGEs with convulsive seizures are most of the time characterized by myoclonia or tonic and/or clonic convulsions [26]. Most syndromes of these IGE start in childhood or adolescence, but some have an adult onset. They usually remain lifelong, although a few are age related [26]. IGEs with convulsive seizures are classically modeled in mice and rats by tonic–clonic seizures induced by electroshock (electroconvulsive seizure (ECS)) or pentylenetetrazole (PTZ) injection [27,28]. Indeed, both protocols induce generally one bilateral and symmetric tonic–clonic seizure associated with a discharge of high-amplitude spikes and spike-and-waves that can be recorded with cortical electrodes (EEG). This seizure is always followed by a flattening of the EEG concomitant with a comatose behavior. These models, which are easy to obtain, have proven to be useful in drug development, as most anticonvulsive compounds are effective. However, several current AEDs did not have effect on them [29]. Most of all, the interest of PTZ and ECS to increase our understanding of the pathophysiology of IGE remains limited and it is very likely that they are not predictive for other forms of epilepsy like focal ones.

The most required features by clinical epileptologists in modeling IGE with convulsive seizures are (1) a similar reactivity to AED and (2) EEG pattern. The similarities of the brain structures involved were also found to be important as well as the genetic mutations and behavior during seizures. Several genetic models (e. g., tottering mouse) with spontaneous generalized convulsive seizures have been reported that have notably increased our knowledge of the role of some mutations in the development of IGE [30]. Indeed, most of these models are monogenic with mutations mainly affecting genes coding for ionic channels [31]. However, in addition to the convulsive seizures, the animals also display a complex phenotype (e.g., dyskinesia) [32]. Although these models are of great interest, the sporadic occurrence of the spontaneous seizures, the difficulties in maintaining the lineage, and the lack of both EEG and pharmacological information make them difficult to use during the preclinical development of a candidate AED.

Rodent strains where seizures are triggered by sensory stimuli have also been described and appear more convenient to use. In particular, abundant data have been collected on the generalized epilepsy prone rat (GEPR) that presents convulsive seizures upon stimulation by a loud sound [33]. In this model, the pharmacological reactivity offers many similarities with the clinical reactivity. However, the type of seizures (mainly tonic) and the structures involved (mainly brainstem) make the data obtained with this model difficult to transpose to human IGE with convulsive seizures or even epilepsies with reflex seizures [34]. New models are being developed in mice that result from different types of gene manipulations, mostly issued from our knowledge on clinical genetic [35]. Although promising, these models will need to be characterized in terms of pharmacological reactivity, EEG patterns, and brain structures involved in order to provide relevant information for the clinicians.

19.4.2
Idiopathic Generalized Epilepsies with Absence Seizures

The prevalence of absence epilepsy is 10–12% in children younger than 16 years of age with epilepsy [36]. Among IGEs, absence epilepsy is an epileptic syndrome characterized by *nonconvulsive* seizures during which a brief unresponsiveness to environmental stimuli and cessation of activity may be accompanied by automatisms or moderate myoclonic components [37,38]. On the EEG, typical absence seizures are associated with bilateral, synchronous, and regular three cycles per second spike-and-wave discharges (SWDs), which start and end abruptly.

This unique EEG pattern along with behavioral arrest was found to be the most relevant feature to model absence epilepsy by clinicians (Guillemain *et al.*, in preparation; [5]). Indeed, SWDs have been EEG recorded in the different genetic models that were described during the past 20 years in both mice [30] and rats [39]. The mandatory use of EEG in these models has rapidly allowed the identification of the brain structures involved (i.e., the cortex and the ventrolateral thalamus) in the initiation and maintenance of the SWD, a feature that is highly required by clinicians in our surveys (Guillemain *et al.*, in preparation; [5]). More recently, the group of van Luijtelaar as well as ours identified the somatosensory cortex as the region where SWDs are bilaterally initiated in both the WAG/Rij and the GAERS [40–42]. Although it is unlikely that the somatosensory cortex *per se* initiates SWD in human patients, the concept of a cortical area of initiation was validated in clinical studies where frontal cortical regions appeared as initiating zones [43]. This concept of "focality" of absence seizures has led to the development of several studies to understand what makes a cortical neuronal network prone to initiate SWD [44,45]. This should lead to the development of new therapeutic targets not only for absence epilepsy but also for other forms of epilepsies that are associated with SWD and, very likely, for their epileptogenesis. Indeed, in both WAG/Rij and GAERS models, a period of several weeks during which SWDs progressively develop has been described and thus they offer a unique approach to understand the etiology of this form of epilepsy [45].

Another important feature that is unique in absence epilepsy and needs to be validated in animal models is the pharmacological reactivity. In human patients, some AEDs (e.g., ethosuccimide) selectively suppress absence seizures, whereas others (e.g., carbamazepine and vigabatrin) aggravate them. In the two rat models of absence epilepsy (i.e., GAERS and WAG/Rij), all antiepileptic compounds that suppress SWD in human patients are effective, whereas AEDs that increase SWD in the clinic aggravate absence seizures. Therefore, GAERS and WAG/Rij offer the possibility to powerfully predict whether a candidate AED will suppress absence seizures or will lead to possible counterindications [39].

WAG/Rij and GAERS should also provide important information on the gene mutations that could lead to the development of absence seizures (also see discussion in Ref. [46]). In both models, several quantitative trait loci have been described [45], but they poorly refer to regions of interest in the human genome. In the GAERS, a single-nucleotide mutation was described on the gene coding for the $Ca_v3.2$ subunit of the low-threshold calcium channel [47]. This mutation was found in all three current GAERS colonies (Grenoble, Melbourne, and Istanbul), but not in the WAG/Rij (K. Powell, personal communication). It may control alternative splicing of one exon that could be associated with a gain of function of this channel and could explain about one third of the phenotypes. Such finding is in agreement with the putative mechanisms of action of ethosuccimide, an AED specific for absence epilepsy and could well lead to the development of new targets for AED able to suppress SWD-type of seizures. In conclusion, these two polygenic rat models offer valuable preparations to study the main features selected by clinicians to understand and treat absence epilepsy.

19.4.3
Focal Epilepsies Associated with Cortical Dysplasia

Cortical dysplasia is the most common cause of drug-resistant focal epilepsies in children [48] and has been described as a pathological substrate for epilepsy [49]. Focal cortical dysplasia is characterized by a disruption of the cortical normal lamination and can vary in severity, ranging from a mild disruption with a normal morphology of neurons to a strong loss of laminar organization of the cortex. The latter is usually accompanied by the appearance of dysmorphic and misoriented neurons, neuronal clustering, giant neurons, and/or balloon cells [50]. According to our survey, histopathology emerged as the most important feature to model focal epilepsies associated with cortical dysplasia (Guillemain *et al.*, in preparation; [5]). The EEG pattern of the seizures and the brain structures involved were also found quite relevant by about half of the clinicians.

Several animal models of cortical dysplasia have been previously described following genetic, fetal, or neonatal manipulations [51]. The fetal insult models are induced by administration of an antimitotic drug (i.e., methylazoxymethanol acetate or MAM) or by fetal irradiation of pregnant rats. Both methods induce multifocal cortical dysplasia in newborn rats [52,53]. One of the most characterized animal models of cortical dysplasia is the *in utero* irradiation model in which offsprings develop cortical malformations with a dose-dependent loss of the normal six-layer cortex [54]. Prenatal exposure to MAM results in offsprings with microcephaly, cortical thinning, multifocal brain malformations, and clusters of misplaced neurons in the hippocampus [52]. Genetic animal models also reproduce some rare cortical dysplasia. The telencephalic internal structural heterotopia (TISH) rat model exhibits a forebrain anomaly similar to the human neuronal disorder of "double cortex" and the spontaneous recurrent electrographic and behavioral seizures [55]. Other genetic models of dysplasia are the reeler mice and the ihara mutant rats [51]. The limitation of these models is the capacity for the induced mutations to lead to changes in brain excitability [51]. Spontaneous seizures have been observed only in genetic models that showed bilateral or diffuse lesions.

Type IIB cortical dysplasia [56] has been modeled by focal loss of cortical lamination, astrogliosis, dysmorphic neurons and glia, and undifferentiated giant cells (analogous to balloon cells). Animal models were generated, based on spontaneous or induced mutations of either the *Tsc1* or *Tsc2* genes, mimicking the pathological features of human tuberous sclerosis complex (TSC) with varying degrees. For example, the Eker rat, which carries a spontaneous germline heterozygous mutation of the *Tsc2* gene, exhibits hamartomatous lesions, especially in subcortical or subependymal regions [57,58]. Similarly, a number of conditional knockout mice have allowed to successfully recapitulate selective cytopathological features of TSC, such as disrupted cortical lamination, cytomegalic neurons, and astrogliosis [59–61]. However, a limitation of these models is the failure to consistently reproduce focal tuber-like lesions.

Although certain pathological aspects of focal cortical dysplasia and TSC can be generated in animal models, does this actually lead to epilepsy? Indeed, animal models display epileptic seizures with great variability. Most of them show evidence of decreased seizure threshold and/or increased neuronal excitability. For example, in MAM rats, a decreased seizure threshold in response to proconvulsant drugs and increased spontaneous or evoked epileptiform activity in hippocampal slices were described [62,63]. More recently, using long-term video-EEG monitoring, spontaneous seizures were observed in irradiation- and MAM-induced models [64]. However, the incidence of seizures is relatively low with only 10–20% of the animals being epileptic. Similarly, Eker rats have a slightly increased susceptibility to convulsing agents, but have not been documented to display spontaneous seizures [65], whereas some knockout mouse models of TSC have frequent and progressive seizures [60,66]. Most of these models have a great potential to develop disease-modifying treatments. However, a better characterization of their seizures and their reactivity to AED is required for developing new compounds.

19.4.4
Modeling Focal Epilepsies Associated with Hippocampal Sclerosis

The mesial temporal lobe epilepsy (MTLE) syndrome, the most common form of intractable epilepsies, is characterized by the recurrence of focal seizures in mesial temporal limbic structures such as the hippocampus [67,68]. In most patients, MTLE is initiated by an initial brain insult (e.g., complex febrile seizures) occurring in early childhood, which is then followed by a latent period of several years before the occurrence of the first spontaneous seizures [67,68]. This latent period corresponds to the progressive development of epilepsy, a process termed epileptogenesis [67,68]. In most cases, even if these seizures are initially controlled with appropriate antiepileptic drug treatments, they become refractory to pharmacological medication and last for the patient's lifetime. Histologically, the MTLE syndrome is associated with a hippocampal sclerosis, mainly characterized by a selective neuronal loss associated with a proliferation of astroglial cells within the Ammon's horn of the hippocampus and the hilus of the dentate gyrus (DG) [69]. In addition, MTLE is associated with several forms of neuroplasticity such as a malpositioning of dentate granule cells in the epileptic hippocampus (termed granule cell dispersion) [70] and a sprouting of mossy fibers, that is, the axons of these granule cells.

It is interesting to note that besides the brain structures involved and the histopathology, the clinicians considered that the recurrence of focal seizures with *mild* behavioral expression and the specificity of the EEG pattern of these seizures are critical to model MTLE (Guillemain *et al.*, in preparation; [5]). On the contrary, none of them considered that the occurrence of *generalized convulsive seizures* was relevant for this form of epilepsy. In addition, an initial *status epilepticus*, comorbidities, or the existence of interictal spikes were not considered as critical to model MTLE. Interestingly, the pharmacological reactivity was not found of high importance, probably because of the limited effects of most AEDs in this form of epilepsy. These results raise an important issue as it appears somewhat paradoxical that the models that are commonly used to study the pathophysiology of MTLE (i.e., systemic pilocarpine or kainate) poorly display the features that emerged from our survey. Indeed, in these models, lesions are observed in the hippocampus and limbic structures, but are bilateral and involved different other structures [71]. Therefore, the histopathology of these models appears more complex than what is generally reported in the clinic [72,73]. More problematic is the fact that *generalized* tonic–clonic seizures are mainly taken into account in these models, whereas focal seizures measured by EEG and/or discrete behavioral signs are rarely quantified. This appears in great contrast with clinical observations where secondary tonic–clonic generalizations are rare in MTLE patients [68]. Indeed, these patients suffer from recurrent focal seizures that are most often characterized by an epigastric sensation, consciousness impairment, oroalimentary and gestural automatisms, and postictal confusion, associated with focal discharges on a few derivations of depth-recording electrodes [74]. Developing drugs that suppress generalized convulsive seizures in systemic models may thus lead to compounds that are inappropriate for focal seizures without secondary generalization in human patients. This may explain why several AEDs developed with such models remain ineffective to treat focal seizures in human patients. There is thus an urgent need to reconsider our preclinical strategy to develop new AED more adapted to focal seizures, taking into account their specificity.

A few models with recurrent focal (temporal) seizures that require EEG depth recordings were developed during the past 10 years in mice and rats. They result from the local application of kainate or from a continuous electrical stimulation that triggers an initial *nonconvulsive* epileptic status – that is much less severe than the one triggered by systemic injection of pilocarpine or kainate [75]. This status generally lasts for several hours and does not require pharmacological interruption (e.g., injection of diazepam). Among these models, our laboratory has developed and characterized a mouse model of MTLE that is obtained by a unilateral injection of kainate in the dorsal hippocampus [76]. In this model, the nonconvulsive hippocampal *status epilepticus* is followed by a period of 2–3 weeks, during which recurrent spontaneous hippocampal paroxysmal discharges and hippocampal sclerosis (cell loss, gliosis, mossy fiber sprouting, and granule cell dispersion) progressively develop [75–77]. Using *in vivo* intracellular recordings, we showed that during such focal seizures, hippocampal neurons display sustained membrane depolarization on which are superimposed rhythmic depolarizations supraliminar for action potential discharge and with typical paroxysmal depolarization shift [24]. As in human patients with MTLE, the recurrent seizures recorded in these mice are mostly confined to the hippocampus and rarely generalized [77]. They are associated with mild behavioral modifications (e.g., chewing, head nodding, or stereotyped grooming) [75]. Finally, in this model, due to the high recurrence of hippocampal discharges, AED can easily be tested during 1–2 h after their injection, but also during a chronic treatment. Most importantly, it allows detecting their efficacy on the recurrence of focal seizures, rather than their rare secondary generalization (Bressand *et al.*, in revision). Such a pharmacological profile should offer a better discrimination between drug candidates for focal epilepsies.

Taken together, this model mimics most of the histopathological, electrophysiological, behavioral, and pharmacological features of human MTLE and thus offers a valuable preparation to increase our understanding of this human disease.

19.5
Translation to Clinics: Limitations and Difficulties

There are many forms of epileptic syndromes, (up to 80) and they may be considered as different diseases. They are mainly characterized by the age of onset, the clinical features during seizures, the EEG pattern, the etiology, and so on. In this chapter, we chose to address only four prototypic forms of epilepsy that may represent a first step toward modeling. However, generalizing data from one model of a given form of epilepsy to other forms of epilepsy is a delicate process. Indeed, different mutations, circuits, and molecular mechanisms underlie the different forms of epilepsy. In addition, they are treated differently, either by different antiepileptic drugs or surgery, or they cannot be treated. This is why we have discussed the advantages and limitations of the most used models separately in different sections. However, irrespective of the type of epilepsy, according to our survey among European clinicians, some common criteria appear mandatory in modeling epileptic syndromes. In particular, irrespective of the type of epilepsy, EEG appears as a decisive feature. The use of EEG to record seizures, when possible at the site of onset, should be mandatory for a better determination of the efficacy of a new compound and to approach the cellular and molecular mechanisms that underlie the considered form of epilepsy. Our survey also points out that some features are not critically relevant to an animal model and/or does not help for a better understanding of the pathology and development of the AED. For instance, it appears more and more unlikely that drugs active on models with generalized convulsive seizures will suppress focal seizures in human patients. Similarly, animal models using normal animals as well as slices where acute seizures are induced by a convulsant may help finding new compounds or understanding ictiogenesis, but are questionable to understand the pathophysiology of a given form of epilepsy. Using animal models with features that are different and/or much more complex than the clinical conditions appears inappropriate and probably misleading in the choice of candidate molecules. Whether additional information such as associated comorbidities could help to better design new models remains, however, an interesting and promising issue.

Animal models have played a very important role in advancing our understanding of epilepsy. With their help, basic mechanisms of epileptogenesis and ictiogenesis are being unraveled. However, it remains extremely difficult to design an animal model that recapitulates all the characteristics of a specific epileptic syndrome. If we aim at discovering new AED that effectively suppresses seizures in refractory epilepsies, it appears urgent to reconsider our preclinical strategy and to use animal models with features that are as reminiscent as possible to what is observed in human patients. This means to take into consideration not only the seizures but also other features that characterize the form of epilepsy to be modeled. In this respect, the opinion of hospital neurologists with a strong expertise in epilepsy and drug development is important to consider in order to revisit the models that are currently used (Guillemain *et al.*, in preparation; [5]).

What general criteria should be satisfied before an animal preparation can be validated as a model for a particular human seizure or epilepsy condition? Three criteria should be taken into consideration: construct validity, face validity, and pharmacological predictivity. Considering the construct validity, the etiology should be similar: genetic mutations should provide the same anomaly to be relevant and if the cause is an injury, it should take part in the model design. The age of onset when relevant should also be taken into account. As for the face validity, the similarity between the EEG patterns in human patients and animal model is probably the most important feature to verify, as often required by the clinicians. Finally, the pharmacology reactivity, that is, the response to known AED, in the animal model should be similar to that in the clinical conditions either when suppressing or when aggravating seizures. In an ideal modeling world, animal models should faithfully reproduce all these three criteria.

References

1 Forsgren, L., Hauser, W.A., Olafsson, E., Sander, J.W.A.S., Sillanpää, M., and Tomson, T. (2005) Mortality of epilepsy in developed countries: a review. *Epilepsia*, **46** (Suppl. 11), 18–27.

2 Sander, J.W. (2003) The epidemiology of epilepsy revisited. *Current Opinion in Neurology*, **16** (2), 165–170.

3 Löscher, W. and Schmidt, D. (2011) Modern antiepileptic drug development has failed to deliver: ways out of the current dilemma. *Epilepsia*, **52** (4), 657–678.

4 Löscher, W. (1997) Animal models of intractable epilepsy. *Progress in Neurobiology*, **53** (2), 239–258.

5 Guillemain, I., Kahane, P., and Depaulis, A. (2012) Animal models to study aetiopathology of epilepsy: what are the features to model? *Epileptic Disorders*, **14** (3), 217–225.

6 Edmonds, H.L., Bellin, S.I., Chen, F.C., and Hegreberg, G.A. (1978) Anticonvulsant properties of ropizine in epileptic and nonepileptic beagle dogs. *Epilepsia*, **19** (2), 139–146.

7 Löscher, W. and Schwartz-Porsche, D. (1986) Low levels of gamma-aminobutyric acid in cerebrospinal fluid of dogs with epilepsy. *Journal of Neurochemistry*, **46** (4), 1322–1325.

8 Parker, L., Howlett, I.C., Rusan, Z.M., and Tanouye, M.A. (2011) Seizure and epilepsy: studies of seizure disorders in *Drosophila*. *International Review of Neurobiology*, **99**, 1–21.

9 Bandmann, O. and Burton, E.A. (2010) Genetic zebrafish models of neurodegenerative diseases. *Neurobiology of Disease*, **40** (1), 58–65.

10 Burg, M.G. and Wu, C.-F. (2012) Mechanical and temperature stressor-induced seizure-and-paralysis behaviors in *Drosophila* bang-sensitive mutants. *Journal of Neurogenetics*, **26** (2), 189–197.

11 Kuebler, D. and Tanouye, M.A. (2000) Modifications of seizure susceptibility in *Drosophila*. *Journal of Neurophysiology*, **83** (2), 998–1009.

12 Lin, W.-H., Günay, C., Marley, R., Prinz, A.A., and Baines, R.A. (2012) Activity-dependent alternative splicing increases persistent sodium current and promotes seizure. *The Journal of Neuroscience*, **32** (21), 7267–7277.

13 Baraban, S.C., Taylor, M.R., Castro, P.A., and Baier, H. (2005) Pentylenetetrazole induced changes in zebrafish behavior, neural activity and c-fos expression. *Neuroscience*, **131** (3), 759–768.

14 Lee, Y., Kim, D., Kim, Y.-H., Lee, H., and Lee, C.-J. (2010) Improvement of pentylenetetrazol-induced learning deficits by valproic acid in the adult zebrafish. *European Journal of Pharmacology*, **643** (2–3), 225–231.

15 Hortopan, G.A., Dinday, M.T., and Baraban, S.C. (2010) Spontaneous seizures and altered gene expression in GABA signaling pathways in a mind bomb mutant zebrafish. *The Journal of Neuroscience*, **30** (41), 13718–13728.

16 Hortopan, G.A., Dinday, M.T., and Baraban, S.C. (2010) Zebrafish as a model for studying genetic aspects of epilepsy. *Disease Models & Mechanisms*, **3** (3–4), 144–148.

17 Heinemann, U., Draguhn, A., Ficker, E., Stabel, J., and Zhang, C.L. (1994) Strategies for the development of drugs for pharmacoresistant epilepsies. *Epilepsia*, **35** (Suppl. 5), S10–S21.

18 Wahab, A., Albus, K., Gabriel, S., and Heinemann, U. (2010) In search of models

of pharmacoresistant epilepsy. *Epilepsia*, **51** (Suppl. 3), 154–159.

19 Khalilov, I., Holmes, G.L., and Ben-Ari, Y. (2003) *In vitro* formation of a secondary epileptogenic mirror focus by interhippocampal propagation of seizures. *Nature Neuroscience*, **6** (10), 1079–1085.

20 Khalilov, I., Le Van Quyen, M., Gozlan, H., and Ben-Ari, Y. (2005) Epileptogenic actions of GABA and fast oscillations in the developing hippocampus. *Neuron*, **48** (5), 787–796.

21 Huberfeld, G., de la Prida, L.M., Pallud, J., Cohen, I., Le Van Quyen, M., Adam, C., Clemenceau, S., Baulac, M., and Miles, R. (2011) Glutamatergic pre-ictal discharges emerge at the transition to seizure in human epilepsy. *Nature Neuroscience*, **14** (5), 627–634.

22 Schröder, W., Hinterkeuser, S., Seifert, G., Schramm, J., Jabs, R., Wilkin, G.P., and Steinhäuser, C. (2000) Functional and molecular properties of human astrocytes in acute hippocampal slices obtained from patients with temporal lobe epilepsy. *Epilepsia*, **41** (Suppl. 6), S181–S184.

23 Wendling, F., Bartolomei, F., Mina, F., Huneau, C., and Benquet, P. (2012) Interictal spikes, fast ripples and seizures in partial epilepsies: combining multi-level computational models with experimental data. *The European Journal of Neuroscience*, **36** (2), 2164–2177.

24 Langlois, M., Polack, P.-O., Bernard, H., David, O., Charpier, S., Depaulis, A., and Deransart, C. (2010) Involvement of the thalamic parafascicular nucleus in mesial temporal lobe epilepsy. *The Journal of Neuroscience*, **30** (49), 16523–16535.

25 Jallon, P. and Latour, P. (2005) Epidemiology of idiopathic generalized epilepsies. *Epilepsia*, **46** (Suppl. 9), 10–14.

26 Panayiotopoulos, C.P. (2005) Idiopathic generalized epilepsies: a review and modern approach. *Epilepsia*, **46** (Suppl. 9), 1–6.

27 Löscher, W. (2011) Critical review of current animal models of seizures and epilepsy used in the discovery and development of new antiepileptic drugs. *Seizure*, **20** (5), 359–368.

28 Mares, P. and Kubova, H. (2006) Electrical stimulation-induced models of seizures, in *Models of Seizures and Epilepsy* (eds A. Pitkanen, P. Schwartzkroin, and S.L. Moshe), Elsevier, Burlington, MA, pp. 153–159.

29 Beydoun, A. and D'Souza, J. (2012) Treatment of idiopathic generalized epilepsy: a review of the evidence. *Expert Opinion on Pharmacotherapy*, **13** (9), 1283–1298.

30 Noebels, J.L. (1999) Single-gene models of epilepsy. *Advances in Neurology*, **79**, 227–238.

31 Lerche, H., Shah, M., Beck, H., Noebels, J., Johnston, D., and Vincent, A. (2013) Ion channels in genetic and acquired forms of epilepsy. *The Journal of Physiology*, **591** (Part 4), 753–764.

32 Helbig, I. and Lowenstein, D.H. (2013) Genetics of the epilepsies: where are we and where are we going? *Current Opinion in Neurology*, **26** (2), 179–185.

33 Jobe, P.C., Mishra, P.K., Nandor, L., and Dailey, J.W. (1991) Scope and contribution of genetic models to an understanding of the epilepsies. *Critical Review of Neurobiology*, **6**, 183–220.

34 Hirsch, E., Maton, B., Vergnes, M., Depaulis, A., and Marescaux, C. (1993) Reciprocal positive transfer between kindling of audiogenic seizures and electrical kindling of inferior colliculus. *Epilepsy Research*, **15** (2), 133–139.

35 Frankel, W.N. (2009) Genetics of complex neurological disease: challenges and opportunities for modeling epilepsy in mice and rats. *Trends in Genetics*, **25** (8), 361–367.

36 Callenbach, P.M., Geerts, A.T., Arts, W.F., van Donselaar, C.A., Peters, A.C., Stroink, H., and Brouwer, O.F. (1998) Familial occurrence of epilepsy in children with newly diagnosed multiple seizures: Dutch Study of Epilepsy in Childhood. *Epilepsia*, **39** (3), 331–336.

37 Loiseau, P., Duché, B., and Pédespan, J.M. (1995) Absence epilepsies. *Epilepsia*, **36** (12), 1182–1186.

38 Panayiotopoulos, C.P. (1999) The benign occipital epilepsies of childhood: how many syndromes? *Epilepsia*, **40** (9), 1320–1323.

39 Depaulis, A. and van Luijtelaar, G. (2005) Genetic models of absence epilepsy in the rat, in *Models of Seizures and Epilepsy* (eds A. Pitkanen, P. Schwartzkroin, and S. Moshe), Academic Press, pp. 233–248.

40 David, O., Guillemain, I., Saillet, S., Reyt, S., Deransart, C., Segebarth, C., and Depaulis, A. (2008) Identifying neural drivers with functional MRI: an electrophysiological validation. *PLoS Biology*, **6** (12), 2683–2697.

41 Meeren, H.K.M., Pijn, J.P.M., Van Luijtelaar, E.L.J.M., Coenen, A.M.L., and da Silva, F.H. L. (2002) Cortical focus drives widespread corticothalamic networks during spontaneous absence seizures in rats. *The Journal of Neuroscience*, **22** (4), 1480–1495.

42 Polack, P.-O., Guillemain, I., Hu, E., Deransart, C., Depaulis, A., and Charpier, S. (2007) Deep layer somatosensory cortical neurons initiate spike-and-wave discharges in a genetic model of absence seizures. *The Journal of Neuroscience*, **27** (24), 6590–6599.

43 Holmes, M.D., Brown, M., and Tucker, D. M. (2004) Are "generalized" seizures truly generalized? Evidence of localized mesial frontal and frontopolar discharges in absence. *Epilepsia*, **45** (12), 1568–1579.

44 Chipaux, M., Charpier, S., and Polack, P.O. (2011) Chloride-mediated inhibition of the ictogenic neurones initiating genetically-determined absence seizures. *Neuroscience*, **192**, 642–651.

45 Cope, D.W., Di Giovanni, G., Fyson, S.J., Orbán, G., Errington, A.C., Lőrincz, M.L., Gould, T.M., Carter, D.A., and Crunelli, V. (2009) Enhanced tonic GABAA inhibition in typical absence epilepsy. *Nature Medicine*, **15** (12), 1392–1398.

46 Crunelli, V. and Leresche, N. (2002) Block of thalamic T-type Ca^{2+} channels by ethosuximide is not the whole story. *Epilepsy Currents*, **2** (2), 53–56.

47 Powell, K.L., Cain, S.M., Ng, C., Sirdesai, S., David, L.S., Kyi, M., Garcia, E., Tyson, J.R., Reid, C.A., Bahlo, M., Foote, S.J., Snutch, T.P., and O'Brien, T.J. (2009) A Cav3.2 T-type calcium channel point mutation has splice-variant-specific effects on function and segregates with seizure expression in a polygenic rat model of absence epilepsy. *Neurobiology of Disease*, **29** (2), 371–380.

48 Harvey, A.S., Cross, J.H., Shinnar, S., Mathern, B.W., and ILAE Pediatric Epilepsy Surgery Survey Taskforce (2008) Defining the spectrum of international practice in pediatric epilepsy surgery patients. *Epilepsia*, **49** (1), 146–155.

49 Taylor, D.C., Falconer, M.A., Bruton, C.J., and Corsellis, J.A. (1971) Focal dysplasia of the cerebral cortex in epilepsy. *Journal of Neurology, Neurosurgery and Psychiatry*, **34** (4), 369–387.

50 Palmini, A., Najm, I., Avanzini, G., Babb, T., Guerrini, R., Foldvary-Schaefer, N., Jackson, G., Lüders, H.O., Prayson, R., Spreafico, R., and Vinters, H.V. (2004) Terminology and classification of the cortical dysplasias. *Neurology*, **62** (6 Suppl. 3), S2–S8.

51 Sarkisian, M.R. (2001) Overview of the current animal models for human seizure and epileptic disorders. *Epilepsy & Behavior*, **2** (3), 201–216.

52 Colacitti, C., Sancini, G., DeBiasi, S., Franceschetti, S., Caputi, A., Frassoni, C., Cattabeni, F., Avanzini, G., Spreafico, R., Di Luca, M., and Battaglia, G. (1999) Prenatal methylazoxymethanol treatment in rats produces brain abnormalities with morphological similarities to human developmental brain dysgeneses. *Journal of Neuropathology and Experimental Neurology*, **58** (1), 92–106.

53 Roper, S.N. (1998) *In utero* irradiation of rats as a model of human cerebrocortical dysgenesis: a review. *Epilepsy Research*, **32** (1–2), 63–74.

54 Kellinghaus, C., Kunieda, T., Ying, Z., Pan, A., Lüders, H.O., and Najm, I.M. (2004) Severity of histopathologic abnormalities and *in vivo* epileptogenicity in the *in utero* radiation model of rats is dose dependent. *Epilepsia*, **45** (6), 583–591.

55 Lee, K.S. *et al.* (1997) A genetic animal model of human neocortical heterotopia associated with seizures. *The Journal of Neuroscience*, **17** (16), 6236–6242.

56 Blümcke, I. and Spreafico, R. (2011) An international consensus classification for focal cortical dysplasias. *Lancet Neurology*, **10** (1), 26–27.

57 Mizuguchi, M., Takashima, S., Yamanouchi, H., Nakazato, Y., Mitani, H., and Hino, O. (2000) Novel cerebral lesions in the Eker rat model of tuberous sclerosis: cortical tuber and anaplastic ganglioglioma. *Journal of Neuropathology and Experimental Neurology*, **59** (3), 188–196.

58 Yeung, R.S., Katsetos, C.D., and Klein-Szanto, A. (1997) Subependymal astrocytic hamartomas in the Eker rat model of

tuberous sclerosis. *The American Journal of Pathology*, **151** (5), 1477–1486.

59 Meikle, L., Talos, D.M., Onda, H., Pollizzi, K., Rotenberg, A., Sahin, M., Jensen, F.E., and Kwiatkowski, D.J. (2007) A mouse model of tuberous sclerosis: neuronal loss of Tsc1 causes dysplastic and ectopic neurons, reduced myelination, seizure activity, and limited survival. *The Journal of Neuroscience*, **27** (21), 5546–5558.

60 Uhlmann, E.J., Wong, M., Baldwin, R.L., Bajenaru, M.L., Onda, H., Kwiatkowski, D.J., Yamada, K., and Gutmann, D.H. (2002) Astrocyte-specific TSC1 conditional knockout mice exhibit abnormal neuronal organization and seizures. *Annals of Neurology*, **52** (3), 285–296.

61 Way, S.W., McKenna, J., Mietzsch, U., Reith, R.M., Wu, H.C.J., and Gambello, M.J. (2009) Loss of Tsc2 in radial glia models the brain pathology of tuberous sclerosis complex in the mouse. *Human Molecular Genetics*, **18** (7), 1252–1265.

62 Baraban, S.C. and Schwartzkroin, P.A. (1996) Flurothyl seizure susceptibility in rats following prenatal methylazoxymethanol treatment. *Epilepsy Research*, **23** (3), 189–194.

63 Chevassus-au-Louis, N., Ben-Ari, Y., and Vergnes, M. (1998) Decreased seizure threshold and more rapid rate of kindling in rats with cortical malformation induced by prenatal treatment with methylazoxymethanol. *Brain Research*, **812** (1–2), 252–255.

64 Harrington, E.P., Möddel, G., Najm, I.M., and Baraban, S.C. (2007) Altered glutamate receptor? Transporter expression and spontaneous seizures in rats exposed to methylazoxymethanol in utero. *Epilepsia*, **48**, 1.

65 Wenzel, H.J., Patel, L.S., Robbins, C.A., Emmi, A., Yeung, R.S., and Schwartzkroin, P.A. (2004) Morphology of cerebral lesions in the Eker rat model of tuberous sclerosis. *Acta Neuropathologica*, **108** (2), 97–108.

66 Erbayat-Altay, E., Zeng, L.-H., Xu, L., Gutmann, D.H., and Wong, M. (2007) The natural history and treatment of epilepsy in a murine model of tuberous sclerosis. *Epilepsia*, **48** (8), 1470–1476.

67 Engel, J. (2001) Intractable epilepsy: definition and neurobiology. *Epilepsia*, **42** (Suppl. 6), 3.

68 Santos, N.F., Sousa, S.C., Kobayashi, E., Torres, F.R., Sardinha, J.A.F., Cendes, F., and Lopes-Cendes, I. (2002) Clinical and genetic heterogeneity in familial temporal lobe epilepsy. *Epilepsia*, **43** (Suppl. 5), 136.

69 Mathern, G.W., Babb, T.L., Micevych, P.E., Blanco, C.E., and Pretorius, J.K. (1997) Granule cell mRNA levels for BDNF, NGF, and NT-3 correlate with neuron losses or supragranular mossy fiber sprouting in the chronically damaged and epileptic human hippocampus. *Molecular and Chemical Neuropathology*, **30** (1–2), 53–76.

70 Houser, C.R. (1990) Granule cell dispersion in the dentate gyrus of humans with temporal lobe epilepsy. *Brain Research*, **535** (2), 195–204.

71 Navarro Mora, G., Bramanti, P., Osculati, F., Chakir, A., Nicolato, E., Marzola, P., Sbarbati, A., and Fabene, P.F. (2009) Does pilocarpine-induced epilepsy in adult rats require status epilepticus? *PloS One*, **4** (6), e5759.

72 Sloviter, R.S. (2008) Hippocampal epileptogenesis in animal models of mesial temporal lobe epilepsy with hippocampal sclerosis: the importance of the "latent period" and other concepts. *Epilepsia*, **49** (Suppl. 9), 85–92.

73 Williams, P.A., White, A.M., Clark, S., Ferraro, D.J., Swiercz, W., Staley, K.J., and Dudek, F.E. (2009) Development of spontaneous recurrent seizures after kainate-induced status epilepticus. *The Journal of Neuroscience*, **29** (7), 2103–2112.

74 Chabardès, S., Kahane, P., Minotti, L., Tassi, L., Grand, S., Hoffmann, D., and Benabid, A.L. (2005) The temporopolar cortex plays a pivotal role in temporal lobe seizures. *Brain*, **128** (Part 8), 1818–1831.

75 Riban, V., Bouilleret, V., Pham-Lê, B.T., Fritschy, J.-M., Marescaux, C., and Depaulis, A. (2002) Evolution of hippocampal epileptic activity during the development of hippocampal sclerosis in a mouse model of temporal lobe epilepsy. *Neuroscience*, **112** (1), 101–111.

76 Suzuki, F., Junier, M.P., Guilhem, D., Sørensen, J.C., and Onténiente, B. (1995) Morphogenetic effect of kainate on adult hippocampal neurons associated with a prolonged expression of brain-derived

neurotrophic factor. *Neuroscience*, **64** (3), 665–674.

77 Heinrich, C., Lähteinen, S., Suzuki, F., Anne-Marie, L., Huber, S., Häussler, U., Haas, C., Larmet, Y., Castren, E., and Depaulis, A. (2011) Increase in BDNF-mediated TrkB signaling promotes epileptogenesis in a mouse model of mesial temporal lobe epilepsy. *Neurobiology of Disease*, **42** (1), 35–47.

20
Lung Diseases

Laurent Boyer, Armand Mekontso-Dessap, Jorge Boczkowski, and Serge Adnot

20.1
Introduction

Experimental animal models of lung diseases have proved very useful in the past for elucidating pathophysiological mechanisms and developing new therapeutic strategies. There is no ideal model replicating all the changes seen in lung diseases as complex as lung fibrosis, chronic obstructive lung disease, pulmonary hypertension (PH), or acute respiratory distress syndrome (ARDS). Over the past years, considerable effort has been made toward developing more sophisticated murine models of lung diseases and also toward elaborating concepts based on studies done in both experimental animals and human tissues. Fruitful information has been derived from studies using genetically engineered mice with significant impact on our understanding of not only specific biological processes spanning cell proliferation to cell death but also critical molecular events involved in the pathogenesis of human disease [1]. Several reviews have focused on the use of gene-targeted mice to study various models of lung disease, including airways diseases such as asthma and chronic obstructive pulmonary disease (COPD) and parenchymal lung diseases such as idiopathic pulmonary fibrosis, pulmonary hypertension, pneumonia, and acute lung injury [1–5].

In this chapter, we will refer to these reviews since it is not possible to specifically refer to the enormous data set derived from seminal studies that used specific gene modifications in mice during the past 30 years. However, most of these studies are still using a few experimental animal models that remain essential when investigating pathophysiological concepts or developing new therapeutic strategies. For instance, therapies currently used for treating pulmonary hypertension, including ET-1 receptor antagonists, PDE5 inhibitors, and inhaled NO or tyrosine kinase inhibitor, have all been tested initially in classical experimental animal models of PH. In this chapter, we will therefore focus on experimental animal models that remain essential when assessing a new pathogenic or therapeutic concept in the setting of lung emphysema, pulmonary hypertension, fibrotic lung diseases, and acute lung injury.

20.2
Animal Models of Lung Emphysema or Chronic Obstructive Pulmonary Disease

Chronic obstructive pulmonary disease is currently the fifth leading cause of death worldwide, and recent estimations suggest that the prevalence is ever-increasing and affects 9–10% of adults over 40 years. In developed countries, smoking is by far the most important factor of risk. Developing animal models in COPD is not an easy task, since human COPD is a complex disease composed of at least four anatomical lesions with different expressions among patients: pulmonary emphysema, small airways remodeling (including goblet cell metaplasia, increased inflammatory cells, luminal narrowing, and obstruction by mucus), and pulmonary hypertension. To further complicate matters, COPD develops slowly and gradually over several years and only a part of subjects exposed to cigarette smoke develops the disease.

20.2.1
Cigarette Smoke-Induced COPD

Given that cigarette smoke is the main cause of the disease, animal models using smoke exposure seem to be the natural choice to study the pathophysiology of the disease. It is the model that reproduces more efficiently the various anatomical lesions of COPD. There are a variety of commercial and home-built smoking machines that have been used with animal models; some systems use nose-only exposures and some use whole-body exposures. Measurement of either serum cotinine (a nicotine metabolite) or blood carboxyhemoglobin (COHb) is useful as a method of confirming the relative amount of smoke exposure.

Most studies target smoke-induced emphysema [5]. This emphysema is characterized by dilation of alveolar ducts, correlated with the degree of cigarette smoke intoxication and are anatomically similar to moderate forms of centrilobular emphysema in humans (Figure 20.1a and b). The lesions can be subtle, even under microscopic examination: Morphometric analysis is needed to assess and quantify the degree of emphysema.

Although moderate attention was paid to wall remodeling of the small airways in animal models, it is now accepted as an important cause of airway obstruction in smokers [5,6] and this is observed in the cigarette smoke model. Morphometric analysis confirms that the small airway wall is thickened in mice and guinea pigs after chronic exposure to cigarette smoke [7,8]. This remodeled wall is composed largely of collagen and fibronectin, and the number of smooth muscle cells (SMCs) was not increased [7,8]. Pulmonary artery hypertension (PAH) is also observed in this model, but it can develop in a dissociate manner with the other manifestations of the disease. A major disadvantage of this model is that induction of COPD manifestation takes several months to develop (about 6 months of exposure), which makes it a very expensive and time-consuming model. The most significant limitation of this model is that it induces a mild disease, probably equivalent to 1–2 stage classification of human disease [9], despite the fact that in humans the

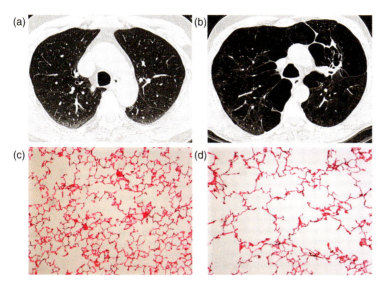

Figure 20.1 Pulmonary emphysema: lung CT scan of a control human subject (a) and of an emphysematous patient (b). Representative photomicrographs (×20 original magnification) of 5 μm thick sections of glutaraldehyde-fixated lung of wild-type mice, 21 days after saline (c) or elastase instillation (d).

majority of the morbidity and mortality due to COPD occur in patients with GOLD stage 3 or 4 (FEV1 <50% predicted).

20.2.2
COPD Induced by Tracheal Elastase Instillation

This model is based on the protease–antiprotease imbalance pathophysiological hypothesis of pulmonary emphysema caused by cigarette smoke [5]. Almost all recent experimental studies have used either pancreatic porcine elastase (PPE) or human neutrophil elastase (HNE) by intratracheal instillation. The emphysema is constituted 21 days after instillation 5 (Figure 20.1c and d). The PPE has the advantages of being inexpensive and easy to obtain. The major drawbacks are centered around two interrelated problems: (i) that elastase and cigarette smoke induced emphysema secondary to proteolytic attack of lung matrix, but mechanisms underlying this process are likely to be very different in the two models, and (ii) the mechanisms leading to elastase-induced emphysema are not clearly defined or are not entirely clear. Indeed, studies using light and electron microscopy [10] showed a rapid degradation of elastin after instillation of elastase, but the disease progresses well after elastase activity has disappeared, suggesting that the model is certainly more complicated than just elastase degradation. Shortly after the administration of the enzyme occur hemorrhage and inflammatory exudate in the lower airways, including neutrophils and macrophages, and an increase in a variety of proinflammatory mediators. The inflammatory process plays an important role in the model because mice deleted for tumor necrosis factor alpha (TNFα) or receptors to IL-1 are almost completely protected against emphysema induced by PPE [11]. Overall, at best, emphysema caused by elastase could be used to screen mechanisms that may apply for smoking subjects, but this approach is far from human exposure to cigarette smoke. The model is also interesting for studies on repair and cellular regeneration when emphysema is constituted.

20.2.3
Genetically Modified Models of COPD

An important part of the recent literature on the COPD pathophysiology is based on models using genetically modified animals. They have the advantage of exploring the effect of a single gene regarding the different COPD alterations. However, most studies using these animals have evaluated the development of emphysema and the researchers were not interested in other COPD alterations [12]. These models should be interpreted with caution because the over or underconstitutive expression of a gene can interfere with lung development and lead to abnormal lung structure similar to those observed in emphysema. Inducible over- or underexpression of a gene in the lung in adulthood using a doxycycline-sensible construction should eliminate the role of the gene in lung development, but some authors have reported that the tetracycline-dependent transactivator used to generate these models can create emphysema *per se* [13]. Finally, doxycycline may inhibit some matrix metalloproteinases (MMPs), which play a role in the pathogenesis of COPD. This set of elements leads to greater caution in the use of inducible transgenic models with need to use all the necessary checks.

20.2.4
Conclusions

Different animal models have been and are used to examine the pathophysiology of COPD. None of these models reproduces all the characteristics of the disease. However, the pattern of exposure to cigarette smoke appears the closest to the human pathology. The elastase model of pulmonary administration keeps its place, especially when it is difficult to develop the exposure to cigarette smoke model. Transgenic models are potentially useful, but the results obtained from their use should be interpreted with caution.

20.3
Animal Models of Pulmonary Hypertension

Pulmonary hypertension is characterized by an increase in pulmonary vascular resistance that impedes the ejection of blood from the right ventricle (RV), ultimately leading to right ventricular failure. For the past three decades, two rodent models have been central to the investigation of human PH: the chronic hypoxia exposure model and the monocrotaline (MCT) lung injury model [3,14]. The MCT rat model continues to be a frequently investigated model of PAH, since it offers technical simplicity, reproducibility, and low cost compared with other models of PAH. Since MCT-induced PH cannot be performed in mice, the hypoxic mouse model is one of the most commonly used to assess PH in genetically engineered mice. Large animal models including primates, (ref), cows (ref), sheep (v), and swine (cc) are also used for specific purposes. For instance, HIV-related PH is better studied in primates: swines have been used as models of PH induced by surgical left to right shunt or of chronic thromboembolic PH; calves develop severe PH when exposed to hypoxia; and ligation of the ductus arteriosus *in utero* in sheep creates a model of primary PH of the newborn for which there is no rodent equivalent [2].

20.3.1
Relevance of Experimental Animal Models of PH to Human PH

Major concerns related to experimental animal models of PH have been addressed. Regarding the pathogenesis of PH, one current criticism is that these models do not recapitulate all the alterations of human PAH, including medial hypertrophy, intimal hyperplasia and adventitial thickening of small pulmonary arteries (PAs), plexiform lesions, and inflammatory cell infiltrates [15]. Moreover, the classification of PH in patients according to the WHO classification in five categories would require animal models using similar taxonomy. Thus, new experimental animal models have emerged in order to reproduce genetic or molecular alterations found in patients with idiopathic PH such as BMPR2 loss of function [16,17] or 5-HTT overexpression [18], to reproduce underlying diseases frequently associated with PH such as schistosomal infection [19], or to combine several pulmonary avascular aggressions such as MCT intoxication and pneumonectomy in rats that were found to aggravate the pulmonary vascular lesions and induce specific alterations of severe PH such as plexiform lesions [20].

An interesting feature shown in recent years is that cultured PA-SMCs derived from remodeled pulmonary vessels from either patients with various types of PH or animal models maintain an abnormal proliferative phenotype *in vitro* [21]. This abnormality was initially considered an intrinsic cell alteration specific to human PH, in analogy with the abnormal behavior of tumor cells [22]. The fact that similar results are obtained with PA-SMCs from animals developing PH after MCT injection or exposure to hypoxia indicates that the proliferative phenotype can be acquired during PH progression [23,24]. The increased PA-SMC growth in both MCT- and hypoxia-induced PH, therefore, suggests that the abnormal proliferative phenotype is independent of the cause of PH.

Regarding the use of these models to test new treatments, the most current criticism is that many therapeutic strategies have been reported to be successful when tested in either the hypoxic or the MCT-PH models that contrast with the paucity of therapeutic strategies shown to be beneficial in human PH. Probably the main reason to explain this ascertainment is that treatments are not tested in patients with PH and in rodent models at the same degree of PH severity. Indeed, treatments in rodents are usually tested when mean pulmonary artery pressure is often in the range of 30–40 mmHg, whereas the usual mean value in patients with PAH is usually higher than 50 mmHg [2]. The rate of PH development also markedly differs between patients and experimental animal models, which can also explain why it may be easier to reverse the rapidly developing pulmonary avascular remodeling process in animals compared with that in humans, which took years to fully develop.

20.3.2
The Monocrotaline Model of Pulmonary Hypertension

A single subcutaneous administration of the pyrrolizidine alkaloid derived from the seeds of the *Crotalaria spectabilis* plant (60–100 mg/kg) reliably results in severe PH within 3–4 weeks and leads to mortality in most rats within 6–8 weeks [2,14]. The MCT alkaloid is activated to the reactive pyrrole metabolite dehydromonocrotaline in the liver, a reaction that is dependent on cytochrome P450 and that occurs in rats but not in mice (Figure 20.2).

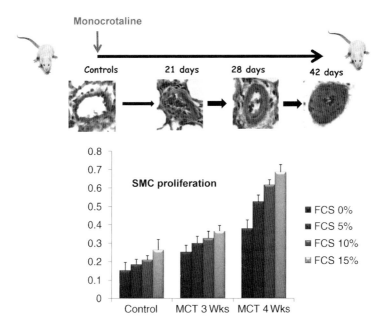

Figure 20.2 Monocrotaline-induced pulmonary hypertension in rats. A single injection of monocrotaline results in the development of major pulmonary vascular remodeling in rats and in severe pulmonary hypertension. As shown in the lower panel, smooth muscle cells collected from pulmonary arteries at various stages of pulmonary hypertension are characterized by a proliferative phenotype that persists *in vitro*.

The rapid progression to death is related to the severity of PH and the subsequent development of RV failure. At lower doses, monocrotaline usually fails to induce PH. Thus, PH severity cannot be controlled and the same batch should be used for repeated experiments.

In most reports, studies are performed in animals with a mean positive airway pressure (PAP) ranging from 35 to 40 mmHg. Studies at higher PAP levels are difficult to conduct due to a great heterogeneity in the tolerance of RV dysfunction and frailty of the animals. Monocrotaline plus pneumonectomy have been shown to induce more severe PH with the development of plexiform-like lesions [20].

20.3.3
Fawn-Hooded Rats

Fawn-hooded rats are characterized by a genetic platelet storage pool disease, which is associated with the inability to store serotonin in platelet granules. Pulmonary hypertension spontaneously develops in this rat strain and is age dependent [25]. Although PH is usually mild in fawn-hooded rats, it can be aggravated by exposure to moderate altitude, as occurs in Denver (elevation 5200 ft). Mechanism at the origin of PH may rely on the increased bioavailability of serotonin in the lung. Other lung abnormalities are associated with PH, including structural abnormalities of the alveoli.

20.3.4
Hypoxic PH

Acute exposure of various mammals to hypoxia results within a few minutes in pulmonary vasoconstriction related to contraction of the SMCs in the distal pulmonary arteries. With chronic exposure, PH is due to not only SMC contraction and polycythemia but also structural remodeling of the pulmonary arteries (Figure 20.3) [26]. Thus, preexisting SMCs in normally muscularized pulmonary arteries undergo hypertrophy and hyperplasia, whereas new SMCs appear in intraacinar arteries that are normally nonmuscularized or muscularized only along part of their circumference. Another component of hypoxia-induced pulmonary artery remodeling is extracellular matrix deposition in the vessel wall, with a buildup of connective tissue proteins such as elastin and collagen [26]. Reversibility is a remarkable feature of chronic hypoxic PH. Although correcting alveolar hypoxia may have little or no effect on PH in the short term, PH caused by chronic hypoxia resolves over several weeks or months after the return to normoxia.

The classic understanding of chronic hypoxic PH is based on the concept that vascular remodeling is a consequence of sustained pulmonary vasoconstriction and increased pulmonary artery pressure [27]. The resulting increase in shear stress is thought to trigger hypertrophy and proliferation of the vascular SMCs. Although this concept remains valid in many aspects, it is no longer viewed as the only pathophysiological mechanism of hypoxic PH [27]. Recent evidence shows that hypoxia-induced pulmonary vascular remodeling can be attenuated despite

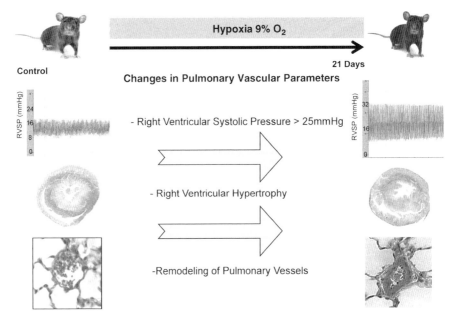

Figure 20.3 Hypoxia-induced pulmonary hypertension in mice. Exposure to chronic hypoxia for 2–3 weeks results in a rise in right ventricular systolic pressure, right ventricular hypertrophy, and remodeling of distal pulmonary vessels.

enhanced hypoxic pulmonary vasoconstriction [28]. This suggests that some of the vasoconstricting substances released in hypoxic lung tissue, most notably endothelin (ET) and serotonin, may serve as growth factors for vascular SMCs or exert other functions independent of both their effects on vascular tone and the severity of pulmonary vasoconstriction. Another recently identified mechanism that may be involved in hypoxia-induced pulmonary vascular remodeling is a direct effect of hypoxia on the expression of specific genes acting on SMCs, endothelial cells, fibroblasts, or extracellular matrix remodeling. Recent studies also suggest that lung infiltration of inflammatory cells play a major role. Inflammatory cytokines are potential targets for therapeutic manipulations of PH [27].

20.3.5
SU5416 Treatment Combined with Hypoxia in Mice

Treatment with the vascular endothelial growth factor receptor (VEGFR) antagonist SU5416 leads to severe PH in rats [29]. Among animal species, mice are very useful for deciphering the pathophysiology of PH, as they offer a variety of tools that are often lacking in other species. PH induction in mice is limited to chronic hypoxia exposure, which fails to replicate the complex vessel lesions seen in human PH. Inhibition of the VEGFR with SU5416 added to 3 weeks of chronic hypoxia was shown by Ciuclan *et al.* to considerably increase the severity of PH compared with hypoxia alone and to produce several specific characteristics relevant to human PH, including complex vascular remodeling with not only medial wall hypertrophy but also concentric neointimal thickening; occlusion of small vessels attributed to endothelial cells; severe right ventricular hypertrophy with right ventricular dysfunction and decreased cardiac output; incomplete reversal after the return to normoxia; and gene expression dysregulation and biomarker alterations mimicking those seen in humans with idiopathic PH [30].

20.3.6
PH Related to COPD or Smoke Exposure

PH due to lung disease and/or hypoxia (group 3 in the PH classification scheme) is considered the most common cause of PH [31]. Most research efforts focused on COPD, with much less attention to interstitial lung diseases. COPD due to cigarette smoke remains one of the leading causes of PH. In experimental animal models of smoke exposure, however, PH precedes the development of emphysema, and drugs targeting both PH and lung parenchymal abnormalities are under investigation [7,8].

20.4
Animal Models of Fibrotic Lung Diseases

Human pulmonary fibrosis is characterized by alveolar epithelial cell injury, areas of type II cell hyperplasia, accumulation of fibroblasts and myofibroblasts, and the deposition of extracellular matrix proteins. The result is a progressive loss of normal lung architecture and impairment in gas exchange. Pertinent features of the human disease include temporal heterogeneity of the fibrotic lesions, progressive nature of the disease, and development of fibrotic foci. No current animal model recapitulates all of these cardinal manifestations of the human disease [4]. However, investigations using murine models have led to the identification of many pathological cells and mediators that are believed to be important in human disease as well [4].

20.4.1
Bleomycin-Induced Pulmonary Fibrosis

The bleomycin model of pulmonary fibrosis is the best-characterized murine model in use today. The drug was originally isolated from *Streptomyces verticillatus*. Bleomycin has been shown to induce lung injury and fibrosis in a wide variety of experimental animals, including mice, rats, hamsters, rabbits, guinea pigs, dogs, and primates. The delivery of bleomycin via the intratracheal route has the advantage that a single injection of the drug produces lung injury and resultant fibrosis in rodents [4]. It initially results in the direct damage of alveolar epithelial cells, followed by the development of neutrophilic and lymphocytic pan-alveolitis within the first week. Subsequently, fibroblast proliferation is noted, and extracellular matrix is synthesized. The development of fibrosis in this model can be seen biochemically and histologically by day 14 with maximal responses generally noted around days 21–28. Bleomycin is thought to induce lung injury via its ability to cause DNA strand breakage and oxidant injury [4]. The development of fibrotic lesions is dependent on the release of chemokines, most notably CCL2 or CCL12 from the injured lung, and the recruitment of inflammatory cells such as monocytes, lymphocytes, and fibrocytes. The profibrotic cytokine, transforming growth factor (TGF)-β1, is also critically involved in the development of bleomycin-induced pulmonary fibrosis.

The advantages of the bleomycin model are that it is well characterized and has clinical relevance. The disadvantage is that the disease may be self-limiting in mice with a resolution of the disease after 90 days.

20.4.2
Other Models

Other models were developed like the FITC-induced model of pulmonary fibrosis that has the advantage of visualizing the areas of the lung where deposition occurs via immunofluorescence imaging for the characteristic green color of the FITC. Models of pulmonary fibrosis induced by irradiation or silica are of interest to study specific causes of the disease. Transgenic models have revealed the pathophysiological fibrotic consequences of increased human or mouse transgenes, such as human collagenase, human TGFα, or IL-13.

20.5
Animal Models of Acute Respiratory Distress Syndrome

Conceptually, ARDS refers to a type of acute diffuse inflammatory lung injury associated with a predisposing risk factor, leading to increased pulmonary microvascular permeability with leakage of fluid into the interstitium and airspace, impairment of alveolar fluid clearance, increased extravascular lung water and lung weight, and loss of aerated lung tissue [32]. The clinical features are hypoxemia and bilateral radiographic opacities, associated with severe ventilation/perfusion mismatching, increased venous admixture, increased physiological dead space, decreased lung compliance, and decreased functional residual capacity. The edema fluid typically exhibits an acute neutrophilic inflammatory response with fibrin-rich proteinaceous exudates and various pro- and anti-inflammatory cytokines [33]. ARDS may lead to extrapulmonary organ damage with acute multiorgan failure and long-term functional disability. The pathologic hallmark of the acute phase is diffuse alveolar damage (with hyaline membrane, edema, inflammation, and/or hemorrhage). Both epithelial and endothelial injuries coexist, with microvascular thrombi and lung vascular dysfunction. In some survivors, the repair phase may be fibroproliferative.

The clinical definition of ARDS has been recently revised (Berlin definition) [32] with diagnostic criteria of timing (within 1 week of a known clinical insult or new or worsening respiratory symptoms), chest imaging (bilateral opacities on chest radiograph or computed tomography scan not fully explained by effusions, lobar/lung collapse, or nodules), origin of edema (respiratory failure not fully explained by cardiac failure or fluid overload, with the need for objective assessment (e.g., echocardiography) to exclude hydrostatic edema if no risk factor present), and hypoxemia (mild ARDS if PaO_2/FIO_2 ratio is between 201 and 300 mmHg with positive end expiratory pressure (PEEP) or continuous positive airway pressure (CPAP) ≥ 5 cmH$_2$O; moderate ARDS if PaO_2/FIO_2 ratio is between 101 and 200 mmHg with PEEP ≥ 5 cmH$_2$O; severe ARDS if PaO_2/FIO_2 ratio is ≤ 100 mmHg with PEEP ≥ 5 cmH$_2$O). This definition points out the complexity of the syndrome and the difficulty in reproducing it in an animal model. Most of the existing models are relevant only for limited aspects of human ARDS (Table 20.1).

Despite 40 years of investigation, the fundamental mechanisms that initiate and propagate lung injury during ARDS have not been defined completely. Animal models of ARDS are often based on risk factors for ARDS [34]. The diversity of causes renders modeling human ARDS difficult. The list of common risk factors for ARDS is extensive, including direct and indirect insults that may overlap: pneumonia, nonpulmonary sepsis, aspiration of gastric contents, pulmonary contusion, inhalational injury, pulmonary vasculitis, drowning, major trauma, pancreatitis, severe burns, noncardiogenic shock, drug overdose, and transfusions. Contrary to newborns, depletion of surfactant is usually a consequence rather than a primary cause of ARDS in adults. Exposure to high concentrations of oxygen eventually results in severe lung injury in most mammalian species, but its association with human ARDS remains questionable. By definition, ARDS is associated with the delivery of supportive mechanical ventilation (noninvasive in the mild ARDS group and invasive in the moderate to severe ARDS groups). Animal models should, therefore, ideally include mechanical ventilation to simulate the primary treatment applied in the clinical scenario. In addition, some mechanical ventilation modalities (excessive tidal volume, for example) may induce or worsen lung injury (ventilator-induced lung injury (VILI)), and the reduction of tidal volume may be associated with improved survival in humans with ARDS.

The main animal models of ARDS reported in the literature use the following insults: mechanical ventilation with injurious strategies (e.g., large tidal volumes), intravenous or intratracheal endotoxin (lipopolysaccharide, a glycolipid present in the outer membrane of Gram-negative bacteria), intravenous or intratracheal live bacteria, intratracheal hydrochloric acid, surfactant depletion by warm saline lavage, hyperoxia, intravenous oleic acid (the most common free fatty acid in mammals), peritonitis, and ischemia reperfusion [34]. Bleomycin administration (an antineoplastic antibiotic drug) is usually considered a model of pulmonary fibrosis, but also shares features of ARDS [34]. The main characteristics of these animal models of ARDS are summarized in Table 20.1. No single model can mimic the full histopathological picture of ARDS. Some of these models have synergistic effects and have been combined in an attempt to scrutinize the complexity of

Table 20.1 Main characteristics of the most common animal models of ARDS.

Insult	Corresponding human disease	Specificities of lung injury	Factors influencing the response variability	Advantages	Limitations
Mechanical ventilation with large tidal volumes	VILI	Alveolar and endothelial tissue damage by mechanical stretch	• Ventilator settings (e.g., tidal volume size, PEEP level, recruitment maneuvers)	Clinical relevance [15]	Complex for small animals and/or prolonged periods
i.v. oleic acid	Fat embolism	• Direct cell necrosis (endothelium > epithelium) • Early and rapidly reversible patchy inflammatory lung injury • Pulmonary fibrosis after repeated doses	• Route of i.v. administration: peripheral vein, central vein, right atrium, or pulmonary artery	Reproducible	• Oleic acid is insoluble in water and requires exclusive i.v. route • Only mimics ARDS due to lipid injury
Endotoxin	Gram-negative sepsis	• Activation of the innate immune response via TLR4 • Entrapment of PMN in pulmonary capillaries • i.v.: endothelial cell apoptosis, systemic signs of sepsis • i.t.: large increase in PMN in airspaces	• Species: higher susceptibility in species with PIM • Strains: higher susceptibility in BALB/c mice, lower susceptibility in C57BL/6 mice • Type of LPS: less pyrogenic with the O-chain • Purity: interaction of contaminants bacterial lipoproteins with TLRs	Easy to use	Do not explore the role of bacterial exotoxins
Live bacteria	Bacteremia (i.v.), pneumonia (i.t.)	• i.v.: major systemic signs of sepsis, lung microvascular injury with PMN sequestration, but little neutrophilic alveolitis	• Route of administration • Size of bacterial inoculum • Bacterial species	Allows the use of bacteria encountered	Requires growth and culturing of live bacteria

20.5 Animal Models of Acute Respiratory Distress Syndrome

Model	Type	Mechanism/Features	Variables	Advantages	Disadvantages
Cecal ligation and puncture	Peritonitis	• i.t.: limited systemic signs of sepsis, severe local pneumonia with epithelial injury Major systemic signs of sepsis with mild lung injury	• Animal species: higher susceptibility in species with PIM • Number and size of holes in the cecum • Type of colonic flora	Closely replicates clinical peritonitis in the clinical setting	Requires surgery
Hydrochloric acid aspiration	Aspiration of gastric content	• Patchy inflammatory lung injury in airways (with increased resistances) and parenchyma (epithelium > endothelium) • Fibroproliferative repair phase	Acid concentration	Reproducible	Do not account for the complexity of human gastric fluid (bacterial cell wall products, cytokines, high osmolarity, higher pH)
Hyperoxia	Pure oxygen lung toxicity	• Oxidation by reactive oxygen species (oxygen-free radicals) • Cell injury (apoptosis and necrosis of endothelium > epithelium) • Fibroproliferative repair phase	• Strains: Fischer rats more susceptible than Sprague-Dawley rats; C57BL/6 mice more susceptible than C3H/HeJ • Preexposure to lower oxygen levels induces tolerance via increase in antioxidant enzymes • Age: neonates and older animals are more tolerant	Reproducible	Limited clinical relevance in humans [13]; requires specialized equipment (sealed cage)
Surfactant depletion	Surfactant deficiency disorder	• The reduction in surfactant lipid concentration in alveolar lining fluid increases alveolar surface tension, facilitating alveolar collapse at low volumes and impairing alveolar host defenses	Volume and number of lavages	Easy for testing ventilatory strategies	Requires sedation, intubation, and mechanical ventilation

(continued)

Table 20.1 (Continued)

Insult	Corresponding human disease	Specificities of lung injury	Factors influencing the response variability	Advantages	Limitations
		Minimal changes in permeability, inflammation, and PMN recruitment			
Bleomycin	Pulmonary fibrosis	• Cell death by oxygen radicals and DNA breaks (endothelium > epithelium) • Neutrophilic alveolitis followed by lymphocytic response, then fibrotic response, without hyaline membranes	• Expression of bleomycin hydrolase, and genes involved in apoptosis and oxidation pathways • Low susceptibility of rabbits, Balb/C, and C3H mice; high susceptibility of C57BL/6 mice	i.t. route is simple and reproducible	More close to pulmonary fibrosis than to ARDS

VILI: ventilator-induced lung injury; i.v.: intravenous; i.t.: intratracheal; PMN: polymorphonuclear neutrophils; TLR: toll-like receptor; PEEP: positive end expiratory pressure; a > b denotes that the condition predominates "b" compared with "a."

human ARDS. Large animal models (dogs, sheep, or pigs) allow prolonged studies with ventilation, but such models are very expensive and laborious (need to create an animal ICU). Smaller animals (rabbits, rats, or mice) allow short-term studies targeting individual pathways, but the generalizability to humans is limited [34]. The broad use of mice models may be explained by the availability of specific reagents and genetically modified animals and recent progresses in the measurement of physiological parameters in small animals [35].

There are important interspecies differences in response to lung injury concerning physiology (lung mechanics and pulmonary circulation) and immunology (bacterial recognition via toll-like receptors, chemokine and chemokine receptor pathways, and presence of pulmonary intravascular macrophages) [34]. Pulmonary intravascular macrophages are resident mature macrophages that adhere to endothelial cells in pulmonary capillaries to phagocyte microorganisms and particles. Their presence in some species (sheep, cattle, pigs, cats, goats, horses, and cetaceans) enhances endotoxin-induced lung injury, whereas their absence in other species (dog, rat, mouse, rabbit, nonhuman, and human primates) mitigates such injury. Important species differences also exist in the nitric oxide pathway, which is important in ARDS pathophysiology [36].

20.6
Translation to Clinics: Limitations and Difficulties

At present, there is no perfect preclinical model that completely recapitulates changes seen in lung diseases as complex as lung fibrosis, chronic obstructive lung disease, pulmonary hypertension, or acute respiratory distress syndrome. The usefulness of such models, however, differs with respect to the types of lung diseases. For instance, pathophysiological concepts or therapeutic strategies developed in the field of pulmonary hypertension are usually assessed and validated while using several approaches, including (a) lung specimens and cells derived from patients with PH and (b) related experimental mice models. Both approaches are needed and interconnected. Concepts in the field of COPD or lung fibrosis are sometimes supported by similar strategies. With regard to COPD, the pattern of exposure to cigarette smoke appears closest to the human pathology. However, animal models are used only to examine specific pathophysiological aspects since none of the models reproduces all the characteristics of the disease. Regarding lung fibrosis, the advantages of the bleomycin model are that it is well characterized and has clinical relevance. The disadvantage is that the disease may be self-limiting in mice with a resolution of the disease after 90 days. ARDS is perhaps the most difficult human lung disease to recapitulate in experimental animal models. As mentioned earlier, the clinical definition of ARDS has been recently revised, pointing out the complexity of the syndrome. Consequently, most of the existing models are relevant only for limited aspects of human ARDS.

References

1 Baron, R.M., Choi, A.J., Owen, C.A., and Choi, A.M. (2012) Genetically manipulated mouse models of lung disease: potential and pitfalls. *American Journal of Physiology. Lung Cellular and Molecular Physiology*, **302** (6), L485–L497.

2 Ryan, J., Bloch, K., and Archer, SL. (2011) Rodent models of pulmonary hypertension: harmonisation with the World Health Organization's categorisation of human PH. *International Journal of Clinical Practice. Supplement*, (172), 15–34.

3 Gomez-Arroyo, J., Saleem, S.J., Mizuno, S., Syed, A.A., Bogaard, H.J., Abbate, A., Taraseviciene-Stewart, L., Sung, Y., Kraskauskas, D., Farkas, D., Conrad, D.H., Nicolls, M.R., and Voelkel, N.F. (2012) A brief overview of mouse models of pulmonary arterial hypertension: problems and prospects. *American Journal of Physiology. Lung Cellular and Molecular Physiology*, **302** (10), L977–L991.

4 Moore, B.B. and Hogaboam, C.M. (2008) Murine models of pulmonary fibrosis. *American Journal of Physiology. Lung Cellular and Molecular Physiology*, **294** (2), L152–L160.

5 Mahadeva, R. and Shapiro, S.D. (2002) Chronic obstructive pulmonary disease * 3: experimental animal models of pulmonary emphysema. *Thorax*, **57** (10), 908–914.

6 Hogg, J.C. (2004) Pathophysiology of airflow limitation in chronic obstructive pulmonary disease. *Lancet*, **364** (9435), 709–721.

7 Wright, J.L. and Churg, A. (2002) Animal models of cigarette smoke-induced COPD. *Chest*, **122** (6 Suppl.), 301S–306S.

8 Wright, J.L., Cosio, M., and Churg, A. (2008) Animal models of chronic obstructive pulmonary disease. *American Journal of Physiology. Lung Cellular and Molecular Physiology*, **295** (1), L1–L15.

9 Fabbri, L., Pauwels, R.A., and Hurd, S.S. (2004) Global strategy for the diagnosis, management, and prevention of chronic obstructive pulmonary disease: GOLD executive summary updated 2003. *COPD*, **1** (1), 105–141, discussion 103–104.

10 Kuhn, C., Yu, S.Y., Chraplyvy, M., Linder, H.E., and Senior, R.M. (1976) The induction of emphysema with elastase. II. Changes in connective tissue. *Laboratory Investigation; a Journal of Technical Methods and Pathology*, **34** (4), 372–380.

11 Lucey, E.C., Keane, J., Kuang, P.P., Snider, G.L., and Goldstein, R.H. (2002) Severity of elastase-induced emphysema is decreased in tumor necrosis factor-alpha and interleukin-1beta receptor-deficient mice. *Laboratory Investigation; a Journal of Technical Methods and Pathology*, **82** (1), 79–85.

12 Kuhn, C., 3rd, Homer, R.J., Zhu, Z., Ward, N., Flavell, R.A., Geba, G.P., and Elias, J.A. (2000) Airway hyperresponsiveness and airway obstruction in transgenic mice: morphologic correlates in mice overexpressing interleukin (IL)-11 and IL-6 in the lung. *American Journal of Respiratory Cell and Molecular Biology*, **22** (3), 289–295.

13 Sisson, T.H., Hansen, J.M., Shah, M., Hanson, K.E., Du, M., Ling, T., Simon, R.H., and Christensen, P.J. (2006) Expression of the reverse tetracycline-transactivator gene causes emphysema-like changes in mice. *American Journal of Respiratory Cell and Molecular Biology*, **34** (5), 552–560.

14 Gomez-Arroyo, J.G., Farkas, L., Alhussaini, A.A., Farkas, D., Kraskauskas, D., Voelkel, N.F., and Bogaard, H.J. (2011) The monocrotaline model of pulmonary hypertension in perspective. *American Journal of Physiology. Lung Cellular and Molecular Physiology*, **302** (4), L363–L369.

15 Morrell, N.W., Adnot, S., Archer, S.L., Dupuis, J., Jones, P.L., MacLean, M.R., McMurtry, I.F., Stenmark, K.R., Thistlethwaite, P.A., Weissmann, N., Yuan, J.X., and Weir, E.K. (2009) Cellular and molecular basis of pulmonary arterial hypertension. *Journal of the American College of Cardiology*, **54** (1 Suppl.), S20–S31.

16 West, J., Fagan, K., Steudel, W., Fouty, B., Lane, K., Harral, J., Hoedt-Miller, M., Tada, Y., Ozimek, J., Tuder, R., and Rodman, D.M. (2004) Pulmonary hypertension in transgenic mice expressing a dominant-negative BMPRII gene in smooth muscle. *Circulation Research*, **94** (8), 1109–1114.

17 Morrell, N.W. (2006) Pulmonary hypertension due to BMPR2 mutation: a

new paradigm for tissue remodeling? *Proceedings of the American Thoracic Society*, **3** (8), 680–686.

18 Guignabert, C., Izikki, M., Tu, L.I., Li, Z., Zadigue, P., Barlier-Mur, A.M., Hanoun, N., Rodman, D., Hamon, M., Adnot, S., and Eddahibi, S. (2006) Transgenic mice overexpressing the 5-hydroxytryptamine transporter gene in smooth muscle develop pulmonary hypertension. *Circulation Research*, **98** (10), 1323–1330.

19 Crosby, A., Jones, F.M., Southwood, M., Stewart, S., Schermuly, R., Butrous, G., Dunne, D.W., and Morrell, N.W. (2010) Pulmonary vascular remodeling correlates with lung eggs and cytokines in murine schistosomiasis. *American Journal of Respiratory and Critical Care Medicine*, **181** (3), 279–288.

20 White, R.J., Meoli, D.F., Swarthout, R.F., Kallop, D.Y., Galaria, I.I., Harvey, J.L., Miller, C.M., Blaxall, B.C., Hall, C.M., Pierce, R.A., Cool, C.D., and Taubman, M.B. (2007) Plexiform-like lesions and increased tissue factor expression in a rat model of severe pulmonary arterial hypertension. *American Journal of Physiology. Lung Cellular and Molecular Physiology*, **293** (3), L583–L590.

21 Adnot, S. (2005) Lessons learned from cancer may help in the treatment of pulmonary hypertension. *Journal of Clinical Investigation*, **115** (6), 1461–1463.

22 Adnot, S. and Eddahibi, S. (2007) Lessons from oncology to understand and treat pulmonary hypertension. *International Journal of Clinical Practice. Supplement*, (158), 19–25.

23 Houssaini, A., Abid, S., Mouraret, N., Wan, F., Rideau, D., Saker, M., Marcos, E., Tissot, CM., Dubois-Rande, J.L., Amsellem, V., and Adnot, S. (2013) Rapamycin reverses pulmonary artery smooth muscle cell proliferation in pulmonary hypertension. *American Journal of Respiratory Cell and Molecular Biology*, **48** (5), 568–577.

24 Krymskaya, V.P., Snow, J., Cesarone, G., Khavin, I., Goncharov, D.A., Lim, P.N., Veasey, S.C., Ihida-Stansbury, K., Jones, P.L., and Goncharova, E.A. (2011) mTOR is required for pulmonary arterial vascular smooth muscle cell proliferation under chronic hypoxia. *The FASEB Journal*, **25** (6), 1922–1933.

25 Sato, K., Webb, S., Tucker, A., Rabinovitch, M., O'Brien, R.F., McMurtry, I.F., and Stelzner, T.J. (1992) Factors influencing the idiopathic development of pulmonary hypertension in the fawn hooded rat. *The American Review of Respiratory Disease*, **145** (4 Part 1), 793–797.

26 Rabinovitch, M., Gamble, W., Nadas, A.S., Miettinen, O., and Reid, L. (1979) Rat pulmonary circulation after chronic hypoxia: hemodynamic and structural features. *The American Journal of Physiology*, **236**, H818–H827.

27 Stenmark, K.R., Fagan, K.A., and Frid, M.G. (2006) Hypoxia-induced pulmonary vascular remodeling: cellular and molecular mechanisms. *Circulation Research*, **99** (7), 675–691.

28 Eddahibi, S., Humbert, M., Fadel, E., Raffestin, B., Darmon, M., Capron, F., Simonneau, G., Dartevelle, P., Hamon, M., and Adnot, S. (2001) Serotonin transporter overexpression is responsible for pulmonary artery smooth muscle hyperplasia in primary pulmonary hypertension. *Journal of Clinical Investigation*, **108** (8), 1141–1150.

29 Taraseviciene-Stewart, L., Kasahara, Y., Alger, L., Hirth, P., Mc Mahon, G., Waltenberger, J., Voelkel, N.F., and Tuder, R.M. (2001) Inhibition of the VEGF receptor 2 combined with chronic hypoxia causes cell death-dependent pulmonary endothelial cell proliferation and severe pulmonary hypertension. *The FASEB Journal*, **15** (2), 427–438.

30 Ciuclan, L., Bonneau, O., Hussey, M., Duggan, N., Holmes, AM., Good, R., Stringer, R., Jones, P., Morrell, N.W., Jarai, G., Walker, C., Westwick, J., and Thomas, M. (2011) A novel murine model of severe pulmonary arterial hypertension. *American Journal of Respiratory and Critical Care Medicine*, **184** (10), 1171–1182.

31 Minai, O.A., Chaouat, A., and Adnot, S. (2010) Pulmonary hypertension in COPD: epidemiology, significance, and management: pulmonary vascular disease: the global perspective. *Chest*, **137** (6 Suppl.), 39S–51S.

32 Ferguson, N.D., Fan, E., Camporota, L., Antonelli, M., Anzueto, A., Beale, R., Brochard, L., Brower, R., Esteban, A., Gattinoni, L., Rhodes, A., Slutsky, A.S., Vincent, J.L., Rubenfeld, G.D., Thompson, B.T., and Ranieri, V.M. (2012) The Berlin definition of ARDS: an expanded rationale, justification, and supplementary material. *Intensive Care Medicine*, **38** (10), 1573–1582.

33 Imai, Y., Parodo, J., Kajikawa, O., de Perrot, M., Fischer, S., Edwards, V., Cutz, E., Liu, M., Keshavjee, S., Martin, T.R., Marshall, J.C., Ranieri, V.M., and Slutsky, A.S. (2003) Injurious mechanical ventilation and end-organ epithelial cell apoptosis and organ dysfunction in an experimental model of acute respiratory distress syndrome. *JAMA*, **289** (16), 2104–2112.

34 Matute-Bello, G., Frevert, C.W., and Martin, T.R. (2008) Animal models of acute lung injury. *American Journal of Physiology. Lung Cellular and Molecular Physiology*, **295** (3), L379–L399.

35 Mekontso Dessap, A., Voiriot, G., Zhou, T., Marcos, E., Dudek, S.M., Jacobson, J.R., Machado, R., Adnot, S., Brochard, L., Maitre, B., and Garcia, J.G. (2011) Conflicting physiological and genomic cardiopulmonary effects of recruitment maneuvers in murine acute lung injury. *American Journal of Respiratory Cell and Molecular Biology*, **46** (4), 541–550.

36 Schneemann, M. and Schoedon, G. (2002) Species differences in macrophage NO production are important. *Nature Immunology*, **3** (2), 102.

21
Heart Failure
Jin Bo Su and Alain Berdeaux

21.1
Introduction

Heart failure (HF) occurs when the heart is unable to produce sufficient pump action to equilibrate adequately cardiac output with the oxygen and metabolic substrate demands of the body. HF can be caused by different cardiovascular diseases, including myocardial ischemia and/or myocardial infarction (MI), dilated cardiomyopathy (DCM), hypertrophic cardiomyopathy (HCM), hypertension, congenital cardiac defect, infective myocarditis, and other less common etiologies. With improvement in cardiovascular medicines and progressive aging of the population, HF tends to become paradoxically a rather common but potentially lethal cardiovascular disease. To study the mechanisms involved in the development and treatment of HF, diverse animal models have been developed according to the etiology of HF. Small animal models, particularly mice, have contributed significantly to insights into the molecular and genetic bases of cardiovascular biology. However, there are significant differences in cardiac characteristics such as heart rate, oxygen consumption, adrenergic receptor ratios, and response to loss of regulatory proteins between mice and humans [1,2]. Moreover, there are significant differences in contractile protein expression, critical to the excitation–contraction coupling process, between these species as indicated by their difference in predominant myosin isoforms [1], in ion channels such as K_{ATP} (ATP-sensitive potassium) channels as evidenced by distinct or indistinct molecular differential pharmacology of atrial versus ventricular K_{ATP} channels [3], and in phenotypic differences between mouse and human stem cells in the cell cycle regulation, control of apoptosis, and cytokine expression [2]. Finally, due to the difference in the heart size, the results obtained in murine models could not be directly extrapolated to humans. For example, if a gene or cellular therapy obtains positive results in a murine model of MI, the first difficulty encountered in reproducing the same protocol in humans is to obtain gene or cell materials in sufficient amount to satisfy their use in the human heart, which is much larger than that in mice even though the percentage of the infarct zone normalized to the whole heart is not larger than that in mice. Therefore, large animal models of HF, which more closely approximate human anatomy, physiology, and function, still remain essential for the preclinical discoveries of new therapies and interventions for HF.

**21.2
Hypertension-Related Heart Failure**

Hypertension is a major risk factor for stroke, heart attack, HF, arterial aneurysm, and peripheral arterial disease and is also a cause of chronic kidney disease. In response to hypertension, the heart works more than under normal arterial pressure and develops left ventricular hypertrophy (LVH). LVH can eventually normalize the increase in wall tension to abrogate the initial stimulus. Although LVH in response to pathological signaling has traditionally been considered as an adaptive response to sustain cardiac output in the face of stress, sustained LVH leads to functional maladaptation associated with an increased risk for sudden death or to HF progression. Different models of hypertension-induced HF have been created in small and large animals, including hypertension induced by chronic infusion of angiotensin II in rats, dogs, and pigs, by mineralocorticoid DOCA (deoxycorticosterone acetate) or aldosterone plus salt [4–7], by chronic inhibition of nitric oxide (NO) synthase alone [8] or combined with high-salt diet in rats [9], and by experimental renal ischemia in rats or dogs. In addition, several genetic hypertensive strains of rats have been widely used for HF studies. These include spontaneously hypertensive rat (SHR), spontaneously hypertensive heart failure prone (SHHP/Mcc-*cp*), and Dahl/Rapp salt-sensitive rats.

Among these models, some are considered as mixed hypertension and hypertrophy models rather than classically defined HF models. For example, the DOCA or aldosterone–salt model showed a depressed renin–angiotensin system and has been used as an angiotensin-independent hypertension model to investigate new antihypertensive compounds. Both the DOCA and aldosterone–salt impair the kidney capacity to eliminate salt, so the salt loading rapidly induces hypertension and cardiac hypertrophy without signs of congestive HF [10]. Nevertheless, mineralocorticoid hyperactivity, especially overproduction of deoxycorticosterone, is rarely observed in humans [6] and is generally the result of a genetic defect [11]. Therefore, the DOCA- and aldosterone–salt-induced hypertension is not a very realistic model for human hypertension and HF.

Chronic angiotensin II infusion in dogs, pigs, and rats using osmotic minipump or catheter inserted in the artery, left atrium, or cerebral ventricle induces significant elevation in arterial pressure, cardiac hypertrophy, and fibrosis. However, the animals chronically receiving angiotensin II do not develop classical HF but so-called HF with preserved ejection fraction. Despite impaired LV relaxation indexes, LV systolic function parameters such as cardiac output, stroke volume, and fraction ejection usually remain in a normal range [12–15]. Interestingly, in pigs receiving chronic angiotensin II infusion, alterations in LV isovolumetric relaxation are accompanied by an abnormal isovolumetric contraction characterized by increased isovolumetric contraction time and increased heart rate [15].

Due to the role of NO, a paracrine vasodilator, in the regulation of vascular tone, myocardial contractile function, and inhibition of platelet aggregation, chronic inhibition of NO synthesis by inhibitors such as L-NAME (N^{ω}-nitro-L-arginine methyl ester) and nitro-L-arginine increases systolic blood pressure and impairs renal function in rats. However, chronic inhibition of NO synthases in conscious dogs does not produce a persistent increase in arterial blood pressure despite a significant increase in peripheral vascular resistance, which is due to a compensatory role of prostaglandins with vasodilator properties [16]. Since the role of decreased NO production in human hypertension is not clearly defined, it is impossible to say whether NO synthase inhibition is an appropriate model of hypertension. However, this model deserves more attention as performing experiments using this model is technically easy and mortality is low. In addition, a variant of this model has been developed by combining NO synthase inhibition and salt diet. This combination induces hypertension, LVH, myocardial fibrosis, and LV dysfunction, which can be detected by echocardiography and expressed as a reduced fractional shortening. The impairment of LV contractile function is correlated with increased oxidative stress as indicated by increased serum TNF-α (tumor necrosis factor-alpha) and cardiac glutathione depletion [9].

The SHR model is commonly used to investigate hypertension, as the model exhibits numerous similarities with human essential hypertension and the compounds lowering blood pressure in SHRs also lower blood pressure in hypertensive humans [17]. In the last 6 months of their 2-year life span, more than a half of SHRs exhibit cardiac decompensation [18]. The transition from compensated hypertrophy to failure in SHRs of advanced age is associated with a marked increase in collagen, a reduction in cardiomyocyte mass due to increased apoptosis, and a reduction in maximum Ca^{2+}-activated myofibrillar force [19]. Rats with HF can be identified outwardly as they become less active and less well groomed and develop occasional tachypnea, which becomes more persistent and turns into labored respiration when HF progresses. LVH is a feature of the young adult SHR, whereas hypertrophy of the right ventricle is a reliable marker of HF in SHRs [18]. SHRs with HF have increased LV diastolic and systolic volume, LV filling pressure, and decreased LV ejection fraction. Because the process of development of HF in SHRs is similar to that in human hypertension-induced HF [17], old SHR is a realistic hypertension-induced HF model.

Originally designated as the congenic strain SHR/N-*cp* (corpulent), the strain of SHHP/Mcc-*cp* rats was developed by backcrossing "Koletsky obese" rats (i.e., rats heterozygous for the *cp* gene) to SHRs [20,21]. SHHP/Mcc-*cp* rats develop hypertension and HF spontaneously. Along with hypertension, 25% SHHP/Mcc-*cp* rats are obese and have hyperinsulinemia and diabetes (males) or abnormal glucose tolerance (females). As compared with SHR, in SHHP/Mcc-*cp* rats HF occurs at a relatively younger age, especially in obese SHHP/Mcc-*cp* rats in whom fatal DCM develops between 10 and 12 months in males and 14 and 16 months in females, whereas lean male SHHP/Mcc-*cp* rats develop hypertension and LVH by 3–5 months and overt HF by 16–20 months of age [20,22,23]. The circulating levels of norepinephrine, renin, aldosterone, and atriopeptin are raised [23,24]. Abnormalities in cardiac structure are biventricular hypertrophy, cardiomyocyte enlargement, and increased interstitial fibrosis. The eccentric hypertrophy is evident in 10–12-month-old non-failing male SHHP/Mcc-*cp* rats, which differ from the concentric hypertrophy in SHRs of the same age [23,25]. This model seems to have many similarities to the human disease: a slow progression of morbidity of hypertension, hyperinsulinemia and diabetes, reduced expression of the genes for the enzymes controlling mitochondrial fatty acid β-oxidation in failing heart but not in unfailing heart of SHHP/Mcc-*cp* rats, which is similar to that in human HF [26], and reduced myocardial β-adrenoceptors but increased β-adrenergic receptor kinase 1 in SHHP/Mcc-*cp* rats [23], which is similar to those occurring in human HF [27]. Because of its natural feature, its time course, and neurohumoral changes in the development of hypertension and HF, which do not need human technical intervention, this model has considerable potential as a model to study the comorbidity factors of HF. The disadvantages of this model are the variable expressions of symptoms and its financial aspects as it is a slowly developing model.

Dahl/Rapp salt-sensitive rats are widely used in evaluating the relationship between salt diet and hypertension [28]. The development of hypertension and HF in the Dahl/Rapp salt-sensitive rat can be controlled by titration of the amount of salt in their diet; the development is more rapid and greater in male than female rats [29]. Dahl/Rapp salt-sensitive rats fed with high-salt diet (8% NaCl) after the age of 6 weeks develop concentric LVH and fibrosis at 11 weeks and marked LV dilatation at 15–20 weeks in association with respiratory dysfunction and LV global hypokinesis. All the Dahl/Rapp salt-sensitive rats died within 1 week due to massive pulmonary congestion [30]. As in human HF, specific organ (heart, lung, and liver) enlargement is also observed in this model. Isometric contractions of the isolated LV papillary muscle of the Dahl/Rapp salt-sensitive rat heart are impaired at baseline and after isoprenaline stimulation [30], a response quite similar to that reported in end-stage human HF. Impaired NO production from L-arginine in the kidney is an abnormality feather of renal hemodynamics and the development of hypertension in salt-sensitive rats [28,31].

21.3
Pressure and Volume Overload-Induced Heart Failure

21.3.1
Pressure Overload-Induced Heart Failure

A simple method to increase LV pressure overload is outflow constriction by aortic banding in different species of animals such as mice, rats, rabbits, dogs, and monkeys. Aortic banding in rats and mice is clearly a model of cardiac hypertrophy rather than a model of HF. However, along with the development of genetic

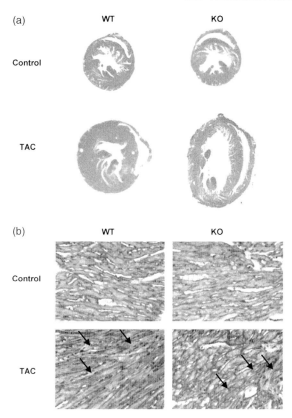

Figure 21.1 In response to transverse aortic constriction (TAC), the transcriptional coactivator peroxisome proliferator-activated receptor-γ coactivator 1α gene knockout (KO) mice developed dilated cardiomyopathy, whereas wild-type (WT) mice developed concentric hypertrophic cardiomyopathy. Hearts from the animals were excised 2 months after TAC. (a) Low-magnification views of transverse sections of the same hearts. (b) Sample higher magnification views of the same hearts as in part (a). Increased streaks in the heart sections of mice with TAC indicate the accumulation of extracellular matrix or fibrosis (magnifications: 20×). (Adapted from Ref. [32].)

manipulation in mice, the aortic constriction has been used in these mice to examine the role of such genetic modification on cardiac function. For example, transverse aortic constriction leads to accelerated HF in mice lacking the transcriptional coactivator peroxisome proliferator-activated receptor-γ coactivator 1α gene (Figure 21.1) [32]. In contrast, aortic banding performed in puppies of 8–10 weeks of age progressively induces LVH in response to pressure overload along with the growth of dogs [33–37]. This model allows us to detail the mechanisms involved in the development of LVH in face of pressure overload and to describe the changes in myocardial structure and function, neurohumoral systems, and cellular and molecular events that occurred during the transition from

LVH to decompensatory HF. This model mimics aortic valve stenosis in humans in which congestive HF is a combination of systolic dysfunction and diastolic dysfunction. However, the high cost limits its use in the screening of drugs, molecules, or genetic strategies with a therapeutic potential for the treatment of HF.

21.3.2
Volume Overload-Induced Heart Failure

In rats, volume overload can be induced by the creation of an arteriovenous fistula between abdominal aorta and vena cava below the renal artery. A marked cardiac hypertrophy occurs in both the left and right ventricles 1 month after the procedure. Despite a short episode of cardiac contractile dysfunction following the creation of such arteriovenous fistula, cardiac function returns to normal and cardiac output is increased after 2 months [38,39]. In rats with aortocaval fistula, LV end-diastolic pressure and pulse arterial pressure increase, but mean arterial pressure remains unchanged, and blood flow to skeletal muscle and cutaneous and splanchnic regions decrease, but cerebral, coronary, and renal blood flows remain unchanged [40]. These rats have elevated plasma epinephrine and norepinephrine levels [40], whereas mitochondrial function remains unchanged [38]. Thus, this model is a particular form of HF.

In large animals, a common approach to produce a volume overload state is generation of mitral regurgitation by chordal rupture of the mitral valve apparatus [41–43]. Chronic volume overload after creation of mitral regurgitation (mitral regurgitation fraction >50%) results in significant LV dilation, eccentric LVH (typical volume overload-induced hypertrophy), and subsequent LV dysfunction and HF, thus recapitulating the volume overload-induced HF phenotype. In this model, the abnormalities at the cellular level such as impaired cardiomyocyte contractile function and progressive neurohumoral activation have been evidenced [41,42,44]. This model has also been used to investigate mechanical and pharmacological strategies to treat mitral regurgitation-induced LV functional and structural alterations [43–45]. Studies performed in this model have provided evidence that β-blockers may be useful in the treatment of volume overload-induced HF and the mechanisms by which β-adrenergic receptor antagonism may operate in the context of volume overload-induced HF [43,44].

21.3.3
Double Pressure and Volume Overload-Induced Heart Failure

In rabbits, volume overload, pressure overload, and their combination are used to induce HF. Aortic valve perforation with a catheter introduced through the carotid artery produces aortic regurgitation associated with LVH, followed by systolic dysfunction. More than 50% of these rabbits develop HF after a period of several months [46]. HF can be more consistently and rapidly induced when aortic regurgitation is followed by aortic constriction performed just below the diaphragm 2 weeks after destroying the aortic valve. HF occurs about 4 weeks after the initial procedure, which is associated with inversion of the force–frequency relation and alteration of post-rest potentiation [47], impaired β-adrenergic system [48,49], and increased protein and mRNA levels of Na^+/Ca^{2+} exchanger, whereas sarcoplasmic reticulum Ca^{2+}-ATPase remains unchanged [50], as observed in failing human hearts [51]. This model closely mimics alterations of myocardial function and molecules regulating intracellular Ca^{2+} movements observed in the end-stage failing human myocardium. Therefore, this model may be suitable for studying changes in excitation–contraction coupling during the development of HF.

21.4
Toxic Molecule-Induced Heart Failure

21.4.1
Adriamycin-Induced Heart Failure in Rats

Adriamycin and other anthracycline molecules are used in the treatment of human cancers. One of their well-known common side effects is cardiotoxicity, which can lead to congestive HF and death [52,53]. Rats treated with adriamycin at a dose of 2 mg/kg/week for 10–12 weeks died from congestive HF characterized by decreased cardiac output, decreased blood pressure, pleural effusion, ascites, and hepatic congestion [54,55]. In this model, there is no change in heart weight, but there are marked pathological changes in cardiomyocytes, including cytoplasmic vacuolation, myofilament disorganization, and necrosis [55]. Although this model is simple to manage, noninvasive, and rather economical to induce HF, it does not mimic any other type of HF nor is it useful for investigating the mechanisms from chronic hypertrophy to HF decompensation.

21.4.2
Monocrotaline-Induced Right Ventricular Heart Failure

In rats, subcutaneous administration of a single dose of *Crotalaria* alkaloid, monocrotaline (60–105 mg/kg), for 4–5 weeks induces right ventricular hypercontractility, pulmonary hypertension, and right ventricular hypertrophy [56–59]. Right ventricular HF develops after 4 weeks of monocrotaline injection [60], and at 6 weeks, HF is severe with labored respiration and often large volumes of fluid in the chest [61]. In rats with right ventricular HF, β-adrenergic agonist-induced inotropic responses are decreased due to selective decreases in $β_1$-adrenoceptor density and adenylate cyclase activity in the right ventricle [62,63], which are similar to human primary pulmonary hypertension [64]. One advantage of this model is its simplicity to induce HF. Although the monocrotaline model is certainly useful in the evaluation of pharmacological molecules for the treatment of pulmonary hypertension-induced right HF, it is difficult to know whether the results obtained in this model can be extended to the majority of patients with HF related to other etiologies such as essential hypertension and coronary artery disease.

21.5
Heart Failure Models Related to Myocardial Ischemia and/or Myocardial Infarction

21.5.1
Myocardial Ischemia and/or Myocardial Infarction

Coronary artery disease results in myocardial ischemia and MI and is the most common cause of HF in developed industrial countries. Different animal models of myocardial ischemia- or MI-related HF have been developed to investigate the mechanisms of the disease and to evaluate diagnostic methods and pharmacological, genetic, and cellular therapies. In large animals, myocardial ischemia can be chronically induced by ameroid constriction to establish initial high-grade coronary stenosis followed by occlusion, which leads to LV dysfunction when oxygen demand and consumption increase, for example, during exercise [65]. However, the HF phenotype is most effectively produced by acute and total coronary artery occlusion inducing MI. The most common model of MI-induced HF used for testing new pharmacological strategies so far is coronary ligature-induced MI in rats because surgical occlusion of the left coronary artery of the rat is a relatively simple, economical technique for producing experimental MI. In this model, changes in myocardial and pump functions are proportional to MI size. Rats with small MI (<30% of LV mass) have no discernible impairment in either baseline hemodynamics or peak indices of pumping and pressure generating ability. Rats with moderate MI (30–50%) have normal baseline hemodynamics but reduced peak flow indices and developed pressure. Rats with MI greater than 50% exhibit congestive HF with elevated filling pressures and reduced cardiac output, and have a minimal capacity to respond to pre- and afterload stresses [66]. Following more and more use of transgenic mice in the experimental studies aimed at determining the functions of specific genes, coronary ligature-induced MI has been established in mice. The advantage of this model is the rapidity with which the symptoms of HF can be induced. However, coronary artery ligation is not analogous to the pathogenesis of coronary artery disease or to MI in humans as the model is built from a normal heart with normal coronary arteries, thus not modeling human HF due to coronary arterial disease related to atherosclerosis [66]. Other problems with this model are the high mortality of the animals and the variation in infarct size depending on the skill of the operator, and the difficulty in studying the progression from compensation to end-stage HF. Nevertheless, the MI-induced HF models in rats and mice are useful in evaluating pharmacological, genetic, or cell therapies of MI. The large animal HF models secondary to MI permit pathological and compensatory mechanisms involved in the development of cardiac dysfunction and transition from the compensatory to decompensatory HF after MI to be deciphered more precisely. Historically, the descriptions of prolonged myocardial ischemia causing myocyte death – which progresses as a transmural wavefront, occurring first in the subendocardial myocardium but ultimately becoming nearly transmural – and the importance of collateral blood flow and early coronary reperfusion in the salvage of myocardial tissue were initially obtained in the canine model of MI [67–69]. These pioneering studies have provided the proof of concept of the current reperfusion treatment guidelines for acute coronary syndromes. In addition to testing pharmacological, genetic, and cellular strategies, the MI models in larger animals also allow the development of novel cardiovascular devices such as coronary stent [70] and gene or cell delivery techniques such as the endoscopic cell delivery [71]. However, the very well developed epicardial collateral vessels in canine hearts make it difficult to predict the optimal size and location of MI and it is a limiting factor for the evaluation of new drugs, gene, and cell therapies. Alternatively, porcine hearts exhibit coronary artery anatomy and gross anatomic structure quite similar to those of humans, including consistent coronary arterial anatomy, lack of preformed epicardial collateral vessels, and distribution of blood supply to particular areas or structures [72]. This makes pigs a reasonable choice for studying myocardial ischemia and LV remodeling after MI [65].

21.5.2
Coronary Microembolization-Induced Heart Failure

In dogs, multiple sequential intracoronary microsphere injections performed over a 10-week period produce progressive myocardial damage indicated by patchy myocardial fibrosis and LVH. Over the subsequent 3 months, LV dysfunction progresses to HF as evidenced by decreased LV ejection fraction and cardiac output, increased LV end-diastolic pressure and volume, and activation of neurohumoral systems, as indicated by increased plasma catecholamine and atrial natriuretic factor [73]. This model has been used for the evaluation of long-term therapeutic effects of different pharmacological agents such as angiotensin-converting enzyme inhibitors, β-blockers, digoxin, and statins [74,75]. Similar to dogs, in anesthetized rats, 150 000–200 000 plastic microspheres of 15 μm diameter can be delivered to the coronaries during a temporary occlusion of the ascending aorta through a catheter placed into the left ventricle by way of the external right carotid artery. Embolized rats have a small decrease in heart rate, stroke volume, and cardiac index, and an increase in total peripheral resistance and LV end-diastolic pressure [76]. It is likely that the model created by this technique has similar characteristics and advantages but also disadvantages to the coronary ligation model. Another way to generate coronary microembolization in rats is the injection of blood clots (prepared with their own blood and sized by filtration through 38 μm screen) into the left ventricle. Indeed, the injection of blood clots during the obstruction of the ascending aorta during a thoracotomy induces MI-featured structural changes, as indicated by diffused myocardial necrosis, fibrosis, myocyte apoptosis, and LV dilation as well as myocardial dysfunction as indicated by reduced LV dP/dt max and ejection fraction [77–79]. This model is also characterized by marked inflammatory response of the myocardium as indicated by an increase in proinflammatory factors such as TNF-α, interleukin-6, and intercellular adhesion molecule-1 [77]. However, it is not clear so far whether the rats develop congestive HF because the studied period was too short in these studies, and even though myocardial dysfunction persists following 4 weeks of coronary microembolization, it is unlikely that this time period is enough to induce a real and definitive HF [78].

21.6
Pacing-Induced Heart Failure

DCM is a disease of heart muscle, leading to progressive ventricular chamber enlargement and contractile dysfunction. DCM is the third most common cause of HF and the most frequent reason for heart transplantation. The tachycardia-induced DCM by rapid ventricular pacing in dogs, sheep, and rabbits, and by rapid left atrial pacing in pigs is the most well-characterized animal model of DCM. The progression and reversal of pacing-induced HF are time, pacing rate, and species dependent. For example, typically, pacing-induced HF in dogs is generally induced by continuous right ventricular stimulation at a pacing rate of 240–260 beats/min for 2–4 weeks, although LV pacing can also be a choice with an initial pacing rate of 210 beats/min for 3 weeks followed by a pacing rate of 240 beats/min for an additional week [80]. In sheep, LV pacing at 220–240 beats/min induces HF [81,82] similar to that induced by right ventricular pacing observed in dogs, whereas right ventricular pacing at 180–190 beats/min induces HF after 5 weeks of initialization of pacing. In pigs, HF can be induced by left atrial pacing at 240 beats/min for 3 weeks [83], whereas in rabbits HF can be established by a stepwise increasing pacing rate starting at 320 beats/min, held for 7 days, and then gradually increased to 380 beats/min, with an increment of 20 beats/min each week [84] or started directly at 350–380 beats/min [85]. In this model, pacing leads are usually fixed on the right/left ventricle or on the left atrium during a thoracotomy or on the apex of the right ventricle through a venous line [86].

Chronic rapid pacing produces a typical congestive HF subsequent to DCM, characterized by signs and symptoms of congestion and fluid retention leading to dyspnea, ascites, and peripheral edema. These pathological HF symptoms are due to elevation of the venous capillary pressure, activation of neurohormonal systems, dilatation of cardiac chambers, ventricular systolic and diastolic dysfunction with low cardiac output (Figure 21.2) [87–92], and alterations in the myocardial β-adrenergic system expressed as decreased responsiveness to β- and α-adrenergic stimulation, decreased β-adrenoceptor density and adenylate cyclase activity, and increased Gi protein level in the myocardium [93,94]. These characteristics are associated with an abnormal intracellular calcium handling indicated by a prolonged decline in the intracellular Ca^{2+} ($[Ca^{2+}]_i$) transient with a similar peak of $[Ca^{2+}]_i$ transient as in cardiomyocytes isolated from normal dogs [95] or decreased peak systolic and diastolic levels and the amplitude of electrically stimulated $[Ca^{2+}]_i$ transients in cardiomyocytes from failing rabbit heart, and reduction in L-type Ca^{2+} current density, Na^+/Ca^{2+} exchanger, and sarcoplasmic reticulum Ca^{2+}-ATPase mRNA [96]. Activation of neurohumoral systems is indicated by significant elevation of plasma catecholamines, atrial and brain natriuretic factors, plasma renin activity, and angiotensins, endothelins, and cytokines such as TNF-α [91,97–100]. Changes in the

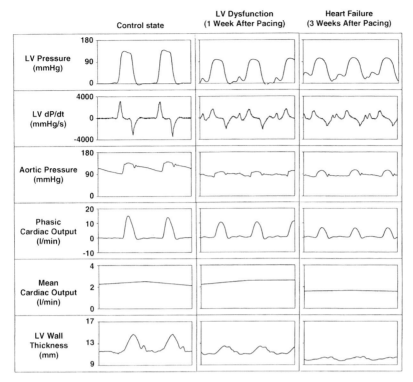

Figure 21.2 Evolution of cardiac function during chronic right ventricular pacing at a rate of 250 beats/min. These representative recordings of LV pressure, first derivative of LV pressure (LV dP/dt), aortic pressure, phasic cardiac output, mean cardiac output, and LV wall thickness were obtained in the same conscious dog in the control state (left panel), in the phase of LV dysfunction (1 week of pacing, middle panel), and in the phase of heart failure (3 weeks of pacing, right panel). LV dysfunction was characterized by an increase in LV end-diastolic pressure and reductions in LV dP/dt max and mean aortic pressure, and a depression in LV systolic wall thickening. At this phase, mean cardiac output was not modified due to accelerated heart rate compared with the control state. At the stage of heart failure, mean cardiac output was reduced and LV systolic wall thickening was further depressed and LV was dilated as indicated by decreased LV end-diastolic wall thickness. (Adapted from Ref. [99].)

myocardial structure are loss of cardiomyocytes replaced by fibrosis and increased volume of remaining viable cardiomyocytes without a significant increase in LV weight [101]. However, although pacing-induced DCM is not accompanied by an increase in LV weight and/or cardiomyocyte volume, right ventricular hypertrophy and increased right ventricular cardiomyocyte volume occur in the swine model [102]. In addition, pacing-induced HF is also associated with marked vascular endothelial dysfunction as indicated by impaired responsiveness to endothelium-dependent vasodilators and reduced NO release related to reduction in endothelial NO synthase gene and protein levels [103–107]. Another important feature of this model is the reversibility of LV functional, structural, and neurohumoral alterations. The abnormalities in cardiac contraction, relaxation, and neurohormones can be nearly normalized after stopping the pacemaker for a sufficient time [108].

Advantages of the rapid pacing-induced HF model include repeatability of HF induction in all animals subjected to rapid pacing, similar alterations in neurohormonal systems to those observed in humans, predictable degrees of LV dilation, and pump dysfunction consistent with those found in patients with DCM. This model is useful for testing pharmacological strategies aimed at stopping or attenuating progression of LV dysfunction to HF. Moreover, compared with the HF model in small animals, this HF model in larger animals allows not only testing of pharmacological strategies and cell and gene therapies but also the development of different devices aimed to improve cardiac function [86]. However, this model does not produce the complete spectrum of HF due to other etiologies, especially the changes in myocardial structure that are different from those observed in HF secondary to myocardial ischemia and volume overload.

21.7
Gene Mutation-Induced Cardiomyopathies

21.7.1
Cardiomyopathic Hamsters

Cardiomyopathic hamster, a representative model of human hereditary cardiomyopathies, has HCM and DCM inbred sublines, both descending from the same ancestor. The pathophysiological basis for cardiomyopathies in the hamster resides in an inherited mutation in the gene encoding for delta-sarcoglycan, a component of the dystrophin complex [109,110]. Two major mechanisms contribute to the development of cardiomyopathies: cardiomyocyte loss due to intrinsic cell defects [111,112], and myocardial ischemia induced by coronary vasospasms due to vascular endothelial dysfunction induced by enhanced renin–angiotensin system-dependent oxidative stress [113–115].

21.7.2
Golden Retriever Muscular Dystrophy Dogs

Duchenne muscular dystrophy (DMD) affects 1/3500 male births and is the most prevalent X-linked genetic disorder in humans. Mutations in the dystrophin gene located on the X chromosome (Xp21) lead to loss of sarcolemmal dystrophin [116–118], disruption of dystrophin–glycoprotein complex, and muscle damage. Cardiac involvement evolves toward cardiomyopathy with dilation of the chambers and LV function depression. It is responsible for death in approximately 40% of patients aged between 10 and 30 years [119–121]. Since the late 1980s, the GRMD (golden retriever muscular dystrophy) dogs have been used as the most relevant model of

DMD [122–124] in preclinical investigations including pharmacological investigation, gene transfers, and cell therapy. Similar to DMD patients, GRMD dogs also develop lethal DCM [124–126]. This dystrophin-deficient cardiomyopathy is characterized by subendocardial dysfunction and patched myocardial necrosis and fibrosis at young age [125] and progressive chamber dilation, wall thinning, subendocardial dysfunction-dominant global dysfunction marked by subendocardial contractile impairment, loss of endo-epicardial length-dependent activation gradient, altered phosphorylation of sarcomeric regulatory proteins, especially in the subendocardium, and reduced myocardial endothelial and neuronal NO synthases in the heart [126]. In addition, GRMD dogs also develop vascular endothelial dysfunction, which may contribute to the pathogenesis of muscular damage and HF [127]. The advantage of the model is that it produces the entire spectrum of the pathology and clinical symptoms of human DMD. The disadvantage is the need of expensive installation and veterinary skills in the daily care of very disabled animals. Therefore, this is a very expensive and limited experimental model.

21.7.3
Genetic Modification-Induced Cardiomyopathies in Mice

Besides the natural gene mutation-induced cardiomyopathies leading to HF and death, genetic modification by addition or deletion of genes in mice produces diverse cardiomyopathies with more or less severe consequences, depending on the gene modified. These models have been used to identify genes that are causative for HF and in the evaluation of molecular mechanisms responsible for the development and progression of the disease. These models can also be used to investigate rescue or repair by knockout or overexpression of specific genes. However, there are a few examples of genetic modifications inducing cardiomyopathies with or without associated HF.

The muscle LIM protein (MLP) is a regulator of myogenic differentiation, and disruption of MLP gene in mice induces DCM associated with myocardial hypertrophy, interstitial cell proliferation, and fibrosis. Adult mice exhibit clinical and hemodynamic signs of HF similar to those in humans, indicating MLP dysfunction as a possible mechanism involved in the development of human DCM and HF [128]. Knockout of the gene encoding cardiac myosin-binding protein C, which is a thick filament-associated protein localized to the crossbridge-containing C zones of cardiac muscle sarcomeres, induces an eccentric LVH with LV contractile dysfunction in homozygote mice at 3–4 months of age [129]. Transgenic expression of a skeletal muscle myogenic regulator in the heart also induces hypertrophic and dilated cardiomyopathy, although the real physiopathological meaning of this genetic manipulation remains unclear [130]. Overexpression of the cardiac $G_s\alpha$ (stimulatory G protein α-subunit) in mice results in sustained sympathetic stimulation, and older mice overexpressing $G_s\alpha$ exhibit LV dilatation and dysfunction and increased mortality [131]. Overexpressing β-adrenergic receptor kinase leads to dampening of myocardial adenylate cyclase activity, β-adrenergic receptor uncoupling, and impaired contractility [132]. Transgenic mice overexpressing tropomodulin, a component of the thin filament proteins that determines sarcomeric actin filament length, exhibit lethal DCM 2–4 weeks after birth with myofibrillar disorganization, reduced contractile function, and ultimately HF [133].

21.8
Translation to Clinics: Limitations and Difficulties

Numerous animal models have been developed for HF studies and a tremendous amount of information regarding alterations in cardiac structure and function, neurohumoral systems, and protein and gene expression has been gained from these models and different therapeutic strategies have emerged from these studies. When translating the data obtained in animal models to clinical situations, we should keep in mind the limitations of animal models as described throughout the chapter for each model in diverse animal species. These limitations are first linked to the species differences in cardiac functional and structural characteristics between humans and animals, for example, between mice and humans as described in Section 21.1. Second, due to the species differences between animal models that are commonly described, it is difficult to predict the real situation in humans when the data obtained in different animal models are not consistent. This may need further research to determine the true situation in humans. For example, treatment with thyroxin increases myocardial β-adrenergic receptor density in rats but not in dogs [134]. Third, the translation of the data obtained in animal models may be related to the extent of similarity in pathologies that can be achieved by an animal model. When an animal model reproduces clinical signs and pathologies similar to those of humans, it is more likely that the data obtained in this animal model are applicable to clinics. Finally, due to the diversity of etiologies involved in the development of HF, the specificity of each cause, and complexity of the mechanisms underlying the development and progression of HF, it must be recognized that there is no one perfect animal model for the study of HF. The choice of an animal model should be individualized based on the targeted goals and must take into account the cost for the experimental facilities and the personal competence needed for the development of such animal models.

References

1 Haghighi, K., Kolokathis, F., Pater, L., Lynch, R.A., Asahi, M., Gramolini, A.O., Fan, G.-C., Tsiapras, D., Hahn, H.S., Adamopoulos, S., Liggett, S.B., Dorn, G.W., 2nd, MacLennan, D.H., Kremastinos, D.T., and Kranias, E.G. (2003) Human phospholamban null results in lethal dilated cardiomyopathy revealing a critical difference between mouse and human. *The Journal of Clinical Investigation*, **111**, 869–876.

2 Ginis, I., Luo, Y., Miura, T., Thies, S., Brandenberger, R., Gerecht-Nir, S., Amit, M., Hoke, A., Carpenter, M.K., Itskovitz-Eldor, J., and Rao, M.S. (2004) Differences between human and mouse embryonic

stem cells. *Developmental Biology*, **269**, 360–380.

3 Fedorov, V.V., Glukhov, A.V., Ambrosi, C.M., Kostecki, G., Chang, R., Janks, D., Schuessler, R.B., Moazami, N., Nichols, C.G., and Efimov, I.R. (2011) Effects of KATP channel openers diazoxide and pinacidil in coronary-perfused atria and ventricles from failing and non-failing human hearts. *Journal of Molecular and Cellular Cardiology*, **51**, 215–225.

4 Schenk, J. and McNeill, J.H. (1992) The pathogenesis of DOCA-salt hypertension. *Journal of Pharmacological and Toxicological Methods*, **27**, 161–170.

5 Crofton, J.T. and Share, L. (1997) Gonadal hormones modulate deoxycorticosterone-salt hypertension in male and female rats. *Hypertension*, **29**, 494–499.

6 Garwitz, E.T. and Jones, A.W. (1982) Aldosterone infusion into the rat and dose-dependent changes in blood pressure and arterial ionic transport. *Hypertension*, **4**, 374–381.

7 McMahon, E.G. and Paul, R.J. (1985) Calcium sensitivity of isometric force in intact and chemically skinned aortas during the development of aldosterone-salt hypertension in the rat. *Circulation Research*, **56**, 427–435.

8 Arnal, J.F., Warin, L., and Michel, J.B. (1992) Determinants of aortic cyclic guanosine monophosphate in hypertension induced by chronic inhibition of nitric oxide synthase. *The Journal of Clinical Investigation*, **90**, 647–652.

9 Bourraindeloup, M., Adamy, C., Candiani, G., Cailleret, M., Bourin, M.-C., Badoual, T., Su, J.B., Adubeiro, S., Roudot-Thoraval, F., Dubois-Rande, J.-L., Hittinger, L., and Pecker, F. (2004) N-Acetylcysteine treatment normalizes serum tumor necrosis factor-alpha level and hinders the progression of cardiac injury in hypertensive rats. *Circulation*, **110**, 2003–2009.

10 De Champlain, J., Krakoff, L.R., and Axelrod, J. (1967) Catecholamine metabolism in experimental hypertension in the rat. *Circulation Research*, **20**, 136–145.

11 White, P.C. (1996) Inherited forms of mineralocorticoid hypertension. *Hypertension*, **28**, 927–936.

12 Fitzgerald, S.M., Stevenson, K.M., Evans, R.G., and Anderson, W.P. (1997) Systemic hemodynamic responses to chronic angiotensin II infusion into the renal artery of dogs. *The American Journal of Physiology*, **273**, R1980–R1989.

13 Bruner, C.A. and Fink, G.D. (1986) Neurohumoral contributions to chronic angiotensin-induced hypertension. *The American Journal of Physiology*, **250**, H52–H61.

14 Vari, R.C., Zinn, S., Verburg, K.M., and Freeman, R.H. (1987) Renal nerves and the pathogenesis of angiotensin-induced hypertension. *Hypertension*, **9**, 345–349.

15 Rienzo, M., Bizé, A., Pongas, D., Michineau, S., Melka, J., Chan, H.L., Sambin, L., Su, J.B., Dubois-Randé, J.-L., Hittinger, L., Berdeaux, A., and Ghaleh, B. (2012) Impaired left ventricular function in the presence of preserved ejection in chronic hypertensive conscious pigs. *Basic Research in Cardiology*, **107**, 298.

16 Puybasset, L., Béa, M.L., Ghaleh, B., Giudicelli, J.F., and Berdeaux, A. (1996) Coronary and systemic hemodynamic effects of sustained inhibition of nitric oxide synthesis in conscious dogs. Evidence for cross talk between nitric oxide and cyclooxygenase in coronary vessels. *Circulation Research*, **79**, 343–357.

17 Mitchell, G.F., Pfeffer, J.M., and Pfeffer, M.A. (1997) The transition to failure in the spontaneously hypertensive rat. *American Journal of Hypertension*, **10**, 120S–126S.

18 Bing, O.H., Brooks, W.W., Robinson, K.G., Slawsky, M.T., Hayes, J.A., Litwin, S.E., Sen, S., and Conrad, C.H. (1995) The spontaneously hypertensive rat as a model of the transition from compensated left ventricular hypertrophy to failure. *Journal of Molecular and Cellular Cardiology*, **27**, 383–396.

19 Li, Z., Bing, O.H., Long, X., Robinson, K.G., and Lakatta, E.G. (1997) Increased cardiomyocyte apoptosis during the transition to heart failure in the spontaneously hypertensive rat. *The American Journal of Physiology*, **272**, H2313–H2319.

20 Ruben, Z., Miller, J.E., Rohrbacher, E., and Walsh, G.M. (1984) A potential model for a human disease: spontaneous cardiomyopathy-congestive heart failure in SHR/N-cp rats. *Human Pathology*, **15**, 902–903.

21 McCune, S.A., Baker, P.B., and Stills, H.F., Jr. (1990) SHHF/Mcc-cp rat: model of obesity, non-insulin-dependent diabetes, and congestive heart failure. *ILAR Journal*, **32** (2), 23–27.

22 Hennes, M.M., McCune, S.A., Shrago, E., and Kissebah, A.H. (1990) Synergistic effects of male sex and obesity on hepatic insulin dynamics in SHR/Mcc-cp rat. *Diabetes*, **39**, 789–795.

23 Anderson, K.M., Eckhart, A.D., Willette, R.N., and Koch, W.J. (1999) The myocardial beta-adrenergic system in spontaneously hypertensive heart failure (SHHF) rats. *Hypertension*, **33**, 402–407.

24 Holycross, B.J., Summers, B.M., Dunn, R.B., and McCune, S.A. (1997) Plasma renin activity in heart failure-prone SHHF/Mcc-facp rats. *The American Journal of Physiology*, **273**, H228–H233.

25 Haas, G.J., McCune, S.A., Brown, D.M., and Cody, R.J. (1995) Echocardiographic characterization of left ventricular adaptation in a genetically determined heart failure rat model. *American Heart Journal*, **130**, 806–811.

26 Sack, M.N., Rader, T.A., Park, S., Bastin, J., McCune, S.A., and Kelly, D.P. (1996) Fatty acid oxidation enzyme gene expression is downregulated in the failing heart. *Circulation*, **94**, 2837–2842.

27 Akhter, S.A., Eckhart, A.D., Rockman, H.A., Shotwell, K., Lefkowitz, R.J., and Koch, W.J. (1999) *In vivo* inhibition of elevated myocardial beta-adrenergic receptor kinase activity in hybrid transgenic mice restores normal beta-adrenergic signaling and function. *Circulation*, **100**, 648–653.

28 Sanders, P.W. (1996) Salt-sensitive hypertension: lessons from animal models. *American Journal of Kidney Diseases*, **28**, 775–782.

29 Dahl, L.K., Knudsen, K.D., Ohanian, E.V., Muirhead, M., and Tuthill, R. (1975) Role of the gonads in hypertension-prone rats. *The Journal of Experimental Medicine*, **142**, 748–759.

30 Inoko, M., Kihara, Y., Morii, I., Fujiwara, H., and Sasayama, S. (1994) Transition from compensatory hypertrophy to dilated, failing left ventricles in Dahl salt-sensitive rats. *The American Journal of Physiology*, **267**, H2471–H2482.

31 He, H., Kimura, S., Fujisawa, Y., Tomohiro, A., Kiyomoto, K., Aki, Y., and Abe, Y. (1997) Dietary L-arginine supplementation normalizes regional blood flow in Dahl-Iwai salt-sensitive rats. *American Journal of Hypertension*, **10**, 89S–93S.

32 Arany, Z., Novikov, M., Chin, S., Ma, Y., Rosenzweig, A., and Spiegelman, B.M. (2006) Transverse aortic constriction leads to accelerated heart failure in mice lacking PPAR-γ coactivator 1α. *Proceedings of the National Academy of Sciences of the United States of America*, **103**, 10086–10091.

33 Gaasch, W.H., Zile, M.R., Hoshino, P.K., Apstein, C.S., and Blaustein, A.S. (1989) Stress-shortening relations and myocardial blood flow in compensated and failing canine hearts with pressure-overload hypertrophy. *Circulation*, **79**, 872–883.

34 Hittinger, L., Shannon, R.P., Bishop, S.P., Gelpi, R.J., and Vatner, S.F. (1989) Subendomyocardial exhaustion of blood flow reserve and increased fibrosis in conscious dogs with heart failure. *Circulation Research*, **65**, 971–980.

35 Hittinger, L., Ghaleh, B., Chen, J., Edwards, J.G., Kudej, R.K., Iwase, M., Kim, S.-J., Vatner, S.F., and Vatner, D.E. (1999) Reduced subendocardial ryanodine receptors and consequent effects on cardiac function in conscious dogs with left ventricular hypertrophy. *Circulation Research*, **84**, 999–1006.

36 Hittinger, L., Mirsky, I., Shen, Y.-T., Patrick, T.A., Bishop, S.P., and Vatner, S.F. (1995) Hemodynamic mechanisms responsible for reduced subendocardial coronary reserve in dogs with severe left ventricular hypertrophy. *Circulation*, **92**, 978–986.

37 Hittinger, L., Shannon, R.P., Kohin, S., Lader, A.S., Manders, W.T., Patrick, T.A., Kelly, P., and Vatner, S.F. (1989) Isoproterenol-induced alterations in myocardial blood flow, systolic and

diastolic function in conscious dogs with heart failure. *Circulation*, **80**, 658–668.
38. Dart, C.H., Jr. and Holloszy, J.O. (1969) Hypertrophied non-failing rat heart, partial biochemical characterization. *Circulation Research*, **25**, 245–253.
39. Liu, Z., Hilbelink, D.R., Crockett, W.B., and Gerdes, A.M. (1991) Regional changes in hemodynamics and cardiac myocyte size in rats with aortocaval fistulas. 1. Developing and established hypertrophy. *Circulation Research*, **69**, 52–58.
40. Flaim, S.F., Minteer, W.J., Nellis, S.H., and Clark, D.P. (1979) Chronic arteriovenous shunt: evaluation of a model for heart failure in rat. *The American Journal of Physiology*, **236**, H698–H704.
41. Kleaveland, J.P., Kussmaul, W.G., Vinciguerra, T., Diters, R., and Carabello, B.A. (1988) Volume overload hypertrophy in a closed-chest model of mitral regurgitation. *The American Journal of Physiology*, **254**, H1034–H1041.
42. Carabello, B.A., Nakano, K., Corin, W., Biederman, R., and Spann, J.F., Jr. (1989) Left ventricular function in experimental volume overload hypertrophy. *The American Journal of Physiology*, **256**, H974–H981.
43. Tsutsui, H., Spinale, F.G., Nagatsu, M., Schmid, P.G., Ishihara, K., DeFreyte, G., Cooper, G., 4th, and Carabello, B.A. (1994) Effects of chronic beta-adrenergic blockade on the left ventricular and cardiocyte abnormalities of chronic canine mitral regurgitation. *The Journal of Clinical Investigation*, **93**, 2639–2648.
44. Tallaj, J., Wei, C.-C., Hankes, G.H., Holland, M., Rynders, P., Dillon, A.R., Ardell, J.L., Armour, J.A., Lucchesi, P.A., and Dell'Italia, L.J. (2003) Beta1-adrenergic receptor blockade attenuates angiotensin II-mediated catecholamine release into the cardiac interstitium in mitral regurgitation. *Circulation*, **108**, 225–230.
45. Spinale, F.G., Ishihra, K., Zile, M., DeFryte, G., Crawford, F.A., and Carabello, B.A. (1993) Structural basis for changes in left ventricular function and geometry because of chronic mitral regurgitation and after correction of volume overload. *The Journal of Thoracic and Cardiovascular Surgery*, **106**, 1147–1157.
46. Magid, N.M., Opio, G., Wallerson, D.C., Young, M.S., and Borer, J.S. (1994) Heart failure due to chronic experimental aortic regurgitation. *The American Journal of Physiology*, **267**, H556–H562.
47. Ezzaher, A., El Houda Bouanani, N., and Crozatier, B. (1992) Force–frequency relations and response to ryanodine in failing rabbit hearts. *The American Journal of Physiology*, **263**, H1710–H1715.
48. Gilson, N., El Houda Bouanani, N., Corsin, A., and Crozatier, B. (1990) Left ventricular function and beta-adrenoceptors in rabbit failing heart. *The American Journal of Physiology*, **258**, H634–H641.
49. Ezzaher, A., El Houda Bouanani, N., Su, J. B., Hittinger, L., and Crozatier, B. (1991) Increased negative inotropic effect of calcium-channel blockers in hypertrophied and failing rabbit heart. *The Journal of Pharmacology and Experimental Therapeutics*, **257**, 466–471.
50. Pogwizd, S.M., Qi, M., Yuan, W., Samarel, A.M., and Bers, D.M. (1999) Upregulation of Na^+/Ca^{2+} exchanger expression and function in an arrhythmogenic rabbit model of heart failure. *Circulation Research*, **85**, 1009–1019.
51. Hasenfuss, G., Schillinger, W., Lehnart, S. E., Preuss, M., Pieske, B., Maier, L.S., Prestle, J., Minami, K., and Just, H. (1999) Relationship between Na^+-Ca^{2+}-exchanger protein levels and diastolic function of failing human myocardium. *Circulation*, **99**, 641–648.
52. Lefrak, E.A., Pitha, J., Rosenheim, S., and Gottlieb, J.A. (1973) A clinicopathologic analysis of adriamycin cardiotoxicity. *Cancer*, **32**, 302–314.
53. Bristow, M.R., Mason, J.W., Billingham, M. E., and Daniels, J.R. (1978) Doxorubicin cardiomyopathy: evaluation by phonocardiography, endomyocardial biopsy, and cardiac catheterization. *Annals of Internal Medicine*, **88**, 168–175.
54. Mettler, F.P., Young, D.M., and Ward, J.M. (1977) Adriamycin-induced cardiotoxicity (cardiomyopathy and congestive heart failure) in rats. *Cancer Research*, **37**, 2705–2713.
55. Ambler, G.R., Johnston, B.M., Maxwell, L., Gavin, J.B., and Gluckman, P.D. (1993) Improvement of doxorubicin induced

cardiomyopathy in rats treated with insulin-like growth factor I. *Cardiovascular Research*, **27**, 1368–1373.

56 Werchan, P.M., Summer, W.R., Gerdes, A. M., and McDonough, K.H. (1989) Right ventricular performance after monocrotaline-induced pulmonary hypertension. *The American Journal of Physiology*, **256**, H1328–H1336.

57 Wanstall, J.C. and O'Donnell, S.R. (1990) Endothelin and 5-hydroxytryptamine on rat pulmonary artery in pulmonary hypertension. *European Journal of Pharmacology*, **176**, 159–168.

58 Ghodsi, F. and Will, J.A. (1981) Changes in pulmonary structure and function induced by monocrotaline intoxication. *The American Journal of Physiology*, **240**, H149–H155.

59 Meyrick, B., Gamble, W., and Reid, L. (1980) Development of *Crotalaria* pulmonary hypertension: hemodynamic and structural study. *The American Journal of Physiology*, **239**, H692–H702.

60 Ceconi, C., Condorelli, E., Quinzanini, M., Rodella, A., Ferrari, R., and Harris, P. (1989) Noradrenaline, atrial natriuretic peptide, bombesin and neurotensin in myocardium and blood of rats in congestive cardiac failure. *Cardiovascular Research*, **23**, 674–682.

61 Brown, L., Miller, J., Dagger, A., and Sernia, C. (1998) Cardiac and vascular responses after monocrotaline-induced hypertrophy in rats. *Journal of Cardiovascular Pharmacology*, **31**, 108–115.

62 Pelá, G., Missale, C., Raddino, R., Condorelli, E., Spano, P.F., and Visioli, O. (1990) Beta 1- and beta 2-receptors are differentially desensitized in an experimental model of heart failure. *Journal of Cardiovascular Pharmacology*, **16**, 839–846.

63 Vescovo, G., Jones, S.M., Harding, S.E., and Poole-Wilson, P.A. (1989) Isoproterenol sensitivity of isolated cardiac myocytes from rats with monocrotaline-induced right-sided hypertrophy and heart failure. *Journal of Molecular and Cellular Cardiology*, **21**, 1047–1061.

64 Bristow, M.R., Minobe, W., Rasmussen, R., Larrabee, P., Skerl, L., Klein, J.W., Anderson, F.L., Murray, J., Mestroni, L., and Karwande, S.V. (1992) Beta-adrenergic neuroeffector abnormalities in the failing human heart are produced by local rather than systemic mechanisms. *The Journal of Clinical Investigation*, **89**, 803–815.

65 White, F.C., Roth, D.M., and Bloor, C.M. (1986) The pig as a model for myocardial ischemia and exercise. *Laboratory Animal Science*, **36**, 351–356.

66 Pfeffer, M.A., Pfeffer, J.M., Fishbein, M.C., Fletcher, P.J., Spadaro, J., Kloner, R.A., and Braunwald, E. (1979) Myocardial infarct size and ventricular function in rats. *Circulation Research*, **44**, 503–512.

67 Reimer, K.A. and Jennings, R.B. (1979) The "wavefront phenomenon" of myocardial ischemic cell death. II. Transmural progression of necrosis within the framework of ischemic bed size (myocardium at risk) and collateral flow. *Laboratory Investigation*, **40**, 633–644.

68 Reimer, K.A., Lowe, J.E., Rasmussen, M. M., and Jennings, R.B. (1977) The wavefront phenomenon of ischemic cell death. 1. Myocardial infarct size vs duration of coronary occlusion in dogs. *Circulation*, **56**, 786–794.

69 Przyklenk, K., Vivaldi, M.T., Schoen, F.J., Malcolm, J., Arnold, O., and Kloner, R.A. (1986) Salvage of ischaemic myocardium by reperfusion: importance of collateral blood flow and myocardial oxygen demand during occlusion. *Cardiovascular Research*, **20**, 403–414.

70 Suzuki, T., Kopia, G., Hayashi, S., Bailey, L. R., Llanos, G., Wilensky, R., Klugherz, B. D., Papandreou, G., Narayan, P., Leon, M. B., Yeung, A.C., Tio, F., Tsao, P.S., Falotico, R., and Carter, A.J. (2001) Stent-based delivery of sirolimus reduces neointimal formation in a porcine coronary model. *Circulation*, **104**, 1188–1193.

71 Chazaud, B., Hittinger, L., Sonnet, C., Champagne, S., Le Corvoisier, P., Benhaiem-Sigaux, N., Unterseeh, T., Su, J., Merlet, P., Rahmouni, A., Garot, J., Gherardi, R., and Teiger, E. (2003) Endoventricular porcine autologous myoblast transplantation can be successfully achieved with minor mechanical cell damage. *Cardiovascular Research*, **58**, 444–450.

72 Weaver, M.E., Pantely, G.A., Bristow, J.D., and Ladley, H.D. (1986) A quantitative study of the anatomy and distribution of coronary arteries in swine in comparison with other animals and man. *Cardiovascular Research*, **20**, 907–917.

73 Sabbah, H.N., Stein, P.D., Kono, T., Gheorghiade, M., Levine, T.B., Jafri, S., Hawkins, E.T., and Goldstein, S. (1991) A canine model of chronic heart failure produced by multiple sequential coronary microembolizations. *The American Journal of Physiology*, **260**, H1379–H1384.

74 Zacà, V., Rastogi, S., Imai, M., Wang, M., Sharov, V.G., Jiang, A., Goldstein, S., and Sabbah, H.N. (2007) Chronic monotherapy with rosuvastatin prevents progressive left ventricular dysfunction and remodeling in dogs with heart failure. *Journal of the American College of Cardiology*, **50**, 551–557.

75 Sabbah, H.N., Shimoyama, H., Kono, T., Gupta, R.C., Sharov, V.G., Scicli, G., Levine, T.B., and Goldstein, S. (1994) Effects of long-term monotherapy with enalapril, metoprolol, and digoxin on the progression of left ventricular dysfunction and dilation in dogs with reduced ejection fraction. *Circulation*, **89**, 2852–2859.

76 Medvedev, O.S. and Gorodetskaya, E.A. (1993) Systemic and regional hemodynamic effects of perindopril in experimental heart failure. *American Heart Journal*, **126**, 764–769.

77 Li, S., Zhong, S., Zeng, K., Luo, Y., Zhang, F., Sun, X., and Chen, L. (2010) Blockade of NF-kappaB by pyrrolidine dithiocarbamate attenuates myocardial inflammatory response and ventricular dysfunction following coronary microembolization induced by homologous microthrombi in rats. *Basic Research in Cardiology*, **105**, 139–150.

78 Lu, Y., Li, L., Zhao, X., Huang, W., and Wen, W. (2011) Beta blocker metoprolol protects against contractile dysfunction in rats after coronary microembolization by regulating expression of myocardial inflammatory cytokines. *Life Sciences*, **88**, 1009–1015.

79 Zhang, F.-L., Chen, L.-L., Li, S.-M., and Wang, W.-W. (2008) Granulocyte colony stimulating factor attenuated myocardial apoptosis via Janus kinase 2/signal transducer and activator of transcription signal transduction pathway in rats with coronary microembolization. *Zhonghua Xin Xue Guan Bing Za Zhi*, **36**, 254–259.

80 Xie, Y.W., Shen, W., Zhao, G., Xu, X., Wolin, M.S., and Hintze, T.H. (1996) Role of endothelium-derived nitric oxide in the modulation of canine myocardial mitochondrial respiration *in vitro*. Implications for the development of heart failure. *Circulation Research*, **79**, 381–387.

81 Fitzpatrick, M.A., Nicholls, M.G., Espiner, E.A., Ikram, H., Bagshaw, P., and Yandle, T.G. (1989) Neurohumoral changes during onset and offset of ovine heart failure: role of ANP. *The American Journal of Physiology*, **256**, H1052–H1059.

82 Rademaker, M.T., Charles, C.J., Espiner, E.A., Frampton, C.M., Nicholls, M.G., and Richards, A.M. (1997) Comparative bioactivity of atrial and brain natriuretic peptides in an ovine model of heart failure. *Clinical Science*, **92**, 159–165.

83 Spinale, F.G., Fulbright, B.M., Mukherjee, R., Tanaka, R., Hu, J., Crawford, F.A., and Zile, M.R. (1992) Relation between ventricular and myocyte function with tachycardia-induced cardiomyopathy. *Circulation Research*, **71**, 174–187.

84 Sun, S.-Y., Wang, W., Zucker, I.H., and Schultz, H.D. (1999) Enhanced peripheral chemoreflex function in conscious rabbits with pacing-induced heart failure. *Journal of Applied Physiology*, **86**, 1264–1272.

85 Tsuji, Y., Opthof, T., Kamiya, K., Yasui, K., Liu, W., Lu, Z., and Kodama, I. (2000) Pacing-induced heart failure causes a reduction of delayed rectifier potassium currents along with decreases in calcium and transient outward currents in rabbit ventricle. *Cardiovascular Research*, **48**, 300–309.

86 Byrne, M.J., Kaye, D.M., Mathis, M., Reuter, D.G., Alferness, C.A., and Power, J.M. (2004) Percutaneous mitral annular reduction provides continued benefit in an ovine model of dilated cardiomyopathy. *Circulation*, **110**, 3088–3092.

87 Armstrong, P.W., Stopps, T.P., Ford, S.E., and De Bold, A.J. (1986) Rapid ventricular pacing in the dog: pathophysiologic studies of heart failure. *Circulation*, **74**, 1075–1084.

88 Wilson, J.R., Douglas, P., Hickey, W.F., Lanoce, V., Ferraro, N., Muhammad, A., and Reichek, N. (1987) Experimental congestive heart failure produced by rapid ventricular pacing in the dog: cardiac effects. *Circulation*, **75**, 857–867.

89 Shannon, R.P., Komamura, K., Stambler, B.S., Bigaud, M., Manders, W.T., and Vatner, S.F. (1991) Alterations in myocardial contractility in conscious dogs with dilated cardiomyopathy. *The American Journal of Physiology*, **260**, H1903–H1911.

90 Komamura, K., Shannon, R.P., Pasipoularides, A., Ihara, T., Lader, A.S., Patrick, T.A., Bishop, S.P., and Vatner, S.F. (1992) Alterations in left ventricular diastolic function in conscious dogs with pacing-induced heart failure. *The Journal of Clinical Investigation*, **89**, 1825–1838.

91 Riegger, A.J. and Liebau, G. (1982) The renin–angiotensin–aldosterone system, antidiuretic hormone and sympathetic nerve activity in an experimental model of congestive heart failure in the dog. *Clinical Science*, **62**, 465–469.

92 Mukherjee, R., Hewett, K.W., Walker, J.D., Basler, C.G., and Spinale, F.G. (1998) Changes in L-type calcium channel abundance and function during the transition to pacing-induced congestive heart failure. *Cardiovascular Research*, **37**, 432–444.

93 Calderone, A., Bouvier, M., Li, K., Juneau, C., De Champlain, J., and Rouleau, J.L. (1991) Dysfunction of the beta- and alpha-adrenergic systems in a model of congestive heart failure. The pacing-overdrive dog. *Circulation Research*, **69**, 332–343.

94 Marzo, K.P., Frey, M.J., Wilson, J.R., Liang, B.T., Manning, D.R., Lanoce, V., and Molinoff, P.B. (1991) Beta-adrenergic receptor–G protein–adenylate cyclase complex in experimental canine congestive heart failure produced by rapid ventricular pacing. *Circulation Research*, **69**, 1546–1556.

95 Perreault, C.L., Shannon, R.P., Komamura, K., Vatner, S.F., and Morgan, J.P. (1992) Abnormalities in intracellular calcium regulation and contractile function in myocardium from dogs with pacing-induced heart failure. *The Journal of Clinical Investigation*, **89**, 932–938.

96 Yao, A., Su, Z., Nonaka, A., Zubair, I., Spitzer, K.W., Bridge, J.H.B., Muelheims, G., Ross, J., and Barry, W.H. (1998) Abnormal myocyte Ca^{2+} homeostasis in rabbits with pacing-induced heart failure. *American Journal of Physiology. Heart and Circulatory Physiology*, **275**, H1441–H1448.

97 Su, J., Renaud, N., Carayon, A., Crozatier, B., and Hittinger, L. (1994) Effects of the calcium channel blockers, diltiazem and Ro 40-5967, on systemic haemodynamics and plasma noradrenaline levels in conscious dogs with pacing-induced heart failure. *British Journal of Pharmacology*, **113**, 395–402.

98 Barbe, F., Su, J.B., Guyene, T.T., Crozatier, B., Ménard, J., and Hittinger, L. (1996) Bradykinin pathway is involved in acute hemodynamic effects of enalaprilat in dogs with heart failure. *The American Journal of Physiology*, **270**, H1985–H1992.

99 Choussat, R., Hittinger, L., Barbe, F., Maistre, G., Carayon, A., Crozatier, B., and Su, J. (1998) Acute effects of an endothelin-1 receptor antagonist bosentan at different stages of heart failure in conscious dogs. *Cardiovascular Research*, **39**, 580–588.

100 Moe, G.W. and Armstrong, P. (1999) Pacing-induced heart failure: a model to study the mechanism of disease progression and novel therapy in heart failure. *Cardiovascular Research*, **42**, 591–599.

101 Kajstura, J., Zhang, X., Liu, Y., Szoke, E., Cheng, W., Olivetti, G., Hintze, T.H., and Anversa, P. (1995) The cellular basis of pacing-induced dilated cardiomyopathy. Myocyte cell loss and myocyte cellular reactive hypertrophy. *Circulation*, **92**, 2306–2317.

102 McMahon, W.S., Mukherjee, R., Gillette, P.C., Crawford, F.A., and Spinale, F.G. (1996) Right and left ventricular geometry and myocyte contractile processes with dilated cardiomyopathy: myocyte growth and beta-adrenergic responsiveness. *Cardiovascular Research*, **31**, 314–323.

103 Kiuchi, K., Sato, N., Shannon, R.P., Vatner, D.E., Morgan, K., and Vatner, S.F. (1993) Depressed beta-adrenergic receptor- and endothelium-mediated vasodilation in

conscious dogs with heart failure. *Circulation Research*, **73**, 1013–1023.

104 Su, J.B., Barbe, F., Houel, R., Guyene, T.T., Crozatier, B., and Hittinger, L. (1998) Preserved vasodilator effect of bradykinin in dogs with heart failure. *Circulation*, **98**, 2911–2918.

105 Tonduangu, D., Hittinger, L., Ghaleh, B., Le Corvoisier, P., Sambin, L., Champagne, S., Badoual, T., Vincent, F., Berdeaux, A., Crozatier, B., and Su, J.B. (2004) Chronic infusion of bradykinin delays the progression of heart failure and preserves vascular endothelium-mediated vasodilation in conscious dogs. *Circulation*, **109**, 114–119.

106 Smith, C.J., Sun, D., Hoegler, C., Roth, B.S., Zhang, X., Zhao, G., Xu, X.B., Kobari, Y., Pritchard, K., Jr., Sessa, W.C., and Hintze, T.H. (1996) Reduced gene expression of vascular endothelial NO synthase and cyclooxygenase-1 in heart failure. *Circulation Research*, **78**, 58–64.

107 Wang, J., Seyedi, N., Xu, X.B., Wolin, M.S., and Hintze, T.H. (1994) Defective endothelium-mediated control of coronary circulation in conscious dogs after heart failure. *The American Journal of Physiology*, **266**, H670–H680.

108 Moe, G.W., Stopps, T.P., Howard, R.J., and Armstrong, P.W. (1988) Early recovery from heart failure: insights into the pathogenesis of experimental chronic pacing-induced heart failure. *The Journal of Laboratory and Clinical Medicine*, **112**, 426–432.

109 Nigro, V., Okazaki, Y., Belsito, A., Piluso, G., Matsuda, Y., Politano, L., Nigro, G., Ventura, C., Abbondanza, C., Molinari, A.M., Acampora, D., Nishimura, M., Hayashizaki, Y., and Puca, G.A. (1997) Identification of the Syrian hamster cardiomyopathy gene. *Human Molecular Genetics*, **6**, 601–607.

110 Sakamoto, A., Ono, K., Abe, M., Jasmin, G., Eki, T., Murakami, Y., Masaki, T., Toyo-oka, T., and Hanaoka, F. (1997) Both hypertrophic and dilated cardiomyopathies are caused by mutation of the same gene, delta-sarcoglycan, in hamster: an animal model of disrupted dystrophin-associated glycoprotein complex. *Proceedings of the National Academy of Sciences of the United States of America*, **94**, 13873–13878.

111 Gertz, E.W. (1973) Animal model of human disease. Myocardial failure, muscular dystrophy. *The American Journal of Pathology*, **70**, 151–154.

112 Ryoke, T., Gu, Y., Mao, L., Hongo, M., Clark, R.G., Peterson, K.L., and Ross, J., Jr. (1999) Progressive cardiac dysfunction and fibrosis in the cardiomyopathic hamster and effects of growth hormone and angiotensin-converting enzyme inhibition. *Circulation*, **100**, 1734–1743.

113 Crespo, M.J. (1999) Vascular alterations during the development and progression of experimental heart failure. *Journal of Cardiac Failure*, **5**, 55–63.

114 Crespo, M.J., Alticri, P.I., and Escobales, N. (2006) Increased vascular angiotensin II binding capacity and ET-1 release in young cardiomyopathic hamsters. *Vascular Pharmacology*, **44**, 247–252.

115 Escobales, N. and Crespo, M.J. (2006) Angiotensin II-dependent vascular alterations in young cardiomyopathic hamsters: role for oxidative stress. *Vascular Pharmacology*, **44**, 22–28.

116 Bonilla, E., Samitt, C.E., Miranda, A.F., Hays, A.P., Salviati, G., DiMauro, S., Kunkel, L.M., Hoffman, E.P., and Rowland, L.P. (1988) Duchenne muscular dystrophy: deficiency of dystrophin at the muscle cell surface. *Cell*, **54**, 447–452.

117 Hoffman, E.P., Brown, R.H., and Kunkel, L.M. (1987) Dystrophin: the protein product of the Duchenne muscular dystrophy locus. *Cell*, **51**, 919–928.

118 Koenig, M., Hoffman, E.P., Bertelson, C.J., Monaco, A.P., Feener, C., and Kunkel, L.M. (1987) Complete cloning of the Duchenne muscular dystrophy (DMD) cDNA and preliminary genomic organization of the DMD gene in normal and affected individuals. *Cell*, **50**, 509–517.

119 Mukoyama, M., Kondo, K., Hizawa, K., and Nishitani, H. (1987) Life spans of Duchenne muscular dystrophy patients in the hospital care program in Japan. *Journal of the Neurological Sciences*, **81**, 155–158.

120 Nigro, G., Comi, L.I., Politano, L., and Bain, R.J. (1990) The incidence and evolution of cardiomyopathy in Duchenne muscular dystrophy. *International Journal of Cardiology*, **26**, 271–277.

121 De Kermadec, J.M., Bécane, H.M., Chénard, A., Tertrain, F., and Weiss, Y. (1994) Prevalence of left ventricular systolic dysfunction in Duchenne muscular dystrophy: an echocardiographic study. *American Heart Journal*, **127**, 618–623.

122 Cooper, B.J., Winand, N.J., Stedman, H., Valentine, B.A., Hoffman, E.P., Kunkel, L. M., Scott, M.O., Fischbeck, K.H., Kornegay, J.N., and Avery, R.J. (1988) The homologue of the Duchenne locus is defective in X-linked muscular dystrophy of dogs. *Nature*, **334**, 154–156.

123 Sampaolesi, M., Blot, S., D'Antona, G., Granger, N., Tonlorenzi, R., Innocenzi, A., Mognol, P., Thibaud, J.-L., Galvez, B.G., Barthélémy, I., Perani, L., Mantero, S., Guttinger, M., Pansarasa, O., Rinaldi, C., Cusella De Angelis, M.G., Torrente, Y., Bordignon, C., Bottinelli, R., and Cossu, G. (2006) Mesoangioblast stem cells ameliorate muscle function in dystrophic dogs. *Nature*, **444**, 574–579.

124 Townsend, D., Turner, I., Yasuda, S., Martindale, J., Davis, J., Shillingford, M., Kornegay, J.N., and Metzger, J.M. (2010) Chronic administration of membrane sealant prevents severe cardiac injury and ventricular dilatation in dystrophic dogs. *The Journal of Clinical Investigation*, **120**, 1140–1150.

125 Chetboul, V., Escriou, C., Tessier, D., Richard, V., Pouchelon, J.-L., Thibault, H., Lallemand, F., Thuillez, C., Blot, S., and Derumeaux, G. (2004) Tissue Doppler imaging detects early asymptomatic myocardial abnormalities in a dog model of Duchenne's cardiomyopathy. *European Heart Journal*, **25**, 1934–1939.

126 Su, J.B., Cazorla, O., Blot, S., Blanchard-Gutton, N., Ait Mou, Y., Barthélémy, I., Sambin, L., Sampedrano, C.C., Gouni, V., Unterfinger, Y., Aguilar, P., Thibaud, J.-L., Bizé, A., Pouchelon, J.-L., Dabiré, H., Ghaleh, B., Berdeaux, A., Chetboul, V., Lacampagne, A., and Hittinger, L. (2012) Bradykinin restores left ventricular function, sarcomeric protein phosphorylation, and e/nNOS levels in dogs with Duchenne muscular dystrophy cardiomyopathy. *Cardiovascular Research*, **95**, 86–96.

127 Dabiré, H., Barthélémy, I., Blanchard-Gutton, N., Sambin, L., Sampedrano, C.C., Gouni, V., Unterfinger, Y., Aguilar, P., Thibaud, J.-L., Ghaleh, B., Bizé, A., Pouchelon, J.-L., Blot, S., Berdeaux, A., Hittinger, L., Chetboul, V., and Su, J.B. (2012) Vascular endothelial dysfunction in Duchenne muscular dystrophy is restored by bradykinin through upregulation of eNOS and nNOS. *Basic Research in Cardiology*, **107**, 240.

128 Arber, S., Hunter, J.J., Ross, J., Jr., Hongo, M., Sansig, G., Borg, J., Perriard, J.C., Chien, K.R., and Caroni, P. (1997) MLP-deficient mice exhibit a disruption of cardiac cytoarchitectural organization, dilated cardiomyopathy, and heart failure. *Cell*, **88**, 393–403.

129 Carrier, L., Knöll, R., Vignier, N., Keller, D. I., Bausero, P., Prudhon, B., Isnard, R., Ambroisine, M.-L., Fiszman, M., Ross, J., Schwartz, K., and Chien, K.R. (2004) Asymmetric septal hypertrophy in heterozygous cMyBP-C null mice. *Cardiovascular Research*, **63**, 293–304.

130 Edwards, J.G., Lyons, G.E., Micales, B.K., Malhotra, A., Factor, S., and Leinwand, L. A. (1996) Cardiomyopathy in transgenic myf5 mice. *Circulation Research*, **78**, 379–387.

131 Iwase, M., Uechi, M., Vatner, D.E., Asai, K., Shannon, R.P., Kudej, R.K., Wagner, T.E., Wight, D.C., Patrick, T.A., Ishikawa, Y., Homcy, C.J., and Vatner, S.F. (1997) Cardiomyopathy induced by cardiac Gs alpha overexpression. *The American Journal of Physiology*, **272**, H585–H589.

132 Koch, W.J., Rockman, H.A., Samama, P., Hamilton, R.A., Bond, R.A., Milano, C.A., and Lefkowitz, R.J. (1995) Cardiac function in mice overexpressing the beta-adrenergic receptor kinase or a beta ARK inhibitor. *Science*, **268**, 1350–1353.

133 Sussman, M.A., Welch, S., Cambon, N., Klevitsky, R., Hewett, T.E., Price, R., Witt,

S.A., and Kimball, T.R. (1998) Myofibril degeneration caused by tropomodulin overexpression leads to dilated cardiomyopathy in juvenile mice. *The Journal of Clinical Investigation*, **101**, 51–61.

134 Crozatier, B., Su, J.B., Corsin, A., and Bouanani, N.el.-H. (1991) Species differences in myocardial beta-adrenergic receptor regulation in response to hyperthyroidism. *Circulation Research*, **69**, 1234–1243.

22
Endocrine Disorders

Thomas Cuny, Anne Barlier, and Alain Enjalbert

22.1
Introduction

Animal models have been developed for more than 50 years, in many fields of medicine. F.G. Banting and J.J.R. Macleod were the pioneers in endocrinology and diabetology by discovering the hormone insulin thanks to diabetic dogs and pacreatic extracts. They were awared with the Nobel Prize for Medicine and Physiology in 1923 (www.nobelprize.org).

In endocrinology, animal models have been developed in two major directions: to improve the understanding of disease pathophysiology and to investigate the effect of new medical therapies. Of note, analyzing the hormonal secretion in addition to classical parameters, such as regression of clinical symptoms, is a specificity of endocrine diseases and is classically used for monitoring the therapeutic efficiency.

The mouse increasingly became a popular choice for developing *in vivo* mammalian models, as it shares many physiological systems and genomic coding regions with humans [1]. The small size of mice coupled with the ability to reproduce similar strains carrying the genetic mutation in a short generation time represents many practical advantages of this model [2].

In this chapter, we briefly summarize animal models currently used or those that have been developed for studying endocrine diseases. Because of the plethora of models, this chapter is organized in three sections; the models used for diabetes mellitus and obesity are, however, not included herein. In the first section, animal models used in autoimmune endocrine diseases have been introduced; in the second section, models of endocrine tumors have been presented; and in the third section, models used in relevant endocrine disorders such as hormonal pituitary deficiencies or polycystic ovary syndrome(PCOS) have been studied. Besides advantages, the limitations of such *in vivo* models have been discussed, particularly the differences that might exist between animals and humans and their consequences in terms of pathophysiological approaches and therapeutic possibilities.

22.2
Animal Models in Autoimmune Endocrine Diseases

Autoimmune diseases affect nearly 10% of population across the world and concern in part the endocrine tissues. More common endocrine autoimmune syndromes in humans (excluding type 1 diabetes) include Hashimoto's thyroiditis, Grave's disease(GD), and, to a lesser degree, Addison's disease (AD) [3]. An exquisite knowledge of the early etiopathogenic stages of the diseases is required. However, these early stages are usually asymptomatic, and hence very difficult to establish in humans. Conversely, animal models can be bred to study and manipulate inheritance [4]. These models exhibit two limitations regarding human conditions: First, the respective immune systems of humans and mice display singular differences [5]. Second, the use of specifically inbred animals to generate homogenous and extreme forms of the autoimmune diseases imperfectly mimics human diseases because endocrine autoimmune diseases are polygenic diseases in which the penetrance of a combination of genes is strongly influenced by environmental factors [3]. In this respect, animal models that spontaneously develop the disease seem to be closest to reality than experimentally induced models, that is, transgenic mice.

22.2.1
Animal Models of Autoimmune Thyroiditis

Among thyroid autoimmune diseases, GD is the one whose pathophysiology remains partially elucidated. The disease results from thyroid-stimulating auto-antibodies (TSAb) mimicking the action of thyrotropin (TSH), by targeting its receptor (TSHR), responsible for autoantigenicity. A thyrotoxic state can subsequently occur, with extrathyroidal manifestations such as severe ophthalmopathy whose treatment is, nowadays, a real challenge. To date, no spontaneous model of the disease has been described, and as a consequence, animal models (mainly mice) have been generated by different protocols of immunization with the TSHR [6]. This has resulted in variable production of TSAb and irregular manifestations of hyperthyroid state, depending on the model used (Table 22.1). Of note, a majority of mice models for GD do not develop extrathyroidal manifestations, especially ophthalmopathy [7], suggesting that expression of TSHR in mice may not be sufficient to mimic the disease [6]. Immunological abnormalities of GD, such as the involvement of regulatory T cells, have been studied in mice with ambiguous data [8,9]. New immunoregulatory therapeutic molecules such as anti-TNF-α or anti-CD20 antibodies have been tested in such models, albeit without significant results. Moreover, although these drugs could improve the severity of orbitopathy, they remain without effect on thyroiditis [10].

In the area of hypothyroidism, obese strain (OS) chickens are known to spontaneously suffer from lymphocytic thyroiditis, mimicking the human Hashimoto's disease [11]. Experimental models of hypothyroidism either by surgery (removal of thyroid gland), radioactive administration, iodine restriction diet, antithyroid drug

22.2 Animal Models in Autoimmune Endocrine Diseases

Table 22.1 Schematic representation of experimentally induced animal models of Grave's disease.

	Injection of TSH-R stably transfected cells				TSAb-transgenic mice (TSAb-Tg mice) — C57BL/6J mice	Human disease	Transient TSH-R expression
	TSHR and MHC II transfection → Fibroblasts → AKR/N mice	TSHR transfection → CHO Ovary cells → Hamster	TSHR transfection → Murine B cell line (M12) → BALB/c mice	TSHR transfection → HEK293 cells → BALB/c mice	B cell clone producing a TSAb from a GD patient; 1. Transgenic construction 2. Microinjection → Fertilized eggs of C57BL/6J mice		TSHR-DNA vaccination (plasmid) or DNA in recombinant adenovirus (Ad-TSHR) → BALB/c mice; TSH-R expression by myoblasts and inflammatory cells
Prevalence of TSHR antibodies[a]	90%	40%	≈100%	≈100%	100%	>95%	67% for vaccination; 70–100% for Ad-TSHR
Frequency of hyperthyroidism[b]	21%	10%	≈100%	≈100%	68%	100%	30% for vaccination; 35–50% for Ad-TSHR
Macroscopical and histological aspects of thyroid gland (from hyperthyroid models)	+ Marked hypertrophy + Thyrocyte hypercellularity + Intrusion into the follicular lumen	+ Goiter + Hypertrophy of follicular epithelial cells + Papillary protrusion and colloid droplet accumulation + Focal lymphocyte infiltration with no follicular destruction	+ Enlargement of thyroid gland + Hypertrophy and enlargement of colloids with thinning of the thyroid epithelium + Focal necrosis and inflammation by lymphocytic infiltration	+ Enlargement of the thyroid gland + Hypertrophy and enlargement of colloids with thinning of the thyroid epithelium + Focal necrosis and inflammation by lymphocytic infiltration	+ Diffuse hypercellularity and follicles with irregular sizes + Vacuoles in the boundary of epithelial cells + Richness of interstitial arterioles – No lymphocyte infiltration	+ Vascular and homogenous thyroid goiter + Infiltration of thyroid by T and B lymphocytes and plasma cells + Hypertrophy of follicular epithelial cells + Colloid droplet accumulation	+ Some models exhibit thyroid lymphocytic infiltrates depending on the vaccination protocol + With Ad-TSHR: hyperplastic thyroid glands + Goiter in both protocols

Main properties of each model in terms of TSH-R antibody production, hyperthyroid state prevalence, and histopathological features of thyroid gland are mentioned.
a) Antibodies with TSH binding inhibition activity.
b) Criteria for thyrotoxic state include elevated serum of T_4 and/or T_3 levels, decrease in TSH, thyroid goiter, and weight loss.

administration, or genetic manipulations attempt to study the peculiar effect of thyroid hormone deficiency on organic functions, during the development. Among them, the drug-induced models have been the most used throughout the literature with relevant information about structural brain damages, cognitive functions impairment, and alterations in conduct such as learning and spatial memory [12]. Advantages and disadvantages of each model have been discussed recently, and even if they seem interesting, their contribution to human pathology is limited to pathophysiological insights [13].

22.2.2
Animal Models for Addison's Disease

Addison's disease is a rare endocrine condition, due to circulating autoantibodies directed against 21-hydroxylase, with a prevalence of 110–140 cases per million [14]. Dogs represent the most reliable model as they can spontaneously develop autoimmune adrenal insufficiency with a form of the disease very similar to human AD in a number of ways [15]. Moreover, the prevalence of the disease is significantly higher in dogs than in humans, ranging from 1.5 to 9%, especially in susceptible breeds such as Portuguese Water Dogs (PWDs) [15]. Models of PWDs have been useful in the understanding of the genetic background of the disease by the identification of two disease-associated loci, orthologs to human MHC and cytotoxic T-lymphocyte antigen-4 (CTLA4) gene regions [16]. These regions are known to be involved in many forms of human autoimmune disorders.

Other models of AD exist such as murine models, developed by using repeated immunization with adrenal extracts and lipopolysaccharide from *Klebsiella* as adjuvant [17]. However, the absence of diffuse atrophy of the adrenal cortex combined with regeneration nodules, usually observed in humans, limits their reliability. In addition, there are very few reports about the occurrence of adrenocortical insufficiency in animals with experimental adrenalitis, whereas it is frequently observed at different degrees in human AD [18].

22.2.3
Animal Models for Other Endocrine Autoimmune Diseases

Other autoimmune endocrine diseases, such as hypophysitis or oophoritis, have been less studied in animals because they remain rare in terms of prevalence and are usually isolated. Conversely, autoimmune hypoparathyroidism may occur alone or in combination with other disorders in the APECED (autoimmune polyendocrinopathy-candidiasis-ectodermal dystrophy) syndrome. The latter is due to inactivating mutations in the gene *AIRE* (autoimmune regulator), localized on chromosome 21q22.3 in humans [19]. Development of *Aire*-deficient mice emphasized the critical involvement of this gene in the thymic T-cell selection, one of the cornerstones of the autoimmunity process [20,21]. Nevertheless, the main interest of study with animal models in APECED syndrome concerns exclusively the understanding of the autoimmunity mechanisms, especially in the early phases, as the clinical manifestations of APECED in humans and mice are significantly different [22].

22.3
Animal Models in Endocrine Tumors

Animal models have provided a considerable range of possibilities for investigations in endocrine tumors. Identification of molecular disruptors playing a role in tumorigenesis as well as new promising therapies has been studied in animals complementary to *in vitro* experimentations. Genetically engineered mice models are once again overrepresented in this section.

22.3.1
Multiple Endocrine Neoplasia Syndromes

Multiple endocrine neoplasia type 1 (MEN1) is an autosomal dominant tumor predisposition syndrome due to mutations in the putative tumor suppressor gene *MEN1* and characterized by the combined occurrence of parathyroid, pancreatic islet, and anterior pituitary tumors [23]. *MEN1* encodes for menin, a 610-amino acid protein that, through multiple pathways, regulates cell growth. The corresponding gene in mouse (called *Men1*) shares 89% analogy with the human gene, indicating a high degree of evolutionary conservation [24]. Mice models heterozygous for *Men1* ($Men1^{-/+}$) develop multiple endocrine tumors mimicking the endocrine manifestations of the syndrome in humans. Nevertheless, depending on the model used, phenotypic differences could be observed as the emergence of gonadal tumors, never described in humans, or the systematic occurrence of thyroid tumors, whereas this remains uncertain in humans [2,25]. Similar to humans, pancreatic islets and pituitary tumors of $Men1^{-/+}$ mice express significant levels of somatostatin receptor subtype 2 and vascular endothelial growth factor receptor, subsequently providing good models for testing targeted therapies such as somatostatin analogs or angiogenesis inhibitors [25].

The pivotal role of menin in the control of growth has been underlined in mice by homozygous inactivation of the gene that resulted in embryonic lethality or severe organic developmental abnormalities [26]. These data differed from those observed in *Drosophila*, where *Mnn1*, the ortholog of *Men1*, seemed rather to act as a gatekeeper on the genome integrity [27]. Whether these functions of the protein can be translated to human cellular physiology remains unknown, and regarding discrepancies between animal models, further investigations are needed.

In addition to conventional knockout (KO) models and because a somatic loss of the wild-type allele is required for tumorigenesis, mice with a conditional KO of *Men1*, that is, in a tissue-specific manner, have been developed in order to establish the direct effect of menin inactivation on the development of endocrine tumors. These models are useful in overcoming homozygous-null ($Men1^{-/-}$) mice lethality. Tissue-specific loss of *Men1* in parathyroid, pituitary, or pancreatic β-cells led to hyperparathyroidism, prolactin pituitary tumors, and multiple pancreatic islets, respectively, with high insulin levels.

Multiple endocrine neoplasia type 2 (MEN2) syndrome is divided into three clinical entities, known as MEN2A, MEN2B, and familial medullary thyroid carcinoma (MTC). Mutations in *RET* (rearranging during transfection) proto-oncogene, known to encode a receptor with tyrosine kinase activity, are responsible for MEN2. In 1974, aged bulls were found to spontaneously develop thyroid neoplasms similar to human medullary thyroid carcinomas and provided the first animal model of the disease [28]. Since then, mice models for MEN2 have been generated through knock-in (KI) strategies (Table 22.2). Three mice models, carrying the Cys634Arg mutation in *RET*, developed MTC with high penetrance and/or thyroid C-cell hyperplasia. However, unlike humans, no adrenal enlargement has been observed [2]. RAS-Erk, Jun kinase, and Src have been identified as canonical molecular pathways of the tumorigenesis in a *Drosophila* model of MEN2 (with targeted mutations in dRet) [29]. Moreover, this model allowed the identification of new critical genes, hitherto unknown, exhibiting LOH in some MEN2-associated human tumors [29]. The therapeutic response to vandetanib, an inhibitor of RET currently used in patients with MTC, is another argument that supports the reliability of *Drosophila* for future pharmacological studies [30].

To conclude, mutations in the *Cdkn1b* gene, encoding for p27Kip1, an inhibitor of cyclin-dependent kinase inhibitor, have been first identified in rat colonies suffering from MEN1-like syndrome (Table 22.2). The discovery of *Cdkn1b* mutations in MENX rats led Pellegata *et al.* to identify a germline nonsense mutation in the human *CDKN1B* gene in a *MEN1* mutation-negative patient. This patient presented pituitary and parathyroid tumors [31]. This new syndrome due to *CDKN1B* gene has been named MEN4 in humans. Although this first report has been confirmed thereafter by similar observations, the contribution of *CDKN1B* to patients with MEN1 phenotype but without mutations in *MEN1* remains modest.

22.3.2
Adrenal Tumorigenesis

The molecular bases of adrenal tumorigenesis remain partially elucidated in humans. Nowadays, three main species have been used to approach adrenocortical cancer (ACC) genesis: the mouse, the ferret, and the dog [32]. Each of them exhibits advantages and limitations compared with each other and with human conditions, and might be, accordingly, considered as a complementary model. In the same direction, it is noteworthy that adrenal tumorigenesis is the typical example of human disease investigations where *in vivo*, *ex vivo*, and *in vitro* conditions have been synergistically used.

Mice models for ACC are divided into three types: (i) models that spontaneously develop tumors after surgical gonadectomy, (ii) those transplanted with NCI-H295 cell line (ACC cell line), and (iii) genetically modified models [33]. Limitations of mice lie in differences in anatomy, enzymatic expression, and hormonal production of adrenal cortex compared with humans. In transgenic mice, the

Table 22.2 Genetic and clinical features of multiple endocrine neoplasia (NEM) syndromes currently known in humans and rodent models.

MEN syndromes	Genetic characteristics		Clinical manifestations		Commentaries
	Human	Mice models	Human	Mice models	
Type 1	Tumor suppressor gene *MEN1* (11q13) >1300 mutations known Loss-of-function mutations predominate	Gene *Men1*, chromosome 19 89% of analogy with human gene Conventional and conditional KO models	Typical: hyperparathyroidism, GEPNETs (gastrinoma) Pituitary adenoma (PRL) Less frequent: adrenal tumor, lipoma	Parathyroids, anterior pituitary, pancreatic, adrenal tumors **Gonadal and thyroid tumors** in male and female	Tissue-specific KO models develop **insulinoma** and PRL
Type 2A	Proto-oncogene *RET* (10q11.2) Missense mutations Cys634Arg and Cys620Arg are the most common	Cys634Arg and Cys620Arg mutations in human *RET* cDNA have been established, than injected in fertilized oocytes of mice or in a tissue-specific manner (KI models)	MTC Pheochromocytoma, paraganglioma Hyperparathyroidism	Thyroid C-cell hyperplasia and MTC with expression of calcitonin **Adrenal tumors are not found**	Mice overexpressing Cys634Arg-RET transgene in pancreas developed cystadenomas and cystadenocarcinomas
Type 2B	Proto-oncogene *RET* (10q11.2) Met918Thr mutations occur in 95% of patients	KI models with the Met918Thr mutation in human *RET* cDNA and the mouse *Ret* gene have been established	MTC Pheochromocytoma, neuromas, and ganglioneuromatosis of the gastrointestinal tract	Mice develop tumors in the sympathetic nervous tissue **except enteric nervous system** C-cell hyperplasia was noted **without development of MTC**	Gradual effect of the MEN2B *Ret* mutations on tumor development is observed in mice, none in humans
Type 4	Tumor suppressor gene *CDKN1B* (12p13) Encodes the cyclin-dependent kinase inhibitor p27kip1 Low proportion of MEN1-like patients carries *CDKN1B* mutations	*Cdkn1b*, chromosome 4 (rat) Encodes the cyclin-dependent kinase inhibitor p27Kip1	MEN1-like phenotype	Parathyroid adenomas, pancreatic islet cell hyperplasia, thyroid C-cell hyperplasia, bilateral pheochromocytomas, paragangliomas, and cataract	Gene has been identified first in a naturally occurring rat model and screened secondarily in humans

GEPNETs: gastroenteropancreatic neuroendocrine tumors; MTC: medullary thyroid carcinoma, PRL: prolactinoma.
Main differences with human diseases are shown in bold.

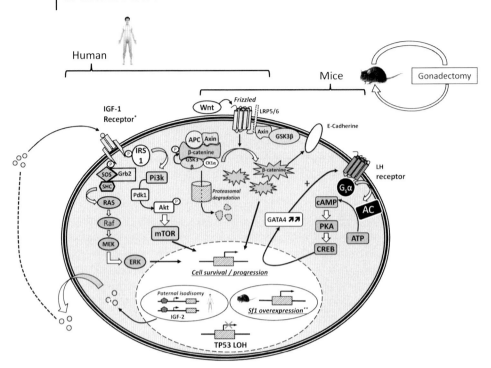

Figure 22.1 Main signaling pathways involved in adrenal tumorigenesis of humans and mice. Note that Wnt/β-catenin pathway has been identified in both humans and mice. LH-R pathway plays a critical role in malignant adrenal tumorigenesis of gonadectomized rodents, whereas the LH-R can be expressed as an illegitimate receptor in human AIMAH (ACTH-independent macronodular adrenal hyperplasia) nucleus. Colored circles define shared genetic factors of tumorigenesis between mice and humans, and empty circles are species specific. *Main effects of IGF-2 in adrenals, included in tumoral tissue, are mediated via IGF-1R. **Sf1 overexpression has been found to trigger adrenocortical tumor growth in children, whereas in adults its expression has been associated with poor prognosis.

Wnt/β-catenin and the IGF-2 pathways, two signaling cascades of transduction strongly involved in human adrenal tumorigenesis, have been investigated. However, IGF2-pathway overactivating does not seem to play a crucial role in ACC tumorigenesis of transgenic mice (Figure 22.1) [34,35]. *Ex vivo* models, namely, immunodeficient mice xenografted with human ACC line NCI-H295, are useful especially for preclinical drug testing [36], as it has been recently showed for new PI3K/mTOR dual inhibitors [37]. The efficiency of such treatments can be easily assessed on tumor (size and weight), hormonal parameters, and survival [33]. Finally, *in vitro* studies using human ACC cell lines incubated with different drugs, such as mTOR inhibitors, are precious for analyzing molecular events (apoptosis, growth arrest, and cell cycle regulation) triggered by the drug, but are unavailable in *in vivo* and *ex vivo* conditions [38].

Subcapsular tumors have been reported so far in the adrenals of various gonadectomized animals such as ferrets, guinea pigs, hamster, goats, and cats [32,39], suggesting shared mechanisms of tumorigenesis that remain partially elucidated. In gonadectomized ferrets, the incidence of adrenocortical neoplasia reaches 15–22%. Although the experimental protocol for promoting tumorigenesis might be interesting for pathophysiological studies, it remains far from reality for translational approach in humans.

Dogs also represent reliable models of ACC insofar it occurs spontaneously with a higher frequency than in humans, estimated to be about 0–2/10 000 dogs/year [32]. Clinical presentation as well as hormonal profile (excess of cortisol rather than androgens) is superimposable on human disease [32]. Moreover, canine ACC models could be of interest for genomic comparative analysis and because they can undergo treatment with o,p′-DDD like humans [32].

Benign adenomas from the adrenal cortex responsible for primary hyperaldosteronism had been reproduced either in experimental models or in genetic models. Nevertheless, observations were more relevant in terms of clinical manifestations, with similarities with human disease, than in pathophysiological conclusions [40]. Animal models of pheochromocytoma comprised mainly athymic nude mice previously injected with mouse pheochromocytoma cell line (e.g., MTT) and rats [41]. Although there are few studies in this field, they can still provide a good model to study new systemic targeted therapies in the so challenging cases of metastatic pheochromocytomas, as recently suggested [42]. Animal models with mutations in the succinate dehydrogenase (SDH) genes, known to predispose to familial pheochromocytoma/paraganglioma syndrome, are lacking. However, previous data support the idea that such models suffer rather from severe and lethal morphological abnormalities than enterochromaffin cell tumors [43].

22.3.3
Thyroid Tumorigenesis

Animal models in thyroid cancer have been mainly developed to improve the understanding of molecular events promoting tumorigenesis. Mutations in *RET*, which predispose to MTC, could presumably elicit emergence of sporadic papillary forms of thyroid cancer as well. Thus, fusion of *RET* (by intrachromosomal rearrangement) in its tyrosine kinase domain to other sequences of protein has been previously described and leads to unregulated activity of the tyrosine kinase domain. These new fusion genes are designated as *RET-PTC* genes. Transgenic mice, expressing *RET-PTC* isoforms, developed thyroid neoplasias, providing good models to investigate the oncogenic activity of the *RET* receptor as well as the molecular pathways involved in the tumorigenesis process. Similarly, mutations in the B-type RAF kinase (BRAF), already known as a critical molecular event of thyroid cancer development in humans, lead to similar phenotype in adult bred mice [44], whereas STAT3 has been recently identified as a pivotal negative regulator of thyroid tumorigenesis in mice [45]. Finally, new targeted therapies

(BRAF and Src inhibitors) have been tested successfully in mice models of human refractory thyroid cancer or anaplastic carcinoma [46,47].

22.3.4
Pituitary Tumorigenesis

In 1982, a pioneer study showed for the first time that subcutaneous transplantation of ACTH-secreting mouse cell lines (AtT-20) in athymic nude mice led to morphological changes roughly similar to those observed in human Cushing's disease [48], paving the way for development of supplemental *ex vivo* models. Recently, a study conducted by Dai *et al.* underlined the complementary approach of *in vitro* and *ex vivo* experimental conditions, using both pituitary adenoma cell line cultures and xenografted-female nude mice, for testing mTOR inhibitors and temozolomide combination effects [49]. Although pituitary cell lines obtained from animals, such as rat somatolactotroph GH4C1 cell line, are essential for studying molecular events and canonical signaling pathways involved in pituitary tumorigenesis [50], *in vivo* models are of interest for testing candidate gene, supposed to promote pituitary tumor formation (Table 22.3). Thus, transfer of the human pituitary tumor transforming gene 1 (PTTG-1), known to be highly expressed in human aggressive pituitary tumors, leads to pituitary focal hyperplasia in mouse [51]. Recently, it appeared that germline mutations in the gene *AIP* (aryl hydrocarbon interacting protein) led to familial isolated pituitary adenoma (FIPA) predisposition in humans, mainly somatotropinomas [52]. Whereas homozygous *Aip* loss in mouse ($Aip^{-/-}$) and attenuated expression of the gene led, respectively, to embryonic lethality (by congenital cardiovascular abnormalities) and patent ductus venosus (with reduced liver size), $Aip^{+/-}$ mice developed, like humans, pituitary adenomas with a predominance of GH adenomas. However, these pituitary tumors do not arise before adulthood, whereas they essentially affect children or young patients in humans. Moreover, the penetrance of the disease, incomplete in humans, reaches ~100% in 15-month-old $Aip^{+/-}$ mice [52].

Another strong difference between humans and mice has been highlighted in the yield of pituitary tumorigenesis: whereas somatic mutations in the *gsp* oncogene, responsible for permanent and unregulated activation of the cAMP pathway within pituitary cells, occurred in 30–40% of patients with GH pituitary adenomas, similar molecular abnormalities only led to pituitary hyperplasia in mice models, hyperplasia never or rarely present in human pituitary adenomas [53].

In transgenic mice, overexpression of *HMGA2* (high mobility group A protein type 2), whose protein product acts usually as a transcriptional regulator of cell cycle, has been associated with a higher occurrence of pituitary adenomas (somatotropinomas and prolactinomas) [54]. Interestingly, a translational approach recently identifies *HMGA2* overexpression as a critical event of GH and PRL pituitary adenomas also in humans [55]. Moreover, HMGA2 abundance seems to be correlated with pituitary adenoma size and proliferation markers in humans, and therefore might be used as a prognosis marker for relapse [56].

For a better understanding of tumor behavior and response to usual treatment, functional studies have been conducted in animals. In canine Cushing's disease

Table 22.3 Main genetic abnormalities identified in human pituitary tumorigenesis.

Gene (human/mouse)	Function	Genetic event(s)	Associated PA features	
			Humans	Mice
Sporadic PA				
RB1/Rb1	Tumor suppressor	Underexpression (PM) or LOH	Invasive pituitary tumors	$Rb1^{+/-}$ mice develop pituitary tumors of the intermediate lobe (age: 12 months)
GADD45/–	Tumor suppressor	Underexpression (PM ≈ 80% cases)	NFPA, PRL, and GH adenomas	Overexpression of GADD45β in LβT2 mouse gonadotrope cells blocked tumor cell proliferation
Cyclin D1 (CCND1)	Oncogene	Overexpression/allelic imbalance	70% of NFPAs and 40% of GH adenomas Aggressive PA	No specific model
GNAS (gsp)	Oncogene	Activating mutations (constitutive activity)	40% of GH adenomas McCune–Albright syndrome	No specific model
HMGA2	Oncogene	Overexpression	PRL and GH adenomas Prognostic marker?	KI models develop GH- and PRL-secreting PA
Pdt-FGFR4	Oncogene	Overexpression	Various PA Invasive growth	90% of transgenic mice developed pituitary tumors by the age of 11 months
PTTG/Pttg1	Oncogene	Overexpression	Various PA Invasive growth	KI models develop pituitary hyperplasia and adenoma formation
Familial PA predisposition (germline mutations)				
MEN1/Men1	Tumor suppressor	Inactivating mutations	Prolactinomas 20% of MEN1	$Men1^{+/-}$: PA in ≈35% cases Conditional KO leads to prolactinoma
AIP/Aip	Tumor suppressor	Inactivating mutations	Isolated GH adenomas in young patients Incomplete penetrance	$Aip^{+/-}$: GH-secreting PA in adult Complete penetrance
PRKAR1A/Prkar1a	Tumor suppressor	Inactivating mutations	GH adenomas or hyperplasia 10% of patients with Carney complex	$Prkar1a^{+/-}$ mice do not present CNC features Conditional KO leads to GH hyperplasia without PA
CDKN1B (p27^{Kip1})/Cdkn1b	CDK inhibitor	Inactivating mutations	MEN1-like phenotype (MEN4) ≈3% of MEN1-negative patient	Cdkn1b mutated rats develop spontaneously PRL (MENX)

When available, the phenotype of corresponding mice model is mentioned. PA: pituitary adenoma(s); PM: promoter methylation; NFPA: nonfunctioning pituitary adenomas.

(CDD), de Bruin *et al.* showed notable difference compared with humans concerning the somatostatin receptor subtype (sst) expression profile. Sst2 was predominant in CCD tissue, with a significant suppression of ACTH release obtained under treatment by the sst2 analog, octreotide [57]. Conversely, sst5 is the predominant subtype in human corticotroph adenoma cells, whereas sst2 is almost unexpressed [58]. Therefore, therapeutic effects obtained with somatostatin analogs in CDD cannot be extrapolated in humans.

In genetically engineered zebrafish that develop corticotroph tumors, cyclin E upregulation and G1/S phase disruption have been observed like in humans [59]. It is noteworthy that cyclin E expression is preferentially upregulated in human corticotroph adenomas compared with tumors arising from other lineages [60]. Both zebrafish and mouse have been subsequently treated with a pharmacological CDK2/cyclin E inhibitor ((R)-roscovitine), resulting in an interesting antiproliferative effect [59]. This drug is currently undergoing clinical trials for several malignancies and its use, regarding relatively mild side effects, might be of interest in Cushing's disease but requires further investigations.

Besides the transgenic mice or spontaneous model, pituitary xenografts have been used by several research teams across the world. Our team successfully used xenograft mouse models of acromegaly, obtained after transplantation of murine

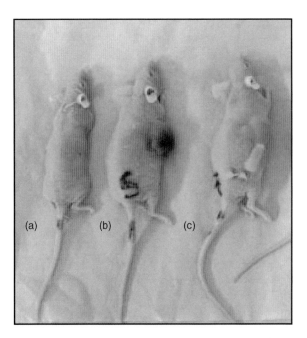

Figure 22.2 Experimentally induced mice models of acromegaly, by subcutaneous xenograft transplantation of GH4C1 murine somatolactotroph cell lines. Note the size differences between the normal nude mouse (a) and nude mouse developing a somatotroph xenograft without treatment (b) and with somatostatin analog treatment (octreotide) delivered by micropump (c).

22.4
Animal Models in Endocrine Physiology: Organogenesis, Reproduction, and Metabolism

22.4.1
Pituitary Development Disorders: Lessons from Animal Models

Several transcription factors involved in the embryological development of the murine pituitary also appear to play a role in human pituitary organogenesis, suggesting that the pituitary development is roughly similar between vertebrates [61]. The Snell dwarf and Jackson dwarf mice, mutated in *Pou1f1* (previously known as *Pit1*), allowed to identify the gene involved in combined pituitary hormone deficiency (CPHD) human phenotypes [62]. Similarly, the description of Ames dwarf (df) mice that spontaneously carry *Prop1* mutations led to identify *PROP1* gene mutations in humans with deficiencies in GH, TSH, and PRL pituitary axis [63]. Thus, there is a remarkable overlap between mouse and human phenotypes in most aspects of pituitary disorders [61], with a correspondence that remains nevertheless imperfect. Indeed, mutations in *Prop1* also lead to a corticotroph deficiency in humans, but not in mice [64]. Similarly, *LHX4* mutations in humans lead to hormonal deficiencies that remain viable with a mechanism of haploinsufficiency [65], whereas mutations in *Lhx4* have been associated with perinatal lethality and a recessive transmission pattern in mice (Figure 22.3). The differences observed between animal and human phenotypes may be the result of species differences in temporal or spatial expression, or different phenotypic manifestations of the same genetic defect due to the influence of other genes that have functional variant alleles segregating in the population [66]. Studying pituitary ontogenesis in mice has been considerably facilitated by targeted disruption of *Sox2*, *Sox3*, *Lhx2*, *Lhx3*, *Lhx4*, and *Tpit*, thanks to molecular biological mutagenesis [61]. Despite undeniable progress, the spectrum of hormone deficiencies is specific of each species and a majority of CPHDs in humans are still unexplained.

In pituitary, the complex genetic background of idiopathic hypogonadotropic hypogonadism (IHH) is still under investigation. In 2003, the *GPR54* gene was identified in both mice and humans as a key gatekeeper of puberty and reproductive function [67]. Several genes involved in differentiation, migration, and function of gonadotroph neurons are still known as putative causes of IHH (Table 22.4) [68].

With a prevalence of 0.2% in the male population, Klinefelter syndrome (KS) is the most common chromosomal disorder causing male infertility. A similar spontaneous karyotype has been described in various species such as cat, bull, and shrew. All of them share symptomatic features that, to a certain extent,

(a)

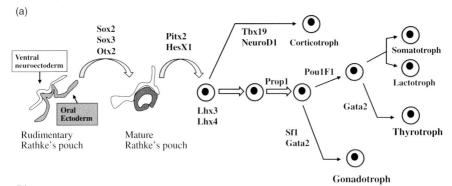

Gene	Human phenotype	Mice phenotype (loss of function)	Inheritance
Responsible for CPHD			
PROP1	GH, LH, FSH, TSH, PRL, and possibly ACTH. Progressive installation. AP size variable	Reduction of GH, LH, FSH, TSH, PRL, ACTH cell populations. Hypoplasia of AP	Recessive in humans and mice
POU1F1	GH, TSH, and PRL deficiencies (severe). Small or normal AP	Reduction of GH, TSH, and PRL cell populations. AP hypoplasia	Recessive/dominant in humans, recessive in mice
PITX2	Rieger syndrome	Homozygous: severe pituitary hypoplasia and lethality. Reduced function: thyrotroph function impairement	Haploinsufficient in humans / uncertain in mice
TBX19	Isolated severe ACTH deficiency with neonatal onset	Severe ACTH and glucocorticoid deficiencies. Adrenal hypoplasia and pigmentation defects	Recessive
Responsible for specific syndrome			
SOX2	LH and FSH deficiencies. Eyes and corpus callosum malformation, esophagal atresia, learning difficulties	Homozygous: embryonic lethality. Heterozygous: poor growth, reduction of all AP cell types, eyes and CNS abnormalities	*De novo* with haploinsufficiency in human. Heterozygous mutation with haploinsufficiency in mice
SOX3	CPHD or IGHD, mental retardation, ectopic posterior pituitary, midline abnormalities. Infundibular hypoplasia	Agenesis of corpus callosum, craniofacial, hypothalamic, and infundibular abnormalities	X-linked recessive in both mice and humans
OTX2	Severe ocular malformations ±CPHD. Hypoplastic AP and ectopic posterior pituitary	Lack of forebrain and midbrain, olfactory and optic placodes	Heterozygous: haploinsufficiency / dominant negative
LHX3	CPHD (GH, TSH, LH/FSH ± ACTH deficiencies). Hypoplasia of AP, short and rigid cervical spine. Sensorineural deafness	Hypoplasia of Rathke's pouch	Recessive in humans and mice
LHX4	CPHD (GH, TSH ± ACTH deficiencies). Cerebellar and skull defects. Hypoplasia of AP and ectopic posterior pituitary	Mild hypoplasia of AP	Dominant in humans / recessive in mice
GLI2	Holoprosencephaly, central incisor, cleft lip, polydactyly. ±CPHD and ectopic posterior pituitary	NA	Haploinsufficiency

Figure 22.3 (a) Schematic embryological steps of pituitary cell development and differentiation in humans. Critical genes involved at each step are mentioned beside the arrow. (b): Summary of genes involved in isolated or combined pituitary hormone deficiencies with phenotypic differences between humans and mice.

Table 22.4 Genetic basis of idiopathic hypogonadotropic hypogonadism with main mechanisms of the defect.

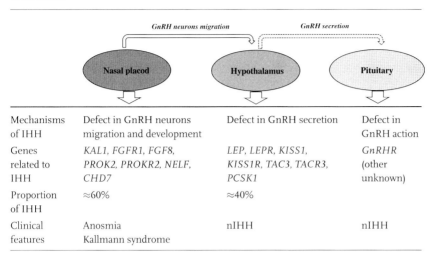

Mechanisms of IHH	Defect in GnRH neurons migration and development	Defect in GnRH secretion	Defect in GnRH action
Genes related to IHH	KAL1, FGFR1, FGF8, PROK2, PROKR2, NELF, CHD7	LEP, LEPR, KISS1, KISS1R, TAC3, TACR3, PCSK1	GnRHR (other unknown)
Proportion of IHH	≈60%	≈40%	
Clinical features	Anosmia Kallmann syndrome	nIHH	nIHH

resemble the aspects of human KS. A correlation between the disturbed karyotype and the early onset of testicular cancer has been suggested even in dogs [69]. To date, two mice models of Klinefelter syndrome, that is, with a supernumerary X chromosome, are available, providing the most reliable model to investigate the human KS [69].

With rodents, the zebrafish also offers new insights into the pituitary physiology because players of endocrine systems previously identified in mammalian systems are conserved in zebrafish [70].

22.4.2
Animal Models and Reproductive Function

Among reproductive disorders, PCOS is the most frequent female endocrine disorder. A range of animal models, including rodents, sheep, and nonhuman primates, have been used to study the origin and pathology of the disease. Prenatal exposure of sheep [71] and nonhuman primates [72] to androgens has provided good models with striking similarities to women with PCOS. Pratically, their utilisation is strongly limited by their very expansive cost. Rodents emerged as reliable *in vivo* models, especially to study clinical and hormonal features of the disease (Table 22.5) [73]. In a complementary manner, a kind of *ex vivo* model – chick eggs grafted with ovarian tissue – provided deepest information about the role of testosterone in early folliculogenesis and its relevance to human PCOS [74].

At present, a convincing whole-animal model regrouping all features associated with human PCOS is still lacking.

In the same direction, a direct role for androgen receptor (AR)-mediated androgen actions has been confirmed by AR–KO mice models [75]. In males, AR–

Table 22.5 Summary of three kinds of experimentally induced rodent models for human polycystic ovary syndrome.

		Similarities with human PCOS — Advantages of the model	Discrepancies with human PCOS — Limitations of the models
Hormonally induced PCOS	Androgen exposure[a] (pre/postnatal)	1. Models exhibit acyclicity and anovulation 2. Polycystic ovaries, hyperandrogenism, and insulin resistance 3. Elevated levels of LH 4. Strong evidences for prenatal exposure to DHT and postnatal exposure to T and TP	1. Development of PCOS phenotype is highly dependent on the period of exposition 2. Risk of vaginal fusion with prenatal exposure 3. Variability in disrupted ovulation phenotype 4. Variability of LH serum levels dependent on the model 5. Decrease in ovary weight
	Estrogen exposure[b]	1. Acyclicity, anovulation, and ovarian atrophy 2. Polycystic ovaries could be observed with metabolic features of PCOS	1. Ovary weight and LH levels decrease 2. Lack of metabolic features
	Aromatase inhibitors	1. Acyclicity, irregular estrous cycles, and anovulation 2. Ovaries with features of PCOS (see above) 3. Increased body weight 4. Elevated levels of LH and T	1. Lack of studies 2. Reduction of E2 observed with the model may interfere with ovaries function
	Antiprogestins (RU486)	1. Acyclicity, irregular estrous cycles, and anovulation 2. Polycystic ovaries with features of PCOS 3. Serum LH, T, and E2 levels increased	1. No metabolic features of PCOS 2. Effect of the drug unknown in mice
Physiologically induced PCOS	Excess of light exposure	1. Chronic anovulation and acyclicity 2. Smaller polycystic ovaries 3. No reduction of E2 activity as observed with hormone inducers	1. LH levels unchanged 2. Androgen levels unknown

Genetically induced PCOS	Leptin mutant rodent strains: Leptin-deficient (*ob/ob*) Leptin receptor-deficient (*db/db*) New Zealand obese mouse (*NZO*) JCR:LA-cp corpulent rat (*cp/cp*)	1. Infertility, acyclicity, and anovulation 2. Increased serum T, E2, and P levels (*ob/ob* and *db/db*) 3. Metabolic features of PCOS: glucose intolerance, hyperinsulinism, and obesity	1. Absence of polycystic ovaries (*ob/ob*, *db/db*, and *NZO* models) 2. LH serum levels unchanged (*ob/ob*) or reduced (*db/db*) 3. Unchanged T levels (*NZO*) 4. Ovaries reduced in weight (*cp/cp*)
	Transgenic mice for LH gene	1. Infertility and anovulation 2. Polycystic ovaries 3. Elevated E2 and T levels 4. Metabolic alterations: obesity, increased abdominal fat, and hyperinsulinism	1. Development of ovarian tumors and enlarged ovaries
	Transgenic mice for plasminogen activator inhibitor 1	1. Evident hyperandrogenism with significant elevated T levels 2. Ovaries with morphological features of PCOS	1. No assessment of metabolic features 2. Hormonal profile needs to be further investigated

Limitations and advantages of each model are mentioned regarding the mimicking of the disease and/or intrinsic limitations of the model.
a) Androgens used: testosterone (T), testosterone propionate (TP), and dihydrotestosterone (DHT).
b) E2 is abbreviation for 17β-estradiol.

KO models provided relevant information about the control of male fertility by androgens and paved the way for new therapeutic strategies in male fertility. In females, AR–KO models clarified the physiological implications of androgens in follicle maturation and growth but also increased the degree of complexity in reproductive function.

22.4.3
Animal Models Used in Calcium Homeostasis Studies

Mice models mimicking pathologies of the calcium receptor (CaSr) have been generated to study the human CaSr gain-of-function familial hypocalciuric hypercalcemia and neonatal severe primary hyperparathyroidism (NHSPT) syndromes. Conversely, loss-of-function CaSr mutations lead to the autosomal dominant hypocalcemia with hypercalciuria (ADHH) syndrome. These models are reliable especially to analyze the direct metabolic consequences of hyperparathyroidism *in vivo*.

The DiGeorge syndrome (DGS), an inherited form of hypoparathyroidism, is related to mutations in the transcription factor *TBX1*, and mice models heterozygous for *Tbx1* showed only partial correlation with the human disease, but exhibited other morphological abnormalities relevant to the role of *Tbx1* in organogenesis [76]. Similarly, hypoparathyroidism, sensorineural deafness, and renal dysplasia (HDR) syndrome is another form of inherited hypoparathyroidism with severe hypocalcemia, due to GATA3 haploinsufficiency [77]. This situation is in contrast to that in heterozygous Gata3-KO ($Gata3^{-/+}$) mice, where no abnormalities associated with the HDR phenotype have been reported so far [78].

To conclude on phosphocalcic metabolism, the pleiotropic effects of vitamin D on immune system of cattle have been recently reviewed. The authors suggested that the bovine model may be useful for understanding vitamin D requirements in humans [79].

22.5
Translation to Clinics: Limitations and Difficulties

Endocrine disorders represent a heterogeneous group of diseases whose pathophysiology and clinical outcomes in humans are still imperfectly known. Animal models have been successfully developed in this field because of strong similarities to human endocrine glands in terms of physiological functions, anatomic properties, embryological development, and pattern of secretion. As already mentioned, pituitary ontogenesis in humans and related disorders such as pituitary deficiency(ies) have been considerably understood, thanks to mice models that display steps of pituitary development quite similar to those in humans. Spontaneous or genetically induced mice models of pituitary deficiency led to the identification of similar genetic background in human corresponding diseases. Moreover, most of the physiological events governed by endocrine systems in animal physiology (growth and reproductive function) imply, more or less, the same ortholog hormones as in humans. It is, therefore, not surprising to find spontaneous endocrine diseases in animals quite similar to those observed in humans, such as Grave's disease in mice or Cushing's disease in dogs. Based on these observations, hormonal therapies issued from animals have been developed with success to treat human hormonal deficiencies. Finally, as in other fields of physiology, the main advantage of animal models over *ex vivo* conditions lies in organism integrity, representing further a model of the whole disease. Taken together, these models may actually appear as perfect *in vivo* models for endocrine diseases. This is, however, not the case at different degrees. Indeed, although patterns of hormonal secretion can be sometimes superimposable in animals and humans, any minute difference may be accompanied by significant differences in hormonal homeostasis in each species. This fine regulation all along the life characterizes the specificity and complexity of endocrine system in each species and should, therefore, carefully extrapolate data from animals to humans. In pituitary, hormonal secretion, such as prolactin in zebrafish, does not share the same circadian rhythm in animals and humans. In parallel, differences exist also in the presentation of endocrine diseases. Although engineered mice suffering from GD usually display features similar to those of human GD, most of them do not exhibit Grave's orbitopathy, which is, in humans, one of the most important issues of the disease. Previous data demonstrated that mice exhibit much more open bony orbit than humans, hampering the local cytokine accumulation responsible for retro-orbital inflammation. Similarly, as it has been discussed in the text for MEN syndromes and pituitary deficiencies, phenotypes can present differently between mice and humans despite a similar genetic defect. It suggests the crucial role of environment and epigenetic phenomena in each species, which should be taken into consideration for translational analysis. In a same pathological condition, differences may also exist between animals and humans at the cellular level. For instance, it has been noted for somatostatin receptor expression in corticotroph cells of dogs and human, underlining the limitations of pharmacological studies in animals for a translational approach in humans. This also suggests that for molecular investigations, human cellular models, mimicking more reliably the molecular aspects of the disease, are strongly required.

In conclusion, complementary to *in vitro* cell cultures and *ex vivo* conditions, which are essential for functional and molecular investigations, animal models provide reliable *in vivo* conditions to enrich the possibility of disease investigations in a complementary way. Although similar features are often noted, animal models remain nevertheless an imperfect approach to mimic human diseases. They have to be used in parallel to human *in vitro* or *ex vivo* studies. The conclusions of these preclinical studies have to be considered with precaution until human clinical studies are performed.

References

1 Mouse Genome Sequencing Consortium (2002) Initial sequencing and comparative analysis of the mouse genome. *Nature*, **420** (6915), 520–569.

2 Piret, S.E. and Thakker, R.V. (2011) Mouse models for inherited endocrine and metabolic disorders. *The Journal of Endocrinology*, **211** (3), 211–230.

3 Anderson, M.S. (2008) Update in endocrine autoimmunity. *The Journal of Clinical Endocrinology and Metabolism*, **93** (10), 3663–3670.

4 Lam-Tse, W.K., Lernmark, A., and Drexhage, H.A. (2002) Animal models of endocrine/ organ-specific autoimmune diseases: do they really help us to understand human autoimmunity? *Springer Seminars in Immunopathology*, **24** (3), 297–321.

5 Mestas, J. and Hughes, C.C. (2004) Of mice and not men: differences between mouse and human immunology. *Journal of Immunology*, **172** (5), 2731–2738.

6 Nagayama, Y. (2007) Graves' animal models of Graves' hyperthyroidism. *Thyroid*, **17** (10), 981–988.

7 Baker, G., Mazziotti, G., von Ruhland, C., and Ludgate, M. (2005) Reevaluating thyrotropin receptor-induced mouse models

of Graves' disease and ophthalmopathy. *Endocrinology*, **146** (2), 835–844.
8 Mao, C., Wang, S., Xiao, Y., Xu, J., Jiang, Q., Jin, M., Jiang, X., Guo, H., Ning, G., and Zhang, Y. (2011) Impairment of regulatory capacity of $CD4^+CD25^+$ regulatory T cells mediated by dendritic cell polarization and hyperthyroidism in Graves' disease. *Journal of Immunology*, **186** (8), 4734–4743.
9 Pan, D., Shin, Y.H., Gopalakrishnan, G., Hennessey, J., and De Groot, L.J. (2009) Regulatory T cells in Graves' disease. *Clinical Endocrinology*, **71** (4), 587–593.
10 Banga, J.P., Nielsen, C.H., Gilbert, J.A., El Fassi, D., and Hegedus, L. (2008) Application of new therapies in Graves' disease and thyroid-associated ophthalmopathy: animal models and translation to human clinical trials. *Thyroid*, **18** (9), 973–981.
11 Dietrich, H.M., Cole, R.K., and Wick, G. (1999) The natural history of the obese strain of chickens: an animal model for spontaneous autoimmune thyroiditis. *Poultry Science*, **78** (10), 1359–1371.
12 Kawada, J., Mino, H., Nishida, M., and Yoshimura, Y. (1988) An appropriate model for congenital hypothyroidism in the rat induced by neonatal treatment with propylthiouracil and surgical thyroidectomy: studies on learning ability and biochemical parameters. *Neuroendocrinology*, **47** (5), 424–430.
13 Argumedo, G.S., Sanz, C.R., and Olguin, H.J. (2012) Experimental models of developmental hypothyroidism. *Hormone and Metabolic Research*, **44** (2), 79–85.
14 Laureti, S., Vecchi, L., Santeusanio, F., and Falorni, A. (1999) Is the prevalence of Addison's disease underestimated? *The Journal of Clinical Endocrinology and Metabolism*, **84** (5), 1762.
15 Pedersen, N.C. (1999) A review of immunologic diseases of the dog. *Veterinary Immunology and Immunopathology*, **69** (2–4), 251–342.
16 Chase, K., Sargan, D., Miller, K., Ostrander, E.A., and Lark, K.G. (2006) Understanding the genetics of autoimmune disease: two loci that regulate late onset Addison's disease in Portuguese Water Dogs. *International Journal of Immunogenetics*, **33** (3), 179–184.
17 Fujii, Y., Kato, N., Kito, J., Asai, J., and Yokochi, T. (1992) Experimental autoimmune adrenalitis: a murine model for Addison's disease. *Autoimmunity*, **12** (1), 47–52.
18 Bratland, E. and Husebye, E.S. (2011) Cellular immunity and immunopathology in autoimmune Addison's disease. *Molecular and Cellular Endocrinology*, **336** (1–2), 180–190.
19 Akirav, E.M., Ruddle, N.H., and Herold, K.C. (2011) The role of AIRE in human autoimmune disease. *Nature Reviews. Endocrinology*, **7** (1), 25–33.
20 Anderson, M.S., Venanzi, E.S., Klein, L., Chen, Z., Berzins, S.P., Turley, S.J., von Boehmer, H., Bronson, R., Dierich, A., Benoist, C., and Mathis, D. (2002) Projection of an immunological self shadow within the thymus by the aire protein. *Science*, **298** (5597), 1395–1401.
21 Pereira, L.E., Bostik, P., and Ansari, A.A. (2005) The development of mouse APECED models provides new insight into the role of AIRE in immune regulation. *Clinical and Developmental Immunology*, **12** (3), 211–216.
22 Hubert, F.X., Kinkel, S.A., Crewther, P.E., Cannon, P.Z., Webster, K.E., Link, M., Uibo, R., O'Bryan, M.K., Meager, A., Forehan, S.P., Smyth, G.K., Mittaz, L., Antonarakis, S.E., Peterson, P., Heath, W.R., and Scott, H.S. (2009) Aire-deficient C57BL/6 mice mimicking the common human 13-base pair deletion mutation present with only a mild autoimmune phenotype. *Journal of Immunology*, **182** (6), 3902–3918.
23 Thakker, R.V. (2010) Multiple endocrine neoplasia type 1 (MEN1). *Best Practice & Research. Clinical Endocrinology & Metabolism*, **24** (3), 355–370.
24 Bassett, J.H., Rashbass, P., Harding, B., Forbes, S.A., Pannett, A.A., and Thakker, R.V. (1999) Studies of the murine homolog of the multiple endocrine neoplasia type 1 (MEN1) gene, men1. *Journal of Bone and Mineral Research*, **14** (1), 3–10.
25 Harding, B., Lemos, M.C., Reed, A.A., Walls, G.V., Jeyabalan, J., Bowl, M.R., Tateossian, H., Sullivan, N., Hough, T., Fraser, W.D., Ansorge, O., Cheeseman, M.T., and Thakker, R.V. (2009) Multiple endocrine neoplasia type 1 knockout mice

develop parathyroid, pancreatic, pituitary and adrenal tumours with hypercalcaemia, hypophosphataemia and hypercorticosteronaemia. *Endocrine-Related Cancer*, **16** (4), 1313–1327.

26 Bertolino, P., Radovanovic, I., Casse, H., Aguzzi, A., Wang, Z.Q., and Zhang, C.X. (2003) Genetic ablation of the tumor suppressor menin causes lethality at mid-gestation with defects in multiple organs. *Mechanisms of Development*, **120** (5), 549–560.

27 Busygina, V., Suphapeetiporn, K., Marek, L.R., Stowers, R.S., Xu, T., and Bale, A.E. (2004) Hypermutability in a *Drosophila* model for multiple endocrine neoplasia type 1. *Human Molecular Genetics*, **13** (20), 2399–2408.

28 Capen, C.C. and Black, H.E. (1974) Animal model of human disease. Medullary thyroid carcinoma, multiple endocrine neoplasia, Sipple's syndrome. Animal model: ultimobranchial thyroid neoplasm in the bull. *The American Journal of Pathology*, **74** (2), 377–380.

29 Read, R.D., Goodfellow, P.J., Mardis, E.R., Novak, N., Armstrong, J.R., and Cagan, R.L. (2005) A *Drosophila* model of multiple endocrine neoplasia type 2. *Genetics*, **171** (3), 1057–1081.

30 Das, T. and Cagan, R. (2010) *Drosophila* as a novel therapeutic discovery tool for thyroid cancer. *Thyroid*, **20** (7), 689–695.

31 Pellegata, N.S., Quintanilla-Martinez, L., Siggelkow, H., Samson, E., Bink, K., Hofler, H., Fend, F., Graw, J., and Atkinson, M.J. (2006) Germ-line mutations in p27Kip1 cause a multiple endocrine neoplasia syndrome in rats and humans. *Proceedings of the National Academy of Sciences of the United States of America*, **103** (42), 15558–15563.

32 Beuschlein, F., Galac, S., and Wilson, D.B. (2012) Animal models of adrenocortical tumorigenesis. *Molecular and Cellular Endocrinology*, **351** (1), 78–86.

33 Hantel, C. and Beuschlein, F. (2010) Mouse models of adrenal tumorigenesis. *Best Practice & Research. Clinical Endocrinology & Metabolism*, **24** (6), 865–875.

34 Berthon, A., Sahut-Barnola, I., Lambert-Langlais, S., de Joussineau, C., Damon-Soubeyrand, C., Louiset, E., Taketo, M.M., Tissier, F., Bertherat, J., Lefrancois-Martinez, A.M., Martinez, A., and Val, P. (2010) Constitutive beta-catenin activation induces adrenal hyperplasia and promotes adrenal cancer development. *Human Molecular Genetics*, **19** (8), 1561–1576.

35 Drelon, C., Berthon, A., Ragazzon, B., Tissier, F., Bandiera, R., Sahut-Barnola, I., de Joussineau, C., Batisse-Lignier, M., Lefrancois-Martinez, A.M., Bertherat, J., Martinez, A., and Val, P. (2012) Analysis of the role of Igf2 in adrenal tumour development in transgenic mouse models. *PLoS One*, **7** (8), e44171.

36 Luconi, M. and Mannelli, M. (2012) Xenograft models for preclinical drug testing: implications for adrenocortical cancer. *Molecular and Cellular Endocrinology*, **351** (1), 71–77.

37 Doghman, M. and Lalli, E. (2012) Efficacy of the novel dual PI3-kinase/mTOR inhibitor NVP-BEZ235 in a preclinical model of adrenocortical carcinoma. *Molecular and Cellular Endocrinology*, **364** (1–2), 101–104.

38 De Martino, M.C., van Koetsveld, P.M., Feelders, R.A., Sprij-Mooij, D., Waaijers, M., Lamberts, S.W., de Herder, W.W., Colao, A., Pivonello, R., and Hofland, L.J. (2012) The role of mTOR inhibitors in the inhibition of growth and cortisol secretion in human adrenocortical carcinoma cells. *Endocrine-Related Cancer*, **19** (3), 351–364.

39 Meler, E.N., Scott-Moncrieff, J.C., Peter, A.T., Bennett, S., Ramos-Vara, J., Salisbury, S.K., and Naughton, J.F. (2011) Cyclic estrous-like behavior in a spayed cat associated with excessive sex-hormone production by an adrenocortical carcinoma. *Journal of Feline Medicine and Surgery*, **13** (6), 473–478.

40 Beuschlein, F. (2010) Animal models of primary aldosteronism. *Hormone and Metabolic Research*, **42** (6), 446–449.

41 Tischler, A.S., Powers, J.F., and Alroy, J. (2004) Animal models of pheochromocytoma. *Histology and Histopathology*, **19** (3), 883–895.

42 Pacak, K., Sirova, M., Giubellino, A., Lencesova, L., Csaderova, L., Laukova, M., Hudecova, S., and Krizanova, O. (2012) NF-kappaB inhibition significantly upregulates the norepinephrine transporter system, causes apoptosis in pheochromocytoma cell lines and prevents metastasis in an animal

model. *International Journal of Cancer*, **131** (10), 2445–2455.

43 Ishii, T., Miyazawa, M., Onouchi, H., Yasuda, K., Hartman, P.S., and Ishii, N. (2012) Model animals for the study of oxidative stress from complex II. *Biochimica et Biophysica Acta*, **1827** (5), 588–597.

44 Charles, R.P., Lezza, G., Amendola, E., Dankort, D., and McMahon, M. (2011) Mutationally activated BRAF(V600E) elicits papillary thyroid cancer in the adult mouse. *Cancer Research*, **71** (11), 3863–3871.

45 Couto, J.P., Daly, L., Almeida, A., Knauf, J.A., Fagin, J.A., Sobrinho-Simoes, M., Lima, J., Maximo, V., Soares, P., Lyden, D., and Bromberg, J.F. (2012) STAT3 negatively regulates thyroid tumorigenesis. *Proceedings of the National Academy of Sciences of the United States of America*, **109** (35), E2361–E2370.

46 Kim, W.G., Guigon, C.J., Fozzatti, L., Park, J.W., Lu, C., Willingham, M.C., and Cheng, S.Y. (2012) SKI-606, an Src inhibitor, reduces tumor growth, invasion, and distant metastasis in a mouse model of thyroid cancer. *Clinical Cancer Research*, **18** (5), 1281–1290.

47 Nehs, M.A., Nucera, C., Nagarkatti, S.S., Sadow, P.M., Morales-Garcia, D., Hodin, R.A., and Parangi, S. (2012) Late intervention with anti-BRAF(V600E) therapy induces tumor regression in an orthotopic mouse model of human anaplastic thyroid cancer. *Endocrinology*, **153** (2), 985–994.

48 Leung, C.K., Paterson, J.A., Imai, Y., and Shiu, R.P. (1982) Transplantation of ACTH-secreting pituitary tumor cells in athymic nude mice. *Virchows Archiv A: Pathological Anatomy and Histology*, **396** (3), 303–312.

49 Dai, C., Zhang, B., Liu, X., Ma, S., Yang, Y., Yao, Y., Feng, M., Bao, X., Li, G., Wang, J., Guo, K., Ma, W., Xing, B., Lian, W., Xiao, J., Cai, F., Zhang, H., and Wang, R. (2013) Inhibition of PI3K/AKT/mTOR pathway enhances temozolomide-induced cytotoxicity in pituitary adenoma cell lines *in vitro* and xenografted pituitary adenoma in female nude mice. *Endocrinology*, **154** (3), 1247–1259.

50 Cuny, T., Gerard, C., Saveanu, A., Barlier, A., and Enjalbert, A. (2011) Physiopathology of somatolactotroph cells: from transduction mechanisms to cotargeting therapy. *Annals of the New York Academy of Sciences*, **1220**, 60–70.

51 Abbud, R.A., Takumi, I., Barker, E.M., Ren, S.G., Chen, D.Y., Wawrowsky, K., and Melmed, S. (2005) Early multipotential pituitary focal hyperplasia in the alpha-subunit of glycoprotein hormone-driven pituitary tumor-transforming gene transgenic mice. *Journal of Molecular Endocrinology*, **19** (5), 1383–1391.

52 Beckers, A., Aaltonen, L.A., Daly, A.F., and Karhu, A. (2013) Familial isolated pituitary adenomas (FIPA) and the pituitary adenoma predisposition due to mutations in the aryl hydrocarbon receptor interacting protein (AIP) gene. *Endocrine Reviews*, **34** (2), 1–39.

53 Burton, F.H., Hasel, K.W., Bloom, F.E., and Sutcliffe, J.G. (1991) Pituitary hyperplasia and gigantism in mice caused by a cholera toxin transgene. *Nature*, **350** (6313), 74–77.

54 Fedele, M., Battista, S., Kenyon, L., Baldassarre, G., Fidanza, V., Klein-Szanto, A.J., Parlow, A.F., Visone, R., Pierantoni, G.M., Outwater, E., Santoro, M., Croce, C.M., and Fusco, A. (2002) Overexpression of the HMGA2 gene in transgenic mice leads to the onset of pituitary adenomas. *Oncogene*, **21** (20), 3190–3198.

55 Palmieri, D., Valentino, T., De Martino, I., Esposito, F., Cappabianca, P., Wierinckx, A., Vitiello, M., Lombardi, G., Colao, A., Trouillas, J., Pierantoni, G.M., Fusco, A., and Fedele, M. (2012) PIT1 upregulation by HMGA proteins has a role in pituitary tumorigenesis. *Endocrine-Related Cancer*, **19** (2), 123–135.

56 Fedele, M., Visone, R., De Martino, I., Troncone, G., Palmieri, D., Battista, S., Ciarmiello, A., Pallante, P., Arra, C., Melillo, R.M., Helin, K., Croce, C.M., and Fusco, A. (2006) HMGA2 induces pituitary tumorigenesis by enhancing E2F1 activity. *Cancer Cell*, **9** (6), 459–471.

57 de Bruin, C., Hanson, J.M., Meij, B.P., Kooistra, H.S., Waaijers, A.M., Uitterlinden, P., Lamberts, S.W., and Hofland, L.J. (2008) Expression and functional analysis of dopamine receptor subtype 2 and somatostatin receptor subtypes in canine

Cushing's disease. *Endocrinology*, **149** (9), 4357–4366.

58 de Bruin, C., Pereira, A.M., Feelders, R.A., Romijn, J.A., Roelfsema, F., Sprij-Mooij, D.M., van Aken, M.O., van der Lelij, A.J., de Herder, W.W., Lamberts, S.W., and Hofland, L.J. (2009) Coexpression of dopamine and somatostatin receptor subtypes in corticotroph adenomas. *The Journal of Clinical Endocrinology and Metabolism*, **94** (4), 1118–1124.

59 Liu, N.A., Jiang, H., Ben-Shlomo, A., Wawrowsky, K., Fan, X.M., Lin, S., and Melmed, S. (2011) Targeting zebrafish and murine pituitary corticotroph tumors with a cyclin-dependent kinase (CDK) inhibitor. *Proceedings of the National Academy of Sciences of the United States of America*, **108** (20), 8414–8419.

60 Jordan, S., Lidhar, K., Korbonits, M., Lowe, D.G., and Grossman, A.B. (2000) Cyclin D and cyclin E expression in normal and adenomatous pituitary. *European Journal of Endocrinology/European Federation of Endocrine Societies*, **143** (1), R1–R6.

61 Kelberman, D., Rizzoti, K., Lovell-Badge, R., Robinson, I.C., and Dattani, M.T. (2009) Genetic regulation of pituitary gland development in human and mouse. *Endocrine Reviews*, **30** (7), 790–829.

62 Li, S., Crenshaw, E.B., 3rd, Rawson, E.J., Simmons, D.M., Swanson, L.W., and Rosenfeld, M.G. (1990) Dwarf locus mutants lacking three pituitary cell types result from mutations in the POU-domain gene pit-1. *Nature*, **347** (6293), 528–533.

63 Wu, W., Cogan, J.D., Pfaffle, R.W., Dasen, J.S., Frisch, H., O'Connell, S.M., Flynn, S.E., Brown, M.R., Mullis, P.E., Parks, J.S., Phillips, J.A., 3rd, and Rosenfeld, M.G. (1998) Mutations in PROP1 cause familial combined pituitary hormone deficiency. *Nature Genetics*, **18** (2), 147–149.

64 Reynaud, R., Gueydan, M., Saveanu, A., Vallette-Kasic, S., Enjalbert, A., Brue, T., and Barlier, A. (2006) Genetic screening of combined pituitary hormone deficiency: experience in 195 patients. *The Journal of Clinical Endocrinology and Metabolism*, **91** (9), 3329–3336.

65 Castinetti, F., Saveanu, A., Reynaud, R., Quentien, M.H., Buffin, A., Brauner, R., Kaffel, N., Albarel, F., Guedj, A.M., El Kholy, M., Amin, M., Enjalbert, S.A., Barlier, A., and Brue, T. (2008) A novel dysfunctional LHX4 mutation with high phenotypical variability in patients with hypopituitarism. *The Journal of Clinical Endocrinology and Metabolism*, **93** (7), 2790–2799.

66 Davis, S.W., Castinetti, F., Carvalho, L.R., Ellsworth, B.S., Potok, M.A., Lyons, R.H., Brinkmeier, M.L., Raetzman, L.T., Carninci, P., Mortensen, A.H., Hayashizaki, Y., Arnhold, I.J., Mendonca, B.B., Brue, T., and Camper, S.A. (2010) Molecular mechanisms of pituitary organogenesis: in search of novel regulatory genes. *Molecular and Cellular Endocrinology*, **323** (1), 4–19.

67 Seminara, S.B., Messager, S., Chatzidaki, E.E., Thresher, R.R., Acierno, J.S., Jr., Shagoury, J.K., Bo-Abbas, Y., Kuohung, W., Schwinof, K.M., Hendrick, A.G., Zahn, D., Dixon, J., Kaiser, U.B., Slaugenhaupt, S.A., Gusella, J.F., O'Rahilly, S., Carlton, M.B., Crowley, W.F., Jr., Aparicio, S.A., and Colledge, W.H. (2003) The GPR54 gene as a regulator of puberty. *The New England Journal of Medicine*, **349** (17), 1614–1627.

68 Han, T.S. and Bouloux, P.M. (2012) Kallmann syndrome and other causes of hypothalamic hypogonadism and related development disorders, in *Handbook of Neuroendocrinology*, Elsevier Ltd., pp. 597–617.

69 Wistuba, J. (2010) Animal models for Klinefelter's syndrome and their relevance for the clinic. *Molecular Human Reproduction*, **16** (6), 375–385.

70 Lohr, H. and Hammerschmidt, M. (2011) Zebrafish in endocrine systems: recent advances and implications for human disease. *Annual Review of Physiology*, **73**, 183–211.

71 Padmanabhan, V. and Veiga-Lopez, A. (2012) Sheep models of polycystic ovary syndrome phenotype. *Molecular and Cellular Endocrinology*, **373** (1–2), 8–20.

72 Abbott, D.H., Dumesic, D.A., Eisner, J.R., Colman, R.J., and Kemnitz, J.W. (1998) Insights into the development of polycystic ovary syndrome (PCOS) from studies of prenatally androgenized female rhesus monkeys. *Trends in Endocrinology and Metabolism*, **9** (2), 62–67.

73 Walters, K.A., Allan, C.M., and Handelsman, D.J. (2012) Rodent models for

human polycystic ovary syndrome. *Biology of Reproduction*, **86** (5), 149, 1–12.

74 Qureshi, A.I., Nussey, S.S., Bano, G., Musonda, P., Whitehead, S.A., and Mason, H.D. (2008) Testosterone selectively increases primary follicles in ovarian cortex grafted onto embryonic chick membranes: relevance to polycystic ovaries. *Reproduction*, **136** (2), 187–194.

75 Walters, K.A., Simanainen, U., and Handelsman, D.J. (2010) Molecular insights into androgen actions in male and female reproductive function from androgen receptor knockout models. *Human Reproduction Update*, **16** (5), 543–558.

76 Garfield, N. and Karaplis, A.C. (2001) Genetics and animal models of hypoparathyroidism. *Trends in Endocrinology and Metabolism*, **12** (7), 288–294.

77 Van Esch, H., Groenen, P., Nesbit, M.A., Schuffenhauer, S., Lichtner, P., Vanderlinden, G., Harding, B., Beetz, R., Bilous, R.W., Holdaway, I., Shaw, N.J., Fryns, J.P., Van de Ven, W., Thakker, R.V., and Devriendt, K. (2000) GATA3 haplo-insufficiency causes human HDR syndrome. *Nature*, **406** (6794), 419–422.

78 Pandolfi, P.P., Roth, M.E., Karis, A., Leonard, M.W., Dzierzak, E., Grosveld, F. G., Engel, J.D., and Lindenbaum, M.H. (1995) Targeted disruption of the GATA3 gene causes severe abnormalities in the nervous system and in fetal liver haematopoiesis. *Nature Genetics*, **11** (1), 40–44.

79 Nelson, C.D., Reinhardt, T.A., Lippolis, J.D., Sacco, R.E., and Nonnecke, B.J. (2012) Vitamin D signaling in the bovine immune system: a model for understanding human vitamin D requirements. *Nutrients*, **4** (3), 181–196.

23
Gastrointestinal Disorders: A Patho-biotechnology Approach to Probiotic Therapy
Roy D. Sleator

23.1
Introduction

Probiotics are commensal organisms that can be harnessed for therapeutic or prophylactic benefit [1], usually exerting their effects by modulating normal microbe–microbe and host–microbe interactions. In acute infections, probiotics may boost the protection afforded by commensal flora through competitive interactions, direct antagonism of pathogens, and/or production of antimicrobial factors [2]. In other clinical conditions, such as chronic infections and immunosuppression, microbe–host signaling is probably more relevant to effective probiotic action. Gut homeostasis, the maintenance of a "balanced" and beneficial flora, requires continual signaling from bacteria within the gut lumen, maintaining the mucosal barrier while at the same time priming the gut for responses to injury [3]. Given these health promoting benefits, improving probiotic stress tolerance and ability to grow and survive in foods prior to ingestion and subsequently within the animal host is an important biological and clinical goal. This is particularly relevant given that many potentially beneficial probiotics often prove to be physiologically fragile – a significant limitation in clinical applications [4].

The patho-biotechnology concept, defined as the exploitation of pathogen-derived stress survival strategies for beneficial applications in food and biomedicine [5–7], seeks to attain this goal. A primary focus of this approach involves equipping nonpathogenic or probiotic bacteria with the genetic elements necessary to overcome the many stresses encountered during the probiotic life cycle (both external and internal to the host) as well as enabling probiotics to better deal with invading pathogens [8,9].

This strategy can be divided into three distinct approaches (Figure 23.1): the first tackles the issue of probiotic storage and delivery. Providing sensitive probiotic strains with pathogen-derived stress survival mechanisms, such as the ability to accumulate compatible solutes (which improve survival at extreme temperatures and water availability), helps counter reductions in viability experienced during manufacture and storage of delivery matrices (food or tablet formulations). The second approach aims to improve host colonization by expression of host-specific

In Vivo Models for Drug Discovery, First Edition. Edited by José M. Vela, Rafael Maldonado, and Michel Hamon.
© 2014 Wiley-VCH Verlag GmbH & Co. KGaA. Published 2014 by Wiley-VCH Verlag GmbH & Co. KGaA.

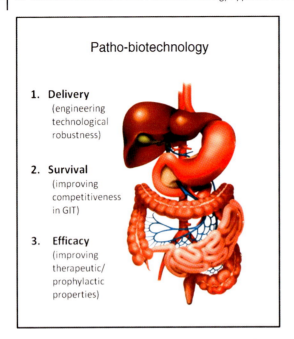

Figure 23.1 The patho-biotechnology concept involves three approaches to generating improved probiotic cultures.

survival strategies (or virulence-associated factors such as the ability to cope with bile – an important part of the physicochemical defense system of the body), thereby positively affecting the efficacy of the probiotic. The final approach involves the development of the so-called designer probiotics – strains that specifically target invading pathogens by blocking crucial ligand–receptor interactions between the pathogen and host cell [10].

23.2
Delivery: Improving Probiotic Resistance to Process-Induced Stresses and Storage Conditions

The most common stresses encountered during production of probiotic delivery matrices (food and/or tablet formulations) are temperature and water availability (a_w) [11]. The ability to cope with such stresses is a particularly desirable trait in the selection of commercially viable probiotic strains. A common strategy employed by a variety of microbes to deal with both low a_w and temperature stress is the accumulation of protective compounds such as betaine, carnitine, and proline. These compatible solutes help to stabilize protein structure and function at low temperatures while preventing water loss from the cell and plasmolysis under low a_w conditions [12].

Improving a strain's ability to accumulate compatible solutes is thus an obvious first step in the development of more robust probiotic strains. Bacteria have evolved sophisticated mechanisms for compatible solute accumulation, including both uptake and synthesis systems [12]. Indeed, the foodborne pathogen *Listeria monocytogenes* (probably the best-studied pathogen in terms of compatible solute accumulation) [13] possesses three distinct uptake systems (BetL, Gbu, and OpuC) and at least one compatible solute synthesis system (ProBA). By placing the *betL* gene (encoding the secondary betaine uptake system BetL) [14] under the transcriptional control of the nisin-inducible promoter P*nisA*, it was possible to assess the role of BetL (and thus betaine accumulation) in contributing to probiotic growth and survival under a variety of stresses likely encountered during food and/or tablet manufacture [8]. Our probiotic of choice, *Lactobacillus salivarius* UCC118, exhibits significantly lower accumulation levels than *L. monocytogenes* and is correspondingly less physiologically robust than the pathogen. As expected, the *betL*-complemented *L. salivarius* strain showed a significant increase in betaine accumulation compared with the wild type (Figure 23.2a). Indeed, sufficient BetL was produced to confer increased salt tolerance, with growth of the transformed strain at significantly higher salt concentrations (7% NaCl) than the parent (Figure 23.2b). In addition to increased osmotolerance, the BetL$^+$ strain showed significantly improved resistance to both chill and cryotolerance (2 logs greater survival than the control at $-20\,°C$ and 0.5 logs greater survival at $-70\,°C$) as well as freeze drying (36% survival compared with 18% for the control strain) and spray drying (1.4% compared with 0.3%) – common stresses encountered during food and/or tablet formulation [8]. Furthermore, the presence of BetL resulted in a significant improvement in barotolerance. This is particularly significant, given that high-pressure processing is gaining increasing popularity as a novel nonthermal mechanism of food processing and preservation [15,16].

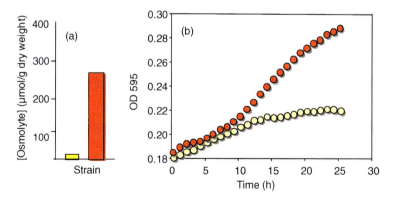

Figure 23.2 (a) [^{14}C]Glycine betaine uptake rates in *L. salivarius* UCC118-BetL$^+$ (yellow bar) and UCC118-BetL$^-$ (red bar). (b) Growth of *L. salivarius* UCC118-BetL$^+$ (red) and UCC118-BetL$^-$ (yellow) in MRS with 7% added NaCl. (Adapted from Ref. [8].)

Thus, improving probiotic stress tolerance significantly improves resistance to stresses encountered during product processing, as well as prolongs survival during subsequent storage.

23.3
Survival: Improving Probiotic–Host Colonization

Besides fighting stresses encountered during processing and storage, probiotic bacteria must also overcome the physiochemical defenses of the host in order to reach the gastrointestinal tract in sufficient numbers to exert a beneficial effect. Recently, we demonstrated that BetL significantly improved the tolerance of the probiotic strain *Bifidobacterium breve* UCC2003 to gastric juice [9]. Interestingly, in support of this observation, Termont *et al.* [17] also reported similar results for a *Lactococcus lactis* strain expressing the *Escherichia coli* trehalose synthesis genes, thus suggesting a novel protective role for compatible solutes in the gastric environment. Furthermore, in line with our previous observations with *L. salivarius* UCC118 [8], a significant osmoprotective effect was observed following the introduction of *betL* into *B. breve*, allowing significantly improved growth of the probiotic in conditions similar to those encountered *in vivo* (1.5% NaCl, equivalent to the osmolarity of the gut). In addition, *B. breve* strains expressing BetL were recovered at significantly higher levels than the wild type in the feces, intestines, and cecum of inoculated animals. Finally, in addition to improved gastric transit and intestinal persistence, the addition of BetL improved the clinical efficacy of the probiotic culture; mice fed *B. breve* UCC2003 (BetL$^+$) exhibited significantly lower levels of systemic infection compared with the control strain following oral inoculation with *L. monocytogenes*. This is, to the best of our knowledge, the first clear evidence of an enhanced prophylactic effect following precise bioengineering of a probiotic strain.

23.4
Efficacy: "Designer Probiotics"

In addition to improving probiotic stress tolerance, recent studies have led to the development of "designer probiotics." Expressing receptor-mimic structures on their surface [10,18–20], these genetically engineered strains specifically target enteric infections by blocking crucial ligand–receptor interactions between the pathogen and host cell [10]. Many of the pathogens responsible for the major enteric infections exploit oligosaccharides on the surface of host cells as receptors for toxins and/or adhesins, enabling colonization of the mucosa and entry of the pathogen or secreted toxins into the host cell. Blocking this adherence prevents infection, whereas toxin neutralization ameliorates symptoms until the pathogen is eventually overcome by the immune system. When administered orally, these probiotics bind to and neutralize toxins in the gut lumen and interfere with pathogen adherence to the intestinal epithelium. One such construct consists of an *E. coli* strain expressing a chimeric lipopolysaccharide (LPS) terminating in a Shiga toxin (Stx) receptor. It has been observed that 1 mg dry weight of this recombinant strain neutralizes >100 μg of Stx1 and Stx2 [18]. Paton *et al.* [19,20] have also constructed probiotics with receptor blocking potential against enterotoxigenic *E. coli* (ETEC) toxin LT and cholera toxin (Ctx). Besides treating enteric infections, "designer probiotics" have also been developed to combat HIV. Rao *et al.* [21] recently described the construction of a probiotic strain of *E. coli*, engineered to secrete HIV-gp41-hemolysin A hybrid peptides, which block HIV fusion and entry into host cells. When administered orally or as a rectal suppository, this "live microbicide" colonizes the gut mucosa and secretes the peptide *in situ*, thereby providing protection in advance of HIV exposure for up to a month. Other anti-HIV probiotics currently being developed include a genetically engineered *Streptococcus gordonii*, which produces cyanovirin-N, a potent HIV-inactivating protein originally isolated from cyanobacterium, and a natural human vaginal isolate of *Lactobacillus jensenii* modified to secrete two-domain CD4, which inhibits HIV entry into target cells [22].

Notwithstanding their *in vitro* and *in vivo* efficacy in animal models, further refinements to the receptor-mimic probiotics might be necessary before commencement of phase I clinical trials. Patho-biotechnology – the introduction of genes to improve resistance to stomach acid, or otherwise promote colonization or survival in the gut, for example – would enable dose regimes to be lowered substantially, providing greater efficacy and further cost benefits.

In addition to infection control, probiotics (and other nonpathogenic bacteria) are also being engineered to function as novel vaccine delivery vehicles that can stimulate both innate and acquired immunity but lack the possibility of reversion to virulence, which exists with more conventional pathogenic platforms. Guimarães *et al.* [23] recently described the construction of a *L. lactis* strain expressing *inlA*, encoding internalin A, a surface protein related to invasion in *L. monocytogenes*. In this instance, the otherwise noninvasive *L. lactis* strain is now capable of invading the small intestine and delivering molecules (DNA or protein) into mammalian epithelial cells, making it a safer and more attractive alternative to attenuated *L. monocytogenes* as an antigen delivery vehicle.

Probiotic vaccine carriers administered by the mucosal route mimic the immune response elicited by natural infection and can lead to long-lasting protective mucosal and systemic responses [24]. Mucosal vaccine delivery (those administered orally, anally, or by nasal spray) also offers significant technological and commercial advantages over traditional formulations, including reduced pain, the possibility of cross-contamination associated with intramuscular injection, and the lack of a requirement for medically trained personnel to administer the vaccine [25].

23.5
Translation to Clinics: Limitations and Difficulties

Probiotics thus have the potential to alleviate the symptoms of chronic gastrointestinal disorders and associated sequelae, fight infection, modulate the immune system, and act as delivery vehicles for bioactive molecules [25]. Notwithstanding these impressive health benefits, probiotic research has really only begun to achieve scientific credibility over the last decade [26], despite the fact that Yakult launched the first probiotic fermented food drink in Japan in 1935 – years before the emergence of the first commercially available antibiotics.

However, with the ever-increasing emergence of antibiotic resistance and the significant decline in isolation and production of new antibacterials, probiotics are now beginning to represent a viable alternative to traditional drug-based therapies. In order to further improve the efficiency and clinical efficacy of probiotic cultures, optimization will be achieved through a number of novel approaches such as the patho-biotechnology concept. Developments in synthetic and systems biology based on the rapidly advancing "omics" technologies have resulted in an ever-increasing number of novel genetic loci with defined additional functions. This coupled with computer-aided bioinformatics and novel tools for genetic modification will ultimately lead to the development of artificial microorganisms [27,28] and eventually to a new class of probiotics, perhaps more correctly termed pharmabiotics, assembled from components of various origins and tailored to fulfill all the requirements of an ideal therapeutic agent. The major difficulty associated with this new generation of probiotic strains is the stringent regulations related to the development and application of genetically modified microbes for human therapeutic applications. Indeed, at present, the legal impediments far outweigh the technological difficulties associated with the development of the field.

Acknowledgment

Roy D. Sleator is coordinator of the FP7 IAPP grant ClouDx-i. This chapter represents a modified version of a paper previously published in *Nutrafoods*, **7** (2/3), 2008.

References

1 Fuller, R. (1989) Probiotics in man and animals. *The Journal of Applied Bacteriology*, **66**, 365–378.
2 Shanahan, F. (2006) Probiotics: promise, problems, and progress. *Gastroenterology & Hepatology Annual Review*, **1**, 41–45.
3 Madara, J. (2004) Building an intestine: architectural contributions of commensal bacteria. *The New England Journal of Medicine*, **351**, 1685–1686.
4 Sleator, R.D. and Hill, C. (2007) Patho-biotechnology: using bad bugs to make good bugs better. *Science Progress*, **90**, 1–14.
5 Sleator, R.D. and Hill, C. (2006) Patho-biotechnology: using bad bugs to do good things. *Current Opinion in Biotechnology*, **17**, 211–216.
6 Sleator, R.D. and Hill, C. (2007) 'Bioengineered Bugs' – a patho-biotechnology approach to probiotic research and application. *Medical Hypotheses*, **70**, 167–169.
7 Sleator, R.D. and Hill, C. (2007) Improving probiotic function using a patho-biotechnology approach. *Gene Therapy & Molecular Biology*, **11**, 269–274.

8 Sheehan, V., Sleator, R.D., Fitzgerald, G., and Hill, C. (2006) Heterologous expression of BetL, a betaine uptake system, enhances the stress tolerance of *Lactobacillus salivarius* UCC118. *Applied and Environmental Microbiology*, **72**, 2170–2177.

9 Sheehan, V.M., Sleator, R.D., Hill, C., and Fitzgerald, G.F. (2007) Improving gastric transit, gastrointestinal persistence and therapeutic efficacy of *Bifidobacterium breve* UCC2003. *Microbiology*, **153**, 3563–3571.

10 Paton, A.W., Morona, R., and Paton, J.C. (2006) Designer probiotics for prevention of enteric infections. *Nature Reviews. Microbiology*, **4**, 193–200.

11 Hill, C., Cotter, P., Sleator, R.D., and Gahan, C.G.M. (2002) Bacterial stress response in *Listeria monocytogenes*: jumping the hurdles imposed by minimal processing. *International Dairy Journal*, **12**, 273–283.

12 Sleator, R.D. and Hill, C. (2002) Bacterial osmoadaptation: the role of osmolytes in bacterial stress and virulence. *FEMS Microbiology Reviews*, **26**, 49–71.

13 Sleator, R.D., Gahan, C.G.M., and Hill, C. (2003) A post-genomic appraisal of osmotolerance in *Listeria monocytogenes*. *Applied and Environmental Microbiology*, **69**, 1–9.

14 Sleator, R.D., Gahan, C.G.M., Abee, T., and Hill, C. (1999) Identification and disruption of BetL, a secondary glycine betaine transport system linked to the salt tolerance of *Listeria monocytogenes* LO28. *Applied and Environmental Microbiology*, **65**, 2078–2083.

15 Smiddy, M., Sleator, R.D., Kelly, A., and Hill, C. (2004) Role for the compatible solutes glycine betaine and L-carnitine in listerial barotolerance. *Applied and Environmental Microbiology*, **70**, 7555–7557.

16 Smiddy, M., O'Gorman, L., Sleator, R.D., Hill, C., and Kelly, A. (2005) Greater high-pressure resistance of bacteria in oysters than in broth. *Innovative Food Science & Emerging Technologies*, **6**, 83–90.

17 Termont, S., Vandenbrouke, K., Iserentant, D., Neirynck, S., Steidler, L., Remaut, E., and Rottiers, P. (2006) Intracellular accumulation of trehalose protects *Lactococcus lactis* from freeze-drying damage and bile toxicity and increases gastric acid resistance. *Applied and Environmental Microbiology*, **72**, 7694–7700.

18 Paton, A.W., Morona, R., and Paton, J.C. (2000) A new biological agent for treatment of Shiga toxigenic *Escherichia coli* infections and dysentery in humans. *Nature Medicine*, **6**, 265–270.

19 Paton, A.W., Morona, R., and Paton, J.C. (2001) Neutralization of Shiga toxins Stx1, Stx2c and Stx2e by recombinant bacteria expressing mimics of globotriose and globotetraose. *Infection and Immunity*, **69**, 1967–1970.

20 Paton, A.W., Jennings, M.P., Morona, R., Wang, H., Focareta, A., Roddam, L.F., Paton, J.C. (2005) Recombinant probiotics for treatment and prevention of enterotoxigenic *Escherichia coli* diarrhea. *Gastroenterology*, **128**, 1219–1228.

21 Rao, S., Hu, S., McHugh, L., Lueders, K., Henry, K., Zhao, Q., Fekete, R.A., Kar, S., Adhya, S., and Hamer, D.H. (2005) Toward a live microbial microbicide for HIV: commensal bacteria secreting an HIV fusion inhibitor peptide. *Proceedings of the National Academy of Sciences of the United States of America*, **102**, 11993–11998.

22 Chang, T.L.-Y., Chang, C.H., Simpson, D.A., Xu, Q., Martin, P.K., Lagenaur, L.A., Schoolnik, G.K., Ho, D.D., Hillier, S.L., Holodniy, M., Lewicki, J.A., and LeE, P.P. (2003) Inhibition of HIV infectivity by a natural human isolate of *Lactobacillus jensenii* engineered to express functional two-domain CD4. *Proceedings of the National Academy of Sciences of the United States of America*, **100**, 11672–11677.

23 Guimarães, V.D., Gabriel, J.E., Lefèvre, F. et al. (2005) Internalin-expressing *Lactococcus lactis* is able to invade small intestine of guinea pigs and deliver DNA into mammalian epithelial cells. *Microbes and Infection*, **7**, 836–844.

24 Holmgren, J. and Czerkinsky, C. (2005) Mucosal immunity and vaccines. *Nature Medicine*, **11**, S45–S53.

25 Sleator, R.D. and Hill, C. (2007) Probiotics as therapeutics for the developing world. *Journal of Infection in Developing Countries*, **1**, 7–12.

26 Chermesh, I. and Eliakim, R. (2006) Probiotics and the gastrointestinal tract:

where are we in 2005? *World Journal of Gastroenterology*, **12**, 853–857.

27 Smith, H.O., Hutchison, C.A., III, Pfannkoch, C., and Venter, J.C. (2003) Generating a synthetic genome by whole genome assembly: φX174 bacteriophage from synthetic oligonucleotides. *Proceedings of the National Academy of Sciences of the United States of America*, **100**, 15440–15445.

28 Lartigue, C., Glass, J.I., Alperovich, N., Pieper, R., Parmar, P.P., Hutchison, C.A., III, Smith, H.O., and Venter, J.C. (2007) Genome transplantation in bacteria: changing one species to another. *Science*, **317**, 632–638.

24
Renal Disorders

Dominique Guerrot, Christos Chatziantoniou, and Jean-Claude Dussaule

24.1
Introduction

The kidneys are essential to homeostasis in mammals. They maintain the volume and composition of the body fluids despite variations in nutritional intakes. Maintenance of the composition of body fluids includes regulation of extracellular osmolarity, electrolytic concentrations, and acid–base balance. The kidneys also play an important role in the functioning of the endocrine system with regard to the synthesis of renin, calcitriol, and erythropoietin.

Functionally, each kidney is divided into three components: glomerular, tubulointerstitial, and vascular. Schematically, glomerular ultrafiltrate circulating in tubules makes possible bidirectional transport between primitive urine and peritubular capillaries. Quantitatively, 180 l of fluid is filtered by human kidneys in 24 h and nearly 99% of this filtration is reabsorbed all along the tubules. Specific transporters of tubular epithelial cells are able to modify not only the quantity but also the composition of urine, their activity being controlled by neuroendocrine factors. Recent discoveries on the molecular structures of transporters have notably increased the knowledge on tubular mechanisms of reabsorption and secretion [1].

At the microscopic level, nephrons (1 million per kidney in humans) are the renal functional units. Each nephron is subdivided into one glomerulus and one tubule, and is surrounded by capillaries. It is difficult to study renal function at the molecular level due to the cellular heterogeneity of nephrons. In glomeruli, four types of cells are present: *parietal cells* on the urinary pole of glomeruli, vascular *endothelial cells* from capillaries that interact with *mesangial cells* and *podocytes*. In tubules, several segments are individualized with different cellular composition and specific functions: proximal tubule, followed by Henle's loop, and convoluted distal, connector, and collector tubules. Interactions between renal resident cells and, in pathological conditions, with fibroblasts and inflammatory cells explain that *in vivo* models are useful in analyzing renal functions and describing renal structures, but are generally inappropriate to figure out cellular mechanisms. *Ex vivo* studies after dissection of renal vasculature, glomerular corpuscles, or tubules can be useful in conjunction with *in vivo* studies [2]. Cultures of resident renal cells are largely used

In Vivo Models for Drug Discovery, First Edition. Edited by José M. Vela, Rafael Maldonado, and Michel Hamon.
© 2014 Wiley-VCH Verlag GmbH & Co. KGaA. Published 2014 by Wiley-VCH Verlag GmbH & Co. KGaA.

for studying the cellular signals but with caution in interpreting data, due to the progressive changes of the phenotypes of epithelial and mesenchymal cells proliferating *in vitro* [3]. Recently, the development of conditional transgenic models with Cre-lox methods provided more accurate insights *in vivo* into the role of specific renal cells in physiological and pathophysiological conditions [4].

Injuries of glomerular, vascular, and tubulointerstitial compartments induce primary nephropathies that, in some cases, lead to renal failure with a complete degradation of renal functions, including endocrine activity (synthesis of erythropoietin and calcitriol). In other cases, a unique function of the kidneys is disturbed such as acid–base balance, electrolytic excretion, or blood pressure regulation. For clinicians and researchers, the presence of proteins in urine is a cardinal sign of renal dysfunction. The second major disturbance determining renal failure is the decrease in glomerular filtration rate. Acute renal failure induces oliguria or anuria with the capacity of recovery of glomerular filtration, whereas renal failure observed in chronic kidney diseases (CKDs) is more insidious and may progress down to an irreversible loss of function associated with the development of renal fibrosis.

24.2
Animal Models

The purpose of using animal models is to reproduce human renal diseases, to test new drugs limiting abnormal renal phenotype in pathological conditions, and to induce the stabilization or the regression of experimental nephropathies with the hope of efficient human translation. Although treatments for human renal diseases have been developed, we still need new therapeutics to limit the progression of CKD down to end-stage renal failure. Two distinct methods are available for developing renal disorders in animals: either by selecting a pathologic genetic trait or by inducing lesions in normal kidneys. Renal injury follows administration of toxics, aggression from hemodynamic, immunological, or infectious origins, or surgical lesions. Some examples of these various models of renal disorders are given in the following sections. Genetic and somatic approaches can be associated to reinforce the degradation of renal function [5]. Before the transgenic revolution that dramatically improved genetic manipulation, both methods were already in concurrence, as demonstrated by the examples of hypertensive models in the fields of cardiovascular and renal diseases. Strains of hypertensive rats were obtained after adequate crossbreeds. These strains, spontaneous hypertensive rats (SHRs), insensitive to salt intake, or Dahl's, Milan, and Sabra rats, becoming hypertensive only in the presence of a rich sodium diet, have been extensively studied in parallel with models of hypertension induced in normal rats by the administration of vasoconstrictors (angiotensin II, nitric oxide antagonists), hormones (DOCA salt), or by surgery (renovascular model of Goldblatt, renal cross-transplantation) [6]. Both methods are complementary: the advantage of hypertensive strains of animals is the duration of the disease that mimics what occurs in human essential hypertension. However, genetic models make it difficult to distinguish between embryonic renal defects and consequences

Table 24.1 Examples of alterations of tubular transports in transgenic mice.

Mice models	Mice phenotypes	Associated human diseases
KO of genes encoding proteins of transport		
NHE3 (transport of sodium and proton in proximal tubule)	Decrease in GFR	
NKCC2 (reabsorption of Na, Cl, and K in Henle's loop)	Lethal (dehydration)	Mutations of NKCC2: Bartter syndrome
ROMK (K channel)	Lethal (dehydration, hydronephrosis)	Mutations of ROMK: Bartter syndrome
NCC (reabsorption of Na and Cl in convoluted distal tubule)	Hypotension	Mutations of NCC: Gitelman syndrome
ClC-5 (chloride proton exchanger)	Fanconi syndrome	Mutations of ClC-5: Dent's disease
HNF1-a (reabsorption of glucose and Na in proximal)	Fanconi syndrome	Mutations of HNF1-a: MODY 3
NDCBE (reabsorption of sodium in distal tubule [7]	Sodium wasting	
Pendrin (reabsorption of chloride in distal tubule)	Chloride wasting hypotension	
ENaC (sodium channel in distal tubule)	Sodium wasting	Liddle syndrome: (familial hypertension) if mutations increase ENaC activity
AQP2 (aquaporin in distal tubule)	Polyuria	Mutations of AQP2: nephrogenic diabetes insipidus
Mutations of PKD1 encoding PC1 (polycystine: ciliary protein)	Polycystic kidney disease	Mutations of PC1: polycystic kidney disease

of chronic hypertension on kidneys in adults. The same remarks may be applicable to the sophisticated transgenic models in mice (mice have been studied more often than other species because of the relative facility of transgenesis), except when the conditional expression of genetic mutations limits the role of development in renal lesions [4].

In the following sections, we will present some usual models of renal injury in mice or rats. In addition, Tables 24.1 and 24.2 present a selection of models that were developed to gain insights into the mechanisms of tubular function in physiological and pathophysiological conditions.

24.2.1
The RenTg Model of CKD

Animal models mimicking CKD are essential for revealing the mechanisms underlying progression of CKD and, most importantly, for the discovery of novel

Table 24.2 KO mice for renin–angiotensin or atrial natriuretic peptide (ANP) systems.

Mice models	Renal phenotypes
KO of genes encoding proteins of RAS or proteins of ANP system	
Angiotensinogen	Hypotension, atrophy of renal inner medulla
Renin	Hypotension, hydronephrosis
AT1 angiotensin II receptor	Hypotension, hydronephrosis
ACE1 (angiotensin-converting enzyme type 1)	Hypotension, hydronephrosis
Atrial natriuretic peptide	Hypertension with sodium-rich diet
Type A receptor of natriuretic peptides	Moderate hypertension

therapeutics. Since CKD results from recurrent or progressive injuries in glomeruli, tubules, interstitium, and/or vasculature, several animal models have been developed, including genetic (renin transgenic model, RenTg, and collagen IV mutations), spontaneous (aging, spontaneous hypertensive rats, and lupus nephritis), and induced models (unilateral ureteral obstruction (UUO), nephrotoxic serum-induced glomerulonephritis, 5/6 nephrectomy, and puromycin or adriamycin administration) [8].

Unfortunately, all animal models have their limitations. Chronic, derived from the Greek word *chronos* (a god personifying time), means that CKD develops slowly over a long period, progressively undermining normal renal structure and function. In contrast, most animal models, for practical and financial reasons, develop rapidly, leading to severe loss of renal function within days or, in best-case scenario, weeks. The RenTg model, a relatively novel model of hypertension-induced chronic disease, may be the answer to the problem of lack of time course correspondence between the slowly progressing human disease and the rapid deterioration of renal function in animal models.

This renin transgenic model of hypertensive nephropathy was created by Caron et al. [9]. Briefly, a synthetic cDNA consisting of parts of the Ren-2 and Ren-1d genes was inserted into a liver-specific locus, driven by a strong and well-characterized albumin promoter/enhancer (AlbP/E) that has previously been shown to be active only in the liver. The construct contains several modifications including glycosylation sites for increased stability, a furin cleavage site to facilitate prorenin to active renin processing in the liver and allow secretion of active renin into the bloodstream, and a c-myc epitope tag for protein immunodetection. The resulting transgene expresses renin ectopically at a constant high level in the liver and leads to elevated plasma levels of prorenin and active renin.

Our laboratory has extensively used the RenTg model as an experimental model of hypertensive nephropathy and has performed time course analysis for several functional and structural parameters affected in CKD [10,11]. RenTg mice display elevated systolic blood pressure from as early as 3 months of age (140 mmHg versus 120 mmHg for age-matched wild-type littermates). Proteinuria was slightly increased at 3 months of age and continued increasing in a time-dependent manner exceeding 150 g/mol albumin/creatinine at 12 months of age. GFR, the basic criterion for classification of CKD, began to decrease at 6–8 months of age and reached 125 µl/min (versus 220 µl/min for wild-type littermates) at 12 months of age. Accordingly, several aspects of renal histology, including sclerotic glomeruli, tubular dilation, and renal fibrosis, developed progressively in a time-dependent manner. Renal inflammation preceded interstitial fibrosis and glomerular damage since endothelial dysfunction and inflammatory markers were highly upregulated from as early as 3 months of age. Overall, 12-month-old mice were hypertensive and proteinuric and showed established lesions typical of hypertensive renal disease such as perivascular and periglomerular inflammation, glomerulosclerosis, mesangial expansion, and tubular dilation as well as cardiac hypertrophy and fibrosis, fully mimicking the characteristics of CKD in humans.

24.2.1.1 Benefits of the RenTg Model

As mentioned earlier, CKD may be caused by diseases that affect any of the renal structures, including vessels, glomeruli, and the tubulointerstitial compartment. The damage can be induced by various diseases with hypertension and diabetes representing the major ones. Renin–angiotensin system (RAS) is a well-established inducer of renal injury, involved in both hypertensive and diabetic nephropathy. RenTg animals express renin at high levels leading to persistently increased angiotensin II, maintained throughout the life of the mice. Therefore, a sustained induction of proinflammatory and profibrotic mediators is achieved, accompanied by elevated blood pressure. All these factors contribute to the slow decline of renal function and structure observed in CKD.

Another important aspect addressed by this model is kinetics. Although speed is very important for practical and financial reasons, studying CKD in models that develop end-stage renal damage within 10 days can stimulate pathophysiological mechanisms that differ from those encountered in a slowly progressive disease. A slow procedure such as progression of CKD is mediated by several mechanisms and signaling pathways. Endothelial dysfunction, inflammation, and fibrosis are induced via shift in the balance of pro- and anti-inflammatory/fibrotic mediators [12]. In each of these tightly regulated procedures, many, yet unidentified, molecules are involved (receptors, transcription factors, miRNAs, etc.). Using models that lead to severe tissue necrosis, glomerular injury, or abrupt reduction of kidney function within a few days (5/6 nephrectomy), the role of several proteins or even of mechanisms could be underestimated or overlooked. An additional limitation is that renal disease is induced in young healthy animals in most experimental models that contrast with the typical development of CKD usually affecting middle-aged or older humans with compromised, to a smaller or a larger extent, health.

The RenTg model can be the answer to such issues. Since disease progresses by age, all stages of the disease, early or late, can be easily studied. This can offer novel information about the extent of involvement of several mediators in each step of the disease. Moreover, potential pharmaceutical targets that could stop the progression or even result in regression of the disease before it reaches end stage could be identified. The RenTg model could be ideal for testing the efficiency of antihypertensive drugs or potential therapeutic molecules against renal disease.

Our studies have shown that renal failure observed in this model is not dependent on blood pressure since normalization of blood pressure, after a certain point, is not sufficient to ameliorate renal disease [10,12]. Therefore, several possibilities can be explored using combinations of antihypertensive and other drugs on animals that already suffer for a long period of time as is usually the case with humans. Finally, the RenTg mouse, although it requires more time than usual experimental models to develop renal disease, offers several benefits to the researcher. It is easily bred and can be easily backcrossed with other transgenic animals, thus creating double transgenes that can be very helpful for studying the role of several proteins in CKD [13] or in pathologies induced by overactivation of the renin–angiotensin system, such as cardiac hypertrophy and fibrosis [14,15]. Blood pressure and proteinuria of transgenic animals can be easily monitored throughout the life of the mice, so the researcher can choose animals with an anticipated degree of renal inflammation and fibrosis. For instance, our laboratory has shown that mice with proteinuria around 100 mg/mmol albumin/creatinine exhibit reduced GFR, perivascular inflammation, several fibrotic foci, and a small degree of glomerular sclerosis. Therefore, it is possible to choose animals with a certain degree of damage in order to perform an experimental protocol and test the protective (or not) effect of a drug administered at certain ages [10,12].

In conclusion, the RenTg model of hypertensive nephropathy is a useful tool for studying CKD since it resembles the slow progression of the human disease. It offers the possibility of studying early, intermediate, and late stages of the disease, whereas monitoring proteinuria can be used as an indication of the degree of renal damage in mice. In addition, it offers the opportunity to crossbreed with other genetically engineered animals to investigate the role(s) of specific genes.

24.2.2
Unilateral Ureteral Obstruction

The experimental model of UUO induces severe renal injury, as can be observed in human acute obstructive nephropathy. It is commonly used to study mechanisms of tubulointerstitial inflammation and fibrosis *in vivo* [16]. Usually, UUO is performed by a ureteral ligation, which leads to a complete obstruction. Alternative models of obstructive nephropathy include UUO/R-UUO (reversal of UUO after a transient obstruction) and incomplete ligation, but are less reproducible and are infrequently reported in the literature, although their pathophysiology better matches that of the human disease.

24.2.2.1 Technical Aspects
This model can be used quite easily by an experienced operator, in both mice and rats, and shows limited strain dependence. After induction of general anesthesia (intraperitoneal injection of pentobarbital 50 mg/kg, or ketamine 100 mg/kg + xylazine 10 mg/kg, for example, in mice), the animal is shaved and placed on the operating table under temperature-controlled conditions. Palpation of the left kidney indicates the location for the flank incision, which should be ∼1 mm

shorter than the kidney length. Once the skin and the fascia are open, the kidney should be carefully popped out through the incision. The needle of a sterile nonabsorbable suture is inserted immediately below the vascular pedicle, between the vein and the ureteropelvic junction. Two separate knots are necessary to reduce the occurrence of incomplete obstruction and variability. The kidney is reinserted and the incision is closed [17].

24.2.2.2 Pathology and Pathophysiology

The renal consequences of the obstruction depend on the completeness and the duration of the obstruction. A complete obstruction of the ureter leads to a rapid elevation of hydrostatic pressure in the kidney pelvis and the tubules [18]. Within 48 h, histological examination shows tubular dilation, related to the flattening and desquamation of the tubular epithelial cells. The lesions produced by UUO involve multiple interrelated pathophysiological mechanisms. In the epithelial cells, early apoptosis is triggered by TGF-β1- and P38-MAPK-dependent mechanisms [19]. The glomerular filtration is rapidly abolished, as a consequence of increasing intratubular hydrostatic pressure and of the activation of the renin–angiotensin system, responsible for intrarenal vasoconstriction, which contributes to parenchymal hypoxia. The increase in angiotensin II also induces renal inflammation, with NF-κB playing a central role in this context [20]. The expression of multiple proinflammatory cytokines by the injured resident cells, including MCP-1 and IL-1β, leads to an early interstitial infiltration by macrophages and T lymphocytes. Profibrotic pathways are then activated and significant peritubular, interstitial, and perivascular deposition of extracellular matrix is evidenced after 7–10 days of UUO. To specifically study fibrosis, the endpoint is usually set between 10 and 30 days of UUO in mice.

24.2.2.3 Clinical Relevance and Limits

Obstructive nephropathy is a relatively frequent cause of renal failure, particularly in childhood. Etiologies can be congenital, as in pyeloureteral junction syndrome or in congenital anomalies of the kidney and urinary tract (CAKUT), or acquired, the ureteral obstruction being usually caused by urolithiasis or cancer. However, renal failure most frequently develops as a consequence of a long-standing incomplete obstruction, in contrast with the classical UUO model. The advantages of the complete UUO model include good reproducibility, limited cost, easy performance, and the presence of the contralateral kidney as a control. The main limitations are the absence of reliability with the duration of human obstructive nephropathies and the lack of functional readouts (plasma creatinine, BUN, and urine analyses are nonrelevant since urine is exclusively excreted by the contralateral kidney, which also compensates the GFR) [8].

24.2.3
Renal Ischemia–Reperfusion

Renal ischemia is a major cause of acute kidney injury(AKI) in humans. Warm renal ischemia–reperfusion (IR) is a commonly used experimental model for studying acute kidney injury. This model can be used in a broad spectrum of animals, but is predominantly used in rats and mice. IR can either be bilateral or unilateral, with removal of the contralateral kidney. The ischemia can be performed by clamping either the renal artery alone or the pedicle.

24.2.3.1 Technical Aspects

Renal IR is a technically simple model. However, it is characterized by an important variability, depending on multiple factors related to the surgery and the perioperative period. It is therefore important that the surgery be performed under standardized conditions by an experienced operator. After induction of general anesthesia (intraperitoneal injection of pentobarbital 50 mg/kg, or ketamine 100 mg/kg + xylazine 10 mg/kg, for example, in mice), the animal is shaved and placed on the thermostatic station. Palpation of the kidney indicates the location for the flank incision, which should be ~1 mm shorter than the kidney length. Once the skin and the fascia are open, the kidney is carefully popped out through the incision. The renal pedicle is exposed and carefully dissected with ultrafine point tweezers. The use of a surgical microscope is suggested for this critical step. Atraumatic neurosurgical clamps are used for the clamping of the renal pedicle or artery. Adequate clamping is confirmed by checking the change in kidney color, which occurs within seconds from the placement of the clamp. A timer is set once the clamp is placed, the ischemia time usually ranging from 15 to 30 min in mice and from 20 to 60 min in bigger animals. After removal of the clamp, the recoloration of the kidney should be ascertained. The kidney is then reinserted and the incision is closed [21].

24.2.3.2 Pathology and Pathophysiology

Ischemia–reperfusion is characterized by the interruption of blood flow in the kidney over a predetermined period of time, and by subsequent reperfusion. The absence of perfusion leads to GFR abolition and anoxia of parenchyma, with a major disequilibrium between the metabolic demand (especially when the kidney remains at body temperature) and the supply. This produces severe lesions in the epithelial cells, which have the most important metabolic activity. Tubular epithelial cells undergo rapid necrosis, which initiates in the S3 segment of the proximal tubule. Histological examination reveals swelling and detachment of epithelial cells in the tubular lumen.

Paradoxically, when the blood flow and the oxygen supply are restored, renal lesions worsen, especially by means of interstitial infiltration with neutrophils [22]. Indeed, the inflammatory response associated with reperfusion is a major contributor to the pathophysiology of IR, in part related to the release of proinflammatory mediators and reactive oxygen species by the injured epithelium.

Renal IR-induced lesions comprise important alterations of the vascular phenotype, for example, increased vascular permeability, proinflammatory and profibrotic phenotype of endothelial cells, loss of the physiological balance between vasodilator and vasoconstrictor mediators, and complement activation.

Renal IR is a classical model of acute kidney injury. Blood urea nitrogen and plasma creatinine increase after 6 h and generally return to baseline within 7–10 days, depending on the time of ischemia [21]. In order to obtain a slight chronic alteration of the GFR in the classical bilateral IR model, the duration of ischemia has to be long enough to ensure severe renal lesions (at least 22–25 min in mice, depending on the strain and the operation conditions). Such an ischemia induces severe tissue damage and subsequent tubulointerstitial microcirculation rarefaction, with hypoxia-driven fibrosis, but is usually associated with a high postoperative mortality rate.

24.2.3.3 Clinical Relevance and Limits

The experimental model of warm IR is often studied to analyze the pathophysiology of AKI. Although some situations in human disease do have clear similarities with the experimental model (renal transplantation, aortic surgery), most cases of AKI are due to toxic factors or hemodynamic disturbances, without complete interruption of the renal blood supply. Therefore, since anoxia and reperfusion-induced injury are a cornerstone of the IR model, clinical relevance in various human settings is questionable.

Furthermore, in pathological interruptions of renal blood flow in humans, the organ is usually protected in a cold milieu, which modifies the consequences of hypoxia. Temperature and transport activity related to persistent GFR are the major factors that determine the metabolic activity of thick ascending limb cells. This tubular segment is the most susceptible to severe injury in human IR, whereas in warm IR in animals, proximal tubular cells are the first cells injured [23].

24.2.4
Experimental Alloimmune Glomerulonephritis

Goodpasture's disease is characterized by rapidly progressive renal failure due to crescentic glomerulonephritis and pulmonary hemorrhage. In this disease, circulating autoantibodies are directed toward an antigen present in the glomerular basement membrane (GBM) and the alveoli. The target antigen has been identified as the NC domain of the alpha-3 chain of type IV collagen [24]. Various models have been developed to study the mechanisms and consequences of the severe glomerular injury observed in Goodpasture's disease. Since the pathogenic mechanisms involved in these models frequently involve additional glomerular target antigens, the term "experimental crescentic autoimmune/alloimmune glomerulonephritis" may be preferred.

24.2.4.1 Technical Aspects

This experimental concept was first described in sheep immunized against human GBM material [25]. Several models have subsequently been developed, in dogs, and mainly in rodents immunized against heterologous GBM or recombinant heterologous alpha-3 chain of type IV collagen preparations [26,27]. This model presents important differences according to the species/strains studied. For instance, the Wistar Kyoto rats develop severe glomerular lesions, whereas the Lewis rats are resistant [28]. In mice, the 129/Sv, BUB/BnJ, and DBA/1J strains develop characteristic glomerular injury [29].

Passive alloimmune glomerulonephritis can be induced in mice by the injection of decomplemented heterologous serum containing immunoglobulins directed against glomerular antigens. The nephrotoxic serum containing the pathogenic immunoglobulins can be obtained from sheep immunized against a preparation of freshly sieved mouse glomeruli [30]. Mice are injected intravenously with a total of 1.5 mg total protein/g body weight, administered over three consecutive days (days 0, 1, and 2). Concentrations of sheep IgG in mouse serum are measured after the three injections, as a control for the amount of circulating alloantibodies.

24.2.4.2 Pathology and Pathophysiology

The injection of heterologous serum, rich in immunoglobulins directed toward glomerular antigens, induces an immediate inflammatory response characterized by the infiltration by cells of the immune system, predominantly polymorphonuclear cells. This first wave of the innate immune response is followed by T- and B-cell activation, which leads to progressive infiltration by $CD4^+$ T cells and macrophages. This model mimics what happens in several human rapidly progressive glomerulonephritis, in which immune deposits induce endocapillary lesions, with or without extracapillary proliferation, associated with direct or collateral podocyte injury. Four days after the first injection of nephrotoxic serum, significant renal inflammation and tubular injury can be observed, associated with glomerular fibrin deposits and beginning of podocyte injury. From day 8, glomerular crescents (extracapillary proliferation) are evident, and nephritic proteinuria is observed, together with decreased GFR and progressive fibrosis. Although most animals survive during the first 2 weeks, the progressive renal injury is usually fatal within 4–6 weeks [31].

24.2.4.3 Clinical Relevance and Limits

The experimental alloimmune antiglomerular basement membrane nephritis is a model commonly used to study mechanisms of crescentic glomerulonephritis, and shares many similarities with human Goodpasture's disease. The main conceptual difference is represented by the alloimmune nature of the disease in the experimental model, as opposed to the autoimmune process involved in Goodpasture's disease. When using alloimmune sera prepared after injecting nonpurified glomerular material, one should be aware that multiple glomerular and endothelial antigens are nonspecifically targeted. In this context, alternative pathogenic mechanisms, including renal and systemic endothelial dysfunctions, may occur, as opposed to what happens in the human Goodpasture's disease.

24.2.5
Angiotensin II-Mediated Hypertensive Nephropathy

Numerous experimental models have been developed to study hypertension and hypertension-associated nephropathy. Models based on direct or indirect increase in components of the renin–angiotensin–aldosterone system represent an important body of the literature [6].

Angiotensin II is a final effector of the renin–angiotensin pathway, which plays a major role in the physiological control of extracellular volume, vasomotor tone, and the vessel structure, and is an important contributor to blood pressure increase, vascular inflammation, and fibrosis in pathological conditions. Angiotensin II-induced hypertension has therefore become a widely used experimental model for hypertension in rodents.

24.2.5.1 Technical Aspects

Angiotensin II can be easily and safely administered via subcutaneous or intraperitoneal osmotic minipumps. The use of intravenous infusion route is also possible. Together with angiotensin II, several factors are classically combined to increase blood pressure and accelerate the development of renal and vascular lesions, especially NaCl-enriched food (5%) or drink (7 g/l), and/or reduction of the nephron mass by nephrectomy.

The concentration of the angiotensin II solution is calculated depending on the infusion rate of the pump, as provided by the manufacturer. In Sv/129 mice, an angiotensin II infusion rate of 1 µg/kg/min is sufficient to increase blood pressure from day 3, and to produce typical hypertension-associated vascular and glomerular lesions from day 14, in association with NaCl-enriched food [32]. In SD rats, similar results are obtained with 200–400 ng/kg/min angiotensin II and NaCl (personal data).

The osmotic minipump is usually inserted subcutaneously, under short general anesthesia (isoflurane or ketamine combined with xylazine are suitable). Once the animal is shaved, an incision corresponding to the diameter of the pump is made in the back, and a subcutaneous tunnel is prepared with bald instruments through the incision, in order to facilitate the insertion of the pump.

24.2.5.2 Pathology and Pathophysiology

Renal lesions induced by angiotensin II occur via systemic hypertension and via direct effects of the peptide on the kidney.

At least in the first days of the experimental model, hypertension predominantly results from the vasoconstrictor effect of the peptide, driven by smooth muscle cell contraction and cytoskeletal remodeling. Hypervolemia due to NaCl reabsorption also contributes to the blood pressure increase.

Angiotensin II has growth factor properties and is a potent proinflammatory and profibrotic mediator. It regulates the expression of proteins of the extracellular matrix, cytokines, adhesion molecules, and other growth factors, thereby constituting a major pathophysiological actor of the target organ damage in the model, independent of blood pressure increase itself. In addition, angiotensin II induces oxidative stress, which further aggravates hypertension and inflammation of parenchyma and fibrosis.

Angiotensin II-induced hypertensive nephropathy is characterized by the rapid onset of significant proteinuria and delayed renal failure, both depending on the severity of the experimental model (dose of angiotensin II, with or without NaCl-enriched diet, with or without uninephrectomy). Histological lesions typically include vascular hypertrophy, glomerular ischemia and sclerosis, perivascular and interstitial inflammation, and fibrosis. If the model is severe, thrombotic microangiopathy lesions can be found in the kidneys.

24.2.5.3 Clinical Relevance and Limits

Overactivation of the renin–angiotensin system contributes to human hypertension in a majority of patients. Therefore, the use of angiotensin II infusion to induce the experimental model is a logical perspective, regarding this simple pathophysiological view. However, due to the multiple renal, neurohormonal, and vascular mechanisms leading to hypertension, this experimental model remains largely different from what actually happens in humans.

When studying the renal consequences of long-standing hypertension (the so-called hypertensive nephropathy or benign nephroangiosclerosis), a major issue is to differentiate between the effects of high blood pressure *per se* and direct effects on the organ, independent of systemic hypertension, as is clearly the case with the angiotensin II infusion model.

24.2.6
L-NAME-Mediated Hypertensive Nephropathy

24.2.6.1 Technical Aspects

The administration of L-NAME, as the infusion of angiotensin II, chronically increases blood pressure and allows studying the renal consequences of hypertension. In this model, hypertension comes from the lack of production of nitric oxide (NO). NO is a paracrine vasodilator agent. It is synthesized in endothelial cells from the metabolism of L-arginine by NO synthase. L-NAME, a structural analog of L-arginine, prevents NO synthase to degrade the amino acid and to produce NO. In kidneys, NO is also produced in the distal renal tubule where it plays a role in sodium reabsorption [1]. The advantage of this model is its simplicity, as L-NAME can be orally administered. A derived model from L-NAME has been used to characterize the deleterious action of an endogenous metabolite of L-Arg, the asymmetric dimethylarginine (ADMA), produced in large quantities during chronic renal failure [33]. Another usefulness of this model is its pharmacological effectiveness in both rats and mice. However, in mice, usual resistance to nephroangiosclerosis requires a prolonged period of administration, nearly 20 weeks (versus 4 weeks in rats), to induce kidney damages and loss of glomerular function [34,35].

24.2.6.2 Pathology and Pathophysiology

In the laboratory, this model has been used to study the factors of progression and regression of renal fibrosis. We first demonstrated by combining L-NAME administration with antifibrotic drugs that the progression of nephropathy was largely independent of the levels of blood pressure. For instance, bosentan, an antagonist of endothelin receptors, protected rats and mice against the nephropathy induced by L-NAME, without altering blood pressure [34,36]. This result was consistent with a transgenic model of endothelin overexpression [37]. These data also provide keys to understand why, in humans, all the classes of antihypertensive drugs do not equally prevent the progression of CKD in hypertensive patients. Although, classically, *in vitro* models are needed to understand the cellular mechanisms of renal diseases, L-NAME was useful for studying the signaling pathways of angiotensin II. We have shown the involvement of EGF receptor activation in the profibrotic action of angiotensin II, which opens new therapeutic perspectives. These experimental results on the EGF receptor implication in CKD were consistent with those obtained in other models, subtotal nephrectomy [38] and crescentic glomerulonephritis [39]. Administration of L-NAME to transgenic KO mice can provide information on the role of deleted genes in the progression of CKD [40].

The simplicity to interrupt L-NAME toxicity, without harming the animals, allowed us to study the mechanisms of regression of this experimental nephropathy in rats when NO synthesis became effective again. This protocol mimicked treatments against human endothelial dysfunction [41]. We observed that, under these conditions, losartan, an antagonist of AT1 receptor of angiotensin II, could entirely reverse renal functional and structural lesions. However, if L-NAME administration was pursued concomitantly, losartan was less effective, which gave us the opportunity to specifically study the notion of nonreturn point of CKD progression. In fact, although it is relatively easy to reverse CKD in rats or mice [42], in human CKD such a therapeutic objective is rarely reached. When we applied a transcriptomic screening to rats whose renal damages were resistant to losartan compared with responder animals, we identified periostin, an extrarenal matrix protein in physiological conditions, as a marker of the uncontrolled progression of their nephropathies [43]. Moreover, we confirmed the unexpected presence of this protein in kidneys coming from human CKD, which opens a new thematic of research about its potential toxicity and usefulness as a biomarker of rapidly progressive nephropathies.

24.2.6.3 Clinical Relevance and Limits

The discovery of NO has changed the mechanistic views on cardiovascular diseases and, more generally, the role of endothelial dysfunction in the development of vascular diseases is well established [44]. Although no human renal syndrome has been described as a direct consequence of NO deprivation, the concept of endothelial dysfunction can be extended to the renal vasculature, which reinforces the relevance of the L-NAME model [45]. However, like previous ones, this experimental model presents some limitations. First, it does not allow distinguishing the consequences of the absence of NO synthesis by tubules and by endothelial cells. This question has been raised for other paracrine or endocrine systems and has been resolved by elegant genetic studies with regard to AT1 receptor of angiotensin II [46]. Second, the heterogeneity of the renal responses of rats and mice, according to their origin or their breeding conditions [47], to L-NAME makes difficult the comparison of data from one laboratory to another.

24.3
Translation to Clinics: Limitations and Difficulties

In 2007, an INSERM meeting in France was devoted to the translational research in the field of renal diseases and several recommendations were proposed as axis of research to improve the models of renal disorders [48]. Although remarkable progress has been observed in the availability of transgenic models since 2007, the conclusions of this meeting are still current. For instance, the models of diabetic nephropathies in mice did not display the same histological damages as human diabetic nephropathies (presently, the most frequent of CKD). An international consortium has been created on this topic [49]. The Kimmelstiel–Wilson nodular lesions, characteristic in humans, are absent in glomeruli from diabetic kidneys of mice. The degree of fibrosis strongly differs between both species in this disease [49]. The absence of valid experimental models is also noted in the field of renal lithiasis, although the incidence of this disease is dramatically increasing in Western countries. Improvement of the models of transplantation to study the mechanisms of chronic allograft rejection would also be necessary [50].

Another serious limitation, already mentioned in the text, is the role of genetic background in the resistance of some strains of mice to renal injury, without any comparison in human diseases. The heterogeneity of the response of remnant renal tissue to subtotal nephrectomy has been reported by Terzi and coworkers [51]. The comparison of the backgrounds of different strains developing or not developing renal fibrosis after 5/6 nephrectomy gave the opportunity to describe an unknown marker of progression, lipocalin.

Finally, at this time, new biomarkers of progression of CKD are still needed. Their discoveries from animal models of CKD [8] or AKI [52] would be useful in improving the medical supervision of patients and in using, in appropriate cases, new drugs suggested by experimental data, such as inhibitors of TGF-β or specific antagonists of tyrosine kinases activated in the course of CKD.

References

1 Fenton, R.A. and Knepper, M.A. (2007) Mouse models and the urinary concentrating mechanism in the new millennium. *Physiological Reviews*, **87** (4), 1083–1112.

2 Fakhouri, F., Placier, S., Ardaillou, R., Dussaule, J.C., and Chatziantoniou, C. (2001) Angiotensin II activates collagen type I gene in the renal cortex and aorta of transgenic mice through interaction with endothelin and TGF-beta. *Journal of the American Society of Nephrology*, **12** (12), 2701–2710.

3 Bens, M. and Vandewalle, A. (2008) Cell models for studying renal physiology. *Pflügers Archiv: European Journal of Physiology*, **457** (4), 1–15.

4 Duffield, J.S. and Humphreys, B.D. (2011) Origin of new cells in the adult kidney: results from genetic labeling techniques. *Kidney International*, **79** (5), 494–501.

5 Terzi, F., Burtin, M., and Friedlander, G. (2011) Using transgenic mice to analyze the mechanisms of progression of chronic renal failure. *Journal of the American Society of Nephrology*, **11** (Suppl. 16), S144–S148.

6 Dornas, W.C. and Silva, M.E. (2011) Animal models for the study of arterial

7 Leviel, F., Hübner, C.A., Houillier, P., Morla, L., El Moghrabi, S., Brideau, G., Hassan, H., Parker, M.D., Kurth, I., Kougioumtzes, A., Sinning, A., Pech, V., Riemondy, K.A., Miller, R.L., Hummler, E., Shull, G.E., Aronson, P.S., Doucet, A., Wall, S.M., Chambrey, R., and Eladari, D. (2010) The Na^+-dependent chloride–bicarbonate exchanger SLC4A8 mediates an electroneutral Na^+ reabsorption process in the renal cortical collecting ducts of mice. *The Journal of Clinical Investigation*, **120** (5), 1627–1635.

8 Yang, H.C., Zuo, Y., and Fogo, A.B. (2010) Models of chronic kidney disease. *Drug Discovery Today. Disease Models*, **7** (1–2), 13–19.

9 Caron, K.M., James, L.R., Kim, H.S., Morham, S.G., Sequeira Lopez, M.L., Gomez, R.A., Reudelhuber, T.L., and Smithies, O. (2002) A genetically clamped renin transgene for the induction of hypertension. *Proceedings of the National Academy of Sciences of the United States of America*, **99** (12), 8248–8252.

10 Huby, A.C., Rastaldi, M.P., Caron, K., Smithies, O., Dussaule, J.C., and Chatziantoniou, C. (2009) Restoration of podocyte structure and improvement of chronic renal disease in transgenic mice overexpressing renin. *PLoS One*, **4** (8), e6721.

11 Huby, A.C., Kavvadas, P., Abed, A., Toubas, J., Rastaldi, M.P., Dussaule, J.C., Chatziantoniou, C., and Chadjichristos, C.E. (2012) The RenTg mice: a powerful tool to study hypertension-induced chronic kidney disease. *PLoS One*, **7** (12), e52362.

12 Kavvadas, P., Weis, L., Abed, A., Feldman, D.L., Dussaule, J.C., and Chatziantoniou, C. (2013) Renin inhibition reverses renal disease in transgenic mice by shifting the balance between profibrotic and antifibrotic agents. *Hypertension*, **61** (4), 901–907.

13 Toubas, J., Beck, S., Pageaud, A.L., Huby, A.C., Mael-Ainin, M., Dussaule, J.C., Chatziantoniou, C., and Chadjichristos, C.E. (2011) Alteration of connexin expression is an early signal for chronic kidney disease. *American Journal of Physiology. Renal Physiology*, **301** (1), F24–F32.

14 Azibani, F., Benard, L., Schlossarek, S., Merval, R., Tournoux, F., Fazal, L., Polidano, E., Launay, J.M., Carrier, L., Chatziantoniou, C., Samuel, J.L., and Delcayre, C. (2012) Aldosterone inhibits antifibrotic factors in mouse hypertensive heart. *Hypertension*, **59** (6), 1179–1187.

15 Azibani, F., Devaux, Y., Coutance, G., Polidano, E., Fazal, L., Merval, R., Carrier, L., Chatziantoniou, C., Samuel, J.L., and Delcayre, C. (2012) Aldosterone induces a unique hypertrophic phenotype in the hypertensive heart. *PLoS One*, **7** (5), e38197.

16 Chevalier, R.L., Forbes, M.S., and Thornhill, B.A. (2009) Ureteral obstruction as a model of renal interstitial fibrosis and obstructive nephropathy. *Kidney International*, **75** (11), 1145–1152.

17 Guerrot, D., Kerroch, M., Placier, S., Vandermeersch, S., Trivin, C., Mael-Ainin, M., Chatziantoniou, C., and Dussaule, J.C. (2011) Discoidin domain receptor 1 is a major mediator of inflammation and fibrosis in obstructive nephropathy. *The American Journal of Pathology*, **179** (1), 83–91.

18 Hsu, C.H., Kurtz, T.W., Rosenzweig, J., and Weller, J.M. (1977) Intrarenal hemodynamics and ureteral pressure during ureteral obstruction. *Investigative Urology*, **14** (6), 442–445.

19 Dai, C., Yang, J., and Liu, Y. (2003) Transforming growth factor-beta1 potentiates renal tubular epithelial cell death by a mechanism independent of Smad signaling. *The Journal of Biological Chemistry*, **278** (14), 12537–12545.

20 Esteban, V., Lorenzo, O., Rupérez, M., Suzuki, Y., Mezzano, S., Blanco, J., Kretzler, M., Sugaya, T., Egido, J., and Ruiz-Ortega, M. (2004) Angiotensin II, via AT1 and AT2 receptors and NF-kappaB pathway, regulates the inflammatory response in unilateral ureteral obstruction. *Journal of the American Society of Nephrology*, **15** (6), 1514–1529.

21 Wei, Q. and Dong, Z. (2012) Mouse model of ischemic acute kidney injury: technical notes and tricks. *American Journal of Physiology. Renal Physiology*, **303** (11), F1487–F1494.

22 Eltzschig, H.K. and Eckle, T. (2011) Ischemia and reperfusion: from mechanism to translation. *Nature Medicine*, **17** (11), 1391–1401.

23 Heyman, S.N., Rosenberger, C., and Rosen, S. (2010) Experimental ischemia–

reperfusion: biases and myths – the proximal vs. distal hypoxic tubular injury debate revisited. *Kidney International*, **77** (1), 9–16.

24 Kalluri, R., Wilson, C.B., Weber, M., Gunwar, S., Chonko, A.M., Neilson, E.G., and Hudson, B.G. (1995) Identification of the alpha 3 chain of type IV collagen as the common autoantigen in antibasement membrane disease and Goodpasture syndrome. *Journal of the American Society of Nephrology*, **6** (4), 1178–1185.

25 Steblay, R.W. (1962) Glomerulonephritis induced in sheep by injections of heterologous glomerular basement membrane and Freund's complete adjuvant. *The Journal of Experimental Medicine*, **116**, 253–272.

26 Salant, D.J. and Cybulsky, A.V. (1988) Experimental glomerulonephritis. *Methods in Enzymology*, **162**, 421–461.

27 Reynolds, J. (2011) Strain differences and the genetic basis of experimental autoimmune anti-glomerular basement membrane glomerulonephritis. *International Journal of Experimental Pathology*, **92** (3), 211–217.

28 Reynolds, J., Albouainain, A., Duda, M.A., Evans, D.J., and Pusey, C.D. (2006) Strain susceptibility to active induction and passive transfer of experimental autoimmune glomerulonephritis in the rat. *Nephrology, Dialysis, Transplantation*, **21** (12), 3398–3408.

29 Xie, C., Sharma, R., Wang, H., Zhou, X.J., and Mohan, C. (2004) Strain distribution pattern of susceptibility to immune-mediated nephritis. *Journal of Immunology*, **172** (8), 5047–5055.

30 Mesnard, L., Keller, A.C., Michel, M.L., Vandermeersch, S., Rafat, C., Letavernier, E., Tillet, Y., Rondeau, E., and Leite-de-Moraes, M.C. (2009) Invariant natural killer T cells and TGF-beta attenuate anti-GBM glomerulonephritis. *Journal of the American Society of Nephrology*, **20** (6), 1282–1292.

31 Kerroch, M., Guerrot, D., Vandermeersch, S., Placier, S., Mesnard, L., Jouanneau, C., Rondeau, E., Ronco, P., Boffa, J.J., Chatziantoniou, C., and Dussaule, J.C. (2012) Genetic inhibition of discoidin domain receptor 1 protects mice against crescentic glomerulonephritis. *The FASEB Journal*, **26** (10), 4079–4091.

32 Flamant, M., Placier, S., Rodenas, A., Curat, C.A., Vogel, W.F., Chatziantoniou, C., and Dussaule, J.C. (2006) Discoidin domain receptor 1 null mice are protected against hypertension-induced renal disease. *Journal of the American Society of Nephrology*, **17** (12), 3374–3381.

33 Mihout, F., Shweke, N., Bigé, N., Jouanneau, C., Dussaule, J.C., Ronco, P., Chatziantoniou, C., and Boffa, J.J. (2011) Asymmetric dimethylarginine (ADMA) induces chronic kidney disease through a mechanism involving collagen and TGF-β1 synthesis. *The Journal of Pathology*, **223** (1), 37–45.

34 Boffa, J.J., Tharaux, P.L., Placier, S., Ardaillou, R., Dussaule, J.C., and Chatziantoniou, C. (1999) Angiotensin II activates collagen type I gene in the renal vasculature of transgenic mice during inhibition of nitric oxide synthesis: evidence for an endothelin-mediated mechanism. *Circulation*, **100** (18), 1901–1908.

35 Boffa, J.J., Lu, Y., Placier, S., Stefanski, A., Dussaule, J.C., and Chatziantoniou, C. (2003) Regression of renal vascular and glomerular fibrosis: role of angiotensin II receptor antagonism and matrix metalloproteinases. *Journal of the American Society of Nephrology*, **14** (5), 1132–1144.

36 Chatziantoniou, C., Boffa, J.J., Ardaillou, R., and Dussaule, J.C. (1998) Nitric oxide inhibition induces early activation of type I collagen gene in renal resistance vessels and glomeruli in transgenic mice. Role of endothelin. *The Journal of Clinical Investigation*, **101** (12), 2780–2789.

37 Hocher, B., Thöne-Reineke, C., Rohmeiss, P., Schmager, F., Slowinski, T., Burst, V., Siegmund, F., Quertermous, T., Bauer, C., Neumayer, H.H., Schleuning, W.D., and Theuring, F. (1997) Endothelin-1 transgenic mice develop glomerulosclerosis, interstitial fibrosis, and renal cysts but not hypertension. *The Journal of Clinical Investigation*, **99** (6), 1380–1389.

38 Lautrette, A., Li, S., Alili, R., Sunnarborg, S.W., Burtin, M., Lee, D.C., Friedlander, G., and Terzi, F. (2005) Angiotensin II and EGF receptor cross-talk in chronic kidney diseases: a new therapeutic approach. *Nature Medicine*, **11** (8), 867–874.

39 Bollée, G., Flamant, M., Schordan, S., Fligny, C., Rumpel, E., Milon, M.,

Schordan, E., Sabaa, N., Vandermeersch, S., Galaup, A., Rodenas, A., Casal, I., Sunnarborg, S.W., Salant, D.J., Kopp, J.B., Threadgill, D.W., Quaggin, S.E., Dussaule, J.C., Germain, S., Mesnard, L., Endlich, K., Boucheix, C., Belenfant, X., Callard, P., Endlich, N., and Tharaux, P.L. (2011) Epidermal growth factor receptor promotes glomerular injury and renal failure in rapidly progressive crescentic glomerulonephritis. *Nature Medicine*, **17** (10), 1242–1250.

40 Haque, M.Z. and Majid, D.S. (2008) Reduced renal responses to nitric oxide synthase inhibition in mice lacking the gene for gp91phox subunit of NAD(P)H oxidase. *American Journal of Physiology. Renal Physiology*, **295** (3), F758–F764.

41 Ochodnicky, P., Vettoretti, S., Henning, R.H., Buikema, H., Van Dokkum, R.P., and de Zeeuw, D. (2006) Endothelial dysfunction in chronic kidney disease: determinant of susceptibility to end-organ damage and therapeutic response. *Journal of Nephrology*, **19** (3), 246–258.

42 Dussaule, J.C. and Chatziantoniou, C. (2007) Reversal of renal disease: is it enough to inhibit the action of angiotensin II? *Cell Death and Differentiation*, **14** (7), 1343–1349.

43 Guerrot, D., Dussaule, J.C., Mael-Ainin, M., Xu-Dubois, Y.C., Rondeau, E., Chatziantoniou, C., and Placier, S. (2012) Identification of periostin as a critical marker of progression/reversal of hypertensive nephropathy. *PLoS One*, **7** (3), e31974.

44 Versari, D., Daghini, E., Virdis, A., Ghiadoni, L., and Taddei, S. (2009) Endothelial dysfunction as a target for prevention of cardiovascular disease. *Diabetes Care*, **32** (Suppl. 2), S314–S321.

45 Guerrot, D., Dussaule, J.C., Kavvadas, P., Boffa, J.J., Chadjichristos, C.E., and Chatziantoniou, C. (2012) Progression of renal fibrosis: the underestimated role of endothelial alterations. *Fibrogenesis Tissue Repair*, **5** (Suppl. 1), S15–S20.

46 Crowley, S.D., Gurley, S.B., Herrera, M.J., Ruiz, P., Griffiths, R., Kumar, A.P., Kim, H.S., Smithies, O., Le, T.H., and Coffman, T.M. (2006) Angiotensin II causes hypertension and cardiac hypertrophy through its receptors in the kidney. *Proceedings of the National Academy of Sciences of the United States of America*, **103** (47), 17985–17990.

47 Ying, L., Flamant, M., Vandermeersch, S., Boffa, J.J., Chatziantoniou, C., Dussaule, J.C., and Chansel, D. (2003) Renal effects of omapatrilat and captopril in salt-loaded, nitric oxide-deficient rats. *Hypertension*, **42** (5), 937–944.

48 Stengel, B., Antignac, C., Baverel, G., Choukroun, G., Cussenot, O., Dussaule, J.C., Friedlander, G., Lang, P., Lelièvre-Pégorier, M., Massy, Z., Monteiro, R., Parini, A., Soulillou, J.P., Baud, L., and Ronco, P. (2007) Renal and urinary tract disease national research program. *Nephrology and Therapeutics*, **3** (4), 157–162.

49 Alpers, C.E. and Hudkins, K.L. (2011) Mouse models of diabetic nephropathy. *Current Opinion in Nephrology and Hypertension*, **20** (3), 278–284.

50 Brown, K., Phillips, R.E., and Wong, W. (2010) What have we learnt from experimental renal transplantation? *Nephron. Experimental Nephrology*, **115** (1), e9–e14.

51 Viau, A., El Karoui, K., Laouari, D., Burtin, M., Nguyen, C., Mori, K., Pillebout, E., Berger, T., Mak, T.W., Knebelmann, B., Friedlander, G., Barasch, J., and Terzi, F. (2010) Lipocalin 2 is essential for chronic kidney disease progression in mice and humans. *The Journal of Clinical Investigation*, **120** (11), 4065–4076.

52 Singh, A.P., Junemann, A., Muthuraman, A., Jaggi, A.S., Singh, N., Grover, K., and Dhawan, R. (2012) Animal models of acute renal failure. *Pharmacological Reports*, **64** (1), 31–44.

25
Genitourinary Disorders: Lower Urinary Tract and Sexual Functions

Pierre Clément, Delphine Behr-Roussel, and François Giuliano

25.1
Introduction

Nonmalignant diseases of the urogenital system and sexual disorders affect a large number of people and can be life-threatening, for example, renal failure due to neurogenic bladder has enormous impact on the quality of life of patients. Preclinical research in urology and sexual medicine undoubtedly improved the clinical management of urogenitosexual dysfunctions. Noninvasive or minimally invasive techniques in humans have provided insights into the normal or pathological physiology of lower urinary tract (LUT) and sexual functions. However, most of our knowledge about pathophysiological and pharmacological mechanisms regarding these functions comes from more invasive exploration in animal paradigms. These paradigms have proven valuable from exploratory, explanatory, and predictive perspectives. The rat has been, and continues to be, the most utilized laboratory animal for preclinical research in functional urology and sexual medicine, as in many other biomedical domains. In this chapter, we present the most commonly used *in vivo* models for exploring urogenitosexual functions and evaluating potential treatments of urogenitosexual dysfunctions.

25.2
Lower Urinary Tract Function

The urinary bladder and the urethra have two main roles: (i) storage of urine (continence) and (ii) periodic release of urine (micturition). Both functions are under the control of the same tightly connected central (brain and spinal cord) and peripheral (autonomic and somatic) components (reviewed in Ref. [1]). The micturition cycle displays particular features compared with many other visceral physiological processes in that (i) underlying mechanisms switch in an all-or-none manner (between continence and micturition) and (ii) micturition is under voluntary control, thereby involving higher brain areas.

25.2.1
Physiology of Micturition

During the continence phase, the bladder smooth muscle (detrusor) is relaxed while the outlet is closed due to contracted bladder neck (junction between bladder and urethra) and urethral sphincters (internal and external). Conversely, during micturition, the detrusor contracts and the bladder neck relaxes preceded by the relaxation of the urethral sphincters. The coordinated activity of the different elements of the LUT necessary for the micturition cycle to occur is organized in the spinal cord and brain, where multiple reflex pathways control the peripheral nervous system innervating the LUT. The central pathways, which function as an on–off switching circuit, integrate somatosensory information and manage reciprocal relationships between bladder and its outlet, which are summarized as follows:

- *Continence phase:* Bladder sensory afferents are silent with sympathetic and somatic outputs to the LUT responsible for detrusor relaxation and bladder sphincters contraction, respectively.
- *Micturition phase:* As bladder fills with urine, sensory inputs increase until a threshold is reached. Then, the spinobulbospinal reflex circuitry is activated, which stimulates the parasympathetic efferent and inhibits both sympathetic and somatic efferents to the LUT, causing detrusor contraction and bladder sphincters relaxation. As a result, urine flows through the urethra with minimal resistance. The voiding reflex is under voluntary control except in certain neuropathological conditions (e.g., spinal cord trauma).

25.2.2
Investigation of Lower Urinary Tract Function

Evaluating spontaneous diuresis in laboratory animals is readily feasible in a physiologically relevant environment in absence of anesthesia and restraint. This method allows continuous collection of data (micturition volume and frequency) over a long period of time and is of value for assessing chronic treatments effect on LUT function/dysfunction. However, the experimental approach is only slightly informative regarding the mechanism of action of tested therapies and is not detailed presently. Most widely used *in vivo* experimental models for mechanistic exploration of LUT are presented in the following sections.

25.2.2.1 Cystometry Evaluation
The bladder behaves like a low-pressure reservoir with intravesical pressure progressively increasing while bladder volume augments until the micturition threshold is reached (Figure 25.1). Then, a voiding reflex is triggered, which generates a peak in intravesical pressure leading to bladder emptying. The principle of measuring changes in intravesical pressure during micturition cycles

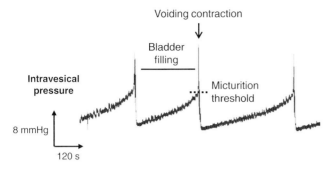

Figure 25.1 Representative cystometry recording in anesthetized rat. Intravesical pressure slowly increases as a solution is infused into the bladder lumen (bladder filling) until a threshold pressure (micturition threshold) is reached to initiate a strong bladder contraction leading to expulsion of bladder content (voiding contraction).

(i.e., cystometry) is the most common means to investigate bladder function in various animal models similarly to humans.

Cystometry experiments consist in monitoring intravesical pressure as a physiological solution is infused at a constant rate into the bladder. This is achieved by inserting a catheter through the bladder dome, which allows bladder perfusion and intravesical pressure recording simultaneously. The method can be applied to anesthetized or conscious animals in normal or pathophysiological models (cf. Section 25.2.3). In conscious animals, the free end of the bladder catheter is tunneled subcutaneously and exteriorized at the back of the neck to allow repeated recordings in unrestrained animals. The endpoints obtained from the cystometry evaluation are (i) micturition threshold pressure, (ii) amplitude of intravesical pressure during voiding, (iii) time interval between voidings, (iv) bladder capacity and compliance, and (v) voiding efficiency.

An alternative to the cystometry procedure already described is the isovolumetric model that consists in measuring, in anesthetized animals, intravesical pressure changes while ureters are tied and bladder outlet blocked, preventing bladder emptying (Figure 25.2). In this model, a solution is slowly infused until bladder contraction is triggered and then the infusion is stopped and bladder reflex contractions reproduce rhythmically. Frequency and amplitude of reflex contractions are the parameters determined during isovolumetric cystometry. Although this method represents a highly extraphysiological model, its use has provided conclusions similar to normal cystometry on some drug effects [2–4].

25.2.2.2 Evaluation of Urethral Function

Bladder outlet function is derived from a complex interplay between pelviperineal striated muscles and urethral wall. Striated muscles include pelvic floor skeletal muscles and external urethral sphincter (EUS), which is part of the urethra wall, together with urethral smooth muscle. Both striated and smooth muscle components contribute to the micturition cycle, so that continence is maintained when intraurethral pressure exceeds intravesical pressure.

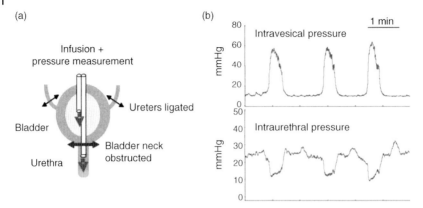

Figure 25.2 Isovolumetric cystometry in anesthetized rat. (a) Two catheters are inserted via the bladder dome. One allows the measurement of intravesical pressure and the perfusion of the bladder (isovolumetric cystometry); the other is inserted into the proximal urethra and allows the measurement of urethral pressure and urethral perfusion. The separation of the bladder and the urethral lumen is performed by a ligature of the urethra by placing a tie just distal to the bladder neck. (b) Recording of intravesical and intraurethral pressures in isovolumetric conditions shows rhythmic contractions of bladder with concomitant relaxation of urethra, reflecting synchronized activity between detrusor and urethral sphincter.

Intraurethral Pressure Intraurethral pressure is created by active mechanisms comprising contractions of striated and smooth muscles. In laboratory animals, intraurethral pressure can be monitored at several levels (consecutively or simultaneously) of the urethra using different techniques, including catheter, balloon, and microtip-type pressure transducers. Intraurethral pressure can be measured in combination with intravesical pressure in isovolumetric conditions by inserting two catheters through the bladder dome (Figure 25.2).

External Urethral Sphincter Electromyogram In human, EUS has an important contribution to intraurethral pressure and plays a major role in urinary continence. In anesthetized animals, EUS rhythmic activity is monitored through micturition cycle by placing recording electrodes into the periurethral striated muscles. Electromyogram (EMG) of EUS can be obtained concomitantly to intravesical pressure in the same animal in order to assess the coordination between the detrusor and the EUS. Frequency and amplitude of contractions are determined as parameters characterizing EUS functioning. This approach is of particular interest in pathophysiological conditions where coordination between detrusor and sphincter is impaired (e.g., neurogenic vesicosphincteric dyssynergia).

25.2.2.3 Bladder Afferent Recording

Vesical somatosensory inputs are essential for normal micturition cycle to occur. Sensory, notably sensation of bladder fullness, and nociceptive information is conveyed to the spinal cord via small myelinated Aδ and unmyelinated C-fibers traveling mainly through the pelvic nerve. Somas of primary sensory neurons innervating the bladder are located in the dorsal root ganglia (sacral and lumbosacral levels in humans and rats, respectively). Recording of bladder afferent firing is feasible in anesthetized or decerebrated animals, in order to eliminate anesthesia as a confounding factor. A bundle of fibers are dissected from the L6 dorsal roots and a single fiber is placed on a recording electrode. Afferent nerve fibers originating in the bladder are identified by applying electrical stimulation to the pelvic nerve or by bladder distension using intravesical catheter (cf. Section 25.2.2.1). Then, the bladder is filled and both the bladder afferent nerve firing and intravesical pressure are recorded simultaneously in order to correlate afferent and detrusor activities [5].

25.2.3
Pathophysiological Models

Lower urinary tract disorders can be schematically classified as disturbances of filling/storage or disturbances of emptying. Malfunction can affect bladder, urethra, or their coordinated activity (e.g., vesicosphincteric dyssynergia following spinal cord injury (SCI)) with, for most of the pathological conditions, multifactorial and unclear etiologies. The latest issue complicates the development of relevant preclinical models for clarifying pathogenesis and testing treatments. Nevertheless, a number of animal paradigms proposed to date have been shown of heuristic value, leading to significant improvement in the understanding of pathophysiology and in the management of LUT disorders in humans.

25.2.3.1 Bladder Outlet Obstruction

LUT associated with benign prostatic hyperplasia (BPH) is a highly prevalent condition in aged men. Enlargement of the prostate can be responsible for urethral obstruction accompanied by a number of voiding and storage symptoms (e.g., urinary urgency, frequency, and small voided volume). Naturally occurring BPH has been reported in dogs and chimpanzees [6,7]. Experimental *in vivo* models of BPH in rodents and rabbits have been developed, which consists in performing bladder outlet obstruction either by physical method (ligature of urethra) or by inducing prostate hyperplasia (testosterone or carcinogen) (reviewed in Ref. [8]). In these models, many of the structural and physiological bladder wall features that are found in BPH–LUT patients progressively appear. In addition, cystometry evaluation in anesthetized or conscious-obstructed animals demonstrates dysfunction similar to the BPH–LUT patients. Among the available models, BPH induced by testosterone in rats more closely mimics the human pathology in that the prostate of 14 days hormonally treated rats displays prostate enlargement as well as stromal and epithelial compartments proliferation [9].

25.2.3.2 Overactive Bladder

Overactive bladder (OAB) exhibits symptoms that are suggestive of urodynamically proven detrusor overactivity (involuntary detrusor contraction) during the filling phase, which may be spontaneous or provoked. This translates in urinary urgency with or without urge incontinence and, usually frequent micturition and nocturia. Overactive bladder can be divided into neurogenic, when there is a relevant neurological condition (cf. Section 25.2.3.3), or nonneurogenic (idiopathic OAB). The main symptom of OAB in humans is urinary urgency, which is associated with involuntary bladder contractions with or without urge urinary incontinence. Involuntary bladder contractions can be induced and monitored by cystometry recordings in animal models of spontaneous or provoked bladder hyperactivity.

Spontaneously Hypertensive Rat This genetic rat model is the most widely used animal model of hypertension. In addition, spontaneously hypertensive rats (SHRs) display abnormal bladder function with neuromorphological and neurochemical changes impacting bladder efferent (notably sympathetic) and afferent [10]. Cystometry evaluation in SHRs evidences features of bladder hyperactivity found in patients with OAB: decreased voided volume, increased urinary frequency, and occurrence of nonvoiding contractions.

Provoked Bladder Hyperactivity Intravesical instillation of a variety of chemicals in anesthetized laboratory animals is widely used to produce acute models of OAB. They include, but are not limited to, prostaglandin E2, agonist of vanilloid receptors (capsaicin and resiniferatoxin), protamine sulfate, and acetic acid [11–14]. These compounds cause bladder irritation or pain through activation of afferent C-fibers resulting in increased detrusor activity and decreased micturition threshold and bladder capacity as demonstrated by cystometry evaluation.

25.2.3.3 Neurogenic Detrusor Overactivity

A variety of neurological pathologies (e.g., multiple sclerosis and Parkinson's disease) may cause OAB, namely, neurogenic detrusor overactivity (NDO) in this context. Spinal cord injury is also responsible for NDO, often associated with detrusor sphincter dyssynergia (DSD). SCI in the rat is an experimental approach that is commonly implemented to study pharmacology of NDO. Lesion of the spinal cord, rostral to lumbosacral levels, can be performed using different procedures (concussion or trans/hemisections). In rats and humans, a spinal micturition reflex progressively develops after SCI that is responsible for NDO. The neurobiological substrate for NDO comprises structural and functional alterations of the bladder wall as well as increased vesical afferent sensory messages [15]. Cystometry measurements in conscious SCI rats show pathophysiological features that resemble NDO in SCI patients (Figure 25.3). Nonvoiding contractions testify OAB and reduced voiding efficiency, and large residual urine volumes are indications of DSD, which can be demonstrated by recording EUS EMG concomitantly to intravesical pressure in anesthetized SCI animals [16].

25.2.3.4 Painful Bladder Syndrome/Interstitial Cystitis

Painful bladder syndrome (PBS) or interstitial cystitis (IC) is characterized by urinary urgency and frequency due to exaggerated sensation of pain or pressure caused by bladder hypersensitivity, in the absence of evident LUT infection. The

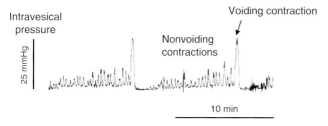

Figure 25.3 Representative cystometry recording in conscious spinal cord injured rat (3 weeks after complete transection). High-frequency small-amplitude ineffective (nonvoiding) bladder contractions occur in the interval between more intense effective (voiding) contractions, reflecting detrusor overactivity.

exact etiology of PBS/IC is unknown, but may include chronic subclinical infection, autoimmunity, or neurogenic inflammation. Several *in vivo* experimental models of PBS/IC have been designed (reviewed in Ref. [17]). Spontaneous PBS/IC can occur in the cat, although it is unclear whether this disorder in cat is analogous to human situation. In addition, occurrence of PBS/IC is not predictable, rendering this model difficult to implement. Features of bladder dysfunction (decreased bladder capacity and intervoiding time intervals) and morphological changes (edema and inflammatory cells infiltration) observed in PBS/IC humans and cats can be reproduced in healthy anesthetized or conscious animals by delivering chemicals or toxins intravesically (e.g., lipopolysaccharide) or systemically (e.g., cyclophosphamide). These standardized experimental approaches are most commonly used in preclinical research.

25.3
Sexual Functions

Sexual functions are unique in that they are not vital, although a major preoccupation, for the individual, but are mandatory for the perpetuation of the species. The human (female and male) sexual response comprises intimately interrelated phases that are desire, excitement, orgasm, and resolution. Each of these phases is controlled by a complex and coordinated interplay of multiple components of the brain, spinal cord, and relevant peripheral organs (reviewed in Ref. [18]).

25.3.1
Physiology of Female and Male Sexual Response

Sexual desire, also termed libido in human or motivation in animals, is defined as the biological need for sexual activity. It involves detection of a suitable mate, approach to it, and establishment of initial contact. What makes the study of sexual desire complex is the fact that corresponding behaviors are highly variable in their expression from one species to another and depend on the context. Sexual desire is mainly controlled by brain mechanisms. In laboratory animals, behavioral manifestations of sexual desire (either innate or learned) can be stereotyped, objectively analyzed, and reliably quantified using standardized experimental paradigms.

Sexual arousal in both humans and animals can be defined as an increase in autonomic activation that prepares the body for sexual activity. In mammals, this translates in physiological modifications in genital organs, but also more globally (heart and respiratory rates, blood pressure, sweat production, etc.). Increased blood flow to genital organs and tumescence of erectile tissues (clitoris and penis) due to blood engorgement are the most specific measurable features of sexual arousal. Sexual arousal also includes a central component that increases neural tone or "awareness" to respond to sexual incentives. Functional investigations have demonstrated that local and global physiological changes associated with sexual arousal result from brain control and spinal reflexes, involving specific centers at different levels of the spinal cord.

Ejaculation terminates sexual interaction in males and is followed by a refractory period during which further sexual stimulation does not produce excitement. Ejaculation comprises two highly coordinated phases (emission and expulsion) and leads to the forceful expulsion of semen out of the body. Occurrence of ejaculation necessitates the process of somatosensory information essentially from the reproductive organs to the spinal cord and the brain. The peripheral synchronized events of ejaculation, which involve sex glands and pelviperineal striated muscles, are organized in a spinal generator identified in the male rat where peripheral and central sexual stimuli are summated.

There are many differences between human and animal sexual behaviors, although homologies and, most often analogies, with mammalian animal models have shed light on the physiology and pharmacology of human sexual functions.

25.3.2
Models for Sexual Behavior

Sexual behavior occurs as a sequence of behavioral events that greatly vary from one species to another. The concept of separating sexual behavior into appetitive (sexual desire/motivation) and consummatory (copulation) aspects has proven valuable. Appetitive behaviors are defined as those bringing the individual into contact with sexual incentives or with sexually meaningful goal objects. These behaviors are flexible, depending on the experience of the individual, and can be learned. Consummatory behaviors are those exhibited by the individual once the sexual incentive or assimilated goal object is reached. Consummatory behaviors are more stereotyped and species and gender specific than appetitive ones. Both aspects of sexual behavior can be investigated during separate or same experimental procedures.

25.3.2.1 Sexual Preference Paradigms
Sexual motivation can be evaluated using sexual preference paradigms that are instrumental responses where preference is instinctive or conditioned. There are

two experimental procedures that have been more widely implemented to measure sexual motivation in laboratory animals (reviewed in Ref. [19]).

Conditioned Place or Partner Preference A neutral cue in the environment, which may be a distinctive feature (e.g., colored area and floor texture) or an odorized partner, for example, is associated with sexual interaction. After conditioning, the animal displays preference for the cue that has been paired with sexual interaction over other(s) that has not. Preference is objectively measured by determining the number of times the subject chooses for or the time it spends with the sex-related cue. Effects of acute and chronic treatment on the interest of the animal for sexual interaction may be assessed in pathophysiological models.

Sexual Incentive Motivation Tests This simple test uses instinctive sexual incentive and, as such does not require conditioning or learning. However, animals must be sexually experienced prior to the sexual incentive motivation test. Sexual motivation is evaluated for an individual placed in an open field where it can choose to interact, without direct physical contact, with a sexual incentive versus a social nonsexual incentive. Sexual preference is evidenced by measuring the higher proportion of time the experimental subject spends in the sexual incentive zone.

25.3.2.2 Copulatory Tests

Copulatory tests investigate both the consummatory and motivational aspects of sexual behavior [20]. Description and measurement of copulatory behavior cannot be summarized here, as it is manifested in its diverse forms from one species to another. We instead present the example of the rat, the most extensively utilized animal model for preclinical studies in sexual medicine.

A sexually receptive female rat engaged in sexual interaction with a male rat displays proceptive and receptive behaviors. Proceptive behaviors (e.g., ear wiggling, hops, and darts) are to solicit attention and approach of the male, whereas receptive behavior is a more passive reaction the female exhibits when the male mounts (i.e., lordosis: back arching). Because lordosis is a postural reflex hormonally dependent and has no counterpart in woman, quantification of proceptivity during standardized copulatory test represents the most transposable measure to the human situation. In the male rat, consummatory behavior consists of mounts, intromissions, and ejaculations that occur in the form of bouts: mounts and intromissions succeed until ejaculation, which is followed by a period of lower activity (refractory period, typically 4–8 min) and then sexual activity resumes. Global sexual performance, but also, more specifically, erectile and ejaculatory performance, as well as sexual motivation, is assessed by determining parameters (number and latency of behavioral events as primary endpoints) of male rat copulatory behavior during standardized tests. Copulatory behavior can be explored using various apparatus; each having advantages and limitations. The bi-level chamber (Figure 25.4) appears the most elegant test that allows reliable, rapid, and repeated evaluation of both motivational and consummatory behaviors in female and male rats.

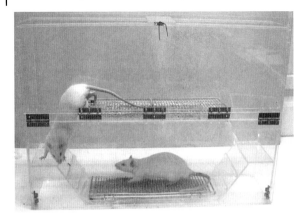

Figure 25.4 Bi-level chamber apparatus for exploration of sexual behavior in the rat. Both motivational and copulatory aspects of sexual behavior can be assessed in female and male rats.

25.3.3
Investigation of the Peripheral Female Sexual Response

There are many similarities in the neuroanatomical organization of female genitalia in mammals, justifying the use of laboratory animals for further understanding of pathophysiology and pharmacology of woman's peripheral sexual response. Genital sexual arousal is characterized by vaginal engorgement with blood. Noninvasive monitoring of blood flow and oxygen partial pressure in the vaginal wall, as well as temperature in the vaginal lumen, is feasible using a microprobe placed in the vagina of anesthetized animals. Vaginal response is elicited by electrical stimulation of the pelvic nerve (parasympathetic innervation) and physiological variables are quantified as objective measures of genital arousal [21]. Stimulation of the genital somatosensory afferents can also induce vaginal blood flow increase through spinal pathways, allowing investigation of the afferent branch of the female genital reflex [22].

25.3.4
Investigation of Erection

Erection is essentially a neurally controlled vascular event depending on the balance between arterial inflow and venous outflow in the penile erectile tissues (corpora cavernosa and corpus spongiosum, including the glans penis). As blood accumulates, the penis gains the rigidity necessary for effective intromission.

25.3.4.1 Penile Reflex
Erection stimulated by touch outside the context of copulation is commonly referred to as reflexive erection. In male rats, reflexive penile erections and movements can be observed in conscious animals restrained on their back if the penile sheath is

retracted with light pressure directed at the base of the penis. The penis shows a characteristic pattern of tumescence and detumescence accompanied by "cups" (the end of the erect glans penis flares out) and "flips" (rapid dorsoflexion of the erect penis). Assessing drugs action on both afferent and efferent arms of the penile reflex in pathophysiological models is feasible using this approach.

25.3.4.2 Erection in Conscious Animals

Erection results in response to sexual cues, that is, olfactory, visual, and auditory stimuli. This type of erection has been termed "psychogenic" and can be studied in conscious rats. Occurrence of erection is observed in the experimental animal in response to sexual stimulus (e.g., estrous odors) or inaccessible female in heat. This so-called noncontact erection model is interesting to implement notably when testing pharmacological manipulation of the brain control of penile erection.

25.3.4.3 Intracavernosal Pressure Measurement

Monitoring pressure variations in the corpus cavernosum (intracavernosal pressure (ICP)) is a quantitative evaluation of erectile function that can be performed in anesthetized or conscious animals. In the male rat, ICP is obtained by inserting a catheter into the proximal shaft of the corpus cavernosum. Recording of ICP in freely moving rats, and even during copulation, is feasible by coupling the catheter with a telemetric device implanted in the animal [23]. Analysis of ICP in different experimental paradigms provides with details on pathophysiological mechanisms and drug mode of action. Whenever feasible, ICP value is expressed as a ratio of mean arterial pressure since ICP is correlated with blood pressure (Figure 25.5) [24].

In-depth investigation of the physiology and pharmacology of penile erection requires the use of anesthetized animals. Then, erection has to be triggered by acting at the central or peripheral nervous system level.

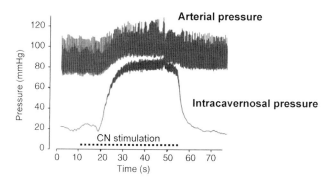

Figure 25.5 Representative recording of intracavernosal and arterial pressures in response to electrical stimulation of the cavernous nerve in anesthetized rat. Stimulation of CN induces rapid rise in ICP followed by a plateau reaching diastolic arterial pressure level (maximal tumescence). As soon as CN stimulation is stopped, ICP rapidly decreases (detumescence) to baseline level (flaccid state).

25.3.4.4 Pharmacologically Induced Erection

The dopamine receptor agonist apomorphine induces erection in anesthetized (and also conscious) male rats by acting in the brain and spinal cord [25]. This agent has been proposed to treat erectile dysfunction in men, although its use is limited because of its side effects. Erectile response to apomorphine systemic injection can be assessed (by monitoring ICP, for instance) in pathophysiological models for evaluating erection-potentiating drugs, using suboptimal dose of apomorphine, or for evidencing potential drug deleterious action on erectile function.

25.3.4.5 Neurally Evoked Erection

Another means to elicit penile erection in anesthetized animal is to perform nerve electrical stimulation. The cavernous nerve (CN) conveys the parasympathetic tone to erectile tissues and its stimulation causes increase in ICP in males of various species. Repeated electrical stimulations of varying intensity (or frequency) are applied to obtain intensity–response curve. Evolution of the curve in pathophysiological models or following treatment gives a precise evaluation of the erectile function. This model has been extensively used to test compounds with facilitatory proerectile effect.

25.3.5
Investigation of Ejaculation

Only the executive mechanisms of ejaculation are addressed; the orgasmic aspect of ejaculation lacks suitable animal model. The emission phase of ejaculation corresponds to the discharge of the different components of semen by accessory sex glands (essentially seminal vesicles and prostate) and epididymis (spermatozoa) into the urethra. The expulsion phase is characterized by rhythmic intense contractions of pelviperineal striated muscles, which propel semen throughout the urethra.

25.3.5.1 Physiological Markers of Emission and Expulsion Phases

Activities in anatomical structures participating in either emission or expulsion can be measured distinctively and simultaneously (Figure 25.6). Sex glands are hollow viscera, with smooth muscle cells that contract (upon stimulation by sympathetic system) during emission resulting in pressure increase. In the anesthetized rat, pressure variations in seminal vesicle or vas deferens (the canal that conduct spermatozoa from the epididymis to the urethra) are quantified by inserting a catheter within the lumen. Striated muscles that are involved in the expulsion phase of ejaculation include ischiocavernosus, levator ani, and more particularly bulbospongiosus (BS) muscles that are commanded by somatic system (pudendal nerve). Recording of EMG is feasible in not only anesthetized but also conscious male rats by placing electrodes into pelviperineal striated muscles.

As for penile erection, the use of *in vivo* models where ejaculation is triggered is key for better understanding the physiology and pharmacology of the ejaculatory process. It is notably possible to explore distinctively emission and expulsion phases of ejaculation as well as their coordination.

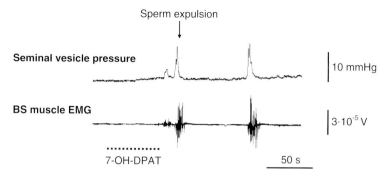

Figure 25.6 Representative recording of pressure into seminal vesicle and electromyogram of bulbospongiosus muscle in response to i.v. injection of 7-OH-DPAT in anesthetized male rat. A peak in seminal vesicle pressure (contraction of the gland) with synchronized burst of contractions of BS muscle, associated or not with sperm expulsion, occurs at several instances following delivery of the dopamine D3 receptor subtype preferential agonist 7-OH-DPAT.

25.3.5.2 Pharmacologically Induced Ejaculation

Ejaculation is obtained in anesthetized male rats by systemic delivery of the amphetamine derivative *p*-chloroamphetamine, which acts in the spinal cord through release of serotonin and noradrenaline [26]. This model is suitable for investigating peripheral modulations. The 7-OH-DPAT model offers the opportunity to study central and peripheral modulations of the ejaculatory process. Indeed, this dopamine D2/D3 receptor subtype agonists act in the brain to provoke ejaculation [27].

25.3.5.3 Lumbar Spinothalamic Neurons Electrical Stimulation

The lumbar spinothalamic neurons have been identified as a fundamental component of the spinal generator for ejaculation and have been characterized in the male rat [28]. These neurons are located around the central canal, mainly in the third and fourth lumbar spinal cord segments, and electrical microstimulation focused in this area triggers ejaculation in the anesthetized male rat. Stimulation is applied by stereotactically descending a microelectrode in the target spinal area. Physiological markers of emission and expulsion are recorded in response to microstimulation of varying intensity, allowing evaluation of lumbar spinothalamic neuron excitability thresholds in pathophysiological models or following treatments (inhibitory or potentiating).

25.3.5.4 Expulsion Spinal Reflex

Expulsion of sperm has long been suggested as a spinal reflex triggered by the peripheral events of emission, although this view is debated. This gave rise to the development of experimental paradigms in anesthetized animals that represented the first rational approaches for studying the neurophysiology and pharmacology of ejaculation.

Urethrogenital Reflex Rhythmic contractions of bulbospongiosus muscle, as evidenced on EMG, are induced by distension of the urethra (liquid accumulation) or stimulation of the sensory branch of the pudendal nerve. The urethrogenital reflex is obtained in anesthetized rats if supraspinal inhibitory tone is suppressed (spinal cord transection or more restricted lesion within the brain) [29].

Pudendal Motoneuron Reflex Discharges The principle of this model is to measure firing in the motor branch of the pudendal nerve in response to electrical stimulation of the dorsal nerve of the penis (sensory branch of the pudendal nerve). Lesion in CNS is not necessary for this reflex to occur in anesthetized rats. Modulation (inhibition or potentiation) of the reflex can be studied in different experimental conditions and notably in treated animals.

25.3.6
Pathophysiological Models

Sexual disorders have a negative impact on the quality of life and may be the cause of significant personal distress. Each aspect of the sexual response (i.e., desire, arousal, and genital function) may be altered, either occasionally or permanently. Sexual dysfunctions are lifelong or acquired and have multiple etiologies that can be primary or secondary. They can also result from the aging process. It follows from this consideration that development of animal pathophysiological models is challenging. Sexual disorders have long been taboos and the field of psychiatrists, but the neurobiological approach that emerged in sexual medicine from the end of the 1980s improved our understanding of human sexual pathophysiologies.

25.3.6.1 Female Sexual Dysfunctions
Female sexual dysfunction prevalence increases at the time of menopause. During the peri- and the postmenopause periods, women may suffer from hypoactive sexual desire disorder, sexual arousal disorder associated with lubrication difficulties, orgasm disorder, or sexual pain disorder associated with vaginal atrophy and dryness. There is a considerable degree of similarity between rats and humans in the neuroendocrine and neurochemical regulation of female sexual functions [30]. Ovariectomized nonhormonally primed females appear relevant for preclinical investigation of treatment effects on sexual dysfunctions in menopausal women. The experimental models of investigation presented in Sections 25.3.2 and 25.3.3 can be implemented to study acute or chronic treatment of the different aspects of menopause-related sexual dysfunctions.

25.3.6.2 Erectile Dysfunction
Multiple factors cause erectile dysfunction, which are in majority from peripheral origin and affect vascularization and/or innervation of erectile tissues. A number of *in vivo* models have been proposed to mimic different clinical conditions leading to erectile dysfunction.

Diabetes Mellitus There is good epidemiological evidence of a causal link between diabetes (insulin or noninsulin dependent) and erectile dysfunction. Both vascular and neural alterations explain the deleterious consequence of diabetes on erectile function. Insulin-dependent diabetes can be induced in rodents by treatment with streptozotocin that is specifically toxic for the insulin-synthesizing pancreatic islet cells. In these animals, impairment of endothelial and neurogenic relaxations of corpora cavernosa as well as penile autonomic neuropathy represents the pathophysiological features of erectile dysfunction.

Cardiovascular Condition As a vascular event, penile erection is particularly sensitive to changes in cardiovascular homeostasis. Notably, hypertension and atherosclerosis may result in erectile dysfunction. SHR was introduced in Section 25.2.3.2 with regard to overactive bladder. These animals also display impaired erectile function due to dysfunction of endothelium in erectile tissue, which occurs before endothelial dysfunction in aortic tissue (Figure 25.7a) [31]. The apolipoprotein E knockout mouse develops over time atherosclerotic lesions that resemble the human situation. Atherosclerosis, due to reduced plasma lipoproteins elimination, can be accelerated in the apolipoprotein E-deficient mice by a lipid-enriched diet. In this pathophysiological model, erectile function is significantly impaired as a consequence of endothelial dysfunction in erectile bodies (Figure 25.7b) [32].

Neurogenic Erectile Dysfunction Radical prostatectomy and cystoprostatectomy are often accompanied by erectile dysfunction. Neural lesion (impacting pelvic plexus or cavernous nerve) is the principal cause. Cavernous nerve crush injury in the rat mimics neural damages associated with pelvic surgeries in the humans. In this model, erectile dysfunction is reported 3–4 weeks after bilateral nerve lesion.

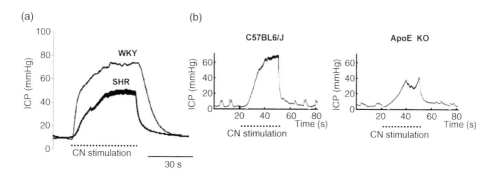

Figure 25.7 Erectile dysfunction in pathophysiological models. (a) Spontaneously hypertensive rats display decreased intracavernosal pressure amplitude in response to cavernous nerve stimulation compared with Wistar Kyoto (WKY) rats, the closest genetic inbred for SHR. (b) Knockout mice for the apolipoprotein E gene (ApoE KO) also exhibit altered ICP response to CN stimulation compared with wild-type C57BL6/J strain.

25.3.6.3 Ejaculatory Disorders

Ejaculatory disorders in men, and more particularly premature ejaculation, are the most common male sexual dysfunctions. In men, biological variation of the intravaginal ejaculation latency time has been observed, which follows a Gaussian distribution. Accordingly, there are men who have short ejaculation latency time, referred to as premature ejaculation, some have retarded ejaculation, and the last category of men who ejaculate in the range of "normal" ejaculation time. Interestingly, a similar distribution of ejaculation latency has been described in male rats [33], thus giving the opportunity to use a relevant animal model of ejaculatory disorders for preclinical researches. In practice, sexually experienced male rats are categorized according to their ejaculatory performance (number and latency of ejaculations) measured during a standardized copulatory test (cf. Section 25.3.2.2). It has been observed that other quantitative parameters of male sexual behavior are comparable from one category to another, notably indicating unchanged sexual motivation. Then, males that exhibit high ejaculatory performance are regarded as "premature" ejaculators, whereas those who have low performance are regarded as "retarded/delayed" ejaculators. Following the categorization, animals can be utilized in various experimental paradigms (cf. Section 25.3.5) for drug investigation.

25.4
Translation to Clinics: Difficulties and Limitations

Translational value of animal findings is optimized when the experimental model used closely resembles the human situation. This requires a comprehensive knowledge of the physiology of urogenitosexual functions and the pathophysiological mechanisms of urogenitosexual dysfunctions. The fact that mammals share a lot of similarities in anatomy, neurophysiology, and neurochemistry of LUT and sexual functions is a valuable benefit for transposing results in animals to humans. However, interspecies differences exist that limit the significance of the findings and have to be considered when interpreting the results.

The major limitation of animal models is when clinical symptoms/signs are subjective in nature. For example, the sensation of urinary urgency in OAB and female hypoactive sexual desire or sexual arousal disorders cannot be ascertained in laboratory animals, requiring the use of surrogate markers. Even if these surrogate markers give incomplete and imperfect views of the human situation, they may share therapeutical options and underlying pathophysiological mechanisms. For instance, the melanocortin receptor agonist bremelanotide has been found to enhance proceptive behavior in female rats and to improve sexual desire and arousal in women with sexual arousal disorder [34,35]. Behavior paradigms are attractive in that they allow animal testing repeatedly in physiological conditions. A potential problem with methods evaluating sexual behavior arises if the investigated drug acts on a process that interferes with the animal's ability to take the behavioral/operant test (e.g., substance impairing locomotion, general arousal, or learning process). On the other hand, potential behavioral side effects can be estimated using such preclinical approaches.

Anesthetized models are less physiological, but they provide further insights into the pathophysiological processes and pharmacological mechanisms. One key point to be examined when implementing anesthetized experiments is the anesthetic used. For example, several anesthetics (injected or inhaled) have been shown to alter LUT function [36]. Alternatively, decerebrated animals can be utilized to avoid influence of anesthesia on bladder function. However, investigation of the role of the brain is impossible in the decerebrated model, which in addition is responsible for drastic changes in the neurophysiological control of LUT. A highly extraphysiological CNS-lesioned paradigm (i.e., urethrogenital reflex) has also been developed for exploration of sexual functions. Although this model has the same limitations as decerebrated animals and focuses on the expulsion phase of ejaculation, it has led to significant progress in our understanding of the ejaculatory process and its control.

Pharmacological models have been developed for exploring urogenitosexual functions and have provided a better description of the neurochemical control of these functions, with demonstrated translation to humans (e.g., proerectile action of apomorphine). However, when such models are implemented for assessing drug effect, interpretation of the results has to be done with regard to the mechanism of action of the tested drug and its possible interaction with the model.

Some urogenitosexual disease models display common features with human conditions, although they are not representative of the human situation, thus questioning their translational value. For example, in bladder hyperactivity induced by irritant substances like acetic acid, inflammation is obtained (a symptom that is not found in patients with OAB) and may represent a confounding factor when drugs are tested. Despite many limitations, these pathophysiological *in vivo* models have proven predictive in demonstrating the potential of pharmacological agents in the treatment of human pathologies.

Animal models in which typical human symptoms are reproduced more closely mimic clinical situation. Translation to human disease is then more straightforward and, in addition, the testing of treatment targeting the disease itself or the concomitant urogenitosexual dysfunction can be performed. For example, the BPH rat model where prostate enlargement is induced by testosterone allows investigation of therapeutical approaches either alleviating urethra obstruction or inhibiting prostatic growth.

In order to increase the translational value of preclinical findings, animal paradigms have to be compared with clinical observations and conclusions of animal studies have to be confirmed in humans whenever feasible, requiring continuous exchanges between basic, applied, and clinical scientific disciplines. Animal models in urogenitosexual research have been developed that are homologous or analogous to human situations, and of which predictive capability has been demonstrated. However, progress is still needed, more particularly in the development of urogenitosexual disease *in vivo* models, which undoubtedly will improve medical management of LUT and sexual dysfunctions.

References

1 Andersson, K.-E. and Arner, A. (2004) Urinary bladder contraction and relaxation: physiology and pathophysiology. *Physiological Reviews*, **84**, 935–986.

2 Giuliani, S., Lecci, A., Tramontana, M., and Maggi, C.A. (1998) The inhibitory effect of nociceptin on the micturition reflex in anaesthetized rats. *British Journal of Pharmacology*, **124**, 1566–1572.

3 Lecci, A., Giuliani, S., Tramontana, M., Criscuoli, M., and Maggi, C.A. (2000) Multiple sites of action in the inhibitory effect of nociceptin on the micturition reflex. *The Journal of Urology*, **163**, 638–645.

4 Cefalu, J.S., Guillon, M.A., Burbach, L.R., Zhu, Q.M., Hu, D.Q., Ho, M.J., Ford, A.P., Nunn, P.A., and Cockayne, D.A. (2009) Selective pharmacological blockade of the TRPV1 receptor suppresses sensory reflexes of the rodent bladder. *The Journal of Urology*, **182**, 776–785.

5 Behr-Roussel, D., Oger, S., Caisey, S., Sandner, P., Bernabé, J., Alexandre, L., and Giuliano, F. (2011) Vardenafil decreases bladder afferent nerve activity in unanesthetized, decerebrate, spinal cord-injured rats. *European Urology*, **59**, 272–279.

6 DeKlerk, D.P., Coffey, D.S., Ewing, L.L., McDermott, I.R., Reiner, W.G., Robinson, C.H., Scott, W.W., Strandberg, J.D., Talalay, P., Walsh, P.C., Wheaton, L.G., and Zirkin, B.R. (1979) Comparison of spontaneous and experimentally induced canine prostatic hyperplasia. *The Journal of Clinical Investigation*, **64**, 842–849.

7 Steiner, M.S., Couch, R.C., Raghow, S., and Stauffer, D. (1999) The chimpanzee as a model of human benign prostatic hyperplasia. *The Journal of Urology*, **162**, 1454–1461.

8 Mahapokai, W., van Sluijs, F.J., and Schalken, J.A. (2000) Models for studying benign prostatic hyperplasia. *Prostate Cancer and Prostatic Diseases*, **3**, 28–33.

9 Lee, J.Z., Omata, S., Tillig, B., Perkash, I., and Constantinou, C.E. (1998) Chronology and urodynamic characterization of micturition in neurohormonally induced experimental prostate growth in the rat. *Neurourology and Urodynamics*, **17**, 55–69.

10 Persson, K., Pandita, R.K., Spitsbergen, J.M., Steers, W.D., Tuttle, J.B., and Andersson, K.-E. (1998) Spinal and peripheral mechanisms contributing to hyperactive voiding in spontaneously hypertensive rats. *The American Journal of Physiology*, **44**, R1366–R1373.

11 Chuang, Y.C., Chancellor, M.B., Seki, S., Yoshimura, N., Tyagi, P., Huang, L., Lavelle, J.P., De Groat, W.C., and Fraser, M.O. (2003) Intravesical protamine sulfate and potassium chloride as a model for bladder hyperactivity. *Urology*, **61**, 664–670.

12 Ishizuka, O., Mattiasson, A., and Andersson, K.-E. (1995) Prostaglandin E2-induced bladder hyperactivity in normal, conscious rats: involvement of tachykinins? *The Journal of Urology*, **153**, 2034–2038.

13 Ishizuka, O., Mattiasson, A., and Andersson, K.-E. (1995) Urodynamic effects of intravesical resiniferatoxin and capsaicin in conscious rats with and without outflow obstruction. *The Journal of Urology*, **154**, 611–616.

14 Caremel, R., Oger-Roussel, S., Behr-Roussel, D., Grise, P., and Giuliano, F.A. (2010) Nitric oxide/cyclic guanosine monophosphate signalling mediates an inhibitory action on sensory pathways of the micturition reflex in the rat. *European Urology*, **58**, 616–625.

15 De Groat, W.C., Kawatatni, T., and Hisamitsu, T. (1995) Mechanisms underlying the recovery of urinary bladder function following spinal cord injury. *Paraplegia*, **33**, 493–505.

16 Behr-Roussel, D., Oger, S., Pignol, B., Pham, E., Le Maux, A., Chabrier, P.E., Caisey, S., Compagnie, S., Picaut, P., Bernabé, J., Alexandre, L., Giuliano, F., and Denys, P. (2012) Minimal effective dose of dysport and botox in a rat model of neurogenic detrusor overactivity. *European Urology*, **61**, 1054–1061.

17 Westropp, J.L. and Buffington, C.A. (2002) *In vivo* models of interstitial cystitis. *The Journal of Urology*, **167**, 694–702.

18 Gelez, H., Clément, P., and Giuliano, F. (2008) Physiology of normal sexual function, in *Textbook of the Neurogenic Bladder*, 2nd edn (eds J. Corcos and E.

Schick), Informa Healthcare, London, pp. 116–145.

19 Agmo, A. (1999) Sexual motivation: an inquiry into events determining the occurrence of sexual behavior. *Behavioural Brain Research*, **105**, 129–150.

20 Giuliano, F., Pfaus, J., Srilatha, B., Hedlund, P., Hisasue, S., Marson, L., and Wallen, K. (2010) Experimental models for the study of female and male sexual function. *Journal of Sexual Medicine*, **7**, 2970–2995.

21 Giuliano, F., Allard, J., Compagnie, S., Alexandre, L., Droupy, S., and Bernabé, J. (2001) Vaginal physiological changes in a model of sexual arousal in anesthetized rats. *American Journal of Physiology. Regulatory, Integrative and Comparative Physiology*, **281**, R140–R149.

22 Tarcan, T., Siroky, M.B., Park, K., Goldstein, I., and Azadzoi, K.M. (2000) Systemic administration of apomorphine improves the hemodynamic mechanism of clitoral and vaginal engorgement in the rabbit. *International Journal of Impotence Research*, **12**, 235–240.

23 Giuliano, F., Bernabé, J., Rampin, O., Courtois, F., Benoit, G., and Rousseau, J.-P. (1994) Telemetric monitoring of intracavernous pressure in freely moving rats during copulation. *The Journal of Urology*, **152**, 1271–1274.

24 Behr-Roussel, D., Gorny, D., Mevel, K., Caisey, S., Bernabé, J., Burgess, G., Wayman, C., Alexandre, L., and Giuliano, F. (2005) Chronic sildenafil improves erectile function and endothelium-dependent cavernosal relaxations in rats: lack of tachyphylaxis. *European Urology*, **47**, 87–91.

25 Allard, J. and Giuliano, F. (2001) Central nervous system agents in the treatment of erectile dysfunction: how do they work? *Current Urology Reports*, **2**, 488–494.

26 Renyi, L. (1985) Ejaculations induced by *p*-chloroamphetamine in the rat. *Neuropharmacology*, **24**, 697–704.

27 Clément, P., Bernabé, J., Denys, P., Alexandre, L., and Giuliano, F. (2007) Ejaculation induced by i.c.v. injection of the preferential dopamine D3 receptor agonist 7-hydroxy-2-(di-*N*-propylamino)tetralin in anesthetized rats. *Neuroscience*, **145**, 605–610.

28 Truitt, W.A. and Coolen, L.M. (2002) Identification of a potential ejaculation generator in the spinal cord. *Science*, **297**, 1566–1569.

29 Gravitt, K. and Marson, L. (2007) Effect of the destruction of cells containing the serotonin reuptake transporter on urethrogenital reflexes. *Journal of Sexual Medicine*, **4**, 322–330.

30 Pfaus, J.G., Kippin, T.E., and Coria-Avila, G. (2003) What can animal models tell us about human sexual response? *Annual Review of Sex Research*, **14**, 1–63.

31 Behr-Roussel, D., Gorny, D., Mevel, K., Compagnie, S., Kern, P., Sivan, V., Bernabé, J., Bedigian, M.P., Alexandre, L., and Giuliano, F. (2005) Erectile dysfunction: an early marker for hypertension? A longitudinal study in spontaneously hypertensive rats. *American Journal of Physiology. Regulatory, Integrative and Comparative Physiology*, **288**, R276–R283.

32 Behr-Roussel, D., Darblade, B., Oudot, A., Compagnie, S., Bernabé, J., Alexandre, L., and Giuliano, F. (2006) Erectile dysfunction in hypercholesterolemic atherosclerotic apolipoprotein E knockout mice. *Journal of Sexual Medicine*, **3**, 596–603.

33 Pattij, T., de Jong, T.R., Uitterdijk, A., Waldinger, M.D., Veening, J.G., Cools, A.R., van der Graff, P.H., and Olivier, B. (2005) Individual differences in male rat ejaculatory behaviour: searching for models to study ejaculation disorders. *The European Journal of Neuroscience*, **22**, 724–734.

34 Diamond, L.E., Earle, D.C., Heiman, J.R., Rosen, R.C., Perelman, M.A., and Harning, R. (2006) An effect on the subjective sexual response in premenopausal women with sexual arousal disorder by bremelanotide (PT-141), a melanocortin receptor agonist. *Journal of Sexual Medicine*, **3**, 628–638.

35 Pfaus, J.G., Shadiack, A., Van Soest, T., Tse, M., and Molinoff, P. (2004) Selective facilitation of sexual solicitation in the female rat by a melanocortin receptor agonist. *Proceedings of the National Academy of Sciences of the United States of America*, **101**, 10201–10204.

36 Matsuura, S. and Downie, J.W. (2000) Effect of anesthetics on reflex micturition in the chronic cannula-implanted rat. *Neurourology and Urodynamics*, **19**, 87–99.

Index

a

acromegaly
– subcutaneous xenograft transplantation of GH4C1 murine
– – somatolactotroph cell lines 484
– xenograft mouse models 484
ACTH-secreting mouse cell lines (AtT-20) 482
acute kidney injury (AKI) 511, 512
– blood urea nitrogen and plasma creatinine 512
– warm renal ischemia–reperfusion (IR) model 511, 512
acute respiratory distress syndrome (ARDS) 431, 440
– animal models, characteristics 442–444
– clinical definition 441
Addison's disease, animal models for 476
adrenal tumorigenesis 478
– mice models, types 478
– signaling pathways, of humans and mice 480
adrenocortical cancer (ACC) genesis. see adrenal tumorigenesis
adriamycin 455
– induced heart failure in rats 455
– in RenTg model of CKD 508
aging 349, 351, 353
– Alzheimer's disease 355
– – APOE4 355, 356
– – APP 355
– – MAPT 356, 357
– – PS1 × APP × MAPT 357
– – PS1, PS2, and PS1 × APP 355, 356
– Down syndrome, TgDyrk1A 360
– Huntington's disease 358
– – R6/2 359
– – tgHD rats 359
– – YAC128 359
– normal 354
– Parkinson's disease 358
– – DJ1(PARK7)KO 358
– – Parkin(PARK2)KO 358
– – α-Syn 358
– role in neuroprotective drug development 408
– TDP43, frontotemporal dementia 359, 360
– and transgenic models 353, 354
AIP gene 482
AIRE gene 476
albumin promoter/enhancer (AlbP/E) 508
aldosterone–salt model 450
algorithms 20, 155
– partial least squares (PLS) 37
allodynia 238, 247, 265, 267, 270–272, 287–289, 306, 308–311, 320
– cold 314, 316, 317, 319, 320
– mechanical 293, 297–299, 310, 312–316, 319, 321
– symptoms in rodent models of neuropathic pain 322, 323
– thermal 69, 244, 315
alloimmune glomerulonephritis, experimental 513
– clinical relevance 514
– limits 514
– pathology 514
– pathophysiology 514
– technical aspects 513, 514
Alzheimer's disease 29
– amyloid-β- and tau-induced toxicity 73
– animal/rodent model 350
– *C. elegans* homologs of human presenilin genes 73
– *Drosophila* as model 69
– familial 355
– humanization of App gene 132
– models, validity 362

American Association for Laboratory Animal Science (AALAS) 100
androgen receptor (AR)-mediated androgen actions 487
anesthetized rat, isovolumetric cystometry 526
angiotensin II-induced hypertensive nephropathy 515
angiotensin-independent hypertension model 450
animal experimental migraine provoking models 242, 245
– glyceryl trinitrate infusion studies 243–245
animal experiments, basic research/medical advancement depend on 28, 29
animal models of human diseases, traditional
– attributes 9
– optimally selected 10
– predictive validity 9, 10
– reliable 9
animals
– appropriate time/age 11
– in biomedicine 3–5
– testing (see animal testing)
– welfare issues 22
Animals (Scientific Procedures) Act of 1986 99
animal testing 4, 107, 108
– *in silico* prediction of compound-related toxicities 108
– for small-molecule pharmaceuticals, adverse effects 108
– – chemistry-related effects 108
– – off-target effects 108
– – on-target effects 108
– *in vitro* models, limitation 108
– *in vivo*, as pivotal component of safety assessment 108
anti-CD20 antibodies 474
antiepileptic drugs (AEDs) 415
anti-NGF therapy 272
antiretroviral drugs, to induce neuropathic pain 315
anxiety disorders 193–195, 201
– animal models 194
– – preclinical anxiety models, and endophenotypes 195, 196
– – preclinical measures of anxiety 194, 195
– anxiety tests 195, 201
– modeling symptoms in rodents 196
anxiolytic drug discovery, tests for 194
anxiolytics 193, 196, 199
aortic banding 452

APECED syndrome, animal models in 476
ApoE alleles 132
App gene 132
ARRIVE (Animal Research: Reporting of *In Vivo* Experiments) guidelines 8, 9
Association for Assessment and Accreditation of Laboratory Animal Care (AAALAC) 100
asymmetric dimethylarginine (ADMA) 516
autoantigenicity 474
autoimmune endocrine diseases
– Addison's disease 476
– autoimmune thyroiditis 474–476
– hypophysitis/oophoritis 476, 477
– tumors 477–485 (*See also* endocrine tumors, animal models)
autosomal dominant hypocalcemia with hypercalciuria (ADHH) syndrome 489

b

Bederson scale 376
bedside-to-bench observations, in human disease 19
behavioral assessment 375
benign nephroangiosclerosis 516
benign prostatic hyperplasia (BPH) 527
betL-complemented *L. salivarius* strain 499
Bifidobacterium breve UCC2003
– BetL, improve tolerance to gastric juice 500
– probiotic–host colonization 500
biomarkers 7, 63, 76, 82
– imaging 150
– markers of major depressive disorder and
– – mouse analogs in chronic mild stress model 201
– progression of CKD 518
– use of 12, 13
biotechnological innovations 131
bipolar disorder (BPD) 65, 199, 200
– characteristics 199
– genome-wide association studies (GWAS) 200
– in mice 200
– mutant rodent strains 200
– reverse translation model 200
bladder outlet function 525
blast injury 373, 374
blood–brain barrier (BBB) 151, 370, 377
BPD. *see* bipolar disorder (BPD)
bradykinesia 387, 394
brain imaging. *See also in vivo* brain imaging in animal models
– choice of right imaging modality 151, 152

– high-resolution PET scanner 151, 152
– magnetic resonance imaging (MRI) 151, 152
β-thalassemia 141
B-type RAF kinase (BRAF) 481, 482
butterfly effect 6

c

Caenorhabditis elegans 71–74, 404, 405
– genome completely sequenced and match with 71
– limitations 74
– novel tools for analyzing
– – amyloid-β- and tau-induced toxicity 73
– – cancer-specific gene mutations 72
– – loss of gene function/protein–protein interactions/transcript levels 72
– – toxicity assessment 72, 73
– in "reverse genetics" approaches 72
– *in vivo* screening, for drug discovery approach in 73
calcium homeostasis studies, animal models used in 489, 490
calcium receptor (CaSr) 489, 490
Canadian Council on Animal Care (CCAC) 100
cancer pain models 270
– analgesic drug used 270
– animal models 271
– – bone cancer pain 271
– – orofacial cancer pain 272
– – visceral cancer pain 271
– cancer-induced pain 270
– pain assessment, in animal models 270, 271
– pain treatment, from bone metastases 270
– pathophysiology 272
– pharmacology 272
– tumor-induced bone pain 270
canine Cushing's disease (CDD) 483, 484
carcinogenicity studies 36, 124
– additional complementary rodent assay 124
– carcinogens operating through genotoxic mechanisms 125
– CHMP guideline 125
– current approaches 126
– current approaches, consolidation 126
– ICH S1B guideline 125
– long-term rodent carcinogenicity study 124
– objective 124
– positive result 125
– rodent-specific mechanisms 126
– transgenic animal models used in 125

cardiac hypertrophy 336, 450, 452, 454, 509, 510
CaSr gain-of-function 489
cavernous nerve (CN) 534
– in anesthetized rat 533
Cdkn1B gene 478
cell death 60, 378, 391, 393, 395, 397–399, 444
c-fos expression 245
chlorpromazine 207, 219
cholera toxin (Ctx) 501
chromosome engineering tools, for manipulation chromosomal regions 140
– to develop mouse models of CGS 140
– – neurodevelopmental disorders 140
– – reciprocal microdeletion and microduplication 140
– – segmental aneuploidies reveal dosage-sensitive gene (*Stat5* gene) 140
– to develop mouse models of polygenic diseases 140
– – identify number of QTLs associated with human diseases 141
– – YACs and BACs, randomly introduced into genome 141
– humanized mouse model carrying freely segregating human chromosome 21
– – generated using MMCT 142
– limitations and difficulties 140–142
– targeted genomic replacement
– – for studying *in vivo* human hematopoiesis, and immune function 142
chronic kidney diseases (CKDs) 506
– biomarkers 518
– in hypertensive patients 517
– RenTg model 507–509
– – benefits 509, 510
chronic obstructive pulmonary disease (COPD) 431
– animal models 432
– – cigarette smoke 432, 433
– – genetically modified models 434
– – smoke exposure 439
– – by tracheal elastase instillation 433, 434
cisplatin, neuropathic pain caused by 317, 318
clinical efficacy 6, 11, 78, 392
– biomarker change 13
– microdosing 81
– probiotic culture 500, 502
clinical trials 6, 7
– first-in-human (FIH) 110
– phase I/II 50, 78, 81, 82, 120
clozapine 212, 215, 218, 221, 222

cognitive function 65, 283, 351, 353, 377, 415, 476
– dysfunction 216, 323, 349, 350, 352
– enhancers 349, 353
– enhancing effects 6
combined pituitary hormone deficiency (CPHD) human phenotypes 485
communication
– pain as central/cognitive perception 301
– between stakeholders 22
competitive advantages, of new drugs 18
complexity
– breeding 135
– and chronicity of schizophrenia 214
– chronic pain in humans 301
– clinical condition 11
– and cognitive impairments in water maze task 357
– endocrine system 490
– etiological, of diseases 13
– heterogeneity and etiological 13
– human gastric fluid 443
– models 185
– stroke and TBI, drugs 377
– and variability of biological system 94, 95
comprehensive reporting 8, 9
computer-aided techniques 19, 33, 34
– CODESSA 36
– CoMFA/CoMSIA techniques 36
– docking 35, 36
– GUSAR 36
– homology modeling 35
– MOLD 36
– molecular dynamics 35
– pharmacophore modeling 35
– prediction of absorption, distribution, metabolism, elimination 35
– quantum mechanics 35
– two- and three-dimensional QSAR 35, 36
– virtual screening
– – ligand-based 35
– – structure-based 35
computer modeling. *see* computer-aided techniques
concordance
– between adverse findings observed
– – in clinical studies and data generated, in preclinical toxicology 112
– between animal and human toxicities 31, 42, 126
– and factors contributing to interspecies differences in toxicodynamics 127

– neurophysiological data, effects of toxin on rate and pattern of neuronal firing 391
– survey conducted by ILSI, assessing 126
conditioned place preference (CPP) 173, 175, 176, 178–180, 184, 185
– biased/unbiased protocol 178
– operant self-administration paradigm, procedure in rodents 180
– properties and experimental conditions of drugs in animals 180
conflict-based test 194
congenital anomalies of kidney and urinary tract (CAKUT) 511
construct/etiological validity 11
contiguous gene syndromes (CGS) 140
control and supervision of experiments on animals (CPCSEA) 101
coronary artery disease 455, 456
cortical spreading depression (CSD) 231, 240, 241
– drug developed for its ability to inhibit 241
– – tonabersat 241
– glutamate, key role in 241
– induced in animals by 240
– measurement 240
– variants of ion channels and pumps 241
corticobasal degeneration (CBG) 387
Council for International Organizations of Medical Sciences (CIOMS) 102
COX inhibitors 265
CPP. *see* conditioned place preference (CPP)
Cre-lox methods 506
crescentic glomerulonephritis 513
cross-species predictability 6
"curative" approaches 12
Cushing's disease 482, 484, 490
cytotoxic T-lymphocyte antigen-4 (CTLA4) gene regions 476

d

Dahl/Rapp salt-sensitive rats 452
Danio rerio 60, 404
decision-making processes 10
dementia 349, 351
– frontotemporal 357, 359
– with Lewy body 387
deoxycorticosterone acetate (DOCA) 450, 506
depression-like behavior 201
– inherently 199
– withdrawal 171
desensitization 12
detrusor contraction 527
detrusor sphincter dyssynergia (DSD) 528

development and reproductive toxicity (DART) studies 122
– aims 122
– designs 123
–– ICH S5(R2) guideline 122
– developmental stages, in reproductive process 122
– minipigs 123
– in NHP 123, 124
– toxicokinetic investigations 124
diabetes 28, 45, 66, 68, 138–141, 305, 336
– genetic models 336, 337
–– db/db mice 336
–– Goto–Kakizaki rats 336
–– ob/ob mice 336
–– Otsuka Long–Evans Tokushima Fatty rats 336
–– Zucker diabetic fatty rats 336
– induced neuropathic pain (see neuropathic pain)
– intrauterine growth-restricted rats 338
DiGeorge syndrome (DGS) 490
dilated cardiomyopathy (DCM) 449
DNA sequencing 131
dopamine (DA) 207
dosing
– appropriate time and 11, 12
– length 344
– ratiometric 48
– and route of administration 406
– schedule 16, 406
Down syndrome 140, 360
– TgDyrk model, validy 362
Drosophila melanogaster 60, 66, 404, 405
– in cancer field 68
–– Ras-driven tumor model 68
– complete sequence of genome 66
– conservation of biological processes 66, 67
– to discover new anti-infective drugs 70
– in genetic/mutation studies 66, 67, 69, 70
– limitations in model 71
– model organism to identify disease-causing genes/proteins 69, 70
– model organism to study obesity and insulin resistance 68
– as model system for drug discovery 67
– in neurodegenerative diseases and psychiatric disorders 69, 70
– nociception and related studies 68, 69
– offers versatile advantages for target discovery and validation 66
– in RNAi technologies, as "knockout" tool 67

– short life cycle and ease and low cost of maintenance 66
– valuable system to model rewarding properties of drugs 70
drug accumulation 15, 16
drug addiction 169
– criteria 169
– diagnosis 169
– DSM criteria 169, 170
drug- and virus-induced neuropathic pain 314
– antiretroviral drugs 315
– caused by anticancer drugs 316–318
–– cisplatin 317
–– oxaliplatin 317
–– paclitaxel 317
–– vincristine 318
– diabetes-inducing drugs 314, 315
–– streptozotocin/alloxan 314
– HIV-related pain 315
– HSV-induced neuropathic pain 316
– postherpetic neuralgia 315, 316
drug delivery systems 7
drug developers 7, 27, 150
drug discrimination 177, 178, 185
drug-induced liver injury (DILI) 42, 43
drug–receptor interaction 12
drug tolerance 172
– cross-tolerance 173
–– between ethanol and cannabinoids 173
–– in rodents 173
– defined at DSM-IV 172
– response to opioids, cannabinoids, and alcohol administration 172, 173
Duchenne muscular dystrophy (DMD) 460
– model 461
dyskinesia 219, 419
– levodopa-induced 393, 395, 400
– tardive 208
dyslipidemia 333, 334, 336–338
dystrophin-deficient cardiomyopathy 461
dystrophin gene mutations 460

e
EAST (epilepsy, ataxia, sensorineural deafness, and tubulopathy) syndrome 65
ejaculation, investigation 534–536
– disorders 538
– executive mechanisms 534
– investigation 534
–– expulsion spinal reflex 535
–– neurons electrical stimulation 535
–– pharmacologically induced 535

– – physiological markers 534
– peripheral synchronized events 530
– *in vivo* models 534
elevated plus maze 194–196, 200, 273
endocrine disorders 473
– autoimmune diseases (*see* autoimmune endocrine diseases)
– limitations/difficulties 490, 491
– physiology (*see* endocrine physiology, animal models)
– tumors (*see* endocrine tumors, animal models)
endocrine physiology, animal models
– in calcium homeostasis studies 489, 490
– phosphocalcic metabolism 490
– pituitary development disorders 485–487
– – organogenesis 485
– reproductive function 487–489
endocrine tumors, animal models
– adrenal tumorigenesis 478–481
– – signaling pathways, in humans and mice 480
– multiple endocrine neoplasia syndromes 477, 478
– pituitary tumorigenesis 482–485
– – experimentally induced mice models of acromegaly 484
– – genetic abnormalities identified in human 483
– thyroid tumorigenesis 481, 482
endophenotypes 195, 196
endothelial dysfunction 509
endothelin-1, 272
endothelin (ET) 438
endothelin-A receptor antagonism 272
enterotoxigenic *E. coli* (ETEC) toxin 501
epilepsy 140, 156, 159, 415
– animal species to use to model 416, 417
– prototypic forms, modeling, idiopathic generalized epilepsies/focal epilepsies 418
– – absence seizures 419, 420
– – convulsive seizures 418, 419
– – cortical dysplasia 420–422
– – hippocampal sclerosis 422, 423
– type of models, providing information on physiopathology 417, 418
erectile dysfunction 536
– cardiovascular condition 537
– diabetes mellitus 537
– neurogenic erectile dysfunction 537
– pathophysiological models 537

ethanol
– behavioral sensitization 173
– cross-tolerance to 173
– reduced sensitivity to 173
– self-administration 182
ethical concerns and positions, on animal research. *see* ethical issues
ethical issues 91, 92
– Declaration of Helsinki 92
– general principles for ethical use of animals in research 95
– – principle of justification 96, 97
– – principle of responsibility 97, 98
– – 3Rs principles 95, 96
– nonhuman primates as research animals 92, 93
etiological validity 11
expulsion spinal reflex 535
– pudendal motoneuron reflex discharges 536
– urethrogenital reflex 536
external urethral sphincter (EUS) 525
– electromyogram 526

f

familial isolated pituitary adenoma (FIPA) 482
Federation of European Laboratory Animal Science Associations (FELASA) 22, 97–100
fibrinolytic activity 377
fibrotic lung diseases
– animal models 439
– bleomycin-induced pulmonary fibrosis 439, 440
functional evaluation, and uses of mouse models 136
– challenges 137, 138
– environmental influences 137
– genetic background 137
– harmonization 136, 137
– new resources 138
– – IKMC 138
– risk assessment 139
– standardization 136, 137
– target identification 138, 139
– translation to humans 138, 139
– – robust protocols, need to 138
– use of GEMs in pharmaceutical industry 139
– – Dmd^{mdx} *(mdx)* mouse model 139
– – XenoMouse 139
functional genomics 131

g

gastrointestinal disorders
– betaine 498
– carnitine 498
– delivery, probiotic resistance to process-induced stresses/storage conditions 498–500
– efficacy, designer probiotics 500, 501
– *Escherichia coli* 500
– limitations/difficulties 501, 502
– patho-biotechnology concept 497, 498
– probiotic storage 497
– proline 498
– survival, improving probiotic–host colonization 500
– virulence-associated factors 498
GATA3 haploinsufficiency 490
GEMMs. *see* genetically engineered, mouse models
gene knockout models 3, 4
gene mutation-induced cardiomyopathies
– cardiomyopathic hamsters 460
– genetic modification, in mouse 461, 462
– golden retriever muscular dystrophy dogs 460, 461
genetic engineering 48, 50, 132, 133, 138, 141, 269, 337, 431, 435, 477
– mouse models 132, 134
genetic medicine, challenges 140
genetic modifications 3, 218, 401, 402, 404, 453, 461, 502
gene–toxin interactions 408, 409
genital sexual arousal 532
genitourinary disorders 523
– animal findings, translational value 538, 539
– lower urinary tract function 523
– – bladder afferent recording 526, 527
– – cystometry evaluation 524, 525
– – micturition, physiology 524
– – pathophysiological models 527–529
– – urethral function, evaluation 525, 526
– sexual functions
– – copulatory tests 531, 532
– – ejaculation, investigation 534–536
– – erection, investigation 532–534
– – female/male sexual response, physiology 529, 530
– – pathophysiological models 536–538
– – peripheral female sexual response 532
– – preference paradigms 530, 531
– – proceptive/receptive behaviors 531
genomic technologies 20

genotoxicity 107, 108
– genetic toxicology studies 120
– – biotechnology-derived pharmaceuticals 120
– – Comet assay 121
– – erythrocyte MN test 120, 121
– – UDS assay 121
– – *in vivo* testing, in rodents 120
– NCE pharmaceuticals, assessement 119
– transgenic animals, used for testing 121
– – advantages 122
– – drawbacks 122
– *in vitro* mammalian cell test 119, 120
Gi protein 458
glomerular basement membrane (GBM) 513
glomerular filtration
– abolished 511
– rate 506
glomerulonephritis
– crescentic 513, 514, 517
– experimental alloimmune (*see* alloimmune glomerulonephritis, experimental)
– nephrotoxic serum-induced 508
glutamate 241
gonadectomized animals, subcapsular tumors 481
Goodpasture's disease 513, 514
Grave's disease (GD) 474, 475
– experimentally induced animal models 475
GTN infusion model 245
guinea pigs 92, 194, 233, 290, 297, 432, 439, 481
– modern preclinical testing 31
– morphometric analysis 432
– penicillin toxicity 31

h

haloperidol 207, 212, 215, 218, 219, 222, 388, 389
– in model, motor aspects of parkinsonism 390
– sensitization in monkeys 220
hamsters
– bleomycin-induced pulmonary fibrosis 439
– cardiomyopathic 460
– under control of hamster prion promoter
– – mutant APP 355
– – mutations, expressing human bAPP695 transgene 355
– penicillin toxicity 31
– TSHR transfection 475
Hashimoto's thyroiditis 474
headache. *see* migraine

heart failure (HF) 449, 455
– adriamycin-induced in rats 455
– cardiac function, evolution 459
– chronic rapid pacing produces 458
– – advantages 460
– double pressure, and volume overload 454, 455
– gene mutation-induced cardiomyopathies
– – cardiomyopathic hamsters 460
– – genetic modification, in mouse 461, 462
– – golden retriever muscular dystrophy dogs 460, 461
– hypertension 450–452
– limitations/difficulties 462
– models related to myocardial ischemia and/or myocardial infarction 456–458
– monocrotaline-induced right ventricular 455
– myocardial ischemia/myocardial infarction 456, 457
– – coronary microembolization 457, 458
– pacing-induced 458–460
– pressure overload 452–454
– toxic molecule 455
– – adriamycin, in rat 455
– – induced 455
– – monocrotaline 455
– volume overload-induced 454
hedonia 198
hepatotoxicity 30, 31, 36, 38, 42, 62, 63
heterogeneity, of diseases 13
heterozygous Gata3-KO ($Gata3^{-/+}$) mice 490
high-affinity selective drug 16
high-content analyses 20
high-risk/high-benefit approach 11
high-throughput screening (HTS) technologies 49, 60
HIV-gp41-hemolysin A hybrid peptides 501
HIV-induced neuropathy 315
HMGA2 gene 482, 483
hormonal pituitary deficiencies 473
human experimental migraine provoking models 241, 242
human neutrophil elastase (HNE) 433
human pituitary tumorigenesis, genetic abnormalities 483
human polycystic ovary syndrome, rodent models 488, 489
human pulmonary fibrosis 439
Huntington's disease 70, 141, 157, 358, 387
– transgenic models
– – rodent models 358, 359
– – validity 362

hyperalgesia 69, 83, 246, 247, 265–268, 272, 273, 287, 301, 306, 311, 312
– capsaicin-induced 288, 289
– carrageenan-induced 287, 288
– complete Freund's adjuvant-induced 288
– mechanical 314, 319
– symptoms in rodemt model of neuropathic pain 322, 323
– thermal heat 313, 314, 316–318, 320, 321
hypertension 333, 334, 336, 342, 378, 432
hypertensive nephropathy 516
– renin transgenic model 508
hypertrophic cardiomyopathy (HCM) 449
hypocalciuric hypercalcemia 489
hypokinetic disorders 387
hypoparathyroidism, sensorineural deafness, and renal dysplasia (HDR) syndrome 490
hypothyroidism 342, 474
hypoxia-induced pulmonary hypertension 438

i

ICP. *see* intracavernosal pressure (ICP)
ICSS. *see* intracranial self-stimulation (ICSS)
idiopathic hypogonadotropic hypogonadism (IHH) 485
– genetic basis 487
immersion tests 264
immunohistochemistry 14, 64
impaired glucose tolerance 333
Indian National Science Academy (INSA) 101
infarct assessment 375
– noninvasive MRI methods 375
– staining 375
innovation 4, 33
– biotechnological 131
– collaborative 43
– medical therapies 6
– open 43
– pharmaceutical 132, 319
– strategies 273
– – anti-NGF 273
"insentient" material 19
in silico models 31, 34
– ADME/toxicity prediction software packages 38–41
– biokinetic modeling 37, 42
– disease- and patient-specific 42, 43
– as prediction models 108
– quantitative structure–activity relationship 34–37

Institutional Animal Ethics Committee (IAEC) 101
insulin resistance 333
International Knockout Mouse Consortium (IKMC) 133
interstitial cystitis (IC) 528
intracavernosal pressure (ICP) 533, 534, 537
intracranial self-stimulation (ICSS) 176, 180, 181, 184, 185, 198
– assessing functional activity of brain's reward pathways 181
– rate-frequency curve 180
– rewarding/aversive effects of drugs of abuse 176
in vitro models 43, 44
– advanced models for prediction of drug toxicity 46, 47
– alternative 44
– hepatocarcinoma cell lines 45
– human hepatocyte imaging assay technology (HIAT) 42
– immortalized cell lines 45
– primary cells, as important tool in 44
– stem cells 45
– – human embryonic stem cells (hESCs) 45, 46
– – human induced pluripotent stem cells (hiPSCs) 45, 46
– – induced pluripotent stem cells (iPSCs) 45, 46
– tumor models (see *in vitro* tumor models)
– using human immortalized cell lines (HICLs) 44
in vitro tumor models 47–50
– commonly used cancer models 49
– cultured human tumor cell lines 47
– proposed approaches to improve anticancer drug development 48
– rodent xenografts models 47
– three-dimensional models 49
– – "co-clinical trial" concept of Pandolfi 50
– – MCTS models 49
– – pharmaceuticals companies, role in development 49, 50
– two-dimensional cell cultures 47
in vivo brain imaging in animal models 149
– role of animal 149
– *in vivo* imaging
– – in animal models and 3R principles 150
– – in animal models in pharmaceutical industry 150
– – as translational approach for basic research 149

in vivo exploratory, and experimental human models 74–76
– exploratory investigational new drug application studies considered by FDA 75
– Phase 0 (exploratory human models) 76–81
– – benefits and limitations, of clinical trials 79
– – microdosing methodology 77, 78, 80
– – regulatory authorities 77
– Phase IB/IIA (proof-of-concept) studies 81–83
– – experimental human models, developed in healthy volunteers 82, 83
– – experimental pain models, under controlled settings 83
– – learning/confirming, activities in clinical development 82
in vivo nonmammalian models 59–61
– *Caenorhabditis elegans* 71–74
– *Drosophila melanogaster* 66–71
– zebrafish 61–66
ischemia–reperfusion, renal 511, 512

j
Jun kinase 478

k
K_{ATP} (ATP-sensitive potassium) channels 449
ketamine 75, 211, 212, 319, 352, 353, 510, 512, 515
kidney
– components 505
– flank incision, palpation 510, 512
– function 506
– thrombotic microangiopathy lesions 516
Klinefelter syndrome (KS) 485, 487
knockout (KO) mice
– atrial natriuretic peptide (ANP) systems 508
– model 4, 6, 10, 132, 399, 400
– phenotypes, for drugs 132
– renin–angiotensin system 508

l
Lactobacillus jensenii 501
– modified to secrete two-domain CD4 501
Lactobacillus salivarius UCC118-BetL$^+$
– [^{14}C]glycine betaine uptake rates in 499
language-impaired "autistic" mouse 6
LD50 test 21
left ventricular hypertrophy (LVH) 450
legislation
– animals protection/prevention, for scientific purposes 31

–– Convention ETS123 and EU Directive 86/609/EEC 21
– animal welfare issues and 22
– guidelines 22
– product assessment 4
– 3Rs principles 19
– and scientists' ability to understand 21
– for testing of chemicals and cosmetics 32
LHX4 mutations 485
Listeria monocytogenes, foodborne pathogen 499
L-NAME administration 516, 517
locomotor responsiveness 6
lower urinary tract (LUT) function 523
– anesthetized models 539
– benign prostatic hyperplasia (BPH) 527
– bladder afferent recording 526, 527
– continence phase 524
– cystometry evaluation 524, 525
– micturition, physiology 524
– pathophysiological models 527–529
–– bladder outlet obstruction 527
–– overactive bladder (OAB) 527, 528
– peripheral nervous system, control 524
– roles 523
– urethral function, evaluation 525, 526
–– external urethral sphincter electromyogram 526
–– intraurethral pressure 526
lung diseases, animal models for
– chronic obstructive pulmonary disease (COPD) 432–434
– fibrotic lung diseases 439, 440
– pulmonary hypertension 434–439
– respiratory distress syndrome, acute 440, 441, 445
–– characteristics, of models 442–444
lung emphysema 432
– animal models 432
– limitations/difficulties 445
lymphocytic thyroiditis 474

m

major depressive disorder (MDD) 197–199
matrix metalloproteinase-9, 377
matrix metalloproteinases (MMPs) 434
medullary thyroid carcinoma (MTC) 478
menin, pivotal role 477
mesial temporal lobe epilepsy (MTLE) syndrome 422
metabolic syndrome 333
– artificially induced, in animals 337, 338
– definitions 334
– obesity, classical animal models 335, 336
– prevalence 335
– treatments used in humans against 339–343
metabolism 16, 485
– drug 42, 80
– glucose 156, 157, 350
– intraneuronal 156
– and kinetics, data role in design and interpretation 116
– L-arginine 516
– neuronal 155, 156
– phosphocalcic 490
– xenobiotics 132, 139
methodologically flawed animal studies 6
methods, alternative 19, 21, 32, 33, 91, 94, 95, 98, 213, 402
– evaluation and validation 32, 33
– OECD guideline 32
– survey report for 3Rs 33
microdosing methodology 77, 78, 80, 81
– *vs.* conventional studies 80
migraine 231
– activation of trigeminovascular system 231
– animal experimental studies 231, 232
– behavioral models 246, 247
–– abnormal eye closures 249
–– allodynia/hyperalgesia 247
–– face grooming 248
–– lateralized head grooming 249
–– photophobia 248, 249
– cortical spreading depression 231
– electrophysiological recordings
–– on primary dural afferents in trigeminal ganglion 237–239
–– in trigeminal nucleus caudalis 239
– histological markers after nociceptive stimulation 239, 240
– neurogenic inflammation model 234, 235
–– effect of inhibitors on dural plasma protein extravasation 235–237
– nociceptive activation 234, 237
– transgenic models 246
– triptans, use in 232
– vascular models 231, 232
– *in vitro* studies 232, 233
– *in vivo* studies 233
Ministry of Science and Technology (MOST) 101, 102
MK-801-induced hyperactivity 222
model addiction, in animals 170
– difficulties to 170–172

modified neurological severity score (mNSS) 376
– description 376
monocrotaline-induced pulmonary hypertension 436
monocrotaline (MCT) lung injury model 435
mood disorders 193, 197. See also anxiety disorders
– endophenotype models of depression 199
– major depressive disorder 197
– preclinical measures of depression 198
– – cognition 199
– – negative affect 198
– – positive affect/hedonia 198
– – socioaffective function 198, 199
mouse analogs in chronic mild stress model 201
mouse defense test battery (MDTB) 195
mouse genetic engineering, improved 133
– CRISPR/Cas strategies 133
– Kymouse strains 133
– nuclease-mediated inactivations 133
– technical developments 133
– tissue/cell-specific inactivation 133
– VelocImmune mouse 133
mouse mutant resource, new 133–136
– Collaborative Cross (CC) 135
– Cre/loxP system 134
– EUCOMMTOOLS 135
– European Mouse Disease Clinic (Eumodic) 133, 135
– International Knockout Mouse Consortium (IKMC) 133
– International Mouse Phenotyping Consortium (IMPC) 134, 135
– large-scale mouse program 135
– pilot programs 133
– Wellcome Trust Sanger Institute Mouse Genetics Project (WTSI-MGP) 134, 135
movement disorders. see Huntington's disease; Parkinson's disease
multicellular tumor spheroid (MCTS) models 49
multiple endocrine neoplasia syndromes
– conventional knockout (KO) models 477
– genetic and clinical features 479
– – syndromes currently known in humans and rodent models 479
– MEN1 syndrome 477
– – knockout (KO) models 477
– – mice models heterozygous 477
– – role of menin 477
– MEN2 syndrome and clinical entities 478
– – Cys634Arg mutation 478
– – mutations in *RET, Cdkn1b* 478
multiple system atrophy (MSA) 387
murine models 271, 431, 476
– in human disease 431, 439, 449
– transgenic, FTLD-TDP research overexpress 359
muscle LIM protein (MLP) 461
musculoskeletal/joint (OA and RA) pain 289
– osteoarthritis pain models 289–293
– rheumatoid arthritis pain models 293–297
mutations 132
– *AIP* gene 482
– *AIRE* gene 476
– A30P and A53T 399
– *BDNF* gene 199
– cancer-specific gene 72
– *CaSr* mutation 489
– conditional 134
– *CRHR1* gene 199
– Cys634Arg 478
– *DISC1* gene 199
– double *APP* 355
– gene mutation-induced cardiomyopathies 460
– *5-HTT* gene 199
– Indiana mutation (V717F) 355
– leptin receptor 336
– *LHX4* gene 485
– *MAPT* gene 357
– *MEN1* gene 478
– monogenic 141
– *Nlgn3* gene 141
– null α-synuclein 402
– null/point 132
– P303L 356
– *Prop1* gene 485
– P303S 356
– random 67
– *RET* gene 478, 481
– R192Q mutation 246
– *SDH* gene 481
– *TBX1* transcription factor 490
– *Tk* gene assay 120
– *TPH2* gene 199
– *Tsc1/2* genes 421
myocardial adenylate cyclase activity 461
myocardial ischemia/myocardial infarction 449, 456, 457. See also heart failure

– coronary microembolization 457, 458
– model of MI-induced HF used for testing 456
– – coronary ligature-induced MI in rats 456, 457
– pacing 458–460

n

National Council for the Control of Animal Experimentation (CONCEA) 102
National Health and Medical Research Council (NHMRC) 101
neonatal severe primary hyperparathyroidism (NHSPT) syndromes 489
nephrotoxic serum-induced glomerulonephritis 508
nerve growth factor (NGF) 272
nerve ligation. *See also* peripheral nerve injury
– infraorbital 313
– peroneal 310
– sciatic 311, 313
– spinal 312–314, 322
neurochemical measurements 14
neurodegenerative diseases 349
neurogenic detrusor overactivity (NDO) 528
neurological severity score (NSS) 376
neuronal death 318, 377, 407
neuropathic pain
– anticancer drugs, caused by 307, 316–318
– central lesions, spinal cord injury, caused by 307, 308
– 2,3-dideoxycytidine-induced 315
– in humans, types 306
– neuropathic-like pain, evoked by chemicals administered 320
– – excitotoxic injury to spinal cord 321
– – intrathecal administration, ATP/BDNF 320
– nociceptive tests (*see* nociceptive pain tests)
– pain in SCI patients, types 308
– – musculoskeletal pain 308
– – neuropathic pain 308, 309
– – visceral pain 308
– peripheral nerve lesions 306
– – caused by anticancer drugs 307
– – diabetes-induced 306
– – HIV-related pain 306, 307
– – postherpetic neuralgia 307
– trigeminal 248
neuroprotectants 392, 408
– effects 64
– efficacy 396, 406
– against excitotoxicity, *in vitro* and *in vivo* models 350

– intracellular mechanisms 388, 394, 395
– in mouse models 73
– STAIR recommendations 375
– strategy for PD 407
– therapies 370
– – assessment 402
neuroprotective drug. *see* neuroprotectants
neuropsychological tests 377
neurotoxins 387, 388, 390, 401, 409
NK1 receptor antagonist, no efficacy in migraine 245
nociceptive pain tests
– phasic pain tests 261
– tonic pain tests 261, 262
nonconventional animal models 114
– juvenile animals 114
– transgenic animal models 114
nonempirical (nontesting) methods 31
nonhuman models 27
NO synthase 451, 461, 516
– inhibition 450, 516
novel pharmacological treatment approaches 6

o

obese strain (OS) chickens 474
obesity 139, 140, 333, 473
– genetic models 336
– – *db/db* mice 336
– – Goto–Kakizaki rats 336
– – *ob/ob* mice 336
– – Otsuka Long–Evans Tokushima Fatty rats 336
– – Zucker diabetic fatty rats 336
– monosodium glutamate-induced 338
objectives
– to assess tolerability and drug exposure 110
– carcinogenicity testing 124
– maximize detection of "system failure," 117
– measurements 14, 531, 532
– microdosing studies 77
– safety pharmacology 118
Office of Laboratory Animal Welfare (OLAW) 100
"omics" approaches 31
osteoarthritis (OA) 289
– pain models 289–293
osteolysis 272
overactive bladder (OAB)
– detrusor contraction 527
– provoked bladder hyperactivity 528
– spontaneously hypertensive rat 528

oxaliplatin, neuropathic pain caused by 317, 318

p

paclitaxel, neuropathic pain caused by 317, 318
pain achievement test 266, 267
pain evaluation, in animal models 283
– capsaicin-induced hyperalgesia 288, 289
– carrageenan-induced hyperalgesia 287, 288
– complete Freund's adjuvant-induced hyperalgesia 288
– formalin test 287
– inflammatory pain 287–289, 302
– in rodents, various components of pain 284–286
painful bladder syndrome (PBS) 528
– *in vivo* experimental models 529
pain in rodents, chronic, modelization 309. *See also* peripheral nerve injury; spinal cord injury
pain models
– cancer (*see* cancer pain models)
– nociceptive tests (*see* nociceptive pain tests)
– osteoarthritis pain models 289–293
– rheumatoid arthritis pain models 293–297
– visceral (*see* visceral pain models)
Parkinson's disease (PD) 387
– classical models with predictive validity 387, 388
– drug/toxin-based models 389
–– haloperidol 390
–– maneb 398
–– MPTP 393–396
–– 6-OHDA 390–393
–– paraquat 398
–– reserpine 389, 390
–– rotenone 396–398
–– trichloroethylene 398
– genetic/functional models 398, 399, 406
–– adult-onset rodent gene-based models 401–403
–– rodent function-based models 403, 404
–– rodent genetic models 399, 400
– limitation, to currently available models 407
– nonrodent genetic models 404, 405
PARP-1 deletion, reducing infarct volume 378
patent
– application 4
– regulatory bodies 4
Pavlovian conditioning 195
penicillin 28, 31
– used in animal models 31

penile erectile tissues 532
perfusion
– bladder 525, 526
– cerebral 155, 368
– and GFR abolition and anoxia 512
– measurement 162
– myocardial 342
– perfusion-weighted imaging 153, 154
peripheral nerve injury 309
– common peroneal nerve injury 312
– dorsal rhizotomy 313
– infraorbital nerve ligation 313
– injury to dorsal root ganglia 314
– laser-induced sciatic nerve injury 312
– nerve compression 310
– nerve lesion procedures 310
– nerve section 309
–– sciatic nerve 309, 310
–– transection of tibial and sural nerves 310
– sciatic nerve
–– complete ligation 310, 311
–– cryoneurolysis 312
–– cuffing 311
–– partial ligation 311
– spared nerve injury 311, 312
– spinal nerve ligation 313, 314
pharmaceutical development
– initiatives aimed at improving 32
– need for alternatives to *in vivo* studies 33
pharmaceutical industry, major challenges for 131
pharmaceutical product 4, 16
pharmacodynamics (PD) 15, 16, 34, 41, 42, 49, 60, 108, 208
pharmacokinetics (PK) 3, 16, 34, 36, 40–42, 48, 75–77, 110, 116, 158, 220
– pharmacodynamic integration 15
– *in vivo*, essential for drug development 68
pharmacological deficit models 349
– cholinergic interventions 350
–– cholinergic antagonists 351, 352
–– cholinergic toxins 350, 351
–– glutamatergic antagonists 352, 353
–– serotonergic intervention 353
– inhibition of energy/glucose metabolism 350
– validity 361
–– construct 361
–– face 361
–– predictive 361
pharmacological effect 9, 15, 16, 18, 40, 75, 77, 156, 178, 516
phenogenomics 131, 142

phototoxicity 108
phylogenetic reduction 19
physical withdrawal syndrome 174, 175
– alcohol withdrawal in rodents 175
– MDMA-maintained rodents 175
– symptoms in humans 174
– THC treatment 175
physicochemical properties 37
– computational tool for predicting 34
– molecules and biological activities 34
– program to calculate 38, 40
pituitary development disorders 485–487
– Ames dwarf (df) mice
– – *Prop1* mutations 485
– embryological steps, in humans 486
– *GPR54* gene 485
– idiopathic hypogonadotropic hypogonadism, genetic basis 487
– mice models of Klinefelter syndrome 487
– pituitary ontogenesis in mice 485
– Snell dwarf and Jackson dwarf mice, mutated in *Pou1f1* 485
plasma protein binding 15
– interaction predictors 37
– prediction software package 38
P38-MAPK-dependent mechanisms 511
polycystic ovary syndrome(PCOS) 473, 487
Portuguese Water Dogs (PWDs) 476
positive airway pressure (PAP) 437
positive end expiratory pressure (PEEP) 441
positron emission tomography (PET) 155
– anesthetized animals 160
– and brain receptors and transporters 156, 157
– effects of anesthesia on imaging 160
– instrumentation 155
– mass effect of injected tracers 162
– multimodal PET–MRI for better clinical translation 162
– and neuronal metabolism 155, 156
– and neurotransmitter release 159
– principles 155
– and receptor occupancy 158
– spatial resolution and sensitivity 160, 161
– translation to clinical applications 159, 160
– without anesthesia, using head fixation devices 160
postoperative pain 297, 298. *See also* pain models
– incisional pain 298, 299
– laparotomy 299
– limitations/difficulties 300–302
– – dynamic weight bearing measurements 301
– – nonopioid drugs 301
– – preclinical validity 301
– – in translation of animal models 300
– morphine and gabapentin, beneficial effects in 300
– ovariohysterectomy 299
– reproducible rat model 300
P/Q channel blockers 241
precision 20, 265
preclinical
– animal data 14
– animal models in biomedical research, 3Ns 3–22
– anxiety models, and endophenotypes 195
– assessment
– – abuse liability 182
– – analgesic drug effects 302
– and clinical imaging results 162
– development process 4, 29
– – candidate AED 419, 423, 424
– discovery approaches on precompetitive level 7
– drug screening 44
– evaluation of new analgesic drugs and 283
– hybrid scanners 162
– interactions 7
– measures
– – anxiety 194
– – depression 198
– models
– – for clarifying pathogenesis and testing treatments 527
– – cognition/memory 221
– – disease and drug-induced states in 65
– – musculoskeletal pain 289
– – for PD 395, 396
– package supporting FIH studies 117
– pharmacological characterization of inhibitors 213
– positron emission tomography 150
– research strategy 7
– safety studies 116
– studies in sexual medicine 531
– testing of drugs targeting, acute and chronic stages of stroke 375
– toxicology studies 112
– translational research on rheumatoid arthritis 297
– validation 77
– – basic pain tests 301
– *in vitro*

– – and animal assays 74
– – preclinical PK data 80
preclinical–clinical translation 7, 19
predictions
– from animal models of human condition 14
predictive validities 11
probiotic–host colonization 500
product assessment legislative 4
progressive supranuclear palsy (PSP) 387
protein X in plasma, overexpression 13
proteomic technologies 20
psychogenic 533
psychostimulants 6
PTTG-1 gene 482
pulmonary emphysema 433
pulmonary fibrosis, bleomycin model 439
pulmonary hemorrhage 513
pulmonary hypertension (PH) 431
– animal models 434
– – fawn-hooded rats 437
– – hypoxic PH 437, 438
– – monocrotaline model 436, 437
– – PH related to COPD 439
– – PH to human PH 435, 436
– – SU5416 treatment combined with hypoxia 438, 439
pyrrolizidine alkaloid 436

q

qualitative assessments, of behavior 14
quantitative pharmacology 15
quantitative structure–activity relationship (QSAR) 34
– modeling 34, 35

r

Rauvolfia serpentina 207
reference drug 11
regulatory framework, for use of animals in research 98
– Australia 101
– Brazil 102
– Canada 100
– China 101, 102
– countries, without specific legal framework 102
– – CIOMS and ICLAS Working Group, guidelines 102
– European Union 98, 99
– India 101
– Japan 100, 101
– the United States 100

regulatory toxicology testing
– animal testing 107, 108
– clinical development program 109
– – ICH M3(R2) guideline 110
– – traditional approach for first-in-human (FIH) clinical trials 110
– national and international guidelines 109
renal disorders 505
– angiotensin II-mediated hypertensive nephropathy 514–516
– animal models, to reproduce human renal diseases 506, 507
– – alterations of tubular transports, in transgenic mice 507
– – KO mice, renin–angiotensin/ANP systems 508
– experimental alloimmune glomerulonephritis 513, 514
– limitations/difficulties 518
– L-NAME-mediated hypertensive nephropathy 516, 517
– renal ischemia–reperfusion 511–513
– RenTg model, benefits 509, 510
– unilateral ureteral obstruction (UUO) 510, 511
renin–angiotensin–aldosterone system 514
renin–angiotensin system (RAS) 509
repeated dose toxicity studies 116
– duration of toxicity studies 117
– – autopsy and microscopic examination 118
– – recommended duration, to support marketing authorization 117
– – shorter-term toxicity studies 117, 118
– ICH M3(R2) guideline 117, 118
– primary goal 116
replacement 19
– acute studies in guidelines 21
– animals in research and testing 33
– mouse gene with human sequence 132
– 3Rs principles 19–22, 95
– for standard lifetime mouse bioassay 125
– targeted genomic 142
– techniques 33
reproductive disorders, animal models
– rodent models for human PCOS 488, 489
reserpine alkaloid 207
respiratory distress syndrome, acute, animal models 440–445
– characteristics, animal models 442–444
RET protooncogene 478
RET-PTC isoforms 481

"reverse translation" approach 18, 19
RNA interfering 10
rofecoxib (Vioxx) 30
route, of administration 16
– oral *vs.* intravenous 18
3Rs in biomedical research 19–22, 95
rt-PA-induced reperfusion 377

s
safety
– acceptable levels 16
– assessment 30, 107, 108, 116
–– drugs 30
–– and toxicology 107
– pharmacology 107, 109–111, 118, 119
schizophrenia 207
– antipsychotic drug (APD) 207, 208, 222
– apomorphine-induced climbing assay in mice 208
– characteristics 207
– chronic phencyclidine (PCP)-induced deficit model 208
– designing, animal model 208
–– based on basal level of PPI 222
– metabolic disorders models 221
–– models for cardiovascular effects 221
– models aimed at, reproducing chronic nature
–– developmental models 216, 217
–– maternal infection/immune challenge 217
–– ventral hippocampal lesion 217, 218
– models amenable to use in screening 209
– models based on genetic manipulations 218
–– dopamine transporter (DAT) knockout mice 218
–– glutamatergic system genetically modified mice 218
–– mice genetically modified for susceptibility genes 218
– models based on use of pharmacological agents 209
–– cannabinoid receptor agonists 212
–– dopaminergic agonists 209–211
–– glycine B receptor antagonists 213
–– 5-HT$_{2A}$ receptor agonists 212
–– muscarinic receptor antagonists 213
–– NMDA/glutamate receptor antagonists 211, 212
– models for side effects 218
–– hyperprolactinemia 220
–– models for cognitive side effects 220, 221
–– models for motor side effects 219
––– catalepsy-associated behavior and haloperidol sensitization in monkeys 220
––– catalepsy in rodents 219
––– paw test in rodents 219, 220
–– sedation and motor incoordination 220
– models more time consuming and/or difficult to implement 214
–– models aimed at reproducing more complex symptoms 214, 215
–– models of cognitive dysfunction 216
–– models of social interaction deficits 215
– models not based on use of pharmacological agents 213
–– conditioned avoidance response 213, 214
–– potentiation of PPI of startle reflex 214
– pharmacotherapy 207
– preclinical models 208
SCI. *see* spinal cord injury
scientific community 4, 93
– challenge to 208
– conceptual reference adopted by 95
– encouraged to accompany, use of animals in 95
– to identify and validate 131
– provide chromosome engineering tools 140
seizures. *See also* epilepsy
– behavioral 421
– convulsive 418, 419
– focal 422–424
– generalized convulsive 422–424
– generalized tonic–clonic 418
– lack of recurrence 417
– nonconvulsive 419
– pharmaco-resistant and pharmaco-sensitive 416
– spontaneous 416, 419, 421
– in zebrafish 64
self-administration procedures 182–184
– intravenous drug self-administration model 182
–– evaluating positive reinforcing effects of compounds 183
– operant 182
– route of administration 182
– schedules of reinforcement 184
sensitization 38, 173, 184, 185
– after surgery 298
– behavioral, defined by 173
– central 238, 247, 287, 298
– C-fiber nociceptors 289, 314
– clinical aspects 301
– haloperidol, in monkeys 220

- incentive sensitization 173
- neuronal 272
- NMDA receptor 321
- peripheral 238, 239
- thermal nociceptive 69
- uterine horn 268
- visceral 266
- visceral afferents 299

sensorimotor deficits 370, 377
serotonin 438
- syndrome 65
sexual behavior models
- appetitive behaviors 530
- conditioned place/partner preference 531
- sexual incentive motivation tests 531
sexual dimorphism 378
sexual functions
- copulatory tests 531, 532
- ejaculation, investigation 534–536, 538
- erection, investigation 532–534
- female/male sexual response, physiology 529, 530
- pathophysiological models 536–538
- peripheral female sexual response 532
- preference paradigms 530, 531
- conditioned place/partner preference 531
- sexual incentive motivation tests 531
Shiga toxin (Stx) receptor 501
simulation
- during drug design 34
- to drug discovery 34
- molecular mechanics-based 35
single-nucleotide polymorphism (SNP) 138
small animal magnetic resonance imaging 152
- magnetic resonance imaging 153, 154
-- anesthetized animals 160
-- mass effect of injected tracers 162
-- spatial resolution and sensitivity 160, 161
- magnetic resonance spectroscopy 152, 153
- principles 152
somatostatin receptor subtype (sst) expression profile 484
spinal cord injury (SCI) 318, 527
- clip compression injury 319
- cystometry measurements 528
- neuropathic pain, caused by central lesions 307, 308
- spinal cord contusion 318
- spinal cord ischemia 319, 320
- spinal cord transection 319
spontaneous hypertensive rats (SHRs) 450, 506

- heart failure prone 450
-- eccentric hypertrophy 452
-- SHHP/Mcc-cp rats 451
state markers, of major depressive disorder 201
stimulus
- chemical 265
- electrical 263, 264
- mechanical 264, 265
- thermal 264
Streptococcus gordonii 501
stroke 367. *See also* seizures
- extravascular models 369
- focal stroke models 369
- global stroke models 368, 369
- intraluminal occlusion model 370
- photothrombosis model 370
- similarities with traumatic brain injury 367, 368
- thromboembolic models 370, 371
structure–activity relationship (SAR) 34, 41, 62, 65
succinate dehydrogenase (SDH) gene 481

t

tachyphylaxis 12
target-driven *vs.* arrow-driven approach 17
target–drug interaction 16
target patient population 16
target product profile 16
target validation 3, 10, 15, 131
TBI. *see* traumatic brain injury (TBI)
teratogenicity 36, 39, 64
therapeutic
- applications 4
- effects 12, 16, 158
-- drug class 12
- indications 16
thymic T-cell selection 476
thyroid autoimmune diseases 474
thyroid cancer, animal models 481
thyroid-stimulating autoantibodies (TSAb) 474
thyroid tumorigenesis 481, 482
thyrotropin 474
time-dependent inhibition (TDI), P450 3A4, 43
tissue cultures 19, 149
tolerance 12
- alcohol 173
- drug (*see* drug tolerance)
- glucose 138, 221, 333, 336, 338
- osmotolerance 499
- probiotic stress 497, 500

toxicokinetic (TK) 16, 116, 124
toxicology studies 114–116
– animal group designs 115
– – high-dose group 115
– – intermediate-dose group 115
– – low-dose group 115
– – vehicle control group 115
– animal species 110, 111
– – nonrodents 112, 113
– – rodents 111, 112
– 2D QSAR models 36
– kinetics and metabolism data
– – role in design and interpretation of preclinical safety 116
– minimal anticipated biological effect level (MABEL) 116
– no observed adverse effect level (NOAEL) 116
– – FIH studies 116
– no observed effect level (NOEL) 115, 116
– repeated dose (*see* repeated dose toxicity studies)
– three-dose level approach 115
– toxicity, acute studies 20, 21
– – LD50 test 21
– toxicity prediction 43
– – networks of collaborators/partners 43
– toxic molecule, heart failure 455
– – adriamycin, in rat 455
– – monocrotaline 455
– use of "positive control" groups, restricted to studies 115
transgenic mice
– alterations of tubular transports in 507
– developing spontaneous cancer 271
– expressing *RET-PTC* isoforms 481
– express MAPT with P303L mutation 356
– IGF2-pathway overactivating 480
– NSE promoter in 357
– overexpressing FTO fed with an enriched diet 138
– overexpressing tropomodulin 462
– overexpression of *HMGA2* 482
– to study epigenetic, physiological, morphological, and behavioral changes 354
– α-synuclein transgenic mice 358, 399
– TSAb-transgenic mice 475
transgenic models. *See also specific models in various disease disorder studies*
– aging 353, 354
– conditional 506
– renin 508

– validity 362
translational medicine 6, 8, 131, 132, 275
translational pharmacology 5
translational research 5, 11, 18, 133, 275, 297, 378, 408, 518
transverse aortic constriction (TAC) 453
traumatic brain injury (TBI) 367
– models with craniotomy
– – controlled cortical impact model 372
– – lateral fluid percussion model 372
– – weight-drop model 372
– models without craniotomy 372
– – acceleration/deceleration model 373
– – impact/acceleration model 373
– – weight-drop model 373
– repetitive 374, 375
troglitazone (Rezulin) 30
tumor necrosis factor alpha (TNFα) 434
"two cultures" problem 6
tyrosine kinase domain 481

u

unbiased design 8
unilateral ureteral obstruction (UUO) 508, 510
– clinical relevance/limits 511
– experimental model 510
– pathology/pathophysiology 511
– technical aspects 510, 511
urinary tract function, lower 523
– bladder afferent recording 526, 527
– cystometry evaluation 524, 525
– micturition, physiology 524
– pathophysiological models 527–529
– – bladder outlet obstruction 527
– – neurogenic detrusor overactivity 528
– – overactive bladder (OAB) 527, 528
– – painful bladder syndrome/interstitial cystitis 528, 529
– urethral function, evaluation 525, 526
urogenitosexual disease models 539

v

validation 3, 4, 10, 249, 266, 271, 315, 321, 323, 420, 445
– acute migraine models 250
– alternative method and incorporate into OECD guideline 32
– animal model 7, 171
– centers for alternative test methods 32
– criterion for novel drug effect 197
– enable acceptance of data 110
– GTN/CGRP rat model need 248

- ICATM, acceptance of new methods 32
- in mammalian models 71
- methodologies require regulatory acceptance as 33
- microdosing as drug development approach 81
- as model for particular human seizure 424
- preclinical/clinical cross-validation 18
- preclinical development 77
- scientific committee for evaluation and 32, 33
- by sequencing 60
- *in silico* techniques in drug development 34
- species differences limiting 142
- spontaneous trigeminal allodynia (STA) model 247
- target 10, 15, 60, 131, 132
- *in vivo* studies 65

vascular endothelial growth factor receptor (VEGFR) antagonist 438
vascular toxicity 377
vasogenic edema 153, 370, 377
ventilator-induced lung injury (VILI) 441
vincristine, neuropathic pain caused by 316–318
visceral motor reflex (VMR), measurement 266
visceral pain models 265
- animal models 267
-- bladder 268
-- colon 269
-- female reproductive organs 267, 268
-- prostate 268
-- ureter 267
- characteristics 265, 266
- measuring electromyographic response 266
- mechanisms 266
- pathophysiology 269, 270
- pharmacology 269, 270
- treatment 266

w

withdrawal, affective manifestations 175–177
- affective symptoms of opioid withdrawal 176
- anxiety and depression-like symptoms 176
- BDNF signaling 177
- drug withdrawal, associated with
-- drug-induced dopamine and 5-HT dysfunction 177
- intracranial electric self-stimulation (ICSS) procedures 176, 185
- withdrawal depression-like behavior 176, 177

writhing test 265

x

xenobiotics 132
xylazine 510, 512, 515

z

zebrafish 60, 491
- embryo screens used in preregulatory phases as 65
- full-length zebrafish cDNAs 61
- gene expression 61
- genetic disease-related screens 61
- genome 61
- inherent advantages for drug screening 62
- limitations and drawbacks in model 65, 66
- model for
-- assessing developmental toxicity 64
-- assessing drug-induced
--- cardiotoxicity 62, 63
--- hepatotoxicity 63
--- neurotoxicity 63, 64
- model for HTS phenotype-based lead discovery 61, 62
- model of seizures 417
- structure–activity relationships (SARs) in 62
- use for research 61
- valuable system for modeling human disease 64, 65